THE YOUNG WOMAN AT THE RISE OF THE 21ST CENTURY

GYNECOLOGICAL AND REPRODUCTIVE ISSUES IN HEALTH AND DISEASE

ANNALS OF THE NEW YORK ACADEMY OF SCIENCES
Volume 900

THE YOUNG WOMAN AT THE RISE OF THE 21ST CENTURY

GYNECOLOGICAL AND REPRODUCTIVE ISSUES IN HEALTH AND DISEASE

Edited by George Creatsas, George Mastorakos, and George P. Chrousos

The New York Academy of Sciences
New York, New York
2000

Library of Congress Cataloging-in-Publication Data

The young woman at the rise of the 21st century: gynecological and reproductive issues in health and disease / editors, George Creatsas, George Mastorakos, George P. Chrousos.
p. cm. — (Annals of the New York Academy of Sciences ; v. 900).
Includes bibliographical references and index.
ISBN 1-57331-266-6 (cloth : alk. paper) — ISBN 1-57331-227-4 (paper : alk. paper).
1. Pediatric endocrinology—Congresses. 2. Adolescent gynecology—Congresses. I. Creatsas, G. II. Mastorakos, George. III. Chrousos, George P. IV. Series.

Q11. N5 vol. 900
[RJ478]
500 s—dc21
[618.1'00835'2] 00-023979

GYAT / BMP
Printed in the United States of America
ISBN 1-57331-226-6 (cloth)
ISBN 1-57331-227-4 (paper)
ISSN 0077-8923

ANNALS OF THE NEW YORK ACADEMY OF SCIENCES

Volume 900
April 2000

THE YOUNG WOMAN AT THE RISE OF THE 21ST CENTURY GYNECOLOGICAL AND REPRODUCTIVE ISSUES IN HEALTH AND DISEASE[a]

Editors and Conference Organizers
GEORGE CREATSAS, GEORGE MASTORAKOS, AND GEORGE P. CHROUSOS

CONTENTS

[a]This volume is the result of a conference entitled **The Young Woman at the Rise of the 21st Century: Gynecological and Reproductive Issues in Health and Disease** held by the Second Department of Obstetrics and Gynecology of the University of Athens, the Hellenic Society of Pediatric and Adolescent Gynecology, and the International Federation of Pediatric and Adolescent Gynecology on November 18 through 21, 1998 in Athens, Greece.

THE YOUNG WOMAN AT THE RISE OF THE 21ST CENTURY
GYNECOLOGICAL AND REPRODUCTIVE ISSUES IN HEALTH AND DISEASE

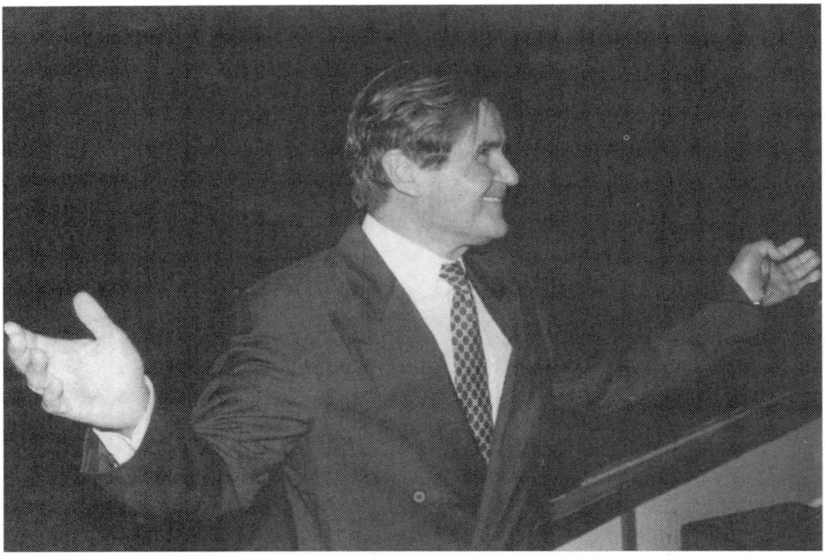

Professor Denis Aravantinos, 1930–1999

Professor Denis Aravantinos

In Memoriam

Professor Denis Aravantinos was a pioneer in the field of obstetrics and gynecology in Greece. He devoted his life to medical research, patients' care, the teaching of students and young doctors, and the demographic situation in Greece.

Professor Aravantinos was born in Athens, where he finished high school. After his graduation from the medical school of the University of Athens, he trained at the Department of Obstetrics and Gynecology of Virchow Hospital, Germany and the Maternité de Beaudelocque of the Port-Royal Hospital, Paris, France. In Greece his career started with the residency at Alexandra Maternity Hospital of Athens where he gradually ascended different posts until 1983, when he became head of the department. In the same year he was elected president of the Hellenic Society of Obstetrics and Gynecology, a position to which he was reelected three times. Professor Aravantinos was elected president of many other medical societies and organizations, including the Hellenic Family Planning Association, the Hellenic Society of Human Reproduction, and the Hellenic Society of Pediatric and Adolescent Gynecology. In addition he was a founder and president of the Hellenic Society of Climacterium and Menopause and of the Hellenic Society of Gynecologic Oncology. In 1985 Professor Aravantinos was elected to the Board of the International Federation of Obstetrics and Gynecology, and in 1988 he became a member of the Education Committee of this organization. From 1987 until 1990, he was a member of the Study Group on the Determinants of Obstetrical Interventions of the World Health Organization. In 1989 he was elected to the Board of the European Association of Gynecologists and Obstetricians, of which he was one of the founders. During the period from 1990 to 1994, he was a member of the deanship at the Ionian University. Since 1990 he had been a member of the AIDS Global Confront Committee. He published a series of books on women's health, including *Female Physiology, Female Pathology*, and *Obstetrics*. He was a member of the Editorial Boards of the *Menopause Digest, European Menopause Journal, European Journal of Obstetrics, Gynecology and Reproductive Biology, International Journal of Prenatal and Perinatal Studies, Cervix and the Lower Female Genital Tract*, and *International Journal of Prenatal and Perinatal Physiology and Medicine*. He organized many Congresses and meetings. He was author or coauthor of more than 380 articles in the field of obstetrics and gynecology in many journals and magazines.

On Tuesday, December 14th, 1999, Professor Denis Aravantinos passed away at the age of 69. Throughout his life, Professor Aravantinos was dedicated to obstetrics and gynecology, the Greek mother, the education of students and young doctors, and medical research. His colleagues, students, and friends will cherish the memory of his creative and original work, his dedication to his patients, and the aura of his warm and generous personality.

Introduction: Setting Reproductive Health Priorities to Meet the Needs of the New Millennium

GEORGE CREATSAS,[a,b] GEORGE MASTORAKOS,[b] AND GEORGE P. CHROUSOS[c]

[b]*2nd Department of Obstetrics and Gynecology, University of Athens, Athens, Greece*

[c]*Developmental Endocrinology Branch, National Institute of Child Health and Human Development, National Institutes of Health, Bethesda, Maryland 28072, USA*

Good reproductive health usually accompanies a safe sexual life and reflects mental, physical, and social well being. International agencies focus their efforts on improving the reproductive health of the Earth's population in the new millennium by establishing priorities, by harmonizing laws affecting public health, and by promoting consensus formation through international conventions. This is a difficult task that has to take into account national, cultural, and religious differences among the different peoples of the world.

The recent developments in preimplantation diagnosis and cloning are examples of the new techniques of molecular biology that already have raised arguments, although some consensus has already been reached. New technologies in assisted reproduction have expanded the possibilities for treating infertility. Over the last decade of the twentieth century, assisted reproduction improved from a set of procedures that were first regarded with skepticism to procedures that are being routinely applied around the world. Subsequently, successful attempts at *in vitro* fertilization and related procedures have increased and offer a higher pregnancy rate compared with surgical management of infertility in cases of endometriosis and tubal damage. In addition, the injection of a single spermatozoon directly into the cytoplasm of an oocyte and the use of immature spermatids open greater possibilities for men with oligospermia, asthenospermia, or testicular dysfunction. At the same time, the application of new ovulation protocols including the use of recombinant FSH has led to the improvement of the fertilization outcome, as have better understanding of endometrial changes through use of electron microscopy procedures and better understanding of the hatching phenomenon.

Today, the population of Europe is estimated to be as much as 850 million and is projected to be 866 million (including the former USSR) in the year 2050, representing 8.6% of the total world population. The fertility decline in southern Europe is characteristicly indicated in Italy and Spain, with 1.19 and 1.22 children per woman, respectively.[1] The phenomenon is even more pronounced in Greece. The asynchronous population development between South and North and the expansion of the population in certain countries in Asia and sub-Saharan regions compared to other

[a]Address for correspondence: Prof. G. Creatsas, M.D., FACS, 9 Kanari Str., 10671 Athens Greece. Phone: +301 7186353; fax: +301 7233330.
e-mail: geocre@aretaieio.uoa.gr

countries produce significant demographic problems that have to be faced through national family planning programs and the relevant world organizations. It is expected that new strategies should be implemented at the beginning of the new millennium, otherwise the situation will deteriorate.

Safe abortions are now the reality in the developed world. Nevertheless, it seems that we are not very close to the wish that every child should be a wanted child. It is estimated that 260,000 unsafe abortions occur in Europe each year (150,000 in southern Europe and 110,000 in eastern Europe). Many of them occur among adolescents.[2,3] The most suitable explanation is the lack of education and the low compliance rate for contraceptive methods, although current scientific findings have increased availability and choices for family planning clients and have made the use of contraceptives more effective.

At the beginning of the new millennium, service delivery practices are expected to improve quality by taking into account the couple's biological and psychosexual needs. Until all these strategies become a reality and offer the expected outcome, however, there is no excuse for the high rate of unwanted pregnancies during adolescence, even in developed countries, or for the high prevalence of sexually transmitted diseases, which present an epidemic in Eastern Europe. "A Call for Help" is the subtitle of an article published three years ago by A. Gromyko in the *Entre Nous*.[4] Recent studies from the same area report that the phenomenon is getting worse because of the increase in prostitution and inadequate protection.

Health care professionals (HCP) are expected to play a role as educators and service providers. They should also cooperate closely with the media and journalists to clear up misunderstandings. Oral contraceptives, for example, have been reported to be safe and the most effective contraceptive method. At the same time, studies mention increased ectopia on the cervical epithelium and a higher relative rate of some STDs including HIV-1 infections among women who use oral contraceptives. This observation provides an example of where an HCP could assist by advising a couple about the best contraceptive methods depending on their needs and avoiding side-effects, misunderstanding, and discontinuation.

Another topic for discussion should be men's sexual behavior. Although many studies have been done on women's sexual activity and lives, related reports on the sexual behavior of men are limited. The condom has become very popular, but even so, it needs to be reemphasized that testicular dysfunction, a common cause of men's infertility, is the result of sexually transmitted diseases. Impotence, on the other hand, presents a rising trend at the end of this decade as a cause of infertility, possibly because of increased stress in men's lives.

The disabled also deserve attention. We all agree that disabled persons should have equal opportunities for a normal reproductive life. Nevertheless, only a limited number of task forces have been organized with this initiative as a focus.

In conclusion, this volume contains the proceedings of the 4th International Congress entitled "The Young Woman at the Rise of the 21st Century," held in Athens in November 1998. In an effort to incorporate all recent knowledge concerning the young woman, this volume presents new scientific information covering broad aspects of gynecology, endocrinology, and reproduction without neglecting to include recent progress in molecular biology and genetics pertaining to reproductive health. It is composed of papers written by internationally known authorities in each field.

Special care has been given to balance basic and clinical information. The papers proposed by the authors were divided into topics covering newly acquired knowledge on the following topics: the neuroendocrinology of the menstrual cycle, the endocrinology of implantation as well as of human gestation and parturition, prenatal diagnosis, the molecular and genetic aspects of reproduction, perinatal care in maternal and fetal well-being and disease, obesity and the polycystic ovary syndrome, the role of anemia in pregnancy and reproduction, the use of oral contraceptives and their effects on the vasculature, the estrogen deficiency syndrome, the role of the endoscopic surgery, the common practice in treatment and detection of sexually transmitted diseases, the fertility potential of young women, the osteoporosis of young women, and the use of GnRH analogues in clinical practice. Thus, this volume explores recent advances in young women's health problems, stratified from basic knowledge and physiology to clinical applications. It is our hope that this volume will be useful for setting reproductive health priorities to address the needs of the new millenium.

At the beginning of this millennium, optimism is appropriate, because humanity has acquired the necessary experience, technology, and scientific imagination to meet the challenges before us. What remains to be done is to apply these tools to solve the puzzle and to adjust our efforts according to changing needs in order to allow future generations to live in a better world, making the year 2000 a year of (r)evolution.

ACKNOWLEDGMENT

We would especially like to thank our assistant, Mrs. Yiota Gkirgkeni, whose invaluable and sustained help with the organization of our editorial tasks made the publication of this volume possible.

REFERENCES

1. SHAH, I. Fertility and contraception in Europe. 1997. Eur. J. Contracept. Rep. Health Care **2:** 53–61.
2. CREATSAS, G. Adolescent sexuality, atool for a safe motherhood. 1997. Int. J. Obstet. Gynecol. **58:** 85–92.
3. THE JOHNS HOPKINS SCHOOL OF PUBLIC HEALTH. Population Reports. 1996. Fam. Plan. Progr. Ser. J. N. **44:** 2.
4. GROMYKO, A. 1999. Sexually transmitted diseases (STDs) epidemic in eastern Europe. A call for help. Entre Nous **33**(Sept.).

Neuropeptides, Neurotransmitters, Neurosteroids, and the Onset of Puberty

A.R. GENAZZANI,[a,b] F. BERNARDI,[b] P. MONTELEONE,[b] S. LUISI,[b] AND M. LUISI[c]

[b]*Department of Reproductive Medicine and Child Development, Section of Gynecology and Obstetrics, University of Pisa, Pisa, Italy*

[c]*CNR, Endocrine Research Unit, Pisa, Italy*

ABSTRACT: Puberty results from withdrawal of the "gonadostat" mechanisms and from increased gonadotropin sensitivity to GnRH. It has been hypothesized that GnRH release may be modulated by a non–steroid-mediated mechanism. Modifications of neuropeptides, neurotransmitters, and neurosteroids may underlie the onset of pubertal processes. Neuropeptides mainly involved in the control of GnRH release are opioids, neuropeptide Y (NPY), galanin, and corticotropin-releasing factor (CRF), whereas neurotransmitters are noradrenaline, dopamine, serotonin, melatonin and γ-aminobutyric acid (GABA). Norepinephrine, epinephrine, and dopamine stimulate GnRH, whereas the effect of serotonin on hypothalamic–pituitary–ovarian axis seems to be norepinephrine-mediated. Neurosteroids are steroid hormones that bind to the GABA-A receptor, synthesized in the brain *de novo* or from blood-borne precursors. DHEA, a GABA-A antagonistic neurosteroid, and allopregnanolone, a GABA-A agonistic neurosteroid, may be important in the onset of gonadarche. In conclusion, the onset of puberty derives from the complex interplay among neuropeptides, neurotransmitters, and neurosteroids that occurs in the awakening of hypothalamic–pituitary–ovarian axis.

INTRODUCTION

The onset of gonadarche most probably results from withdrawal of the "gonadostat" mechanisms and from increased gonadotropin sensitivity to GnRH. Recent data have shown that GnRH release may be modulated by a non–steroid-mediated central mechanism. It has been hypothesized that modifications of neuropeptides, neurotransmitters and neurosteroids may underlie the onset of pubertal processes.

Neuropeptides mainly involved in the control of GnRH release are opioids, neuropeptide Y (NPY), galanin, and corticotropin-releasing factor (CRF), whereas the neurotransmitters are noradrenaline, dopamine, serotonin, melatonin, and γ-aminobutyric acid (GABA) (TABLE 1). It has been hypothesized that β-endorphin stimulates adrenal steroidogenic activity during prepubertal period, but this peptide is not necessary for the onset of adrenarche. NPY and galanin, both neuropeptides whose secretion is modulated by gonadal steroids, influence central behavior and neuroen-

[a]Address for correspondence: Prof. A.R. Genazzani, Department of Reproductive Medicine and Child Development, Section of Gynecology and Obstetrics, University of Pisa, Via Roma 35, Pisa, Italy. Phone: +50 992809; fax: +50 553410.

TABLE 1. Neuropeptides, neurotransmitters and neurosteroids that are able to modulate GnRH release

Neurotransmitters	Noradrenaline Dopamine Acetylcholine Serotonine Melatonin
Neuropeptides	Opioid peptides Neuropeptide Y (NPY) Galanin Corticotropin-releasing factor (CRF)
Neurosteroids	Allopregnanolone DHEAS

docrine functions by stimulating pulsatile GnRH release and gonadotropins. A decrease in melatonin production may remove suppression of hypothalamic–pituitary–ovarian axis activity, thus determining the onset of gonadarche.

Norepinephrine, epinephrine, and dopamine stimulate GnRH release according to a steroid milieu, whereas the effect of serotonin on the hypothalamic–pituitary–ovarian axis seems to be norepinephrine mediated.

Neurosteroids are steroid hormones that bind to the GABA-A receptor and are synthesized in the brain *de novo* or from blood-borne precursors. DHEA, a GABA-A antagonistic neurosteroid, and allopregnanolone, a GABA-A agonistic neurosteroid, positively correlate with Tanner's stage, both in boys and girls. A correlation between allopregnanolone and DHEA throughout pubertal development has been also described.

In conclusion, the onset of puberty derives from the complex interplay between neuropeptides, neurotransmitters, and neurosteroids that occurs in the awakening of hypothalamic–pituitary–ovarian axis (FIG. 1).

NEUROPEPTIDES

Opioidergic System

Endogenous opioid peptides exert an important role in the modulation of reproductive function, as indicated by the fact that morphine abuse is often associated with infertility. There are three families of endogenous opioids: endorphins, enkephalins, and dinorphins. The endorphins, β-endorphin being the most significant, act by binding to μ and ε receptors, while enkephalins and dinorphins have a greater affinity for κ and σ receptors, respectively. Much evidence indicates that endogenous opioid peptides and their receptors are implicated in the modulation of gonadotropin secretion; β-endorphin is the one most involved in controlling LH secretion. In fact, a β-endorphin antiserum injection in the arcuate nucleus of rats increases LH levels much more than enkephalins or dinorphins.[1–2] Moreover, naloxone, a potent μ receptor antagonist, is more efficient than κ and σ receptor antagonists in augmenting LH levels. Although there is evidence that endogenous opioid peptides do not modify LH response to GnRH *in vitro* or *in vivo*,[3] it has been demonstrated that β-endorphin exerts a direct effect on LH secretion.[4]

Recent data have demonstrated that long-term treatment with naltrexone can positively influence LH plasma levels and LH pulsatile secretion in women affected by hypothalamic amenorrhea.[5] The fact that GnRH antagonists neutralize the naloxone-induced LH increment indicates that GnRH is one of the targets for endogenous opioids. Because naloxone loses its potency if the median eminence is lesioned, it seems that this is the site of action of β-endorphin on GnRH secretion. Because β-endorphin plasma variations do not determine changes in LH levels in various experimental models, it seems that only central β-endorphin exerts a major role in the modulation of LH secretion in the median eminence.[6]

Endogenous opioids control LH secretion through the mediation of some neurotransmitters. In fact, the increment in basal levels and peak amplitude of LH induced by naloxone is annulled by the administration of NA/A receptor agonists and serotonin receptor antagonists.[7,8] Moreover, opioids and their antagonists are able to modify the turnover of monoaminergic neurotransmitters, thus exerting an important role in the neuromodulation of GnRH secretion.

Both sexual steroids and CRF can influence the opioidergic regulation of LH secretion. In rats, LH response to naloxone varies with the estrous cycle and is reduced in castrated animals, thus indicating that opioids integrate information "originating" in the gonads at the central level.[9] Moreover, it seems that endogenous opioids mediate the inhibitory action of CRF on LH levels in rats. It has been demonstrated that CRF is capable of stimulating β-endorphin secretion, and it has been hypothesized that the CRF/β-endorphin system is involved in reducing LH levels in response to stress.

β-Endorphin exerts an important role in the regulation of the hypothalamic–pituitary–gonadal axis under the clinical influence of sex steroids, fully integrated with other neuropeptidergic systems. It seems that POMC-derived hormones, such as β-endorphin, are not directly involved in suppressing the "gonadostat" and are therefore incapable of influencing the onset of puberty. It does though seem that these hormones are involved in determining the onset of adrenarche.

Corticotropin-Releasing Factor

An intracerebroventricular corticotropin-releasing factor (CRF) injection in rat produces a decrease in LH levels; this inhibitory effect is present in adrenalectomized rats as well, suggesting that CRF modulates LH secretion at the central level.[10] CRF reduces GnRH levels in the pituitary portal system in female rats and GnRH secretion in hypothalamic explants. It has been demonstrated that the CRF-induced decrease in LH secretion is mediated by endogenous opioids. In fact, the administration of β-endorphin antiserum or β-endorphin antagonists neutralizes the inhibitory effect of CRF on circulating LH levels.[11] Moreover, it seems that CRF stimulates β-endorphin secretion and, through this mechanism, inhibits the sexual function of the female rat.

The CRF/β-endorphin system plays an important role in reducing LH levels during stress. In fact, there is much experimental evidence indicating that both CRF and β-endorphin are stimulated under stressful conditions: the use of CRF antagonists or anti-β-endorphin antiserum neutralizes the inhibitory effect of foot-shock test on LH

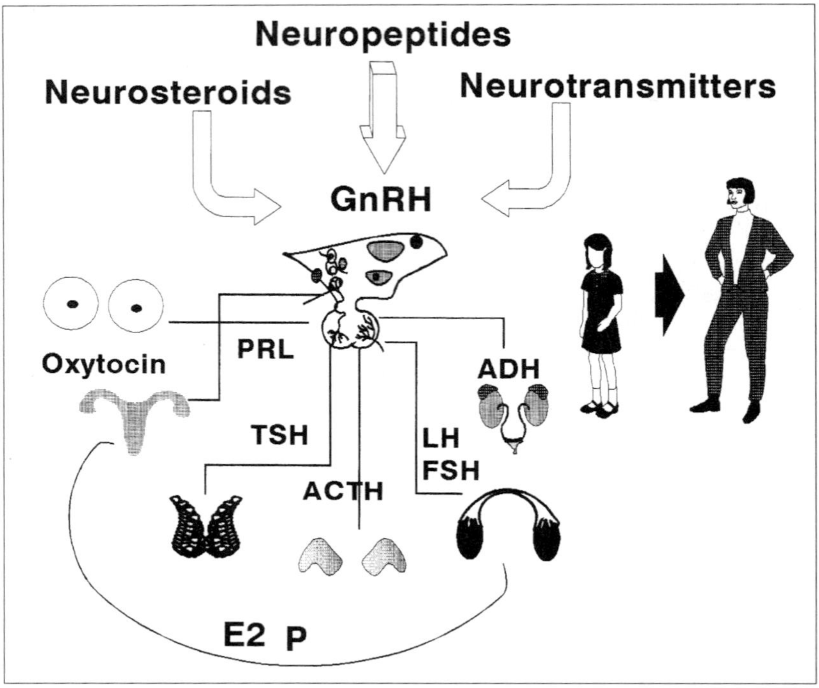

FIGURE 1. The modifications in GnRH release, modulated by a central mechanism involving the secretion of neuropeptides, neurotransmitters, and neurosteroids, are an important factor underlying the onset of pubertal processes.

levels.[11,12] As for β-endorphin, the role of CRF seems to be more important in the induction of adrenarche rather than in the onset of puberty.

Neuropeptide Y and Galanin

In rats, NPY is among the most important hypothalamic excitatory signals for the control of phasic LH secretion.[13,14] The role of NPY at the hypothalamic level is not quite clear because this neuropeptide reduces GnRH secretion in castrated rats, whereas under the influence of estrogens, it exerts an NE-like stimulatory action on LH release.

Studies focusing on the neuroendocrine effects of NPY administration at the central level in castrated male rats have indicated that the inhibitory effect of NPY on LH secretion is mediated by the activation of low-affinity NPY receptors. Sexual steroids seem to have an inhibitory action on these receptors. It has been hypothesized that stress-induced hypogonadism is partly due to the activation of NPY-containing neurons in the arcuate nucleus, leading to prolonged activation of tuberoinfundibular dopaminergic neurons and inhibition of GnRH release.

On the other hand, the activation of high-affinity receptors for NPY stimulates LH release as a consequence of the reduced activity of dopaminergic tubero-infundibular neurons.[15] Sexual steroids are capable of increasing the high-affinity receptor sensitivity to NPY, and it has been hypothesized that the excitatory effect of NPY on LH release is mediated by NPY high-affinity receptors localized in the preoptic area, where NPY may influence GnRH neuron activity through synapses containing NPY or NPY/E or NPY/NE. NPY may therefore act as a co-modulator at the NE neuronal terminals and stimulate CRF release. Moreover, it seems that some NPY neurons present in the arcuate nucleus regulate β-endorphin secretion, thus indicating that this system is important in controlling GnRH secretion.

The peptide galanin stimulates ovulation by acting on the hypothalamus and pituitary gland. *In vivo* studies suggest that galanin stimulates LH release in a dose-dependent manner in ovariectomized rats treated with estrogens, but, unlike NPY, it has no effect in ovariectomized animals treated with estrogens.

Although galanin also stimulates GnRH release at the hypothalamic level, the mechanism of action seems to be different from that of NPY. Moreover, galanin-containing neurons respond to modifications of the estrogenic milieu, thus transmitting appropriate signals for the control of GnRH release.[14]

Besides having a neuromodulatory role at the hypothalamic level, NPY acts directly at the pituitary level, enhancing LH response to GnRH in pituitary cell cultures. These data allow us to hypothesize that NPY exerts a direct effect on gonadotropic cells and explains the mechanism by which NPY may possibly influence ovulation.[16]

There is little information in the literature regarding NPY and galanin and the onset of puberty, although one may hypothesize that these two peptides have some role in this phenomenon, considering their effect on GnRH release.

NEUROTRANSMITTERS

Catecholamines and Serotonin

Among the neurotransmitters involved in regulating LH secretion are epinephrine (E) and norepinephrine (NE). GnRH-releasing neurons receive catecholaminergic inputs from brain stem nuclei. Changes in E and NE turnover observed in the medial preoptic region, which is sexually dimorphic, have been correlated to hormonal events and behavioral patterns characteristic of the reproductive cycle. The stimulating or inhibiting effects of catecholamines on the hypothalamic–pituitary–gonadal axis seem to depend totally on the steroidal milieu. It has been demonstrated that NE suppresses GnRH release in ovariectomized rats, whereas it stimulates GnRH and LH secretion in ovariectomized rats treated with estrogen/progestagens.

If adrenergic antagonists, noradrenergic antagonists, or α-blockers are used, the preovulatory LH peak does not appear. In ovariectomized rats, intermittent subministration of NE stimulates LH secretion, which is mediated by a rapid desensitization of α-adrenergic receptors; on the other hand, continued NE subministration inhibits LH release.

Although it is generally accepted that NE and E facilitate ultradian and cyclic LH secretion (and of GnRH), it is not clear whether they are necessary for these hormonal events. Pharmacological studies have demonstrated that the stimulatory action of NE on the hypothalamic–pituitary–gonadal axis is mediated prevalently by α_1-receptors, whereas there is a mild inhibitory effect mediated by β-receptors.[17]

Recently, the role of dopamine on the hypothalamic–pituitary–gonadal axis has been studied, and it has been demonstrated that dopamine agonists and antagonists can stimulate, inhibit, or have no effect on LH secretion according to the experimental conditions, specificity of the drug, and steroid milieu. The most credited hypothesis is that dopamine is able to stimulate hypothalamic GnRH release through a cAMP-mediated mechanism. This hypothesis is in accordance with the observation that treatment with cAMP analogues or adenylatecyclase stimulators increases the amplitude and length of GnRH pulses.[17]

As for serotonin, the subministration of serotonin antagonists inhibits the secretion of LH in rats; however, it seems improbable that serotonin is involved in determining the LH peak in that the lesion of serotoninergic fibers by a specific neurotoxin is compatible with a normal LH peak. It seems that the effect exerted by some serotonin antagonists on LH secretion is mediated by an adrenal mechanism that is independent from serotonin.[18] Finally, a recent work has shown that in rats with delayed puberty, serotoninergic activation in the hypothalamus–preoptic area is lower that in normal rats in puberty and that dopaminergic activation in the hypothalamus–preoptic area negatively affects initiation of puberty.[19]

Melatonin

In rats, melatonin, a pineal gland hormone, determines a tonic inhibition of the hypothalamic–pituitary–gonadal axis.[20] In female rats, melatonin delays sexual maturation, reduces the number of GnRH binding sites in the pituitary gland, and reduces secretion of gonadotropins. A reduction in amplitude and frequency of LH peaks was observed in rats treated with melatonin.[20]

The first studies concerning the effects of melatonin on ovulation in humans have yielded contradictory results: some have reported that melatonin increases the amplitude of LH pulses without altering their frequency, while others have reported that this hormone has no effect on circulating levels of GnRH and LH.[22] Further studies are necessary in order to clarify this hormone's true role in the female reproductive cycle. While melatonin may play a role in the altered timing of puberty associated with pineal tumors and in the pathophysiology of central precocious puberty, there is no evidence that it is important in the physiologic onset of normal puberty in humans.[21] The decline in the nocturnal surge of melatonin, thought to have been exclusively related to pubertal conversion, was observed to begin in infancy and progressively decline through pubescence.[22,23] Pinealectomy in agonadal primates does not prevent the inhibition of FSH and LH seen during transition from infancy to childhood nor the return of gonadotropins with the advent of puberty.[24]

NEUROSTEROIDS

The GABA-mediated modulation of the hypothalamic–pituitary–gonadal axis has recently incited great interest. In fact, it has been demonstrated that some steroids produced at the central level (allopregnanolone, dehydroepiandrosterone, etc.), which act through a GABA A–mediated mechanism, exert an important role in the regulation of reproductive function.

Our recent studies have demonstrated that allopregnanolone, a GABA-A agonist, modulates the activity of hypothalamic–pituitary–gonadal axis. In fact, the cerebral content of allopregnanolone in female rats varies according to the estrous cycle phase. Moreover, the intracerebroventricular injection of allopregnanolone inhibits ovarian function in female rats, whereas the injection of antiallopregnanolone antiserum induces ovulation.[25]

Considering these data and the fact that hypothalamic allopregnanolone decreases at ovulation, we hypothesized that allopregnanolone controls ovulation by enhancing GABAergic activity in the hypothalamus and pituitary gland. The evidence that allopregnanolone levels vary in women, according the menstrual cycle phase and during pregnancy, led us to hypothesize that mood changes that occur during a woman's reproductive life may be correlated to fluctuating levels of neurosteroids.[26, 27]

Recently, our preliminary data have shown that an age-related increase in allopregnanolone serum levels occurred throughout puberty. We have also found allopregnanolone levels to be positively correlated to Tanner's stage. The increase in allopregnanolone levels may be caused by the onset of adrenal steroidogenesis. Circulating levels of DHEA, a GABA-agonistic neurosteroid, also vary from birth to adulthood.[28] There are, in fact, high levels at birth, but levels of this hormone progressively decrease and reach a plateau between ages 2 and 6, then reach a peak concentration at age 6–7, and progressively increase during puberty in accordance with Tanner's stage. During adrenarche, the increment in DHEA begins before that of testosterone and is not regulated by ACTH or cortisol. Increasing levels of both allopregnanolone and DHEA may simply represent an epiphenomenon of pubertal development and play an important role in awakening the "gonadostat."

CONCLUSIONS

We can deduce that the neuroendocrine mechanism involved in regulating and/or modulating hypothalamic–pituitary activity is very complex. The presence of so many stimulating or inhibiting hormones acting on the reproductive axis makes it very difficult to find the true factors involved in the onset of puberty and alterations of pubertal timing.

REFERENCES

1. Schultz, R., A. Wilhelm, K.M. Pirke, *et al.* 1981. β-Endorphin and dynorphin control serum LH level in immature female rats. Nature **294:** 757–759.
2. Forman, L.J., W.E. Sonntag & J. Meites. 1983. Elevation of plasma LH in response to systemic injection of β-endorphin antiserum in adult male rats. Proc. Soc. Exp. Biol. Med. **173:** 14–17.
3. Cicero, T.J., B.A. Schainker & E.R. Meyer. 1979. Endogenous opioids participate in the regulation of hypothalamic–pituitary–luteinizing hormone axis and testosterone negative feed-back control of luteinizing hormone. Endocrinology **104:**1286–1289.
4. Blank, M.S., A. Fabbria, K.J. Catt & M.L. Du Fau. 1986. Inhibition of luteinizing hormone release by morphine and endogenousopiates in cultured pituitary cells. Endocrinology **118:** 2097–2101.

5. PETRAGLIA, F., A.E. PANERAI, C. RIVIER, *et al.* 1988. Opioid control of gonadotropin secretion. *In* The Brain and Reproductive Function. A.R. Genazzani, U. Montemagno, C. Nappi & F. Petraglia, Eds.: 65. Parthenon Publishing. New York.
6. KALRA, S.P. & J.W. SIMPKINS. 1982. Evidence for noradrenergic mediation of opioid effects on luteinizing hormone secretion. Endocrinology **109:** 776–779.
7. IEIRI, T., H.T. CHEN & J. MEITES. 1980. Naloxone stimulation of luteinizing hormone release in prepubertal female rats: role of serotoninergic system. Life Sci. **36:** 1269–1274.
8. PETRAGLIA, F., V. LOCATELLI, F. FACCHINETTI, *et al.* 1986. Oestrus cycle-related LH responsiveness to naloxone: effect of high oestrogen levels on the activity of opioid receptors. J. Endocrinol. **108:** 89–94.
9. PETRAGLIA, F., W. VALE & C. RIVIER. 1983. Opioids act centrally to modulate stress-induced decrease of LH secretion in the rat. Endocrinology **112:** 2209–2213.
10. RIVIER, C., J. RIVIER & W. VALE. 1986. Stress-induced inhibition of reproductive functions: role of endogenous corticotropin-releasing factor. Science **131:** 607–609.
11. LOPEZ, F.J. & A. NEGRO-VILAR. 1990. Galanin stimulates luteinizing hormone-releasing hormone secretion from arcuate nucleus-median eminence fragments in vitro: involvement of an α-adrenergic mechanism. Endocrinology **127:** 2431–2436.
12. ARISAWA, M., L. DEPALATIS, R. HO, *et al.* 1990. Stimulatory role of substance P on gonadotropin release in ovariectomized rats. Neuroendocrinology **51:** 523–529.
13. KALRA, S.P. 1993. Mandatory neuropeptide–steroid signaling for the preovulatory luteinizing hormone-releasing hormone discharge Endocr. Rev. **14:** 507–538.
14. FUXE, K., A. HARFSTRAND, P. ENEROTH, *et al.* 1988. Neuropeptide Y mechanisms in neuroendocrine regulation. Focus on neuropeptide Y-catecholamine interactions in regulation of LH and prolactin secretion. *In* The Brain and Reproductive Function. A.R. Genazzani, U. Montemagno, C. Nappi & F. Petraglia, Eds.: 45. Parthenon Publishing. New York.
15. RIVIER, C. & W. VALE. 1984. Influence of corticotropin-releasing factor on reproductive function in the rat. Endocrinology **114:** 914–918.
16. PETRAGLIA, F., W. VALE & C. RIVIER. 1983. Opioids act centrally to modulate stress-induced decrease of LH secretion in the rat. Endocrinology **112:** 2209–2213.
17. GENAZZANI, A.R., M.A. PALUMBO, A.A. DE MICHEROUX, *et al.* 1995. Evidence for a role for the neurosteroid allopregnanolone in the modulation of reproductive function in female rats. Eur. J. Endocrinol. **133:** 375–380.
18. MAJEWSKA, M.D. 1992. Neurosteroids: endogenous bimodal modulators of the GABA-A receptor. Mechanism of action and physiological significance. Prog. Neurobiol. **38:** 379–395.
19. ANTONIOU, K., Z. PAPADOPOULOU-DAIFOTIS, K. KANELAKIS, *et al.* 1997. Relationship between the thymus and neurochemical changes in the hypothalamus–preoptic area and prefrontal cortex in female rats with delayed puberty (abstract). Int. J. Dev. Neurosci. **15:** 911.
20. MASSOBRIO, M., D. GUIDETTI, A. REVELLI, *et al.* 1993. Melatonin in human reproduction. *In* Neuroendocrinology of Female Reproductive Function. U. Montemagno, C. Nappi, F. Petraglia & A.R. Genazzani, Eds.: 73. Parthenon Publishing. New York.
21. WALDHAUSER, F. & P.A. BOEPPLE. 1990. The puberal growth spurt in 8 patients with true precocious puberty and growth hormone deficiency: evidence for a direct role of sex steroids. J. Clin. Endocrinol. Metab. **71:** 975.
22. ATTANASIO, A., P. BORRELLI & D. GUPTA. 1985. Circadian rhythms in serum melatonin from infancy to adolescence. J. Clin. Endocrinol. Metab. **61:** 388.
23. CAVALLO, A., G.E. RICHARDS & E.R. SMITH. 1992. Relation between nocturnal melatonin profile and hormonal markers of puberty in humans. Horm. Res. **37:** 185.
24. PLANT, T.M. & D.S. ZORUB. 1986. Pinealectomy in agonadal infantile male rhesus monkeys does not interrupt initiation of the prepubertal hiatus in gonadotropin secretion. Endocrinology **118:** 227.
25. MELLON, S.H. 1994. Neurosteroids: biochemistry, modes of action, and clinical relevance. J. Clin. Endocrinol. Metab. **78:** 1003–1008.
26. RIVEST, R.W., U. LANG, M.L. AUBERT & P.C. SIZONENKO. 1988. Melatonin and female sexual maturation: control of pulsatile LH secretion and ovulation in the rat. *In* Neu-

roendocrinology of Female Reproductive Function. U. Montemagno, C. Nappi, F. Petraglia & A.R. Genazzani, Eds.: 263. Parthenon Publishing. New York.

27. CAGNACCI, A., J.A. ELLIOT & S.S.C. YEN. 1991. Amplification of pulsatile LH secretion by exogenous melatonin in women. J. Clin. Endocrinol. Metab. **1:** 210–212.

28. DE PERETTI, E. & M.G. FOREST. 1976. Unconjugated DHEA serum levels in normal subjects from birth to adolescence in human: the use of a sensitive radioimmunoassay. J. Clin. Endocrinol. Metab. **43:** 982.

Ovarian Regulators of Gonadotropin Secretion

IOANNIS E. MESSINIS[a]

Department of Obstetrics and Gynaecology, University of Thessalia, Medical School, 41222 Larissa, Greece

ABSTRACT: Great progress in the ovarian mechanisms that control gonadotrophin secretion in women has recently been achieved. Estradiol (E_2) is the main component of the ovarian negative effect on basal gonadotropin secretion during the normal menstrual cycle. However, nonsteroidal substances such as inhibins and activins that can affect follicle-stimulating hormone (FSH) secretion *in vitro* may also participate in the control of FSH secretion *in vivo*. Recent evidence has shown that the ovaries also produce another nonsteroidal substance, named gonadotropin surge-attenuating factor (GnSAF), that specifically attenuates GnRH-induced LH secretion and the endogenous LH surge in superovulated women. It is possible that during the normal menstrual cycle GnSAF controls the amplitude of the midcycle LH surge by antagonizing the stimulating effect of E_2 on the pituitary.

INTRODUCTION

Over the last 15 years, it has become evident that the ovaries produce, in addition to steroids, various nonsteroidal hormones, such as inhibins, activins, and follistatin.[1] Although these substances can affect the secretion of follicle-stimulating hormone (FSH) *in vitro*, it is not clear whether they participate in the regulation of gonadotropin secretion *in vivo*. Accumulated evidence has indicated that the ovaries also produce another nonsteroidal substance, named "gonadotropin surge-attenuating factor" (GnSAF), which may play a role in the control of the midcycle luteinizing hormone (LH) surge in women.[2–5] In this article, the role of steroidal and nonsteroidal ovarian substances in the regulation of gonadotropin secretion in women will be discussed.

BASAL GONADOTROPIN SECRETION

The Role of Estrogen

Several studies examined the effect of exogenous estrogen on basal gonadotropin secretion during the normal menstrual cycle. In one of them,[6] estradiol (E_2) benzoate was injected into normal women in increasing doses during the early follicular phase of the cycle in order to achieve preovulatory concentrations of E_2 in the blood. As a result of the estrogen administration, a marked decline in the levels of both FSH and LH was seen and the percentage of decrease was similar for both of them.[6] This demonstrates the ability of exogenous estrogen to suppress endogenous gonadotropins and suggests that FSH and LH are equally sensitive to the negative effect of E_2. Not only exogenous but also endogenous estrogen can affect the secretion of gonadotropins, and this is evident during superovulation induction with the injection of gona-

[a]Address for correspondence: Department of Obstetrics and Gynaecology, University of Thessalia, Medical School, 22 Papakiriazi Street, 41222 Larissa, Greece.

dotropins. In one study,[2] the administration of pure FSH to normal women at the dose of 225 IU per day during the follicular phase of the cycle resulted in a significant increase in serum FSH and E_2 concentrations. The increase in serum E_2 values was followed by a marked decline in basal LH levels, which occurred within two days from the onset of treatment with FSH. The inverse relationship between E_2 and LH in that study[2] was even more clear in another study in which serum E_2 values in blood increased for only a certain period of time.[7] In particular, the administration of a single dose of 450 IU FSH i.m. to normal women on day 2 of a normal menstrual cycle increased serum FSH values significantly for the next three days. This was followed by a significant increase in serum E_2 values, which reached on average a level of 600 pmol/l on cycle day 4 and returned to basal level on cycle day 6. At the same time, LH values declined significantly, and the decrease lasted for the period of the E_2 increase. Endogenous E_2, therefore, when increasing during the follicular phase of the cycle can suppress endogenous LH secretion. In these studies, endogenous FSH secretion was not evaluated due to the exogenous administration of FSH. Another way to assess the importance of endogenous estrogen for the control of basal gonadotropin secretion is to minimize the levels of circulating E_2, as it happens after bilateral ovariectomy. Such experiments have shown a gradual increase in basal FSH and LH values following the operation performed either in the follicular or the luteal phase of the cycle.[8] It is clear from these studies that E_2 is the main component of the mechanism through which the ovaries control basal gonadotropin secretion during the follicular phase of the cycle. Certainly, during the luteal phase of the cycle the effect of progesterone in addition to that of E_2 is also important.[8]

The Role of Inhibin and Related Peptides

Inhibin is a glypoprotein consisting of two subunits termed α and β (inhibin A and inhibin B). It decreases both the synthesis and the secretion of gonadotropins, preferentially that of FSH.[9] Activins are dimeric products of the P subunit of inhibin (activins A, AB, and B), whereas follistatin is a single-chain glycosylated polypeptide, structurally unrelated to inhibin.[9] Follistatin shows inhibin-like activities on FSH secretion *in vitro*, and activins stimulate the secretion of FSH. These proteins have been purified from the follicular fluid of various species including human. Efforts have been made by several investigators to develop immunoassays for the measurement of these substances in peripheral circulation. The immunoassays initially developed for inhibin showed significant cross reaction with the free α subunit which, however, is not biologically active. Recently, two-site enzyme immunoassays for measurement of dimeric inhibins have been developed. According to these, serum inhibin A and inhibin B values show different patterns of changes during the normal menstrual cycle. In particular, values of inhibin A are low during the follicular phase and markedly high during the luteal phase of the cycle, indicating that inhibin A is mainly produced by the corpus luteum.[10] In contrast to inhibin A, inhibin B increases gradually from the early to midfollicular phase, declining thereafter.[11] Inhibin B shows a peak one day after the midcycle LH peak and is very low during the luteal phase of the cycle.[11] This indicates that inhibin B is mainly produced by the follicle.

It is well known that serum FSH, apart from the peak at midcycle, also increases during the intercycle period, that is, during the luteal–follicular transition.[12,13] This rise in FSH starts 2–3 days before the onset of the menstrual period and continues throughout the early follicular phase of the cycle. The so-called "FSH window" is responsible for the recruitment and selection of the dominant follicle. Until recently, the intercycle rise of FSH was thought to be the result of the release of the pituitary from the negative feedback effect of circulating ovarian steroids, the levels of which decline towards the late luteal phase. However, measurement of dimeric inhibin during the mentrual cycle with the new immunoassays has provided evidence that this substance may participate in the control of FSH secretion. In fact, serum values of inhibin A decline from mid- to late luteal phase, and this precedes the intercycle rise of FSH.[10] On the other hand, inhibin B starts to increase one or two days after the onset of the FSH intercycle rise, and as its levels increase a gradual decrease in FSH concentrations occurs at a time when serum E_2 values do not show a substantial increase.[11] These results suggest that inhibin A participates in the initiation and inhibin B in the termination of the FSH window and in that way both inhibins may play a role in the selection of the dominant follicle during the cycle. In addition, these results demonstrate that FSH is the main stimulator of inhibin B secretion, and this is further supported by a recent study demonstrating that, under a certain experimental design using treatment with pulsatile GnRH, inhibin B increases in proportion to the increase of FSH values.[14]

Activins have been also measured in blood during the normal menstrual cycle by a two-site enzyme immunoassay.[15] The results have shown an increase in activin A concentrations from midluteal phase to midfollicular phase of the next cycle.[15] A significant but smaller increase also occurs at midcycle. The fact that the increase in activin A values during the second half of the luteal phase precedes the increase in FSH values indicates that activin A may also play a role in the development of the FSH window and, therefore, may participate in the selection of the dominant follicle. One has to take into consideration, however, that the assay used for measurement of activin A does not differentiate between total activin and free activin, and therefore the values may not represent the biologically active form of this hormone. Improvements in the assay, therefore, are needed for a better assessment of the role of activin A during the normal mesntrual cycle. Regarding activin B, there is only one study, however, in which measurements were made only in two blood samples (one in the follicular and one in the luteal phase of the normal menstrual cycle) with no significant difference in activin B values between the two phases.[16] Finally, follistatin does not show any significant changes throughout the normal mentrual cycle, suggesting that this substance may not exert a specific biological effect *in vivo.*[17] It is possible that follistatin acts as a carrier protein for activins in the circulation, inactivating them and facilitating their action at the tissue level.

Although the studies mentioned in this article indicate that inhibins and activins may participate in the control of gonadotropin secretion *in vivo*, further research is required to clarify the precise role of these substances during the normal menstrual cycle.

GnRH-INDUCED LH SECRETION

It has been established that the midcycle LH surge in women is the result of the positive feedback effect of E_2 on the hypothalamic–pituitary system. E_2 sensitizes the pituitary to GnRH by increasing GnRH receptors on the gonadotropes. The sensitizing effect of E_2 on the pituitary is evident in women at different stages during the normal menstrual cycle after the i.v. injection of two submaximal pulses of GnRH 2 hours apart. In these experiments, in the presence of increased serum E_2 levels, the response of LH to the second GnRH pulse is substantially greater than the response to the first pulse, and this represents the self-priming effect of GnRH on the pituitary.[18] On the other hand, a maximal response to the first pulse occurs at 30 minutes, and this represents the first pool of gonadotropes or the pituitary sensitivity, whereas the whole area under the curve represents the second pool of gonadotropes or the pituitary reserve.[18] It has been suggested that the increase both in sensitivity and reserve of the gonadotropes from the early to late follicular phase of the cycle is important for the occurrence of the midcycle LH surge.

During the last 10 years, evidence has been provided that the ovaries, apart from inhibin, produce another nonsteroidal substance, named gonadotropin surge attenuating factor (GnSAF), which affects the amplitude of the LH surge.[2] This is based on the observation that in women superovulated for *in vitro* fertilization, the endogenous LH surge is markedly attenuated as compared to that in spontaneous cycles.[19] At the same time, the response of LH to GnRH is also markedly reduced.[20] These results suggest that GnSAF attenuates the endogenous LH surge in superovulated women through the reduction of LH response to GnRH. So far, substances with GnSAF activity have been isolated from rat Sertoli cell–enriched medium,[21] from porcine follicular fluid,[22] and very recently from human follicular fluid.[23] There are, however, discrepancies regarding the NH_2-terminal sequence and the molecular weight of the isolated substances that suggest more than one protein may be involved in the control of LH secretion from the pituitary via the suppression of GnRH-induced LH secretion. In women superovulated with FSH, both the first (releasable) and the second (reserve) pools of the gonadotropes as well as the self-priming effect of GnRH on the pituitary are reduced by GnSAF.[24] In these experiments, the response of LH to GnRH at 30 minutes has been used as an *in vivo* bioassay to assess the activity of GnSAF during superovulation induction.

Although GnSAF activity is present during superovulation induction, it is still unclear whether this factor plays a physiological role during the normal menstrual cycle. A recent study has addressed this issue and has provided evidence that GnSAF may participate in the control of LH secretion in women.[25] In that study, normally cycling women were treated with either purified FSH or recombinant FSH (Gonal-F) in two different cycles. In both cycles, pituitary sensitivity, that is, the 30-minute response to 10 μg GnRH,[18,24] was investigated on a daily basis during the whole follicular phase of the cycle; and the results were compared with those in a spontaneous cycle of the same women. According to the results, the response of LH to GnRH was markedly attenuated within 12 hours from the onset of both FSH treatments and remained low up to midfollicular phase.[25] At that stage, the response of LH to GnRH increased significantly and became similar to that in the spontaneous cycles in which, however, LH response had remained stable during the same period of time.[25]

These results suggest that treatment with FSH initially attenuated the response of LH to GnRH via the production of GnSAF from the ovaries, while around the midfollicular phase, the rising concentrations of E_2 were able to overcome the attenuating effect of GnSAF and increase pituitary sensitivity to GnRH. The increased pituitary sensitiviy in the midfollicular phase of the FSH-treated cycles, however, was not further enhanced in the late follicular phase despite the continuous rise in E_2 values.[25] It is suggested that eventually GnSAF was able to overcome the sensitizing effect of E_2. In contrast to the FSH-treated cycles, in the spontaneous cycles LH response to GnRH did not change significantly from early to midfollicular phase and showed a marked increase only during the preovulatory period up to the onset of the LH peak.[25] It is clear, therefore, that during the early and midfollicular phase of the normal menstrual cycle the ovaries antagonize the sensitizing effect of E_2 on the pituitary via GnSAF.

Another interesting finding of that study was that, although in the midfollicular phase of the FSH-treated cycles, LH response to GnRH was similar to that in the spontaneous cycles and E_2 values had already exceeded the threshold level for the positive feedback effect, an LH surge did not occur.[25] This confirms previous data that endogenous LH surge can be blocked in superovulated cycles[26] and suggests that the blockage of the surge is not controlled by GnSAF. Alternatively, however, if GnSAF is a blocking factor, it affects the positive feedback effect of E_2 through multiple mechanisms.

Based on these results as well as on those of previous studies, a hypothesis was developed regarding the physiological role of GnSAF during the normal menstrual cycle. According to this hypothesis, circulating activity of GnSAF is high during the early to midfollicular phase, thus maintaining the pituitary in a state of low responsiveness to GnRH. A decline in the production of GnSAF towards the preovulatory stage releases the pituitary from the break and enhances the sensitizing effect of the increasing concentrations of E_2 on pituitary gonadotropes. Thus, a maximal response of the pituitary to GnRH occurs at that stage resulting in full expression of the endogenous LH surge. It is clear from these results that GnSAF does not block the positive feedback effect of E_2 and therefore does not control the time of onset of the midcycle LH surge, but it controls the amplitude of the surge by a negative effect. In fact, an LH surge occurs whenever at any stage during the follicular phase of the cycle serum E_2 values exceed the threshold level for the positive feedback effect. Although in the early follicular phase the LH surge is attenuated,[27] in the late follicular phase the surge is normal.[28]

In conclusion, E_2 is the main component of the negative ovarian control of basal FSH and LH secretion during the normal menstrual cycle. Nonsteroidal ovarian hormones, such as inhibins and activins, may also participate. Although E_2 is also the principal stimulator of the midcycle LH surge, its effect on the amplitude of the surge is antagonized by the action of GnSAF.

REFERENCES

1. Wallace, E.M. & D.L. Healy. 1996. Inhibins and activins: roles in clinical practice. Br. J. Obstet. Gynaecol. **103:** 945–956.
2. Messinis, I.E. & A.A. Templeton. 1989. Pituitary response to exogenous LHRH in superovulated women. J. Reprod. Fertil. **87:** 633–639.
3. Messinis, I.E. & A.A. Templeton. 1991. Evidence that gonadotrophin surge-attenuating factor exists in man. J. Reprod. Fertil. **92:** 217–223.
4. Messinis, I.E., D. Lolis, L. Papadopoulos, *et al.* 1993. Effect of varying concentrations of follicle stimulating hormone on the production of gonadotrophin surge attenuating factor (GnSAF) in women. Clin. Endocrinol. **39:** 45–50.
5. Messinis, I.E., D. Lolis, K. Zikopoulos, *et al.* 1996. Effect of follicle stimulating hormone or human chorionic gonadotrophin treatment on the production of gonadotrophin surge attenuating factor (GnSAF) during the luteal phase of the human menstrual cycle. Clin. Endocrinol. **44:** 169–175.
6. Messinis, I.E. & A.A. Templeton. 1990. Effects of supraphysiological concentrations of progesterone on the characteristics of the oestradiol-induced gonadotrophin surge in women. J. Reprod. Fertil. **88:** 513–519.
7. Messinis, I.E., D. Lolis, K. Zikopoulos, *et al.* 1994. Effect of an increase in FSH on the production of gonadotrophin-surge-attenuating factor in women. J. Reprod. Fertil. **101:** 689–695.
8. Alexandris, E., S. Milingos, G. Kollios, *et al.* 1997. Changes in gonadotrophin response to gonadotrophin releasing hormone in normal women following bilateral ovariectomy. Clin. Endocrinol. **47:** 721–726.

9. BURGER, H.G. 1992. Inhibin. Reprod. Med. Rev. **1:** 1–20.
10. GROOME, N.P., P.J. ILLINGWORTH, M. O'BRIEN, *et al.* 1994. Detection of dimeric inhibin throughout the human menstrual cycle by two-site enzyme immunoassay. Clin. Endocrinol. **40:** 717–723.
11. GROOME, N.P, P.J. ILLINGWORTH, M. O'BRIEN, *et al.* 1996. Measurement of dimeric inhibin B throughout the human menstrual cycle. J. Clin. Endocrinol. Metab. **81:** 1401–1405.
12. ROSEFF, S.J., M.L. BANGAH, L.M. KETTEL, *et al.* 1989. Dynamic changes in circulating inhibin levels during the luteal–follicular transition of the human menstrual cycle. J. Clin. Endocrinol. Metab. **69:** 718–728.
13. MESSINIS, I.E., D. KOUTSOYIANNIS, S. MILINGOS, *et al.* 1993. Changes in pituitary response to GnRH during the luteal–follicular transition of the human menstrual cycle. Clin. Endocrinol. **38:** 159–163.
14. WELT, C.K., K.A. MARTIN, A.E. TAYLOR, *et al.* 1997. Frequency modulation of follicle-stimulating hormone (FSH) during the luteal–follicular transition: evidence for FSH control of inhibin B in normal women. J. Clin. Endocrinol. Metab. **82:** 2645–2652.
15. MUTTUKRISHNA, S., P.A. FOWLER, L. GEORGE, *et al.* 1996. Changes in peripheral serum levels of total activin A during the human menstrual cycle and pregnancy. J. Clin. Endocrinol. Metab. **81:** 3328–3334.
16. VIHKO, K.K., M. BLAUER, E. KUJANSUU, *et al.* 1998. Activin B: detection by an immunoenzymometric assay in human serum during ovarian stimulation and late pregnancy. Hum. Reprod. **13:** 841–846.
17. KETTEL, L.M., L.V. DEPAOLO, A.J. MORALES, *et al.* 1996. Circulating levels of follistatin from puberty to menopause. Fertil. Steril. **65:** 472–476.
18. WANG, C.F., B.L. LASLEY, A. LEIN & S.S.C. YEN. 1976. The functional changes of the pituitary gonadotrophs during the menstrual cycle. J. Clin. Endocrinol. Metab. **42:** 718–728.
19. MESSINIS, I.E., A. TEMPLETON & D.T. BAIRD. 1985. Endogenous luteinizing hormone surge during superovulation induction with sequential use of clomiphene citrate and pulsatile human menopausal gonadotropin. J. Clin. Endocrinol. Metab. **61:** 1076–1080.
20. MESSINIS, I.E. & A.A. TEMPLETON. 1990. In vivo bioactivity of gonadotrophin surge attenuating factor (GnSAF). Clin. Endocrinol. **33:** 213–218.
21. TIO, S., D. KOPPENAAL, C.W. BARDIN & C.Y. CHENG. 1994. Purufication of gonadotrophin surge-inhibiting factor from Sertoli cell–enriched culture medium. Biochem. Biophys. Res. Commun. **199:** 1229–1236.
22. DANFORTH, D.R. & C.Y. CHENG. 1995. Purification of a candidate gonadotrophin surge inhibiting factor from porcine follicular fluid. Endocrinology **136:** 1658–1665.
23. PAPPA, A., K. SEFERIADIS, TH. FOTSIS, *et al.* 1999. Purification of a candidate gonadotrophin surge attenuating factor (GnSAF) from human follicular fluid. Hum. Reprod. **14:** 1449–1456.
24. MESSINIS, I.E. & A. TEMPLETON. 1991. Attenuation of gonadotrophin release and reserve in superovulated women by gonadotrophin surge attenuating factor (GnSAF). Clin. Endocrinol. **34:** 259–263.
25. MESSINIS, I.E., S. MILINGOS, K. ZIKOPOULOS, *et al.* 1998. Luteinizing hormone response to gonadotrophin-releasing hormone in normal women undergoing ovulation induction with urinary or recombinant follicle stimulating hormone. Hum. Reprod. **13:** 2415–2420.
26. MESSINIS, I.E. & A.A. TEMPLETON. 1987. Endocrine and follicle characteristics of cycles with and without endogenous luteinizing hormone surges during superovulation induction with pulsatile follicle-stimulating hormone. Hum. Reprod. **2:** 11–16.
27. TAYLOR, A.E., H. WHITNEY, J.E. HALL, *et al.* 1995. Midcycle levels of sex steroids are sufficient to recreate the follicle-stimulating hormone but not the luteinizing hormone midcycle surge: evidence for the contribution of other ovarian factors to the surge in normal women. J. Clin. Endocrinol. Metab. **80:** 1541–1547.
28. MESSINIS, I.E. & A.A. TEMPLETON. 1987. Effect of high dose exogenous oestrogen on midcycle luteinizing hormone surge in human spontaneous cycles. Clin. Endocrinol. **27:** 453–459.

Progesterone Is an Autocrine/Paracrine Regulator of Human Granulosa Cell Survival *in Vitro*

A. MAKRIGIANNAKIS,[a,c] G. COUKOS,[a] M. CHRISTOFIDOU-SOLOMIDOU,[b] S. MONTAS,[a] AND C. COUTIFARIS[a]

[a]*Division of Human Reproduction, Department of Obstetrics and Gynecology and the Center for Research on Reproduction and Women's Health, and*
[b]*Department of Medicine, University of Pennsylvania Medical Center, Philadelphia, Pennsylvania 19104, USA*

ABSTRACT: Ovarian follicles are composed of granulosa cells (GC), which undergo apoptosis within 24 hours of culture in serum-free medium. The present study was designed to assess the role of progesterone in regulating human GC survival. Human GC were isolated from follicular aspirates of women undergoing *in vitro* fertilization. GC were then cultured for 24 hours in serum-free media supplemented with progesterone and/or the progesterone antagonist RU486 and dexamethasone. Cells were then fixed and assessed for apoptosis by in situ end labeling of DNA fragments, cell cycle analysis of DNA content, and electron microscopy. When compared with controls, progesterone reduced and RU486 increased the percentage of apoptotic GC (*$p < 0.05$*), whereas dexamethasone had no effect. In addition, RU486 inhibited the protective effect of progesterone on GC survival (*$p < 0.05$*). Taken together, these data indicate that progesterone inhibits human GC apoptosis, and this effect is mediated through the progesterone receptor.

INTRODUCTION

Follicular atresia and luteolysis are important events ensuring ovarian cyclicity, and they are achieved by selective degeneration of follicular and luteal cells. The endocrine and paracrine factors controlling ovarian function have been studied extensively. However, the intracellular events that control this degeneration have not been fully characterized. Recent observations suggest that elimination of follicular and luteal cells is mediated via programmed cell death, termed "apoptosis."[1,2] Typical morphologic and biochemical events of apoptosis, including chromatin condensation and fragmentation of DNA, have been observed in primary rat and human granulosa cells (GC).[3–5]

GC die by an apoptotic mechanism, which can be induced by placing the GC in serum-free culture medium for 24 hours.[3,5] By this *in vitro* system, the apoptotic

[c]Current address for correspondence: Antonis Makrigiannakis, M.D., Ph.D., Department of Reproductive Medicine, IVF Unit, Institute of Obstetrics and Gynecology, Institute of Obstetrics and Gynecology, Imperial College School of Medicine, Hammersmith Hospital, Du Cane Road, W12, OHS, London, UK. Phone 181-3838160; fax: 208-3838534.
a.makrygiannakis@ic.ac.uk

pathway was shown to be inhibited by several different growth factors, including epidermal growth factor (EGF),[6] basic fibroblast growth factor (bFGF),[6] insulin-like growth factor-I (IGF-I),[7] and insulin.[7] The hormonal regulation of apoptosis in follicular and luteal cells appears very complex.[7,8] It has been proposed that intrafollicular-derived IGF-I, and paracrine factors produced by theca interstitial cells, such as transforming growth factor α (TGFα), keratinocyte growth factor, and hepatocyte growth factor (HGF), mediate the suppression of apoptosis by gonadotropins and other endocrine factors in GC of antral follicles.[6–8] Furthermore, there is some evidence that growth factors may affect apoptosis in rat GC via progesterone (P4), which may function as a local mediator of their action.[9]

The concept that P4 may act as an intraovarian autocrine/paracrine factor has been proposed for nearly 20 years.[10] Since then, numerous studies have demonstrated the direct effect of P4 on GC function *in vitro*. P4 enhances the ability of cultured rat GC to respond to follicular stimulating hormone (FSH), an effect associated with increased production of cAMP.[11] Moreover, the synthetic progestin R5020 increases FSH- and luteinizing hormone (LH)-induced P4 secretion *in vitro*.[12,13]

Although considerable research has focused on the effect of various growth factors on GC survival, to date little consideration has been given to progesterone as a potential autocrine/paracrine modulator of human GC apoptosis. It is possible that progesterone acts directly on GC and luteal cells, because these cells possess progesterone receptors.[14,15] The present studies were designed to test this hypothesis by characterizing the ability of progesterone to regulate human GC survival *in vitro*. We herein show that progesterone acts through the progesterone receptor to inhibit GC/luteal cell apoptosis.

MATERIALS AND METHODS

Reagents

All reagents were of analytic grade and were purchased from Sigma Chemical Company (St. Louis, MO) unless otherwise stated.

Cell Culture and Treatments

Human GC were isolated from seven patients aged 25–43 years undergoing *in vitro* fertilization/embryo transfer. These cells had been exposed *in vivo* to a follicular recruitment regimen including a gonadotropin-releasing hormone (GnRH) agonist (Lupron, TAP Pharmaceuticals) for pituitary suppression and by purified FSH (Metrodin or Fertinex, Serono, Randolph, MA) for follicular stimulation. Moreover, all patients had received a single dose of purified human chorionic gonadotropin (hCG) 36 hours prior to follicular aspiration. The follicular fluid was collected and centrifuged. The sedimented cells were resuspended in Ca^{2+}-Mg^{2+}-free Hanks balanced salt solution (Gibco BRL, Life Technologies, NY), overlayed on Ficoll-Hypaque (Organon Technica, Durham, NC), and centrifuged at 400 *g* for 30 minutes. The cells were collected from the interphase. The isolated human GC were suspended, washed twice with Ca^{2+}-Mg^{2+}-free Hanks salt solution, and cultured in Hams F-12:DMEM media (1:1. v/v, Gibco, Grand Island, NY) supplemented with 10% fetal bovine serum (FBS), penicillin (10 U/ml), streptomycin (0.05 mg/ml), and fungizone (0.25 mg/ml). Contamination with monocytes, identified with flow cytometry by the anti-CD14 monoclonal antibody (Becton Dickinson, Lincoln Park, NJ), was <2%. Depending on the experimental design, P4 (10^{-6}–10^{-10} M) or dexamethasone was added to the cultures. All steroids were dissolved in ethanol and then diluted in DMEM/F12 without serum to the desired final concentration. RU 486 (provided by Roussel-UCLAF, Romainville, France) was used at a concentration of (10^{-6} M). Each experiment was performed at least three times with different cell preparations to ensure consistency of the findings.

Electron Microscopy

Routine Embedding in Epoxy Resin for Conventional TEM. Cells grown on human plasma fibronectin-coated (25 µg/ml; Sigma) plastic coverslips were fixed in ice cold fixative (2% paraformaldehyde/0.5% glutaraldehyde) in 0.1 M cacodylate buffer pH 7.4 for 10 minutes. After washing in cacodylate (3 times), coverslips were postfixed in 1% OsO4 in the same buffer for 10 minutes and washed. Cells were then washed 3 times with 0.05 M maleate buffer (pH = 5.2) followed by 1% uranyl acetate in the same buffer (pH = 6.0). The cells were dehydrated in a series of graded alcohols (70%, 95%, and 100% [3x]) for 10 minutes in each step. Sections were infiltrated with resin and allowed to polymerize at 60°C in special slide molds (EMS, Pennsylvania).

Ultrathin Sectioning. Ultrathin sections (100 nm) were cut with a diamond knife (Diatome, Switzerland) on a Leica (Chicago, IL) ultramicrotome. Resin sections were collected on uncoated 150-mesh copper grids (EMS, Pennsylvnia) postcontrasted with 20% uranyl acetate (Amersham)/0.5% lead citrate and viewed on a Hitachi H-600 transmission electron microscope (Nissey Sangyo, Gaithersburg, MD) at 75 kv.

In Situ *Detection of Apoptosis*

Terminal Deoxynucleotidyl Transferase (TdT)-Mediated dUTP-Biotin Nick End Labeling (TUNEL) Assay. Apoptosis was detected by in situ 3′-end labeling of DNA fragments *in vitro*. DNA fragments were labeled and detected by use of the reagents and procedures provided in the ApopTag in situ apoptosis detection kit (Oncor, Gaithersburg, MD). Briefly, GC were fixed in 10% buffered formalin and washed twice in phosphate-buffered saline solution. Cells were then incubated in a humidified chamber at 37°C for 1 hour in the presence of terminal deoxynucleotidyl transferase (TdT) and digoxigenin-11 dUTP and dATP. Cells were washed with buffer and incubated with antidigoxigenin-fluorescein antibody for 30 minutes at room temperature. Cells were then washed with buffer and observed under epifluorescence and brightfield optics. The nuclear structures of individual cells were stained with propidium iodide.

Electron Microscopy. To induce apoptosis *in vitro*, cells were incubated in serum-free media for 24 hours. Cells undergoing apoptosis were identified by electron microscopic examination of epoxy-embedded tissue.

Flow Cytometric Analysis of DNA Content (Cell Cycle Analysis). Trypsin-generated cell suspensions (including floating cells) (minimum 10^6 cells) were fixed in

70% ETOH for at least 16 hours, treated with RNase A (Sigma, 500 μg/ml for 30 minutes at room temperature), stained with propidium iodide (PI 20 μg/ml), and analyzed using an EPICS XL flow cytometer (Coulter Corporation, Hialeah, Florida). Data were analyzed using a Cellfit program. Cells with less than 2n DNA content in the cell cycle analysis profile were considered to be apoptotic.[16]

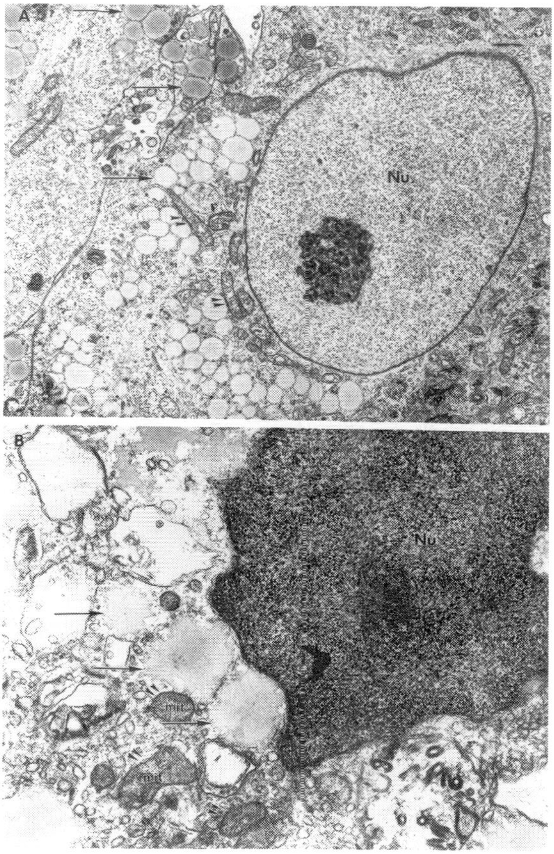

FIGURE 1. Electron microscopy of normal and apoptotic granulosa cells. (**A**) Human granulosa cells, cultured in the presence of serum, show no signs of apoptosis as judged by the physiologic ultrastructure. The nuclei (Nu) and cell organelles are intact. Note the osmiophilic lipid droplets (*arrow*) and intact internal membranes of the numerous mitochondria (*double arrowheads*). (**B**) Granulosa cells in serum-free media have a pathologic ultrastructure. Chromatin is condensed in the nuclei (nu) and the internal structure of mitochondria is damaged or nonexistent (*double arrowheads*). Lipid droplets have a jagged membrane (*arrow*). (Magnifications: **A,** 10,500×; **B,** 45,000×.)

Statistical Analysis

All experiments were conducted in duplicate and repeated at least three times. Percentage data were analyzed by either one-way ANOVA followed by Student-Newman-Keuls multiple range test or Student's *t* test. Only $p < 0.05$ was considered significant.

RESULTS

Serum Deprivation Induces Apoptosis in Human Granulosa Cells

To define the role of serum deprivation in modulating GC apoptosis, we used transmission electron microscopy. Cell ultrastructural morhology was analyzed in GC cultured in the presence of serum or under serum-free conditions. In the presence of serum, GC displayed well developed mitochondria and numerous round osmiophilic lipid-containing secretory droplets characteristic of steroidogenic cells (FIG. 1A). Moreover, the organization of the cytoplasm and other organelles appeared normal. The matrix of the nuclei appeared physiologic, with normal chromatin condensation (FIG. 1A). By contrast, many of the GC cultured in serum-free conditions displayed increased chromatin condensation in the nucleus. The cytoplasm contained damaged mitochondria, with ruptured internal membranes, damaged lipid droplets, and autophagic vesicles (FIG. 1B).

To further confirm the occurrence of apoptosis under serum-free conditions, we performed in situ TUNEL assay (FIG. 2A and B) and flow-cytometric cell cycle analysis of DNA content (FIG. 2C and D). Incubation of GC under serum-free conditions for 24 hours significantly increased apoptosis ($p < 0.05$) (FIG. 2E).

Progesterone Acts through Its Receptor to Promote Survival in Human Granulosa Cells

To assess the role of P4 in GC survival, cells were subjected to conditions inducing apoptosis, such as serum deprivation, and subsequently exposed to P4. Incubation of GC with different doses of progesterone (P4) in the absence of serum-inhibited apoptosis of GC in a dose-dependent manner, with a minimum effective dose of 10^{-8} M, as assessed by TUNEL and flow-cytometric cell cycle analysis of DNA content ($p < 0.05$) (FIG. 3). By contrast, dexamethasone had no effect on GC apoptosis (FIG. 4). The ability of P4 to suppress apoptosis was attenuated by the progesterone receptor antagonist RU 486 (FIG. 4), suggesting that this is mediated through the progesterone receptor. In contrast to P4, RU 486 increased the percentage of apoptotic cells ($p < 0.05$) (FIG. 4).

DISCUSSION

The present study confirms that under serum-free culture conditions, human GC die via an apoptotic mechanism and that programmed cell death occurs in human ovary,[5] as recently observed in rat cells.[3,4] In addition, the present study demonstrates for the first time that P4 inhibits human GC apoptosis. This antiapoptotic action of P4 could not be mimicked by dexamethasone, indicating that it is not

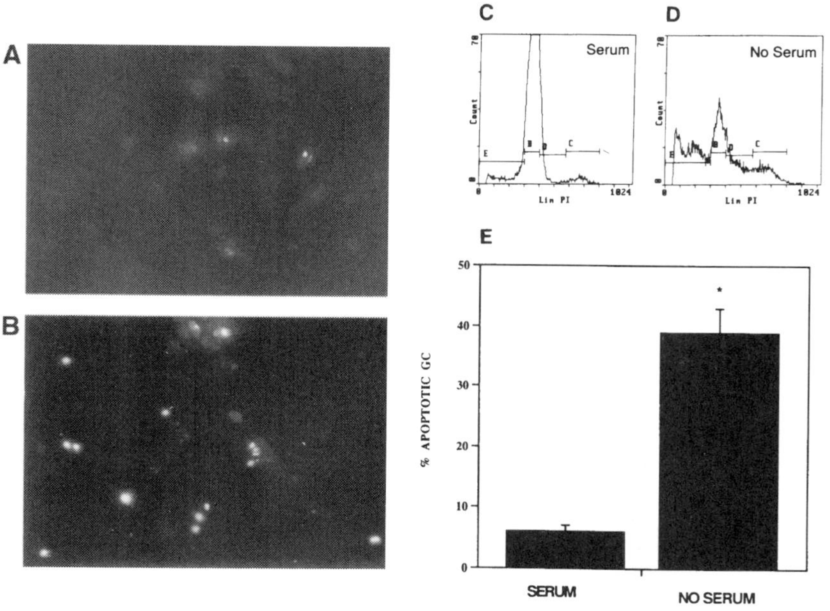

FIGURE 2. Effect of serum deprivation in human granulosa cell (GC) apoptosis. (**A,B**) Granulosa cells observed under fluorescent optics to detect the presence of free 3'OH ends of DNA fragments (TUNEL). Note that many of the GC collected after 24 hours of culture in the absence of serum fluoresce (**B**), indicating that they possess fragmented DNA and are undergoing apoptosis, in contrast to GC cultured in the presence of serum (**A**). (**C,D**) Cell cycle flow cytometric analysis of DNA content of one representative experiment, showing the increase in apoptosis (region **E**) in serum-free culture (**D**) compared to control (serum) (**C**). (**E**) Values represent the mean (standard error of the mean) of three separate experiments (TUNEL). In each experiment, 300–400 cells were observed for each treatment and used to calculate percentage of cells within apoptotic nuclei. *Asterisk* indicates that a value is significantly different from the control value ($p < 0.05$).

mediated by the ovarian glucocorticoid receptor. Because RU 486, a P4 receptor antagonist, attenuates P4 action, it is likely that P4 acts through the progesterone receptor to enhance GC survival. Furthermore, P4 appears to be essential to GC survival, because antagonizing the action of the endogenously produced P4 with RU 486 results in over 70% of GC dying within 24 hours. Moreover, we demonstrated that the concentrations of P4 required for human GC survival are not pharmacologic, suggesting that the ability of P4 to inhibit apoptosis may be physiologically important when P4 secretion is activated within the ovary.

We demonstrated that P4 prevents whereas RU 486 triggers apoptosis in human GC. A similar antiapoptotic effect of P4 was observed in other progesterone-sensitive cell types in humans[17] and other species.[18] More specifically, P4 inhibits rat GC apoptosis,[18,19] whereas a decline in P4 secretion precedes apoptotic changes within luteal cells.[20] Moreover, P4 prevents and RU 486 triggers apoptosis within the uter-

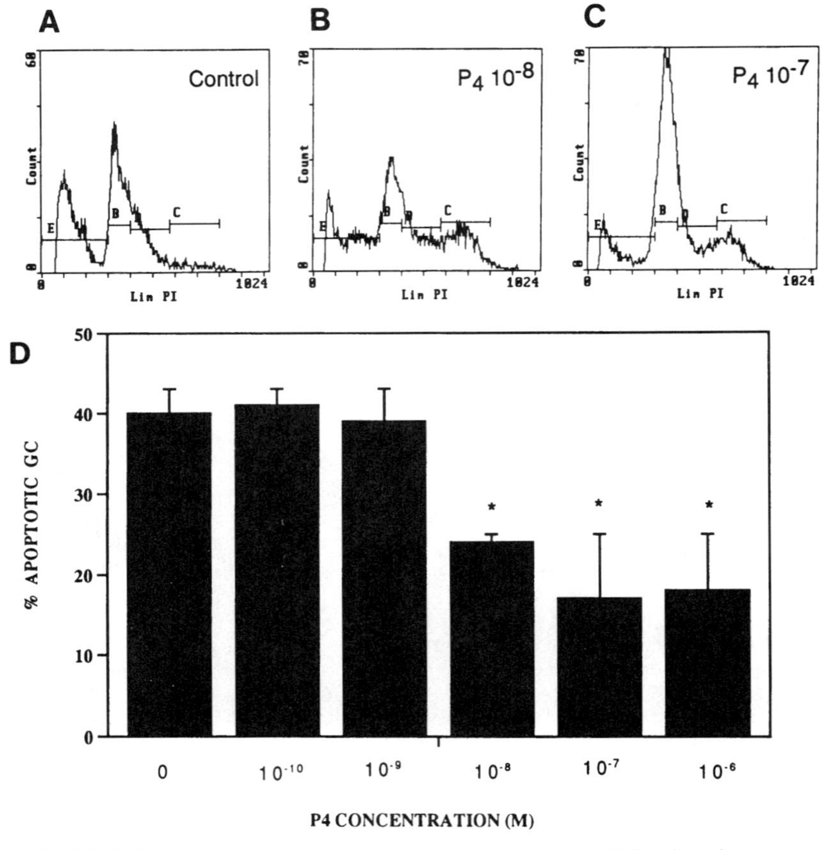

FIGURE 3. Dose response effect of P4 on the percentage of GC undergoing apoptosis. (**A,B,C**) Cell cycle flow cytometric analysis of DNA content of one representative experiment, showing the decrease in apoptosis (region **E**) in the presence of P4 (**B,C**) compared to control (**A**). (**D**) Dose response effect of P4 on the percentage of GC undergoing apoptosis as assessed by in situ DNA staining (TUNEL). Values shown represent the mean (SE). *Asterisk* indicates that a value is significantly different from the control value ($p < 0.05$).

ine epithelium.[17] These studies indicate that P4 acts as an autocrine/paracrine factor to maintain cell viability within the ovary and uterus and that factors that inhibit P4 secretion ultimately induce apoptotic changes in these cells.

Although previous work has shown that a decline in serum P4 precedes apoptosis within the corpus luteum and uterine epithelium, serum P4 levels increase as the GC of hCG-induced preovulatory follicles undergo DNA fragmentation.[2] This contradiction most likely occurs because 3β-hydroxysteroid dehydrogenase (3β-HSD), the enzyme responsible for the conversion of pregnenolone to P4, is expressed in GC of healthy preovulatory follicles as well as thecal and interstitial, but not in GC of follicles undergoing atresia.[21] This selective loss of 3β-HSD within the GC of atretic

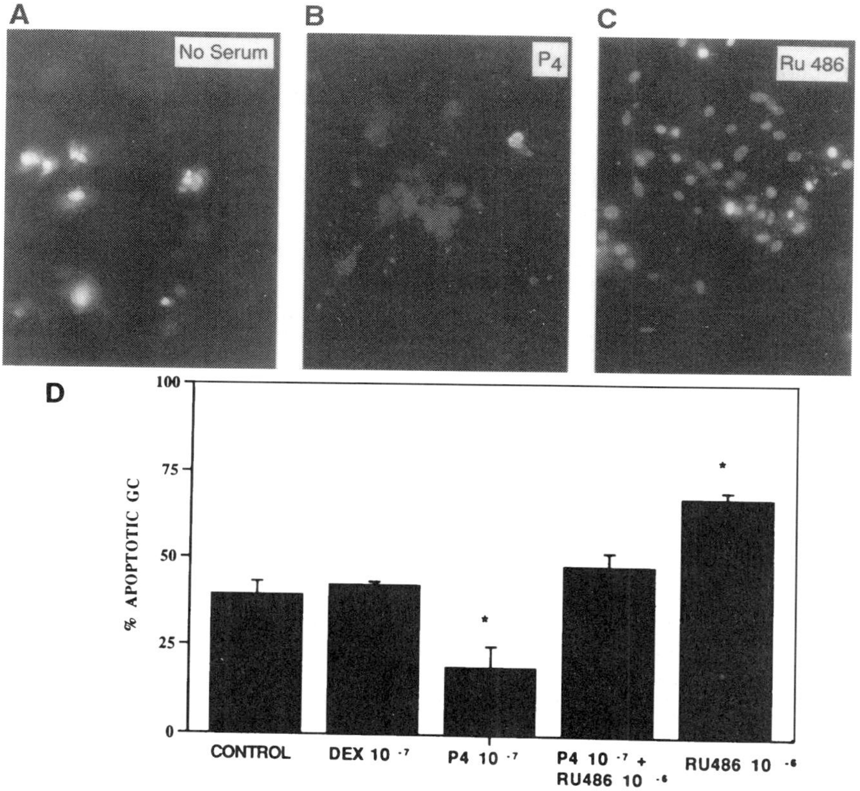

FIGURE 4. Effect of Dex, P4, and/or RU 486 in GC apoptosis. (**A,B,C**) GC undergoing apoptosis in the absence of serum as seen by the fragmented nuclei shown by TUNEL (**A**). Effect of P4 (**B**) and RU 486 (**C**) on GC apoptosis in serum-free culture for 24 hours. Note the decrease in the number of apoptotic nuclei of GC by P4 and the increase in the number of apoptotic nuclei by RU 486 (**C**). (**D**) The effect of Dex (10^{-7} M), P4 (10^{-7} M), and/or RU 486 (10^{-6} M) on the percentage of GC undergoing apoptosis after 24 hours of culture in serum-free media as judged by cell cycle analysis of DNA content. Values represent the mean (SEM) of three separate experiments. In each experiment, 10,000 cells were observed for each treatment and used to calculate percentage of cells within apoptotic nuclei. *Asterisk* indicates that a value is significantly different from the control value ($p < 0.05$).

follicles could result in a decrease in P4 in the GC component of the follicle. Because P4 maintains GC viability *in vitro*, the putative decline in P4 within the the GC layers could result in a corresponding increase in GC DNA fragmentation, even in the presence of elevated P4 levels.

GC undergo apoptosis within 24 hours of serum deprivation *in vitro*. This is prevented by different growth factors such as EGF or bFGF.[6] EGF and its functional homolog TGFα are produced in the ovary,[22,23] whereas both growth factors stimulate P4 secretion.[9] In addition, EGF's antiapoptotic action is inhibited by both RU 486 and aminoglutethamide, which reduces basal and EGF-induced P4 secretion,[9] suggesting that P4 synthesis is an essential part of the mechanism through which EGF and presumably TGFα maintain GC viabililty. Moreover, recent observations suggest that prostaglandin F_{2a} (PGF_{2a}), a known luteolysin in many species, is one factor that has been implicated in the process of apoptosis in the corpus luteum.[24] One action of PGF_{2a} in rat luteal cells appears to involve increased generation of reactive oxygen species,[25] an event that has been linked to both a loss of progesterone biosynthesis[26] and the induction of apoptosis.[27] By comparison, the luteotrophic factor hCG enhances expression of antioxidant factors, such as superoxide dismutase, in the rat corpus luteum[28] and prevents apoptosis in rabbit luteal tissue.[29] The ability of hCG to protect luteal cells from reactive oxygen species may also involve paracrine mediators, such as progesterone, which directly inhibits superoxidase radical generation by mononuclear phagocytes in the rat corpus luteum.[30]

In summary, the present data support the concept that P4 acts through the progesterone receptor to inhibit GC apoptosis. We propose that progesterone is critical for normal follicular development and/or the mophogenesis and survival of the human corpus luteum, one of the most important features in successful human reproduction.

ACKNOWLEDGMENTS

This work was supported by National Institutes of Health grant HD (CC) and by the Alexander Onassis Foundation (AM). The authors wish to thank Valerie Baldwin for help in the preparation of this manuscript.

REFERENCES

1. Hseuh, A.J. *et al.* 1994. Ovarian follicle atresia: a hormonally controlled apoptotic process. Endocrinol. Rev. **15:** 707–724.
2. Hughes, F.J. & W.C. Gorospe. 1991. Biochemical identification of apoptosis (programmed cell death) in granulosa cells: evidence for a potential mechanism underlying follicular atresia. Endocrinology **129:** 2415–2422.
3. Tilly, J.L. *et al.* 1991. Involvement of apoptosis in ovarian follicular atresia and postovulatory regression. Endocrinology **129:** 2799–2801.
4. Makrigiannakis, A. *et al.* 1999. *N*-Cadherin-mediated human granulosa cell adhesion prevents apoptosis. A role in follicular atresia and luteolysis? Am J. Pathol. **154:** 1391–1406.
5. Makrigiannakis, A. *et al.* 2000. Regulated expression and potential roles of p53 and Wilms' tumor suppressor gene (WT1) during follicular development in the human ovary. J. Clin. Endocrinol. Metab. **85:** 449–459.
6. Tilly, J.L. *et al.* 1992. Epidermal growth factor and basic fibroblast growth factor suppress the spontaneous onset of apoptosis in cultutred rat ovarian granulosa cells and follicles by a tyrosine kinase-dependent mechanism. Mol. Endocrinol. **6:** 1942–1950.
7. Chun, S.Y. *et al.* 1994. Gonadotropin suppression of apoptosis in cultured preovulatory follicles: mediatory role of endogenous insulin-like growth factor-I. Endocrinology **135:** 1845–1853.
8. Tilly, J.L. *et al.* 1995. Role of intrafollicular growth factors in maturation and atresia of rat ovarian follicles. Biol. Reprod. (Suppl. 1) **52:** 159.
9. Luciano, A.M. *et al.* 1994. Epidermal growth factor inhibits large granulosa cells apoptosis by stimulating progesterone synthesis and regulating the distribution of intracellular free calcium. Biol. Reprod. **51:** 646–654.

10. Schreiber, J.R. & A.J.W. HSEUH. 1979. Progesterone "receptor" in rat ovary. Endocrinology **105:** 915–925.
11. GOFF, A.K. *et al.* 1979. Stimulatory action of follicle-stimulating hormone and androgen on the responsiveness of rat granulosa cells to gonadotropin in vitro. Endocrinology **104:** 1124–1129.
12. FANJUL, L.F. *et al.* 1983. Progestin augmentation of gonadotrophin stimulated progesterone production by cultured rat granulosa cells. Endocrinology **112:** 405–407.
13. FORTUNE, J.E. & S.E. VINCENT. 1983. Progesterone inhibits the induction of aromatase activity in rat granulosa cells in vitro. Biol. Reprod. **28:** 1078–1089.
14. IWAI, T. 1990. Immunohistochemical localization of oestrogen and progesterone receptors in the human ovary throughout the menstrual cycle. Virchows Arch. [A] **417:** 369–375.
15. GREENBERG, L.H. *et al.* 1990. Are human lutetnizing granulosa cells a site of action for progesterone and relaxin? Fertil. Steril. **53:** 446–453.
16. McGahon, A.J. *et al.* 1995. The end of the (cell) line: methods for the study of apoptosis in vitro. Methods. Cell. Biol. **46:** 153–185.
17. Rotello, R. *et al.* 1992. Characterization of uterine epithelium apoptotic cell death kinetics and regulation by progesterone and RU486. Am. J. Pathol. **140:** 449–456.
18. PELUSO, J.J. & A. PAPPALARDO. 1994. Progesterone and cell-cell adhesion interact to regulate rat granulosa cell apoptosis. Biochem. Cell. Biol. **72:** 547–551.
19. PELUSO, J.J. & A. PAPPALARDO. 1998. Progesterone mediates its anti-mitogenic and anti-apoptotic actions in rat granulosa cells through a progesterone-binding protein with Gamma Aminobutyritic Acid A receptor-like features. Biol. Reprod. **58:** 1131–1137.
20. JUENGEL, J.L. *et al.* 1993. Apoptosis during luteal regression in cattle. Endocrinology **132:** 249–254.
21. TEERDS, K.J. & J.H. DORRINGTON. 1993. Immunohistochemical localization of 3β-hydroxysteroid hydrogenase in the rat ovary during follicular development and atresia. Biol. Reprod. **49:** 989–996.
22. MARUO, T. *et al.* 1993. Expression of epidermal growth factor and its receptor in the human ovary during follicular growth and regression. Endocrinology. **132:** 924–931.
23. YEH, J. *et al.* 1993. Presence of transforming growth factor-alpha messenger ribonucleic acid (mRNA) and absence of epidermal growth factor mRNA in rat ovarian granulosa cells, and the effects of these factors on steroidogenesis in vitro. Biol. Reprod. **48:** 1071–1081.
24. ORLICKY, D.J. *et al.* 1992. Immunohistochemical localization of PGF 2a receptor in the rat ovary. Prostaglandins. Leukotrienes. Essential. Fatty Acids **46:** 223–229.
25. SAWADA, M. & J.C. CARLSON. 1991. Rapid plasma membrane changes in superoxide radical function, fluidity, and phospholipase A2 activity in the corpus luteum of the rat during induction of luteolysis. Endocrinology **128:** 2992–2998.
26. MUSICKI, B. *et al.* 1994. Inhibition of protein synthesis and hormone sensitive steroidogenesis in response to hydrogen peroxide in rat luteal cells. Endocrinology **134:** 588–595.
27. TILLY, J.L. & K.I. TILLY. 1995. Inhibitors of oxidative stress mimic the ability follicle-stimulating hormone to suppress apoptosis in cultured rat ovarian follicles. Endocrinology **136:** 242–252.
28. LALORAYA, M. *et al.* 1988. Changes in the levels of superoxide anion radical and superoxide dismutase during the estrous cycle of Rattus norvegicusand induction of superoxide dismutase in the rat ovary by lutropin. Biochem. Biophys. Res. Commun. **157:** 146–153.
29. Dharmarajan, A.M. *et al.* 1994. Apoptosis during functional corpus luteum regression: evidence of a role for chorionic gonadotropin in promoting luteal cell survival. Endocrine J. (Endocrine) **2:** 295–303.
30. SUGINO, N. *et al.* 1996. Progesterone inhibits superoxide radical production by mononuclear phagocytes in pseudopregnant rats. Endocrinology **137:** 749–754.

A Clinical Understanding of the Estrogen Receptor

LEON SPEROFF

Department of Obstetrics and Gynecology, Oregon Health Sciences University, Portland, Oregon 97201, USA

INTRODUCTION

There has been a tremendous increase in the understanding of steroid hormone receptors based upon basic research from the world of molecular biology. This new information makes it possible to understand a series of questions that have been puzzling clinicians: (1) Even though there is only one mechanism, how can the same estrogen have different effects in different cells? (2) How can a weak effect in one target tissue be a strong effect in another? (3) Are all estrogens the same? (4) How can a drug be an agonist in one organ and an antagonist in another?

The early model of steroid hormone action was too simple to give answers to these questions. Given the requirements for different actions in different tissues (e.g., both inhibition and stimulation), it is not surprising that more complex mechanisms are operative. This review summarizes the new information, providing an understanding for clinicians to answer these questions.

MECHANISM OF ACTION

The specificity of the reaction of tissues to sex steroid hormones is due to the presence of intracellular receptor proteins. Different types of tissues, such as liver, kidney, and uterus, respond in a similar manner. The mechanism includes: (1) steroid hormone diffusion across the cell membrane, (2) steroid hormone binding to receptor protein, (3) interaction of a hormone-receptor complex with nuclear DNA, (4) synthesis of messenger RNA (mRNA), (5) transport of the mRNA to the ribosomes, and finally (6) protein synthesis in the cytoplasm that results in specific cellular activity.[1] The steroid hormone receptors primarily affect gene transcription, but also regulate posttranscriptional events and nongenomic events. *Steroid receptors regulate gene transcription through multiple mechanisms, not all of which require direct interactions with DNA.*

Each of the major classes of the sex steroid hormones, including estrogens, progestins, and androgens, has been demonstrated to act according to this general mechanism. Glucocorticoid, mineralocorticoid, and probably androgen receptors, when in the unbound state, reside in the cytoplasm and move into the nucleus after hormone-receptor binding. Estrogens and progestins are transferred across the nuclear membrane and bind to their receptors within the nucleus.

Steroid hormones are rapidly transported across the cell membrane by simple diffusion. The factors responsible for this transfer are unknown, but the concentration of free (unbound) hormone in the bloodstream seems to be an important and influential determinant of cellular function. Once in the cell, the sex steroid hormones bind to their individual receptors.[2–4] During this process, *transformation or activation* of the receptor occurs. Transformation refers to a conformational change of the hormone-receptor complex, revealing or producing a binding site that is necessary in order for the complex to bind to the chromatin. In the unbound state, the receptor is associated with heat shock proteins that stabilize and protect the receptor and maintain the DNA binding region in an inactive state. Activation of the receptor is driven by hormone binding that causes a dissociation of the receptor-heat shock protein complex.

The hormone-receptor complex binds to specific DNA sites (*hormone-responsive elements*) that are located upstream of the gene. The specific binding of the hormone-receptor complex with DNA results in RNA polymerase initiation of transcription. Transcription leads to translation, mRNA-mediated protein synthesis on the ribosomes. The principal action of steroid hormones is the regulation of intracellular protein synthesis by means of the receptor mechanism.

Biologic activity is maintained only while the nuclear site is occupied with the hormone-receptor complex. The dissociation rate of the hormone and its receptor as well as the half-life of the nuclear chromatin-bound complex are factors in the biologic response, because the hormone response elements are abundant and, under normal conditions, are occupied only to a small extent.[5] Thus, an important clinical principle is the following: duration of exposure to a hormone is as important as dose. One reason only small amounts of estrogen need be present in the circulation is the long half-life of the estrogen hormone-receptor complex. Indeed, a major factor in the potency differences among the various estrogens (estradiol, estrone, and estriol) is the length of time the estrogen-receptor complex occupies the nucleus. The higher rate of dissociation with the weak estrogen (estriol) can be compensated for by continuous application to allow prolonged nuclear binding and activity. Cortisol and progesterone must circulate in large concentrations because their receptor complexes have short half-lives in the nucleus.

An important action of estrogen is the modification of its own and other steroid hormone activity by affecting receptor concentrations. Estrogen increases target tissue responsiveness to itself and to progestins and androgens by increasing the concentration of its own receptor and that of the intracellular progestin and androgen receptors. This process is called *replenishment*. Progesterone and clomiphene, on the other hand, limit tissue response to estrogen by blocking the replenishment mechanism, thus decreasing over time the concentration of estrogen receptors. Replenishment is very responsive to the available amount of steroid and receptors. Small amounts of receptor depletion and small amounts of steroid in the blood activate the mechanism.

THE RECEPTOR SUPERFAMILY

Recombinant DNA techniques have permitted the study of the gene sequences that code for the synthesis of nuclear receptors. Steroid hormone receptors share a common structure with the receptors for thyroid hormone, 1,25-dihydroxy vitamin D_3, and retinoic acid; thus, these receptors are called a superfamily.[6] Each receptor contains characteristic domains that are similar and interchangeable. Therefore, it is not surprising that the specific hormones can interact with more than one receptor in this family. Analysis of these receptors suggests a complex evolutionary history during which gene duplication and swapping between domains of different origins occurred.[7] This family now includes about 150 proteins, present in practically all species, from worms to insects to humans. Many are called *orphan receptors* because specific ligands for these proteins have not been identified.

THE ESTROGEN RECEPTORS

Two estrogen receptors have been identified, designated as estrogen receptor-alpha (ER-α) and estrogen receptor-beta (ER-β).[8,9] Estrogen receptor-alpha was discovered about 1960, and the amino acid sequence was reported in 1986.[10–12] Estrogen receptor-alpha is translated from a 6.8-kilobase mRNA that contains 8 exons derived from a gene on the long arm of chromosome 6.[13] It has a molecular weight of approximately 66,000 with 595 amino acids. The receptor-alpha half-life is approximately 4–7 hours; thus, estrogen receptor-alpha is a protein with a rapid turnover. The more recently discovered estrogen receptor-beta is encoded by a gene localized to chromosome 14,q22-q24, in close proximity to genes related to Alzheimer's disease.[14]

The estrogen receptors are divided into 6 regions in 5 domains, labeled A to F. The ER-β is 97% homologous in amino acid sequence with the alpha estrogen receptor in the DNA-binding domain and 59% homologous in the hormone-binding domain.[9,14]

The following discussion represents information derived from studies of ER-α. The hormone binding characteristics of ER-α and ER-β are similar, indicating that they respond in a comparable manner to the same hormones.[15] There are differences however; for example, phytoestrogens have a greater affinity for ER-β than for ER-α. Different genetic messages can result not only because of differences in binding affinity, but also through variations in the mechanisms to be discussed, notably differences in conformational shape and cellular contexts. In addition, because the regulatory domains differ in the two receptors, ER-β may be incapable of activating gene transcription by means of TAF-1 (to be discussed).

A/B Region, the Regulatory Domain

The amino acid terminal is the most variable in the superfamily of receptors, ranging in size from 20 amino acids in the vitamin D receptor to 600 amino acids in the mineralocorticoid receptor. In the ER-α, it contains several phosphorylation sites and the *transcription activation function called TAF-1*. TAF-1 can stimulate transcription in the absence of hormone binding. The regulatory domain is considerably different in the two estrogen receptors, and in ER-β, TAF-1 is either significantly modified or absent.

C Region, the DNA-Binding Domain

The middle domain binds to DNA and consists of 100 amino acids with 9 cysteines in fixed positions, the two *zinc fingers*. This domain is essential for activation of transcription. Hormone binding induces a conformational change that allows binding to the hormone-responsive elements in the target gene. This domain is very similar in each member of the steroid and thyroid receptor superfamily; however, the genetic message is specific for the hormone that binds to the hormone-binding domain. The DNA-binding domain controls which gene will be regulated by the receptor and is responsible for target gene specificity and high-affinity DNA binding. The specificity of receptor binding to its hormone-responsive element is determined by the zinc finger region, especially the first finger. The specific message can be changed by changing the amino acids in the base of the fingers. Substitutions of amino acids in the fingertips lead to loss of function. Functional specificity is localized to the second zinc finger in an area designated the d (distal) box. Different responses are due to the different genetic expression of each target cell (the unique activity of each cell's genetic constitution allows individual behavior).

D Region, the Hinge

The region between the DNA-binding domain and the hormone-binding domain contains a signal area that is important for the movement of the receptor to the nucleus following synthesis in the cytoplasm. This nuclear localization signal must be present for the estrogen receptor to remain within the nucleus in the absence of hormone. This region is also a site of rotation (hence the hinge designation) in achieving conformational change.

E Region, the Hormone-Binding Domain

The carboxy end of estrogen receptor-alpha is the hormone-binding domain (for both estrogens and antiestrogens), consisting of 251 amino acids (residues 302–553). In addition to hormone binding, this region is responsible for *dimerization* and contains the *transcription activation function called TAF-2*. This is also the site for binding by heat shock proteins (specifically hsp 90), and it is this binding to the heat shock proteins that prevents dimerization and DNA binding. In contrast to TAF-1 activity, TAF-2 depends on hormone binding for full activity. The hormone-binding domain of the steroid receptors contains a characteristic structure, containing helices that form a pocket (also referred to as a sandwich fold).[16] After binding with a hormone, this pocket undergoes a conformational change that creates new surfaces with the potential to interact with coactivator and corepressor proteins.

F Region

The F region of ER-α is a 42 amino acid C-terminal segment. This region modulates gene transcription by estrogen and antiestrogens, having a role that influences antiestrogen efficacy in suppressing estrogen-stimulated transcription.[17] The conformation of the receptor-ligand complex is different with estrogen and antiestrogens, and this conformation is different with and without the F region. The F region is not required for transcriptional response to estrogen; however, it affects the magnitude of ligand-bound receptor activity. It is speculated that this region affects conformation in such a way that protein interactions are influenced. Thus, it is appropriate that the effects of the F domain vary according to cell type and protein context. The F region affects the activities of both TAF-1 and TAF-2, which is what we would expect if the effect is on conformation.[18]

HOW THE ESTROGEN RECEPTOR WORKS

The steroid family receptors are predominantly in the nucleus even when not bound to a ligand, except for the androgen, mineralocorticoid, and glucocorticoid receptors where nuclear uptake depends on hormone binding. The estrogen receptor, however, does undergo what is called *nucleocytoplasmic shuttling*. The estrogen receptor constantly diffuses out of the nucleus and is rapidly transported back in. When this shuttling is impaired, receptors are more rapidly degraded in the cytoplasm. Agents that inhibit dimerization (e.g., the pure estrogen antagonists) inhibit nuclear translocation and thus increase cytoplasmic degradation.

Prior to binding, the estrogen receptor is an inactive complex that includes a variety of proteins, including the heat shock proteins. Heat shock protein 90 appears to be a critical protein, and many of the others are associated with it. This heat shock protein is important not only for maintaining an inactive state, but also for causing proper folding for transport across membranes. "Activation" or "transformation" is the dissociation of heat shock protein 90.[19]

Imagine the unoccupied steroid receptor as a loosely packed, mobile protein complexed with heat shock proteins. The steroid family of receptors exists in this complex and cannot bind to DNA until union with a steroid hormone liberates the heat shock proteins and allows dimerization. The conformational change induced by hormone binding involves a dissociating process to form tighter packing of the receptor. The hormone-binding domain contains helices that form a pocket (also referred to as a sandwich fold).[16] After binding with a hormone, this pocket undergoes a conformational change that creates new surfaces with the potential to interact with coactivator and co-repressor proteins. *Conformational shape is an important factor in determining the exact message transmitted to the gene.* Conformational shape is slightly but significantly different with each ligand; estradiol, tamoxifen, and raloxifene each induce a distinct conformation that contributes to the ultimate message of agonism or antagonism.[20,21] The estrogen activity of estriol is weak because of its altered conformation shape when combined with the estrogen receptor in comparison with estradiol.[22]

The hormone-binding domain of the estrogen receptors contains a cavity surrounded by a wedge-shaped structure, and it is the fit into this cavity that is so effectove in influencing the genetic message. The size of this cavity on the estrogen receptor is relatively large, larger than the volume of an estradiol molecule, explaining the acceptance of a large variety of ligands. Thus, estradiol, tamoxifen, and raloxifene each bind at the same site within the hormone-binding domain, but the conformational shape with each is not identical.

Conformational shape is a major factor in determining the ability of a ligand and its receptor to interact with coactivators and corepressors. Conformational shapes are not simply either "on" or "off," but intermediate conformations are possible, providing a spectrum of agonist/antagonistic activity.

Molecular modeling and physical energy calculations indicate that binding of estrogen with its receptor is not a simple key and lock mechanism. It involves conversion of the estrogen-receptor complex to a preferred geometry dictated, to a major degree, by the specific binding site of the receptor. The estrogenic response depends on the final bound conformation and the electronic properties of functional groups that contribute energy. The final transactivation function is dependent on these variables.[23]

Estrogen, progesterone, androgen, and glucocorticoid receptors bind to their response elements as dimers, one molecule of hormone to each of the two units in the dimer. The estrogen receptor-alpha can form dimers with other alpha receptors (homodimers) or with an estrogen receptor-beta (heterodimer). Similarly, estrogen receptor-beta can form homodimers or heterodimers with the alpha receptor. This creates the potential for many pathways for estrogen signaling, alternatives that are further increased by the possibility of utilizing various response elements in target genes. Cells that express only one of the estrogen receptors would respond to the homodimers; cells that express both could respond to a homodimer and a heterodimer.

The similar amino acid sequence of the DNA-binding domains in this family of receptors indicates evolutionary conservation of homologous segments. An important part of the conformational pattern consists of multiple cysteine-repeating units found in two structures, each held in a finger-like shape by a zinc ion, the so-called zinc fingers.[24] The zinc fingers on the various hormone receptors are not identical. These fingers of amino acids are thought to interact with similar complementary patterns in the DNA. Directed changes (experimental mutations) indicate that conservation of the cysteine residues is necessary for binding activity, as is the utilization of zinc.

The DNA-binding domain is specific for an enhancer site (called the hormone-responsive element) in the gene promoter, located in the 5′ flanking region. The activity of the hormone-responsive element requires the presence of the hormone-receptor complex. Thus, this region is the part of the gene to which the DNA-binding domain of the receptor binds. There are at least four different hormone-responsive elements, one for glucocorticoids/progesterone/androgen, one for estrogen, one for vitamin D_3, and one for thyroid/retinoic acid.[25] These sites significantly differ only in the number of intervening nucleotides.

Binding of the hormone-receptor complex to its hormone-responsive element leads to many changes, only one of which is a conformational alteration in the DNA. Although the hormone-responsive elements for glucocorticoids, progesterone, and androgens mediate all of these hormonal responses, there are subtle differences in the binding sites, and there are additional sequences outside the DNA-binding sites that influence activation by the three different hormones. The cloning of complementary DNAs for steroid receptors has revealed a large number of similar structures of unknown function. It is believed that the protein products of these sequences are involved in the regulation of transcription initiation that occurs at the TATA box.

There are three different RNA polymerases (designated I, II, and III), each dedicated to the transcription of a different set of genes with specific promoters (the site of polymerase initiation of transcription). *Transcription factors are polypeptides, complexed with the polymerase enzyme, that modulate transcription either at the promoter site or at a sequence further upstream on the DNA.*[1] The steroid hormone receptors, therefore, are transcription factors. The polymerase transcription factor complex can be developed in sequential fashion with recruitment of individual polypeptides or transcription can result from interaction with a preformed complete complex. The effect can be either positive or negative, activation or repression.

In most cases, therefore, the steroid hormone receptor activates transcription in partnership with several groups of polypeptides including:[1]*other transcription factors*— peptides that interact with the polymerase enzyme and DNA; *coactivators and corepressors*—peptides that interact with the transcriptional activation function

(TAF) areas of the receptor, also called adaptor proteins; *chromatin factors*—structural organizational changes that allow an architecture appropriate for transcription response.

The steroid-receptor complex regulates the amount of mRNA transcripts emanating from target genes. The estrogen-occupied receptor binds to estrogen response elements in the 5' flanking regions of estrogen-regulated genes, allowing efficient induction of RNA transcription. This can occur by direct binding to DNA and interaction with the estrogen response element or by protein interactions with *coactivators* between the estrogen receptor and DNA sites. *Coactivators and corepressors are intracellular proteins (called adaptor proteins) that activate or suppress the TAF areas by acting either on the receptors or on DNA.*[26–28] Most of the genes regulated by estrogens respond within 1–2 hours after estrogen administration. Only a few respond within minutes. This time requirement may reflect the necessity to synthesize regulating proteins.[29]

Transcriptional activation function is the part of the receptor that activates gene transcription after binding to DNA. Ligand binding produces a conformation that allows TAFs to accomplish their tasks. TAF-1 can stimulate transcription in the absence of hormone when it is fused to DNA; however, it also promotes DNA binding in the intact receptor. TAF-2 is affected by the bound ligand, and the estrogen receptor depends on estrogen binding for full activity. TAF-2 consists of a number of dispersed elements that are brought together after estrogen binding. The activities of TAF-1 and TAF-2 vary according to the promoters in target cells. These areas can act independently or with one another.

Thus, the differential activities of the TAFs account for different activities in different cells. In addition to the binding of the dimerized steroid receptor to the DNA response element, steroid hormone activity is modulated by other pathways (other protein transcription factors and coactivators/corepressors) that influence transcription activation.[30] This is an important concept, the concept of cellular context. The same hormone can produce different responses in different cells according to the cellular context of protein regulators.

The concentration of coactivators/corepressors can affect the cellular response, and this is another explanation for strong responses from small amounts of hormone. A small amount of receptor but a large amount of coactivator/corepressor and the cell can be very responsive to a weak signal.

Phosphorylation of specific receptor sites is an important method of regulation, as is phosphorylation of other peptides that influence gene transcription. Phosphorylation can be regulated by cell membrane receptors and ligand binding, thus establishing a method for cell membrane-bound ligands to communicate with steroid receptor genes.

Cyclic AMP and protein kinase A pathways increase transcriptional activity of the estrogen receptor by phosphorylation. In some cases, phosphorylation modulates the activity of the receptor; in other cases, phosphorylation regulates the activity of a specific peptide or coactivator/corepressor that, in turn, modulates the receptor. The steroid receptor superfamily members are phosphoproteins. Phosphorylation follows steroid binding and occurs in both cytoplasm and nucleus. This phosphorylation is believed to enhance activity of the steroid receptor complex.

Phosphorylation of the receptor increases the potency of the molecule to regulate transcription. Growth factors can stimulate protein kinase phosphorylation that can produce synergistic activation of genes or even ligand-independent activity. Epidermal growth factor (EGF), IGF-I, and TGF-α can activate the estrogen receptor in the absence of estrogen. This response to growth factors can be blocked by pure antiestrogens (suggesting that a strong antagonist locks the receptor in a conformation that resists ligand-independent pathways). The exact mechanism of growth factor activation is not known, but it is known that a steroid receptor can be activated by means of a chemical signal (a phosphorylation cascade) originating at the plasma membrane. *The recruitment of kinase activity is specific for specific ligands; thus, not all ligands stimulate phosphorylation.*

Another explanation for strong responses from small amounts of steroids is a positive feedback relationship. Estrogen activates its receptor, gene expression stimulates growth factors (EFG, IGF-I, TGF-α, and FGF), and the growth factors in an autocrine fashion further activate the estrogen receptor.[31]

Summary of Steps in the Steroid Hormone–Receptor Mechanism:

Binding of the hormone to the hormone-binding domain that has been kept in an inactive state by various heat shock proteins.

Activation of the hormone-receptor complex, by *conformational change,* follows the dissociation of the heat shock proteins.

Dimerization of the complex.

Binding of the dimer to the hormone-responsive element on DNA by the zinc finger area of the DNA-binding domain.

Stimulation of transcription, mediated by transcription activation functions (TAFs), and influenced by the protein (other transcription factors and coactivators/corepressors) *context of the cell,* and by *phosphorylation.*

Summary of Factors That Determine Biologic Activity:

Affinity of the hormone for the hormone-binding domain of the receptor.

Target tissue differential expression of the receptor subtypes (e.g., ER-α and ER-β).

Conformational shape of the ligand-receptor complex, with effects on two important activities: dimerization and modulation of adapter proteins.

Differential expression of target tissue adaptor proteins and phosphorylation.

DIFFERENT ROLES FOR ER-α AND ER-β

Male and female mice have been developed that are homozygous for disruption of the alpha estrogen receptor gene, "estrogen receptor-alpha knockout mice."[32] Both sexes with this knockout are infertile. Spermatogenesis in the male is reduced and the testes undergo progressive atrophy, a result of a testicular role for estrogen, because gonadotropin levels and testicular steroidogenesis remain normal. Sexual mounting behavior is not altered, but intromission, ejaculation, and aggressive behaviors are reduced. Female mice with the alpha estrogen receptor gene disrupted do not ovulate, and the ovaries do not respond to gonadotropin stimulation. These female animals have high levels of estradiol, testosterone, and luteinizing hormone. Follicle stimulating hormone (FSH) β-subunit synthesis is increased, but FSH secretion is at normal levels, indicating different sites of action for estrogen and inhibin. Uterine development is normal (due to a lack of testosterone in early life), but growth is impaired. Mammary gland ductal and alveolar development is absent. Female mice with absent alpha estrogen receptor activity do not display sexual receptive behaviors. This genetically engineered line of mice demonstrates essential activities for the alpha estrogen receptor. Relatively normal fetal and early development suggests that the beta estrogen receptor plays a primary role in these functions. For example, the fetal adrenal gland expresses high levels of ER-β and low levels of ER-α.[33] However, nongenomic actions of estrogen are also possible and can explain some of the estrogenic responses in a knockout model.

Differential expression of the alpha and beta receptors is likely in various tissues (e.g., ER-β is the prevalent estrogen receptor in certain areas of the brain and the cardiovascular system), resulting in different and selective responses to specific estrogens. Human granulosa cells from the ovarian follicle contain *only* ER-β mRNA; the human breast expresses both ER-α and ER-β.[14] Some parts of the rat brain contain only ER-β, others only ER-α, and some areas contain both receptors.[34]

The estrogen story is further complicated by the fact that the same estrogen binding to the alpha and beta receptors can produce opposite effects. For example, estradiol can stimulate gene transcription with ER-α and a given site of the estrogen response element, whereas estradiol inhibits gene transcription with ER-β in this same system.[35] Different and unique messages, therefore, can be determined by the specific combination of (1) a particular estrogen, (2) the alpha or beta receptor, and (3) the targeted response element. To some degree, differences with ER-α and ER-β are influenced by activation of TAF-1 and TAF-2; agents that are capable of mixed estrogen agonism and antagonism produce agonistic messages via TAF-1 with ER-α, but because ER-β lacks a similar TAF-1, such agents can be pure antagonists in cells that respond only to ER-β. ER-α and ER-β affect the peptide context of a cell, especially coactivators and corepressors, differently.

NONGENOMIC ACTIONS OF STEROID HORMONES

The genomic effects of steroid hormones are characterized by a relatively slow response time of 1 hour or longer. However, some steroid hormone effects are immediate, within a few seconds, and nongenomic mechanisms must be operative in order to achieve such rapid responses.[36] These rapid responses are also unaffected by inhibitors of gene transcription or protein synthesis. Rapid actions have been reported for all steroid hormones and include calcium and sodium transport across membranes, neural effects, and certain oocyte and sperm reactions. The messenger and effector systems utilized vary from cell to cell and from steroid to steroid. Specific cell membrane receptors have been identified for various steroids; however, it has been difficult to demonstrate physiologic roles for these binding sites. Nevertheless, investigation thus far indicates that steroid hormones can bind to membrane receptors and trigger rapid changes in electrolyte transport systems.[37] Estrogen-induced vasodilatation in the coronary arteries is believed to be mediated, at least in part, through a nongenomic calcium flux mechanism.[38]

ANTIESTROGENS

Currently, there are two groups of antiestrogens, pure antiestrogens and compounds with both agonistic and antagonistic activities. The mixed agonist–antagonist compounds include both the triphenylethylene derivatives (the nonsteroidal estrogen relatives such as clomiphene and tamoxifen) and the nonsteroidal sulfur-containing agents (the benzothiophenes, such as raloxifene). The pure antiestrogens have a bulky side chain that, with only a little imagination, can be pictured as an obstruction to appropriate conformational changes. An ideal antiestrogen would have the following properties: (1) A compound that would be a pure antagonist on proliferating breast carcinoma cells. (2) Development of resistance that would be rare or require long exposure. (3) High affinity for the estrogen receptor so that therapeutic doses could easily be achieved. (4) No interference with the beneficial actions of estrogens. (5) No toxic or carcinogenic effects.

THE ANTIESTROGEN TAMOXIFEN

Tamoxifen is very similar to clomiphene (in structure and actions), both being nonsteroidal compounds structurally related to diethylstilbestrol. Tamoxifen, in binding to the estrogen receptor, competitively inhibits estrogen binding. *In vitro*, the estrogen binding affinity for its receptor is 100–1000 times greater than that of tamoxifen. Thus, tamoxifen must be present in a concentration 100–1000 times greater than that of estrogen to maintain inhibition of breast cancer cells. *In vitro* studies demonstrate that this action is not cytocidal, but, rather, cytostatic (and thus its use must be long-term). The tamoxifen-estrogen receptor complex binds to DNA, but whether an agonistic, estrogenic message or an antagonistic, antiestrogenic message predominates is determined by what promoter elements are present in specific cell types.

Serum protein changes reflect the estrogenic (agonistic) action of tamoxifen. This includes decreases in antithrombin III, cholesterol, and LDL cholesterol, whereas HDL cholesterol and sex hormone-binding globulin (SHBG) levels increase (as do other binding globulins). The estrogenic activity of tamoxifen, 20 mg daily, is nearly as potent as 2 mg estradiol in lowering FSH levels in postmenopausal women, 26% versus 34% with estradiol.[39] The estrogenic actions of tamoxifen include the stimulation of progesterone receptor synthesis, an estrogen-like maintenance of bone, and estrogenic effects on the vaginal mucosa and the endometrium. Tamoxifen increases the frequency of hepatic carcinoma in rats at very large doses. This is consistent with its estrogenic, agonistic action, but this effect is unlikely to be a clinical problem (and it has not been observed) at doses currently used.[40] Tamoxifen causes a decrease in antithrombin III, and there has been a small increase in the incidence of thromboembolism observed in tamoxifen-treated patients compared with controls.[41,42] However, in the world overview of randomized trials, no significant cardiac or vascular increase in mortality was noted in tamoxifen-treated women.[40]

There now have been many reports of endometrial hyperplasia, endometrial polyps, and endometrial cancer in women receiving tamoxifen treatment.[43,44] In addition, tamoxifen has been associated with major flareups in endometriosis. Tamoxifen, therefore, has a variety of side effects that indicate both estrogenic activity and antiestrogenic activity. How can tamoxifen be both an estrogen agonist and an estrogen antagonist?

TAMOXIFEN MECHANISM OF ACTION

TAF-1 and TAF-2 areas can both activate transcription, but TAF-2 activates transcription only when it is bound by estrogen. The individual transactivating abilities of TAF-1 and TAF-2 depend on the promoter and cell context. Tamoxifen's agonistic ability is due to activation of TAF-1; its antagonistic activity is due to competitive inhibition of the estrogen-dependent activation of TAF-2.

An estrogen-associated protein binds to the right-hand side of TAF-2. Estrogen binding induces binding of this protein, which then activates transcription. This protein recognizes only an activated conformation of the estrogen receptor, the result of estrogen binding. Tamoxifen binding to the TAF-2 area does not activate this domain because, in at least one explanation, the conformational change does not allow binding of the estrogen-associated protein, the activating factor.[26,45]

The activity of TAF-2 is negligible in the presence of tamoxifen. In cells in which TAF-1 and TAF-2 function independently of each other, tamoxifen would be chiefly an antagonist in cells where TAF-2 predominates and an agonist where TAF-1 predominates, and in some cells, mixed activity is possible.[46]

Even though tamoxifen can block estrogen-stimulated transcription of many genes, its degree of antagonistic activity varies among different animals, different cell types, and different promoters within single cells. These differences are due to differences in the relative activities of the TAFs. Thus, the extent to which an antiestrogen inhibits an estrogen-mediated response depends on the degree to which that response is mediated by TAF-2 activity as opposed to TAF-1 activity, or mixed activity.[47] In some cell lines TAF-1 is dominant; in others, both are necessary. No cells in which TAF-2 is dominant have yet been identified.

In most cell types, TAF-1 is too weak to activate transcription by itself, but there are now well-known exceptions: endometrium, bone, and liver. In these tissues, the promoter context is right. Tamoxifen is a significant activator of estrogen receptor-mediated induction of promoters that are regulated by the TAF-1 site. Antiestrogens have no effects on TAF-1 dependent transcription in breast cells.[48]

This explanation may not be the same for other mixed agonists and antagonists. Raloxifene may activate an estrogen-responsive gene through a response element separate from the estrogen response element, an action that requires specific activating peptides.[49] Estrogen metabolites also can interact with response elements other than the classical estrogen response element. The bottom line is that there are multiple pathways to gene activation. The estrogen receptor, depending on the ligand, can regulate more than one response element. Thus, estrogen and antiestrogen actions in various tissues can reflect the presence of different response elements.

THE PURE ANTIESTROGENS

Binding with the pure antiestrogens prevents DNA binding. Because the site responsible for dimerization overlaps with the hormone-binding site, it is believed that pure antiestrogens sterically interfere with dimerization and thus inhibit DNA binding. In addition, these compounds increase the cellular turnover of estrogen receptor, and this action contributes to its antiestrogen effectiveness. Estrogen and progesterone receptors exit the nucleus but are rapidly transported back. When this shuttling is impaired, receptors are more rapidly degraded in the cytoplasm. Agents that inhibit dimerization inhibit nuclear translocation and thus increase cytoplasmic degradation. The half-life of the estrogen receptor when occupied with estradiol is about 5 hours; when occupied with a pure antiestrogen, it is less than 1 hour. This mechanism may be due to interference with nuclear localization exerted by the hinge region. Thus, newly synthesized receptors cannot be efficiently transported into the nucleus and those in the nucleus will leak back into the cytoplasm.

Another possible mechanism for pure antiestrogens involves a binding protein for the insulin-like growth factors. In a breast cancer cell line, ICI 182,780 inhibited growth and increased transcription of the IGFBP-3 gene. Estradiol did the opposite. In the uterus, tamoxifen and estrogen suppress IGFBP-3 production, whereas the ICI antagonist markedly increases IGFBP and causes uterine involution.[50]

Because these agents function in a different manner from tamoxifen, it is not surprising that tamoxifen-resistant tumors respond to these agents.[51]

SELECTIVE ESTROGEN AGONISTS/ANTAGONISTS (SELECTIVE ESTROGEN RECEPTOR MODULATORS)

Agents such as raloxifene and droloxifene have antiestrogenic activity in the uterus as well as in the breast, and at the same time exert agonistic effects in certain target tissues.[52–54] Raloxifene inhibits bone resorption and improves lipids (although there is no effect on HDL cholesterol). By virtue of variations in conformational changes in the drug-receptor complex and the cellular context of specific tissues, drugs such as these can be developed to produce beneficial effects in certain target systems (such as bone) and to avoid unwanted actions (such as endometrial stimulation).

REFERENCES

1. Beato, M. & A. Sánchez-Pacheco. 1996. Interaction of steroid hormone receptors with the transcription initiation complex. Endocr. Rev. **17:** 587–609.
2. King, W.J. & & G.L. Greene. 1984. Monoclonal antibodies localize oestrogen receptor in the nuclei of target cells. Nature **307:** 745.
3. Welshons, W.V., M.E. Lieberman & J. Gorski. 1984. Nuclear localization of unoccupied oestrogen receptors. Nature **307:** 747.
4. Press, M.F. & G.L. Greene. 1988. Localization of progesterone receptor with monoclonal antibodies to the human progestin receptor. Endocrinology **122:** 1165.
5. Webb, P., G.N. Lopez, G.L. Greene *et al.* 1992. The limits of the cellular capacity to mediate an estrogen response. Mol. Endocrinol. **6:**.157.
6. Evans, R.M. 1988. The steroid and thyroid hormone receptor family. Science **240:** 889–895.
7. Laudet, V., C. Hanni, J. Coll *et al.* 1992. Evolution of the nuclear receptor gene superfamily. EMBO J. **11:**1003–1013.
8. Kuiper, G., E. Enmark, M. Pelto-Huikko *et al.* 1996. Cloning of a novel estrogen receptor expressed in rat prostate and ovary. Proc. Natl. Acad. Sci. USA **93:** 5925–5930.
9. Mosselman, S., J. Polman & R. Dijkema. 1996. ER-β: identification and characterizaiton of a novel human estrogen receptor. FEBS Lett. **392:** 49–53.

10. Jensen, E.V. & H.I. Jacobson. 1962. Basic guides to the mechanism of estrogen action. Rec. Prog. Horm. Res. **18:** 387–314.
11. Green, S., P. Walter, G. Greene *et al.* 1986. Cloning of the human oestrogen receptor cDNA. J. Steroid Biochem. **24:** 77–83.
12. Greene, G.L., P. Gilna, M. Walterfield *et al.* 1986. Sequence and expression of human estrogen receptor cDNA. Science **231:** 1150–1154.
13. Parker, M.G. 1993. Structure and function of the oestrogen receptor. J. Neuroendocrinol. **5:** 223–228.
14. Enmark, E., M. Pelto-Huikko, K. Grandien *et al.* 1997. Human estrogen receptor β-gene structure, chromosomal localization, and expression pattern. J. Clin. Endocrinol. Metab. **82:** 4258–4265.
15. Kuiper, G.G.J.M., B. Carlsson, K. Grandien *et al.* 1997. Comparison of the ligand binding specificity and transcript tissue distribution of estrogen receptors α and β. Endocrinology **138:** 863–870.
16. Wurtz, J.M., W. Bourguet, J.P. Renaud *et al.* 1996. A canonical structure for the ligand-binding domain of nuclear receptors. Nat. Struct. Biol. **3:** 87–94.
17. Teutsch, G., F. Nique, G. Lemoine *et al.* 1995. General structure-activity correlations of antihormones. Ann. N.Y. Acad. Sci. **761:** 5–28.
18. Montano, M.M., V. Müller, A. Trobaugh & B.S. Katzenellenbogen. 1995. The carboxy-terminal F domain of the human estrogen receptor: role in the transcriptional activity of the receptor and the effectiveness of antiestrogens as estrogen antagonists. Molec. Endocrinol. **9:** 814–825.
19. Parker, M.G. 1995. Structure and function of estrogen receptors. Vitamins Hormones **51:** 267–287.
20. Brzozowski, A.M., A.C.W. Pike, Z. Dauter *et al.* 1997. Molecular basis of agonism and antagonism in the oestrogen receptor. Nature **389:** 753–758.
21. Tanenbaum, D.M., Y. Wang, S.P. Williams & P.B. Sigler. 1998. Crystallographic comparison of the estrogen and progesterone receptor's ligand binding domains. Proc. Natl. Acad. Sci. USA **95:** 5998–6003.
22. Melamed, M., E. Castraño, A.C. Notides & S. Sasson. 1997. Molecular and kinetic basis for the mixed agonist/antagonist activity of estriol. Molec. Endocrinol. **11:** 1868–1878.
23. Wiese, T.E. & S.C. Brooks. 1994. Molecular modelling of steroidal estrogens: novel conformations and thei role in biological activity. J. Steroid Biochem. Molec. Biol. **50:** 61–73.
24. Freedman, L.P. 1992. Anatomy of the steroid receptor zinc finger region. Endocr. Rev. **13:** 129–145.
25. O'Malley, B.W. & M.-J. Tsai. 1992. Molecular pathways of steroid receptor action. Biol. Reprod. **46:** 163–167.
26. Halachmi, S., E. Marden, G. Martin *et al.* 1994. Estrogen receptor-associated proteins: possible mediators of hormone-induced transcription. Science **264:** 1455–1458.
27. Cavaillès, V., S. Dauvois, F. L'Horset *et al.* 1995. Nuclear factor RIP140 modulates transcriptional activtion by the estrogen receptor. EMBO J. **14:** 3741–3751.
28. Horwitz, K.B., T.A. Jackson, D.L. Bain *et al.* 1996. Nuclear receptor coactivators and corepressors. Mol. Endocrinol. **10:** 1167–1177.
29. Ciocca, D.R. & L.M. Vargas Roid. 1995. Estrogen receptors in human nontarget tissues: biological and clinical implications. Endocr. Rev. **16:** 35–62.
30. Hyder, S.M., G.L. Shipley & G.M. Stancel. 1995. Estrogen action in target cells: selective requirements for activation of different hormone response elements. Molec. Cell Endocrinol. **112:** 35–43.
31. O'Malley, B.W., W.T. Schrader, S. Mani *et al.* 1995. An alternative ligand-independent pathway for activation of steroid receptors. Rec. Prog. Horm. Res. **50:** 333–347.
32. Lindzey, J. & K.S. Korach. 1997. Developmental and physiological effects of estrogen receptor gene disruption in mice. Trends Endocrinol. Metab. **8:** 137–145.
33. Brandenberger, A.W., M.K. Tee, J.Y. Lee *et al.* 1997. Tissue distribution of estrogen receptos alpha (ER-α) and beta (ER-β) mRNA in the midgestational human fetus. J. Clin. Endocrinol. Metab. **82:** 3509–3512.

34. SHUGHRUE, P.J., M.V. LANE & I. MERCHENTHALER. 1997. Comparative distribution of estrogen receptor-alpha and -beta mRNA in the rat central nervous system. J. Comp. Neurol. **388:** 507–525.
35. PAECH, K., P. WEBB, G.G. KUIPER *et al.* 1997. Differential ligand activation of estrogen receptors ERalpha and ERbeta at AP1 sites. Science **277:** 1508–1510.
36. REVELLI, A., M. MASSOBRIO & J. TESARIK. 1998. Nongenomic actions of steroid hormones in reproductive tissues. Endocr. Rev. **19:** 3–17.
37. MORLEY, P., J.F. WHITFIELD, B.C. VANDERHYDEN *et al.* 1992. A new, nongenomic estrogen action: the rapid release of intracellular calcium. Endocrinology **131:** 1305–1312.
38. CHESTER, A.H., C. JIANG, J.A. BORLAND *et al.* 1995. Oestrogen relaxes human epicardial coronary arteries through non-endothelial-dependent mechanisms. Coron. Artery Dis. **6:** 417–422.
39. HELGASON, S., N. WILKING, K. CARLSTROM *et al.* 1982. A comparative study of the estrogenic effects of tamoxifen and 17β–estradiol in postmenopausal women. J. Clin. Endocrinol. Metab. **54:** 404–408.
40. EARLY BREAST CANCER TRIALISTS' COLLABORATIVE GROUP. 1998. Tamoxifen for early breast cancer: an overview of the randomised trials. Lancet **351:** 1451–1467.
41. SAPHNER, T., D.C. TORMEY & R. GRAY. 1991. Venous and arterial thrombosis in patients who received adjuvant therapy for breast cancer. J. Clin. Oncol. **9:** 286.
42. FISHER, B., J. DIGNAM, J. BRYANT *et al.* 1996. Five versus more than five years of tamoxifen therapy for breast cancer patients with negative lymph nodes and estrogen receptor-positive tumors. J. Natl. Cancer Inst. **88:** 1529–1542.
43. KEDAR, R.P., T.H. BOURNE, T.J. POWLES *et al.* 1994. Effects of tamoxifen on uterus and ovaries of postmenopausal women in a randomized breast cancer prevention trial. Lancet **343:** 1318–1321.
44. FISHER, B., J.P. COSTANTINO, C.K. REDMOND *et al.* 1994. Endometrial cancer in tamoxifen-treated breast cancer patients: findings from the National Surgical Adjuvant Breast and Bowel Project (NSABP) B-14. J. Natl. Cancer Inst. **86:** 527–537.
45. LANDEL, C.C., P.J. KUSHNER & G.L. GREENE. 1994. The interaction of human estrogen receptor with DNA is modulated by receptor-associated proteins. Molec. Endocrinol. **8:** 1407–1419.
46. BERRY, M., D. METZGER & P. CHAMBON. 1990. Role of the two activating domains of the oestrogen receptor in the cell type and promoter context dependent agonistic activity of the antioestrogen 4-hydroxytamoxifen. EMBO J. **9:** 2811–2818.
47. TZUKERMAN, M.T., A. ESTY, D. SANTISOMERE *et al.* 1994. Human estrogen receptor transactivational capacity is determined by both cellular and promoter context and mediated by two functionally distinct intramolecular regions. Molec. Endocrinol. **8:** 21–30.
48. WEBB, P., G.N. LOPEX, R.M. UHT & P.J. KUSHNER. 1995. Tamoxifen activation of the estrogen receptor/AP-1 pathway: potential origin for the cell-specific estrogen-like effects of antiestrogens. Molec. Endocrinol. **9:** 443–456.
49. YANG, N.N., M. VENUGOPALAN, S. HARDIKAR & A. GLASEBROOK. 1996. Identification of an estrogen response element activated by metabolites of 17ß-estradiol and raloxifene. Science **273:** 1222–1224.
50. HUYNH, H., X. YANG & M. POLLAK. 1996. Estradiol and antiestrogens regulate a growth inhibitory insulin-like growth factor binding protein 3 autocrine loop in human breast cancer cells. J. Biol. Chem. **271:** 1016–1021.
51. HOWELLM, A., D. DEFRIEND, J. ROBERTSON *et al.* 1995. Response to a specific antioestrogen (ICI 182780) in tamoxifen-resistant breast cancer. Lancet **345:** 29–30.
52. HASMAN, M., B. RATTEL & R. LÖSER. 1994. Preclinical data for droloxifene. Cancer Lett. **84:** 101–116.
53. JORDAN, V.C. 1995. Alternate antiestrogens and approaches to the prevention of breast cancer. J. Cell. Biochem. (Suppl) **22:** 51–57.
54. GEISLER, J., H. HAARSTAD, S. GUNDERSEN *et al.* 1995. Influence of treatment with the anti-oestrogen 3-hydroxytamoxifen (droloxifene) on plasma sex hormone levels in postmenopausal patients with breast cancer. J. Endocrinol. **146:** 359–363.

Molecular Defects Causing Ovarian Dysfunction

SOPHIA N. KALANTARIDOU [a,b] AND GEORGE P. CHROUSOS[c,d]

[a]*Section on Women's Health Research, Developmental Endocrinology Branch, and* [b]*Section on Pediatric Endocrinology, Pediatric and Reproductive Endocrinology Branch, National Institute of Child Health and Human Development, National Institutes of Health, Bethesda, Maryland 20892, USA*

ABSTRACT: The functions of the hypothalamic-pituitary-ovarian and -adrenal axes are intertwined, and molecular defects in either axis may cause ovarian dysfunction. Advances in molecular genetics have allowed new insights into the pathophysiology of ovarian disorders. Specific gene mutations causing delayed puberty and/or ovarian failure, and heterosexual or isosexual precocious puberty have recently been described. The molecular insights gained into ovarian dysfunction have already led to rational therapies for some of these conditions.

INTRODUCTION

The functions of the hypothalamic-pituitary-ovarian and -adrenal axes are intricately intertwined, and molecular defects in either axis may cause ovarian dysfunction.[1] Advances in molecular genetics have provided new insights into the pathophysiology of ovarian and/or adrenal dysfunction. We summarize briefly the molecular defects that influence ovarian function and cause hypogonadotropic or hypergonadotropic hypogonadism or precocious puberty in TABLES 1, 2, and 3, respectively.

Autosomally inherited gonadotropin-releasing hormone (GnRH) receptor gene mutations[2] and X-linked *KAL* gene (Kallmann syndrome)[3,4] and *DAX-1* gene (adrenal hypoplasia congenita) mutations[5] cause hypogonadotropic hypogonadism expressed as failure of affected girls to enter puberty (TABLE 1).

Mutations in the follicle-stimulating hormone (FSH) receptor gene result in hypergonadotropic primary or early secondary amenorrhea and anovulation, with variable development of secondary sex characteristics.[6,7] Mutations of the luteinizing hormone (LH) receptor gene also cause primary or secondary amenorrhea and anovulation, yet they allow development of normal secondary sex characteristics.[8–10] Mutations of the β-subunit of FSH cause primary amenorrhea with poorly developed secondary sex characteristics and infertility.[11,12] whereas mutations of the β-subunit of LH have only been reported in a male with delayed puberty[13] (TABLE 2).

[c]Recipient of scholarship by the "Alexandros S. Onassis" Public Benefit Foundation/Group T-034.

[d]Corresponding author. National Institutes of Health, Building 10, Room 9D42, 10 Center Drive, MSC 1583, Bethesda, MD 20892–1583, USA. Phone: + 301-496-5800; fax: + 301-402-0884.

ChrousoG@exchange.nih.gov

TABLE 1. Molecular defects causing hypogonadotropic hypogonadism

Defect	Characteristics
Gonadotropin-releasing hormone receptor gene mutations[2]	Autosomally inherited hypogonadotropic hypogonadism. One heterozygous female patient received pulsatile GnRH for 46 days but failed to ovulate, whereas her sister (also heterozygous) ovulated with exogenous gonadotropins[2]
KAL gene mutations (Xp22.3)[3,4]	X-linked hypogonadotropic hypogonadism and anosmia or hyposmia[3,4]
DAX-1 gene mutations[5]	X-linked adrenal hypoplasia congenita and idiopathic hypogonadotropic hypogonadism (only families with 46,XY affected members have been reported thus far)[5]

Two genes (*POF1* and *POF2*), important for ovarian function, are localized to Xq21.3-q27 and Xq13.3-q21.1, respectively.[14,15] Also, at least eight different genes in Xq21 are involved in ovarian function.[16] Furthermore, defects in the human diaphanous gene may cause ovarian failure.[17] Several studies have found an increase in the familial incidence of ovarian failure in females with fragile X premutations, suggesting that the *FMR1* gene (Xq27.3) may play a role in ovarian function[18,19] (TABLE 2).

In autoimmune polyglandular failure type 1, also known as autoimmune polyendocrinopathy-candidiasis-ectodermal dystrophy (APECED), ovarian failure develops in up to 60% of cases.[20,21] APECED is an autosomal recessive disease caused by a single gene defect on chromosome 21q22.3.[20,21] In APECED, associated disorders include adrenal failure, hypothyroidism, hypoparathyroidism, and mucocutaneous candidiasis.[20,21]

Steroidogenic enzyme deficiencies, such as those of cholesterol desmolase, 17α-hydroxylase, and 17-20 desmolase, impair estrogen synthesis and cause amenorrhea and failure to develop secondary sex characteristics despite the presence of developing follicles.[22,23] Galactosemia, due to a deficiency in the enzyme galactose-1-phosphate uridyl transferase (GALT), is a rare autosomal recessive disorder, causing mental retardation, cataracts, hepatocellular and renal damage, and ovarian failure; the latter is believed to result from galactose toxicity[24] (TABLE 2).

Congenital adrenal hyperplasia due to 21-hydroxylase, 11-hydroxylase, and 3β-hydroxysteroid dehydrogenase deficiency is associated with heterosexual precocious puberty,[25] whereas the McCune-Albright syndrome and the familial aromatase excess syndromes result in isosexual precocious puberty in girls.[26] The McCune-Albright syndrome results from activating somatic mutations of the α-subunit of the Gs protein and increased cAMP concentrations.[26] The familial aromatase excess syndrome is a genetically heterogeneous disorder that can be inherited in different ways.[27] In both of these conditions, aromatase inhibitors are employed for treatment (TABLE 3).

Our laboratory recently reported on two mechanisms causing ovarian dysfunction. The first is ovarian resistance caused by inactivating mutations of the LH-receptor gene,[8,9] and the second is excessive aromatization of androgens in the context of the aromatase excess syndrome.[27] The latter was associated with isosexual

TABLE 2. Molecular defects causing hypergonadotropic hypogonadism

Defect	Characteristics
Follicle stimulating hormone (FSH) receptor gene mutations[6,7]	Hypergonadotropic primary or early secondary amenorrhea and anovulation with variable development of secondary sex characteristics [6,7]
Luteinizing hormone (LH) receptor gene mutations[8–10]	Primary or secondary amenorrhea and anovulation, yet normal development secondary sex characteristics[8–10]
Mutations in the β-subunit of FSH[11,12]	Primary amenorrhea with poorly developed secondary sex characteristics and infertility.[11,12] One patient conceived after treatment with FSH.[11]
Mutations in the long arm of the X chromosome [*POF1* gene (Xq21.3-q27) [14]; *POF2* gene (Xq13.3-q21.1)[15]; *DIA* gene (Xq22)[17]; Xq21 region[16]; *FRAXA* gene (Xq27.3)[18,19]	Premature ovarian failure (cessation of ovarian function before the age of 40)
Autoimmune polyglandular failure type 1 due to mutations in 21q22.3 (APECED)[20,21]	Autosomal recessive disease characterized by premature ovarian failure (in 60% of cases), Addison's disease, hypothyroidism, hypoparathyroidism, mucocutaneous candidiasis, and others[20,21]
Enzyme deficiencies (cholesterol desmolase, 17α-hydroxylase, and 17-20 desmolase)[22,23]	Impaired estrogen synthesis; amenorrhea and failure to develop secondary sex characteristics despite the presence of developing follicles[22,23]
Galactosemia (due to deficiency in the enzyme galactose-1-phosphate uridyl transferase [GALT]) (24)	Rare autosomal recessive disorder causing mental retardation, cataracts, hepatocellular and renal damage, and ovarian failure (24)

precocious puberty and autosomal dominant transmission of aberrant P450 aromatase gene transcription.[27] We focus mainly on these two molecular defects in the current presentation.

OVARIAN RESISTANCE TO LUTEINIZING HORMONE

Normally, during the late follicular phase, LH stimulates androstenedione production by the ovarian theca cells, which is then aromatized to estradiol by the granulosa cells. During its midcycle surge, LH promotes oocyte and follicular maturation and leads to ovulation and induction of corpus luteum formation by granulosa and theca cells. Subsequently, under the influence of LH the corpus luteum secretes progesterone. The human LH receptor belongs to the G-protein–coupled seven-transmembrane domain receptors superfamily.[28] Latronico *et al.*[8] described inactivating mutations of the LH receptor gene causing ovarian failure. They reported two novel homozygous inactivating nonsense and missense mutations of the LH receptor gene from two unrelated kindreds, causing amenorrhea in a genetic 46,XX female, and defects in the differentiation of the external genitalia in genetic males (male

TABLE 3. Molecular defects causing precocious puberty

Defect	Characteristics
Congenital adrenal hyperplasia (due to 21-hydroxylase, 11-hydroxylase, and 3β-hydroxysteroid dehydrogenase deficiencies[25]	Heterosexual precocious puberty in girls
McCune-Albright syndrome (due to activating somatic mutations of the α-subunit of the Gs protein and increased cAMP concentrations)[26]	Isosexual precocious puberty in girls
Familial aromatase excess syndrome (genetically heterogeneous disorder that can be inherited in an autosomal dominant fashion. The genetic defect is possibly located in the 5′-region of the P450arom gene)[27]	Isosexual precocious puberty in girls

pseudohermaphroditism).[8] The genetically female patient had a homozygous nonsense mutation ($Arg^{554}\rightarrow$Stop codon) in the third cytosolic loop of the LH receptor gene in exon 11 and was probably completely devoid of functional LH receptor.[8] Another inactivating mutation of the LH receptor gene, causing substitution of an alanine residue by a proline at position 593, was also reported.[10]

Women with a normal 46,XX karyotype and mutations of the LH receptor gene have primary or secondary amenorrhea, but normal secondary sex characteristics.[8–10] Levels of LH are elevated and levels of FSH are normal to moderately elevated, with a high LH:FSH ratio. Estradiol levels are normal in the early follicular phase. On ultrasound, the uterus is slightly hypoplastic and the ovaries may be enlarged and contain several cysts.[9] Ovarian biopsy revealed primordial, preantral, and antral follicles in these patients, whereas no preovulatory follicles, corpora lutea, or corpora albicans were seen.[8–10] The ovarian cysts corresponded to antral follicles, with proliferative activity of theca and granulosa cells.[9] Of note, theca cell changes, such as increased size, abundant cytoplasm, and a typical steroid secretory pattern, are seen on ovarian biopsy despite the absence of any LH activity.[9] Although the two-cell/two-gonadotropin hypothesis suggests that both LH and FSH are required for normal steroidogenesis,[29] the presence of normal early follicular estradiol levels in these patients reveals that FSH alone can stimulate sufficient estrogen production for normal pubertal feminization. It therefore appears that in girls, LH does not have a major role in pubertal development.

AROMATASE EXCESS SYNDROME

Aromatase, the last enzyme in estrogen biosynthesis, catalyzes the conversion of androgens to estrogens. It is composed of aromatase cytochrome P450 (P450arom) and flavoprotein NADPH-P450 reductase.[30] Stratakis *et al.*[27] recently reported a kindred with the aromatase excess syndrome associated with clinical manifestations in females. The disorder was inherited in an autosomal dominant fashion, in which affected females had isosexual precocious puberty and/or macromastia and affected males had heterosexual precocious puberty and/or gynecomastia. Symptoms were manifested around the time of adrenarche with greatly advanced bone age and accelerated growth. At 7.5 years of age, one affected girl had elevated plasma estrogen levels and the height and weight of 9.5 and 12-year-old girls, respectively. Breast development and pubic hair were at Tanner stage III with absence of clitoromegaly. Her brother presented at 9 years of age with gynecomastia. The father had undergone bilateral mastectomy for severe gynecomastia at the age of 15, and the paternal grandmother reportedly had macromastia.

The HCG and ACTH stimulation tests and a 3-year followup evaluation of family members suggested that most of the aromatization took place in extragonadal tissues, which included the breast and probably the adrenal glands.[27] The source appeared to be nongonadal conversion of adrenal androgens to estrogens. Markedly increased aromatase activity was found in fibroblasts and Epstein-Barr virus-transformed lymphocytes from the patients. A new 5′-splice variant was present in the P450arom messenger ribonucleic acid, revealing another first exon of this gene, which appeared to be aberrantly expressed in this family. Because of the predicted short final height, both young patients were treated with an aromatase inhibitor and a GnRH analog, which successfully delayed skeletal and pubertal development.

CONCLUSIONS

Advances in molecular genetics have provided new insights into the pathophysiology of ovarian dysfunction. Specific gene mutations, causing delayed puberty and/or ovarian failure and heterosexual or isosexual precocious puberty have recently been described. The molecular insights gained into ovarian dysfunction have already led to rational therapies for some of these conditions.

REFERENCES

1. Chrousos, G.P., D.J. Torpy & P.W. Gold. 1998. Interactions between the hypothalamic-pituitary-adrenal axis and the female reproductive system: clinical implications. Ann. Int. Med. **129:** 229–240.
2. Layman, L.C., D.P. Cohen, M. Jin *et al.* 1998. Mutations in gonadotropin-releasing hormone receptor gene cause hypogonadotropic hypogonadism. Nature Genet. **18:** 14–15.
3. Franco, B., S. Guioli, A. Pragliola *et al.* 1991. A gene deleted in Kallmann's syndrome shares homology with neural cell adhesion and axonal path-finding molecules. Nature **353:** 529–536.
4. Legouis, R., J.P. Hardelin, J. Levilliers *et al.* 1991. The candidate gene for the X-linked Kallmann syndrome encodes a protein related to adhesion molecules. Cell **67:** 423–435.
5. Zanaria, E., F. Muscatelli, B. Bardoni *et al.* 1994. An unusual member of the nuclear hormone receptor superfamily responsible for X-linked adrenal hypoplasia congenita. Nature **372:** 635–641.
6. Aittomäki, K., J.L.D. Lucena, P. Pakarinen *et al.* 1995. Mutation in the follicle-stimulating hormone receptor gene causes hereditary hypergonadotrophic ovarian failure. Cell **82:** 959–968.
7. Aittomäki, K., R. Herva, U.H. Stenman *et al.* Clinical features of primary ovarian failure caused by a point mutation in the follicle-stimulating hormone receptor gene. J. Clin. Endocrinol. Metab. **81:** 3722–3726.
8. Latronico, A.C., J.N. Anasti, I.J.P. Arnhold *et al.* 1996. Brief report: testicular and ovarian resistance to luteinizing hormone caused by inactivating mutations of the luteinizing hormone-receptor gene. N. Engl. J. Med. **334:** 507–512.
9. Arnold, I.J.P., A.C. Latronico, M.C. Batista *et al.* 1997. Ovarian resistance to luteinizing hormone: a novel cause of amenorrhea and infertility. Fertil. Steril. **67:** 394–397.

10. TOLEDO, S.P.A., H.G. BRUNNER, R. KRAAIJ *et al.* 1996. An inactivating mutation of the luteinizing hormone receptor causes amenorrhea in a 46,XX female. J. Clin. Endocrinol. Metab. **81:** 3850–3854.
11. MATTHEWS, C.H., S. BORGATO, P. BECK-PECCOZ *et al.* 1993. Primary amenorrhoea and infertility due to a mutation in the beta-subunit of follicle-stimulating hormone. Nature Genet. **5:** 83–86.
12. LAYMAN, L.C., E.J. LEE, D.B. PEAK *et al.* 1997. Delayed puberty and hypogonadism caused by mutations in the follicle-stimulating hormone beta-subunit gene. N. Engl. J. Med. **337:** 607–611.
13. WEISS, J., L. AXELROD, R.W. WHITCOMB *et al.* 1992. Hypogonadism caused by a single amino acid substitution in the β subunit of luteinizing hormone. N. Engl. J. Med. **326:** 179–183.
14. KRAUSS, C.M., R.N. TURKSOY, L. ATKINS *et al.* 1987. Familial premature ovarian failure due to an interstitial deletion of the long arm of the X chromosome. N. Engl. J. Med. **317:** 125–131.
15. POWELL, C.M., R.T. TAGGART, T.C. DRUMHELLER *et al.* 1994. Molecular and cytogenetic studies of an X;autosome translocation in a patient with premature ovarian failure and review of the literature. Am. J. Med. Genet. **52:** 19–26.
16. SALA, C., G. ARRIGO, G. TORRI *et al.* 1997. Eleven X chromosome breakpoints associated with premature ovarian failure (POF) map to 15-Mb YAC conting spanning Xq21. Genomics **40:** 123–131.
17. BIONE, S., C. SALA, C. MANZINI *et al.* 1998. A human homologue of the Drosophila diaphanous gene is disrupted in a patient with premature ovarian failure: evidence for conserved function in oogenesis and implications for human sterility. Am. J. Med. Genet. **62:** 533–541.
18. SCHWARTZ, C.E., J. DEAN, P.N. HOWARD-PEEBLES *et al.* 1994. Obstetrical and gynecological complications in fragile X carriers: a multicenter study. Am. J. Med. Genet. **51:** 400–402.
19. CONWAY, G.S., N.N. PAYNE, J. WEBB *et al.* 1998. Fragile X premutation screening in women with premature ovarian failure. Hum. Reprod. **13:** 1184–1187.
20. THE FINNISH-GERMAN APECED CONSORTIUM. 1997. An autoimmune disease, APECED, caused by mutations in a novel gene featuring two PHD-type zinc-finger domains. Nature Genet. **17:** 399–403.
21. NAGAMINE, K., P. PETERSON, H.S. SCOTT *et al.* 1997. Positional cloning of the APECED gene. Nature Genet. **17:** 393–398.
22. KATER, C.E. & E.G. BIGLIERI. 1994. Disorders of steroid 17 alpha-hydroxylaxion deficiency. Endocrinol. Metab. Clin. North Am. **23:** 341–357.
23. ZACHMANN, M. 1995. Defects in steroidogenic enzymes: discrepancies between clinical steroid research and molecular biology results. J. Steroid Biochem. Mol. Biol. **53:** 159–164.
24. WAGGONER, D.D., N.R.M. BUIST & G.N. DONNELL. 1990. Long-term prognosis in galactosemia: results of a survey of 350 cases. J. Inherit. Metab. Dis. **13:** 802–818.
25. PANG, S. 1997. Congenital adrenal hyperplasia. Baillieres Clin. Obstet. Gynaecol. **11:** 281–306.
26. WEINSTEIN, L.S., A. SHENKER, P.V. GEJMAN *et al.* 1991. Activating mutations of the stimulatory G protein in the McCune-Albright syndrome. N. Engl. J. Med. **325:** 1688–1695.
27. STRATAKIS, C.A., A. VOTTERO, A. BRODIE *et al.* 1998. The aromatase excess syndrome is associated with feminization of both sexes and autosomal dominant transmission of aberrant P450 aromatase gene transcription. J. Clin. Endocrinol. Metab. **83:** 1348–1357.
28. MINEGISHI, T., K. NAKAMURA, Y. TAKAKURA *et al.* 1990. Cloning and sequencing of human LH/hCG receptor cDNA. Biochem. Biophys. Res. Commun. **172:** 1049–1054.
29. MCNATTY, K.P., A. MAKRIS, C. DEGRAZIA *et al.* 1979. The production of progesterone, androgens, and estrogens by granulosa cells, theca tissue, and stromal tissue from human ovaries in vitro. J. Clin. Endrocrinol. Metab. **49:** 687–699.
30. SIMPSON, E.R., M.S. MAHENDROO, G.D. MEANS *et al.* 1994. Aromatase cytochrome P450, the enzyme responsible for estrogen biosynthesis. Endocr. Rev. **15:** 342–355.

Follicular Atresia and Luteolysis

Evidence of a Role for N-Cadherin

ANTONIS MAKRIGIANNAKIS,[a] GEORGE COUKOS,[b] OREST BLASCHUK,[c] AND CHRISTOS COUTIFARIS[a,d]

[a]*Divisions of Human Reproduction and* [b]*Gynecologic Oncology, Department of Obstetrics and Gynecology, University of Pennsylvania Medical Center, Philadelphia, Pennsylvania 19104, USA*

[c]*Department of Surgery, McGill University, Montreal, Quebec H3A 1A1, Canada*

ABSTRACT: **Studies suggest that cell–cell interactions may regulate apoptosis; and, in particular, the calcium-dependent cell adhesion molecule N-cadherin has been shown to be capable of modulating this process. Here, we review the evidence that N-cadherin is expressed by human granulosa cells (GCs) and mediates cell–cell adhesion between GCs. There is strong correlation between N-cadherin expression by granulosa or luteal cells and follicular survival in isolated follicles and archival tissue sections. There exists a strong expression of the molecule by GCs in follicles of the resting pool, of growing antral follicles, and of healthy corpora lutea. In contrast, the molecule is lost in degenerating GCs of atretic follicles and in luteal cells of the late luteal phase. Further, the experimental evidence demonstrates that cell–cell adhesion is critical to the survival of GCs and that N-cadherin–mediated cell–cell adhesion is a critical mediator of survival signals and inhibits apoptosis in these cells. Possible mechanisms by which apoptosis may be triggerred in GCs include the downregulation of N-cadherin, which is mediated, at least in part, through the enzymatic cleavage of the extracellular domain of the molecule. Collectively, these observations suggest that downregulation of N-cadherin or the absence of a functional extracellular domain of the molecule prevent GC aggregation and is associated with GC apoptosis. We propose that N-cadherin–mediated GC signaling plays a central role in follicular and luteal cell survival.**

INTRODUCTION

Although several hundred thousands of primordial and primary follicles are present in the mammalian ovary before puberty, only very few will fully mature and ovulate. The others will be eliminated by atresia, a process that exhibits both the biochemical and morphological features of programmed cell death.[1–4] Moreover, in each reproductive cycle, a corpus luteum will form and eventually degenerate by luteolysis, which is also an apoptotic process.[5–8] The primary follicular constituents that undergo apoptosis are the granulosa cells (GCs).[9] Because follicular degenera-

[d]Address for correspondence: Christos Coutifaris, M.D., Ph.D., Division of Human Reproduction, Department of Obstetrics and Gynecology, University of Pennsylvania Medical Center, 3400 Spruce Street, 101 Dulles Building, Philadelphia, Pennsylvania 19104. Phone: 215-662-3378; fax: 215-349-5512.
e-mail: ccoutifaris@obgyn.upenn.edu

tion, or corpus luteum regression, is associated with loss of cell–cell adhesion sites,[4] it can be hypothesized that cell adhesion molecules (CAMs) are implicated in GC survival and death. In addition to cell–cell adhesion, recent studies suggest that an interaction with extracellular matrix proteins plays an important role in regulating cell survival.[10] The extracellular matrix proteins appear to mediate their action by binding to cellular adhesion molecules such as integrins.[10] In addition to their role as adhesion receptors, integrins also function as signaling receptors and have been shown to regulate reorganization of the cytoskeleton, intracellular ion transport, lipid metabolism, kinase activation, and gene expression. Importantly, recent evidence suggests that some yet-unidentified integrin-regulated pathways prevent cells from undergoing apoptosis.[11–13]

CELL–CELL CONTACT THROUGH CADHERINS

Cell-to-cell contact is mediated by a great diversity of cell adhesion molecules including some integrins, the immunoglobulin supergene family, selectins, and cadherins. The expression of these adhesion molecules is cell-specific, with cadherins involved in mediating calcium-dependent cell-to-cell adhesion in virtually all solid tissues of multicellular organisms.[14,15] The classical cadherins possess an extracellular domain that contains five tandemly arranged cadherin repeats (EC1 to EC5). The NH_2-terminal repeat contains the adhesive domain that is involved in cadherin-specific adhesion.[16] The first extracellular domain (EC1) contains the classical cadherin adhesion recognition (CAR) sequence, HAV (His-Ala-Val). Recently, Gour and Blaschuk have developed high-affinity cyclic peptides containing the CAR sequence (i.e., N-Ac-CHAVC-NH_2, N-Ac-CHGVC-NH_2), which are potent inhibitors of CAD-dependent processes (PCT patent WO 98/02452). The cytoplasmic domain of cadherins is highly conserved and functions to bind catenins to the cytoskeleton.[17,18] In addition to anchoring the cytoskeleton, there is an increasing body of evidence to suggest that cadherins are also involved in regulating signal transduction pathways.[17] This cadherin-mediated signal transduction pathway likely accounts for the ability of cell-to-cell contact to maintain cell viability.

EXPRESSION OF CADHERIN IN THE OVARY

The human ovary is an excellent model system to assess the role of cadherins in regulating apoptosis. First, apoptotic cell death is a major physiological event within the ovary. Of the 400,000 follicles a woman is endowed with at puberty, the majority will degenerate by a process known as atresia. The GCs, which make up the follicle, undergo modifications that resemble the pathologic features characteristic of programmed cell death or apoptosis, including cytoplasmic shrinkage and chromatin condensation.[7,9] Second, GCs in primordial, primary, and early secondary follicles (FIG. 1) as well as in healthy antral follicles are connected by N-cadherin–mediated adhesion.[7] Luteal cells are also strongly positive for N-cadherin in the early luteal and mid-luteal phase, whereas there is only weak N-cadherin staining during late

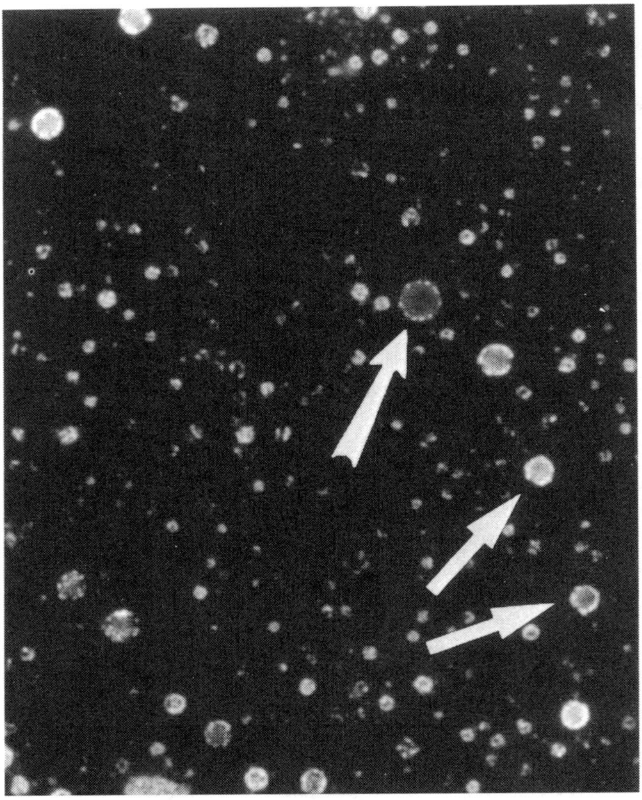

FIGURE 1. Immunolocalization of N-cadherin in isolated preantral human follicles. Human preantral follicles were isolated from ovarian biopsy specimens and immunostained for N-cadherin. Multiple preantral follicles of varying sizes (*arrows*) can be seen surrounded by N-cadherin–positive cells. It can be clearly seen that the oocytes are negative for N-cadherin while remaining/adherent granulosa cells stain intensely for N-cadherin (*arrows*).

luteal phase.[7] As the follicle degenerate, the expression of N-cadherin decreases, and GCs ultimately dissociate.[7] In addition, apoptosis does not occur in preantral follicles and is very low in the early luteal phase, whereas it increases significantly in the late luteal phase.[4,7,19] These observations suggest (a) that the expression of N-cadherin is regulated in human GCs *in vivo* during follicular maturation and corpus luteum formation and (b) that there is a direct correlation between the presence of the N-cadherin molecule and the absence of features characteristic of cellular apoptosis. Although this loss of cell–cell contact has been documented, these relatively old observations provide a physiological rationale to investigate the relationship between N-cadherin–mediated cell contact and GCs survival.

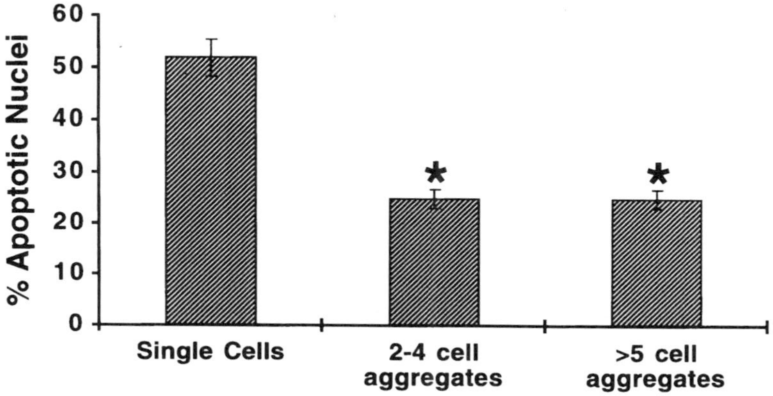

FIGURE 2. Granulosa cell aggregation and apoptosis. Quantitative analysis of TUNEL assay showing the marked decrease (*$p < 0.05$) in apoptotic nuclei (TUNEL positive) when cells were in small (2–4 cell) or large (≥ 5 cells) aggregates, compared to single cells.

CELL–CELL CONTACT INHIBITS HUMAN GRANULOSA CELL APOPTOSIS

Cell–cell contacts promotes GC survival, because single GCs are twice as likely to be apoptotic than GCs engaged in cell–cell interactions (FIG. 2).[7,20] However this observation does not establish a causal relationship between cell contact and cell survival. First, it can be assumed that GCs that do not form cell–cell contacts are dead before culture and therefore unlikely to establish cell contacts *in vitro*. However, almost all GCs are viable before culture.[7] In addition, without exposure to various survival factors such as progesterone,[21] about 50% of single GCs undergo apoptosis. The ability of progesterone to prevent GCs from undergoing apoptosis *in vitro* attests to their initial viability.[21] Another explanation is that aggregated GCs may secrete more progesterone than single GCs. However, culturing human GCs in the presence of aminoglutethimide does not alter the relationship between GC apoptosis and cell adhesion but completely blocks progesterone synthesis.[22] This suggests that endogenous progesterone levels do not account for the enchanced viability of aggregated cells. Similar studies with neutralizing antibodies to other GCs survival factors, such as basic fibroblast growth factor (bFGF),[23] also suggest that endogenous levels of growth factors promoting survival in an autocrine and/or paracrine manner do not explain the relationship between cell contact and cell survival.

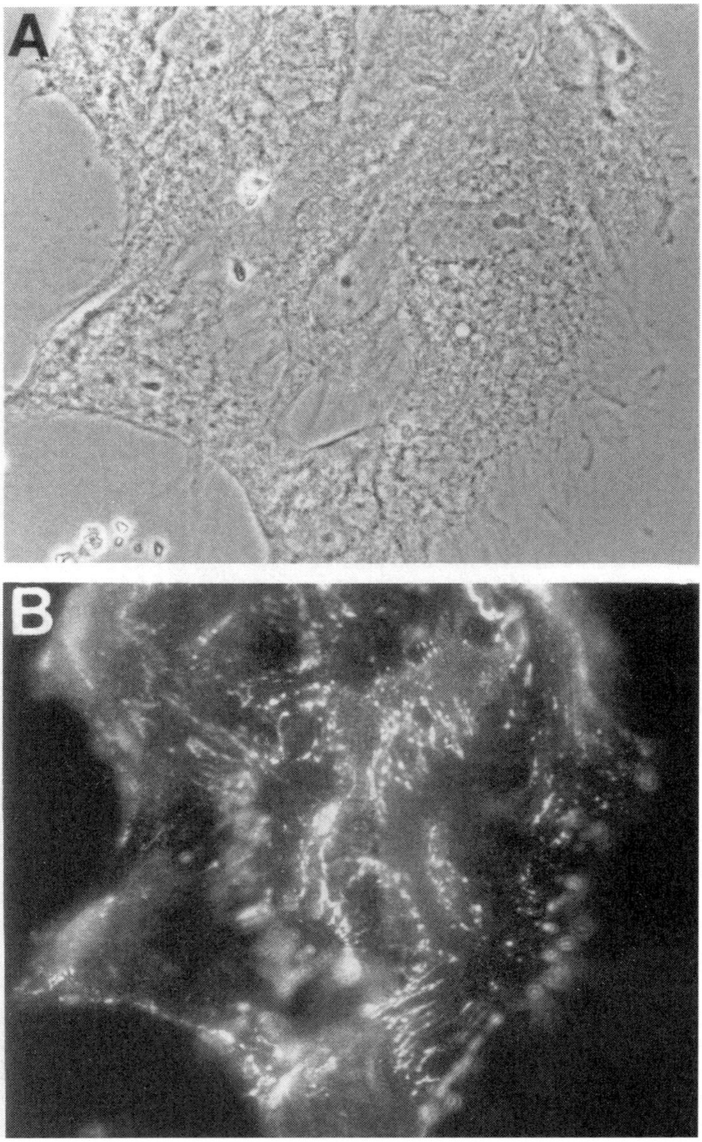

FIGURE 3. N-cadherin expression in isolated human granulosa cells. Phase contrast (**A**) and indirect immunofluorescence (**B**) for N-cadherin of human granulosa cells (GCs) at 24 hours of culture. Note the distribution of N-cadherin at the points of cell–cell contact.

N-CADHERIN–MEDIATED CELL–CELL ADHESION INHIBITS AGGREGATION AND PROMOTES APOPTOSIS IN HUMAN GRANULOSA CELLS

An essential component of adhesion-type junctions is N-cadherin, which is expressed by human GCs (FIG. 3).[7] If N-cadherinœ–mediated GCs aggregation plays an important role in promoting cell survival, then it would be expected that disruption of N-cadherin–mediated cell–cell adhesion would promote apoptosis. We have clearly shown that N-cadherin–neutralizing antibodies or peptides not only inhibited GC aggregation, but also increased apoptosis in these cells; thus strongly suggesting a direct link between N-cadherin–mediated GC adhesion and cell survival. Nevertheless, it should also be noted that, in spite of the presence of a blocking antibody[24,25] or the N-Ac-CHAVC-NH_2 peptide, 25–34% of GCs formed at least a single cell–cell contact, suggesting that other cell adhesion molecules may mediate adhesion between human GCs.[26] We found a higher degree of disruption of human GCs incubated with the N-Ac-CHAVC-NH_2 cyclic peptide compared to the blocking antibody (GC4).[7] This may be due to the smaller size of the peptide, which allows it to penetrate better in the intercellular spaces and disrupt cell–cell adhesion. Of note is that our data showed a higher inhibition of aggregation in human GCs compared to what has been demonstrated in rat GCs.[27] This may be due to species differences or, alternatively, to our use of a different function-blocking peptide. N-Ac-CHAVC-NH_2 (HAV) was designed as a cadherin adhesion recognition (CAR) sequence homologue, which could act as an inhibitor of cell adhesion. In order to serve as effective CAR sequence homologues, peptides must be able to bind to the cadherin molecule with high affinity. Cyclic peptides display enhanced affinity for their ligands and have proven more effective in the study of adhesion molecule function. The information necessary for cadherin-mediated adhesion resides with the HAV motif. Differential antagonistic activities of differently constrained HAV-containing peptides can be explained by the relative orientations of the His and Val side chains. Consequently, in order to retain biological activity, cyclic constructs must influence the backbone conformation without compromising the crucial side chain interaction with the ligand molecule. When this is accomplished, incorporation of the HAV sequence into a cyclic structure restricts the conformations available to the peptide backbone and leads to dramatic increases in potency when compared to the linear analogues. This is the case with N-Ac-CHAVC-NH_2.

PUTATIVE MECHANISMS THROUGH WHICH N-CADHERIN–MEDIATED CELL ADHESION PREVENTS APOPTOSIS IN HUMAN GRANULOSA CELLS

Recent reports have indicated that N-cadherin interacts with the FGF receptor, and this interaction promotes signal transduction through the FGF receptor.[28] In rat GCs, FGF receptors are tyrosine-phosphorylated in serum-free medium in the absence of bFGF.[23] This is likely due to the homophilic binding of N-cadherin between adjacent cells, since exposure to an N-cadherin antibody reduces the level of tyrosine-phosphorylated FGF receptor by 50%.[23] Additionally, FGF receptor antibody studies demonstrate that the FGF receptor is required for cell contact to prevent rat

GCs apoptosis.[23] These data indicate that homophilic binding of N-cadherin promotes the tyrosine phosphorylation of the FGF receptor, thereby triggering a signal transduction pathway that prevents apoptosis.

An alternative pathway for the modulation of cell surface expression and function of N-cadherin is its processing through cleavage of the extracellular domain of the molecule. This led us to hypothesize that one mechanism of regulation of N-cadherin function in GCs could be through proteolytically mediated turnover at the cell surface. Metalloproteinases (MMP) are able to cleave the extracellular domain of cadherins. Specifically, metalloproteinase activity at the cell surface has been shown to cleave the N-cadherin molecule in the rat retina and to release a "soluble" 97-kDa NH_2-terminal fragment in the culture medium.[29] Of particular interest is that MMP-2 and MMP-9 have been identified in human luteinized GCs.[30] MMP activity is regulated by tissue inhibitors of metalloproteinases (TIMPs).[31] A TIMP-like protein has been identified in human follicular fluid with increasing activity during follicular maturation,[30,32] and TIMP-1 mRNA has also been identified in preovulatory human GCs.[31] TIMP-1 and TIMP-2 have also been proposed to play a regulatory role in ovarian connective tissue remodeling.[30] We have shown that, under apoptosis-inducing conditions (serum-free), N-cadherin is cleaved; and its cleavage is inhibited by 1-10 phenanthroline, an MMP inhibitor (FIG. 4).[7] Immunoblot studies using an antibody against the cytoplasmic domain of N-cadherin showed the presence of a

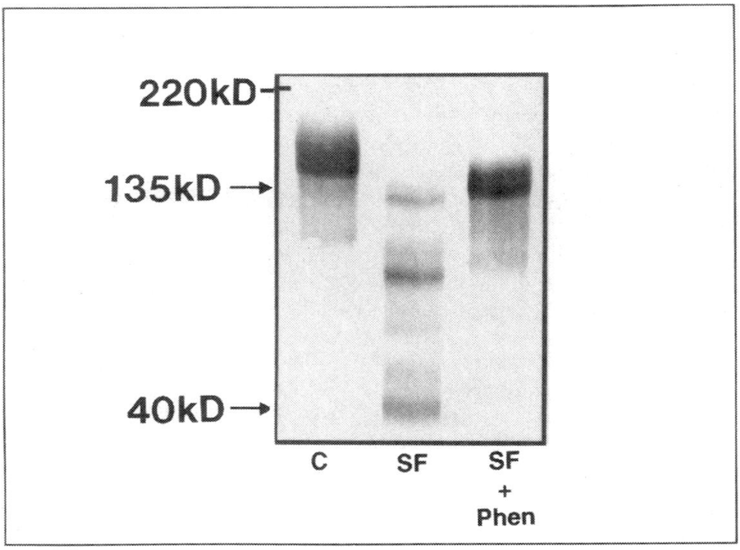

FIGURE 4. Effect of 1–10 phenanthroline on N-cadherin expression and apoptosis on granulosa cells in culture. Immunoblotting for N-cadherin by utilizing the 13A9 antibody against the cytoplasmic domain of N-cadherin. Note the reduction of the 135-kDa N-cadherin protein in GCs in the absence of serum (SF) and the appearance of lower molecular weight fragments. In contrast, 1-10 phenanthroline reverses this effect (SF+Phen).

135-kDa product in the presence of serum and a 40-kDa fragment, representing the cytoplasmic domain (FIG. 4). A third fragment of approximately 90 kDa was identified in the absence of serum, which could represent the intracellular domain and a portion of the extracellular domain (FIG. 4).[7] This suggests that an alternative cleavage site (and thus inactivation) of the N-cadherin molecule may exist in GCs. When an antibody against the extracellular domain of the molecule was used for immunoblotting, a decrease in the detectable membrane-associated N-cadherin was observed.[7] This finding is also in line with cleavage of the extracellular domain of the molecule under apoptosis-inducing conditions. It should be kept in mind that the "soluble," cleaved fragment may be functionally active in culture and contribute to further inhibition of the binding of N-cadherin molecules between GCs still possessing intact molecules on their cell surface. In support of our findings is the observation that VE-cadherin was shown recently to be involved in endothelial cell survival and specifically that shedding of the molecule from the cell surface promoted apoptosis.[33] Thus, GCs apoptosis is associated with the cleavage of the extracellular domain of the N-cadherin molecule, whereas prevention of this molecular event is specifically capable of preventing apoptosis as assessed by a number of independent experimental methods.[7] The signaling cascade(s) following the homotypic/homophilic interactions between N-cadherin molecules on aggregating GCs remains to be elucidated. Despite the variability of the extracellular domain between different cadherins, all members of this family possess a highly conserved cytoplasmic domain that functions as a binding site for catenins, which mediate binding to the cytoskeleton. It is possible that occupation of the cell recognition site on the extracellular domain is followed by activation of signal transduction pathways ultimately leading to upregulation of survival factors. In support of this hypothesis is the interaction of N-cadherin with catenins, which was recently shown to promote cell viability.[34] Alternatively, it is possible that occupation of the extracellular domain of N-cadherin induces conformational changes in the cytoskeleton and cell shape, which might provide nonspecific signals promoting cell survival. Cleavage of the molecule by metalloproteinases may result in the withdrawal of these nonspecific supporting mechanisms, leading the cell to apoptosis. In any case, regulation of N-cadherin expression by extracellular proteolysis provides for a number of theoretical possibilities for the modulation of cell adhesive interactions participating in the survival of human GCs. If the expression and/or the activity of an N-cadherin cleaving protease can be controlled locally, this could provide an additional mechanism through which the survival GCs could be regulated. Taken together, N-cadherin may be intimately involved in determining the fate of follicles and of the corpus luteum. Specifically, we propose that N-cadherin–mediated GC-GC adhesion initiates a signal transduction cascade that can modulate, at least in part, apoptosis of follicular and luteal cells.

FUTURE STUDIES

In the present report we focused on reviewing the role of N-cadherin to mediate cell–cell contacts and regulate human GC survival. It is becoming increasingly clear, however, that cadherin-mediated cell contacts are involved in regulatory pathways in different cell types. Additionally, early embryonic development and organogenesis are modulated by cadherin-mediated cell contacts. Future studies are likely to reveal essential physiological pathways that are influenced by cadherin-mediated cell-to-cell contacts.

ACKNOWLEDGMENTS

This work was supported by a grant from the National Institutes of Health, H.D.-31903(CC) and the Alexander Onassis Foundation (AM). The authors wish to thank Valerie Baldwin for her help in the preparation of this manuscript.

REFERENCES

1. Tilly, J.L. *et al.* 1991. Involvement of apoptosis in ovarian follicular atresia and postovulatory regression. Endocrinology **129:** 2799–2801.
2. Tilly, J.L. *et al.* 1992. Epidermal growth factor and basic fibroblast growth factor suppress the spontaneous onset of apoptosis in cultured rat ovarian granulosa cells and follicles by a tyrosine kinase-dependent mechanism. Mol. Endocrinol. **6:** 1942–1950.
3. Hurwitz, A. & E.Y. Adashi. 1992. Ovarian follicular atresia as an apoptotic process: a paradigm for programmed cell death in endocrine tissues. Mol. Cell. Endocrinol. **84:** C19–C23.
4. Yuan, W. & L. Giudice. 1997. Programmed cell death in human ovary is a function of follicle and corpus luteum status. J. Clin. Endocrinol. Metab. **82:** 3148–3155.
5. Amsterdam, A. *et al.* 1992. Structure–function relationships during differentiation of normal and ongogene-transformed granulosa cells. Biol. Reprod. **46:** 513–522.
6. Keren-tal, J. *et al.* 1995. Involvment of p53 expression in cAMP-mediated apoptosis in immortalized granulosa cells. Exp. Cell. Res. **218:** 283–295.
7. Makrigiannakis, A. *et al.* 1999. N-cadherin mediated human granulosa cell adhesion prevents apoptosis: a role in follicular atresia and luteolysis? Am. J. Pathol. **154:** 1391–1406.
8. Aharoni, D. *et al.* 1995. cAMP-mediated signals as determinants for apoptosis in primary granulosa cells. Exp. Cell. Res. **218:** 271–282.
9. Breckwoldt, M. *et al.* 1996. Expression of Ad4-BP/cytochrome 450 side chain clevage enzyme and induction of cell death in long-term cultures of human granulosa cells. Mol. Hum. Reprod. **6:** 391–400.
10. Ruoslahti, E. & J.C. Reed. 1994. Ancorage dependence, integrins, and apoptosis. Cell **77:** 477–478.
11. Frisch, S.M. & H. Francis. 1994. Disruption of epithelial cell–matrix interactions induces apoptosis. J. Cell Biol. **124:** 619–626.
12. Meredith, J.E. *et al.* 1996. The regulation of growth and intracellular signalling by integrins. Endocrinol. Rev. **17:** 207–220.
13. Clark, E.A & J.S. Brugge. 1995. Integrins and signal transuction pathways: the road taken. Science **268:** 233–239.
14. MacCalman, C.D. *et al.* 1994. Estradiol regulates E-cadherin mRNA levels in the surface epithelium of the mouse ovary. Clin. Exp. Metastasis **12:** 276–282.
15. Munro, S.B. & O.W. Blaschuck. 1996. The structure, function and regulation of cadherins. *In* Cell Adhesion and Invasion in Cancer Metastasis. Pnina Brodt, Ed.: 17–34. RG Landes. Austin, TX.
16. Blaschuk, O.W. *et al.* 1990. Identification of a cadherin cell adhesion recognition sequence. Dev. Biol. **139:** 227–229.
17. Gumbiner, B.M. 1993. Proteins associated with cytoplasmic surface of adhesion molecules. Neuron **11:** 551–564.
18. Knudsen, K.A. *et al.* 1995. Interaction of α-actinin with the cadherin cell–cell adhesion complex via α-catenin. J. Cell Biol. **130:** 67–77.
19. Hsueh, A.J. *et al.* 1996. Gonadal cell apoptosis. Recent. Prog. Horm. Res. **51:** 433–455.

20. PELUSO, J.J. & A. PAPPALARDO. 1994. Progesterone and cell–cell adhesion interact to regulate rat granulosa cell apoptosis. Biochem. Cell. Biol. **72:** 547–551.
21. MAKRIGIANNAKIS, A. *et al.* 1999. Progesterone is an autocrine/paracrine regulator of human granulosa cell survival *in vitro*. Ann. N.Y. Acad. Sci. This volume.
22. MAKRIGIANNAKIS, A. *et al.* 1999. N-cadherin–mediated cell–cell adhesion and progesterone regulate human granulosa cells apoptosis. J. Soc. Gyn. Inv. **5:** 1, 103A.
23. TROLICE, M.P. *et al.* 1997. bFGF and N-cadherin maintain rat granulosa cell and ovarian surface epithelial cell viability by stimulating the tyrosine phosphorylation of the FGF receptor. Endocrinology **138:** 107–113.
24. VOLK, T. & B. GEIGER. 1984. A 135-kD membrane protein of intercellular adherens-junctions. EMBO J. **3:** 2249–2260.
25. VOLK, T. *et al.* 1990. Cleavage of A-CAM by endogenous proteinases in cultured lens and developing chick embryos. Dev. Biol. **139:** 314–326.
26. MAYERHOFFER, A. *et al.* 1994. Expression and alternative splicing of the neural cell adhesion molecule NCAM in human granulosa cells during leuteinization. FEBS Lett. **346:** 207–212.
27. PELUSO, J.J. *et al.* 1996. N-cadherin-mediated cell contact inhibits granulosa cell apoptosis in a progesterone-independent manner. Endocrinology **137:** 1196–1203.
28. WILLIAMS, E.J. *et al.* 1994. Activation of the FGF receptor underlies neurite outgrowth stimulated by L1, N-CAM and N-cadherin. Nmeuron **13:** 583–594.
29. PARADIES, N.E. & G.B. GRUNWALD. 1993. Purification and separation of NCAD90, a soluble endogenous form of N-cadherin, which is generated by proteolysis during retinal development and retains adhesive and neurite-promoting funtion. J. Neurosci. Res. **36:** 33–45.
30. STAMOULI, A. *et al.* 1996. Suppression of matrix metalloproteinase production by hCG in cultures of human leuteinized granulosa cells as a model for gonadotropin-induced luteal rescue. J. Reprod. Fertil. **105:** 235–239.
31. RAPP, G. *et al.* 1990. Characterization of three abundant mRNAs from human ovarian granulosa cels. DNA Cell. Biol. **40:** 1170–1178.
32. CURRY, T.E. *et al.* 1988. Identification and characterization of metalloproteinase inhibitor of activity in human ovarian follicular fluid. Endocrinology **123:** 1611–1618.
33. HERREN, B. *et al.* 1998. Cleavage of β-catenin and plakoglobin and shedding of VE-cadherin during endothelial apoptosis: evidence for a role for caspases and metalloproteinases. Mol. Biol. Cell **9:** 1589–1601.
34. HERMISTON, M.L. & J.J. GORDON. 1995. In vivo analysis of cadherin function in mouse intestinal epithelium: essential roles in adhesion, maintenance of differentiation, and regulation of programmed cell death. J. Cell Biol. **129:** 489–506.

Molecular Basis of Gynecological Cancer

D.A. SPANDIDOS,[a] D.N. DOKIANAKIS, G. KALLERGI, AND E. AGGELAKIS

Laboratory of Virology, Medical School, University of Crete, Heraklion 71409, Crete, Greece

ABSTRACT: Alterations in the cellular genome affecting the expression or function of genes controlling cell growth and differentiation are considered to be the main cause of cancer. Genes that cause cancer are of two distinct types: oncogenes and onco-suppressor genes. The normal proto-oncogene can be converted into an active oncogene by deletion or point mutation in its coding sequence, gene amplification, and by specific chromosome rearrangements. Mutations and abnormal expression in *ras*, *myc*, *c-erb*B-2, and other oncogenes have been reported in several types of gynecological cancer. Onco-suppressor genes are involved in gynecological cancer, their functions are localized in different phases of the cell cycle. Structural changes and deletions of these genes can cause cancer. Mutations in the *p53*, *BRCA1*, *DCC*, and *PTEN* genes have been reported in gynecological cancers such as ovarian, cervical, and endometrial cancer. Human papillomaviruses are of major interest because specific types (HPV-16, -18, and several others) have been identified as causative agents in at least 90% of cancers of the cervix. In this study we summarize the available information regarding the implication of specific oncogenes, onco-suppressor genes, and HPV in the development of female genital malignancies.

INTRODUCTION

Gynecological cancer is a common cause of death. Cervical cancer is considered to be a sexually transmitted disease and has been correlated with human papillomavirus (HPV) infection and with other sexually transmitted factors. Endometrial cancer is the most common gynecological malignancy in many parts of the Western world, nevertheless causing only 13% of deaths related to gynecological cancer because of early diagnosis of the disease.

Molecular studies in all types of gynecological cancers have revealed the implication of certain genes that are altered, activated (oncogenes), or inactivated (onco-suppressor genes). These alterations may occur at the beginning of the progress of neoplastic events, and detection of these alterations in certain genes may be of clinical importance for the early diagnosis and the evaluation of the course of malignancy. Recently, another type of genetic alteration has been described, microsatellite instability (MI), which reflects damage in the DNA replication and repair systems of the cell. Finally, viral infections, mostly by HPV, is one of the major causes of female gynecological cancers.

[a]Address for correspondence: Professor D.A. Spandidos, Laboratory of Virology, Medical School, University of Crete, Heraklion 71409, Crete, Greece. Phone/fax: 30-1-7227809.

ONCOGENES IN GYNECOLOGICAL CANCERS

Cervix

Cancer of the uterine cervix is the second most common cancer in women worldwide and is particularly common in less developed countries, where 80% of the world's cervical cancer occurs. A number of prognostic factors have been linked to the progression of cervical cancers, including depth of stromal invasion, lesion depth, and nodal involvement. Current data implicate the *ras* gene family in cervical cancer, although mutations of this family of genes have been reported at a low frequency in gynecological malignancies. These mutations occur mostly in codon 12 of the K-*ras* gene. In our recent studies on women of the Greek population, mutations of K-*ras* were detected in 17% and mutations of the H-*ras* and N-*ras* genes were found in 3.5%. The *ras* gene mutations were also detected in nonmalignant lesions, indicating that the *ras* genes play an important role in the initial stages of carcinogenesis of the cervix.

Elevated expression of *ras* p21, as demonstrated by the use of specific antibodies, has been found in malignant as opposed to benign or premalignant lesions. In the small-cell type of squamous cell carcinomas, tumors with elevated expression of *ras* p21 were shown to have a better prognosis than negative tumors. Expression of *ras* p21 together with histological type may therefore be of prognostic significance in carcinomas of the cervix in specific histological types.[1] Mutations in codon 12 of the H-*ras* gene have also been found in cervical cancer and in one study were correlated with poor prognosis.[1]

Amplification and overexpression of *myc* has been shown to be frequent in advanced cervical tumors. In some studies overexpression was detected in 35% of the cases. This overexpression was not reported as a consequence of amplification, which was seen in only 8% of the cases. Expression correlates with appearance of the more severe forms of cervical intraepithelial carcinoma (CIN types II and III). However, there was an eightfold greater risk of relapse for patients with overexpression of *myc*, which outweighed even nodal status as a prognostic factor.[1]

Endometrium

The majority of endometrial cancers are adenocarcinomas. They develop from atypical endometrial hyperplasia in the setting of excess estrogenic stimulation. In contrast, serous carcinomas are representative of endometrial cancers in older women who have endometrial atrophy and lack the typical endometrial cancer risk factors reflecting unopposed estrogen exposure.[2] Overexpression of HER-2/NEU occurs in 10% of endometrial adenocarcinomas and correlates with intraperitoneal spread of disease and poor survival. *Myc* has been found to be amplified in 10% of the cases. Point mutations in codon 12 of K-*ras* have also been reported in some endometrial hyperplasias, which may represent an early event in the development of some endometrial cancers. The overexpression of c-*erb*B-2 is often observed in patients with advanced-stage disease and deep myometrial invasion. Overexpression in endometrial cancer of *c-fms*, a proto-oncogene that codes for the colony-stimulating factor-1 (CSF-1) receptor, may delineate a group of high-risk tumors.

Ovary

K-*ras* mutations appear to play a minor role in the pathogenesis of invasive ovarian carcinomas; their role might be more important in borderline ovarian tumors that exhibit low malignant potential.[3] Overexpression of the *HER-2/NEU* oncogene also occurs in approximately 30% of ovarian cancers, and increased expression is correlated with poor survival.[4] Amplification of *akt2* has been detected in 12.1% of samples of ovarian carcinomas. Overexpression of akt2 can also occur in ovarian carcinomas negative for *akt2* amplification. Alterations in *akt2* may therefore play a specific role in ovarian oncogenesis and appear to be associated with a poor prognosis for ovarian cancer patients.

ONCO-SUPPRESSOR GENES AND GYNECOLOGICAL CANCER

Cervical Cancer

p53 is an onco-suppressor gene related to different kinds of tumors. People who inherit one functional copy of *p53*, or who have mutations in the nucleotide sequence of this gene show propensity for many kinds of cancer. *p53* binds to DNA and induces transcription of other regulatory genes whose products bind to the complexes of G_1 cyclin with Cdk2 protein, thus passing the G_1 checkpoint. *p53* blocks kinase activity and prevents a cell from progressing into the S phase and replicating its DNA. The normal function of *p53* is to enable cells to repair themselves after DNA damage. *p53* acts as check on cell proliferation in stressful situations. Mutations of *p53* are present in more than 50% of all cases of cancers. Highly conserved exons 5–8 are the most common mutation targets. *p53* mutations have been found in cervical cancer, generally combined with HPV infections.

p16 is an onco-suppressor gene involved in different kinds of gynecological tumors.[5] The function of this gene product is to prevent cell cycle progression by directly interfering with cyclin/cyclin-dependent kinase (CDK) activation.[6] *p16* is located on the 9q21 chromosomal region and is a potent inhibitor of the cyclin D/kinase 4 complex. There are studies showing low expression of this gene product in patients with cervical cancer, often with mutations in DNA sequence of the *p16* gene.[7] Therefore, it is possible that underexpression of *p16* may play an important role in this type of cancer.

Endometrial Cancer

Mutations or deletions of the *p53* gene have been frequently reported in endometrial cancer. It can also be a prognostic factor.[8] The onco-suppressor gene *PTEN* is probably involved in various kinds of cancer. Deletions in chromosome 10q23 were found in many tumors, resulting in discovery of the *PTEN* gene. Its protein has tyrosine kinase and tensin action; mutations of this gene are reported in glioblastoma, in thyroid, breast, kidney, and gynecological cancers. Mutations and deletions of the *PTEN* gene have been found in many studies of endometrial cancer and have been shown to be involved also in neoplastic transformation of endometrial cells.[9]

Ovarian Cancer

It has been reported that loss of function and mutations of *p53* are involved in ovarian cancer, and possibly these alterations can be used as a prognostic factor.[10] evidence also indicates that *PTEN* is not substantially involved in ovarian cancer.

*BRCA*1 is a tumor suppressor gene located on 17q-23q.[11] This gene is probably involved in DNA damage and repair in cell cycle regulation and in differentiation of cells.[12] Since the cloning of BRCA1 in 1994, much has been learned about the function of the gene. The size of the protein of *BRCA*1 and the variety of transcripts have shown the complexity of the functions of this gene.

Women with mutations in this gene show a high propensity for ovarian and breast cancer. New data have shown that patients with inherited ovarian and breast cancer have the same replacement of five nucleotides in exon 5.[13] The involvement of this gene in other gynecological cancers remains to be established.

MICROSATELLITE INSTABILITY IN GYNECOLOGIC CANCER

Microsatellite instability (MI), since the initial description in 1993 in hereditary nonpolyposis colorectal carcinoma (HNPCC), has been identified in a wide variety of human cancers, both familial and sporadic.[14] The functional role or the role of MIN in human carcinogenesis is not clear.

The human genome is punctuated with repetitive nucleotide sequences or microsatellites. These repetitive di-, tri-, and tetra-nucleotides are frequently, but not invariably, located between genes and have been classified as "junk" DNA. Microsatellites are also called SSLP (simple sequence-length polymorphisms) or STRs (short tandem repeat polymorphisms). The highly polymorphic microsatellite DNA is composed of repetitive sequences of 2–6 bp, highly variable in size. Usually, the nucleotide sequences are repeated 15–30 times. There are 35,000–100,000 (dA–dC)n copies in the human genome.

Microsatellites are the vestigial product of abortive evolution of genes, and the maintenance of repetitive DNA has a negative impact on evolution.[15] It is also assumed that repetitive DNA does not contain only perfect repeats. Instead, they are interrupted by base substitutions that may act as a barrier to homologous recombination. In cancer cells, the expansion of these sequences could break down this barrier to recombination and permit chromosomal exchanges, which are a common finding in most tumors.

In recent descriptions of MI, and in trying to relate one series to another, it is important to distinguish (i) whether the tumors were sporadic or familial; (ii) which category of microsatellite markers were used (di-, tri-, or tetranucleotide markers; (iii) how many microsatellite markers were used; and (iv) whether the MI data were derived from primary tumors or established cell lines, and if the former, what was the histopathology of the tumors included in the analysis.[16]

Families with HPNCC are delineated as those that have elevated incidence of cancers of endometrium, stomach, gall bladder, pancreas, and urinary tract (the so-called extended HNPCC spectrum, the Lynch Cancer Family II syndrome). These tumors may also exhibit MI; MI is prevalent in many familial tumors. An overall assessment of the studies on sporadic cancers indicates that MI is not limited to tumors associated with HNPCC.

If certain loci appear highly unstable in a specific type of cancer, then these loci can be considered as MI hot spots.[17] To determine whether instability at these hot spots is confined to a specific type of cancer or characterizes a broader spectrum of human malignancies, it is necessary to compare MI frequencies at the designated loci among different types of cancer.[16] Furthermore, instability may not be confined to a single repetitive sequence, but may be differentially distributed along particular regions of individual chromosomes (hot spot chromosomal region) and may differ between tumor types.[18] The pattern of distribution of DNA instability could be significantly correlated with tumorigenesis. If MI reflects generalized genomic instability, then genes important for the development of the cancer could be randomly affected. If MI is localized, it would result either in a DNA sequence alteration without functional significance (in the case of microsatellite sequences located outside genes) or in changes in an adjacent gene, possibly involved in carcinogenesis (in the case of microsatellite sequences in the promoter, exon–intron boundaries or the coding region of the genes). Nearly 50% of the MI+[19] presumed sporadic colorectal carcinomas in patients age <35 years were found to carry constitutional hMSH2/hMLH1 mutations. Constitutional mutations are rarely reported in other MI+ tumor types such as endometrial[19] or ovarian tumors.[20]

There is consensus in the literature about the number of markers one must examine before labeling a tumor as MI+ or MI–. MI has been described for tumors in both early and late stages of progression, and therefore there is no consensus about when in the course of the tumorigenesis MI develops, but it is generally accepted that genomic instability is a dynamic process during cell proliferation in MI+. In sporadic breast tumors, MI is described as a late event.[21] Data for "early" breast cancers support the suggestion that microsatellite instability may be an early event in the genesis of some sporadic breast cancers. It is suggested that early or late detection of MI could reflect the number of cell divisions after the inactivation of the human DNA mismatch repair gene activity in the tumor (MMR/hMSH2, hMLH1, hPMS1, and hPMS2).

MI has been used as a diagnostic and prognostic tool for HNPCC–associated as well as non-HNPCC cancer. Microsatellite DNA helps to identify HNPCC patients who would have been excluded by clinical criteria alone[22] and to determine whether a tumor is heritable or sporadic when it occurs in a member of the Lynch II family.

Breast carcinoma, uncommon in the Lynch II syndrome, is heritable or sporadic when it occurs. In breast carcinoma there is a significant correlation between the presence of MI and poor prognosis.[23] Borderline ovarian tumors have been reported to exhibit a significantly higher frequency of MI when compared with invasive epithelial ovarian tumors.[24] Loss of heterozygosity on chromosome 17 in endometrioid ovarian carcinoma may indicate transition to a more aggressive tumor.[25] Endometrial carcinoma is the second most common tumor type in women with HNPCC. MI has been observed in approximately 20% of sporadic cases of inherited form (HNPCC) of endometrial carcinoma.

TABLE 1. Lesions of the female reproductive system caused by different human papillomavirus types

Type of lesion	Location	HPV type
Condyloma acuminatum	Cervix, vulva	6, 11, 54
Bowenoid lesions	Cervix	16, 55
CIN	Cervix	6, 11, 16, 18, 31, 34, 40, 42, 44, 57, 58
Carcinoma	Cervix	16, 18, 33, 35, 39, 45, 51, 52, 56

ABBREVIATIONS: HPV, human papillomavirus; CIN, cervical intraepithelial carcinoma.

HPV IN GYNECOLOGICAL CANCER

Recent data suggest that approximately 15% of all cancers have a viral cause.[26] Infection by these viruses is not sufficient, but it is identified as the first step of a multistep process that leads to cancer. Human papillomaviruses belong to the Papovavıridae family of viruses. These viruses are nonenveloped, and they have ecosedric symmetry. Full particles contain the double-stranded, closed circular DNA genome. The genome consists of 7200–8000 base pairs containing up to 10 open reading frames (ORF). These viruses show a high tropism for the mucosal or cutaneous epithelium.[26]

The papillomavirus family represents a remarkably heterogeneous group of viruses. At present, 77 distinct genotypes have been identified in humans, and partial sequences have been obtained from more than 30 putative novel genotypes. In humans, papillomavirus infections cause a variety of benign proliferations: warts, epithelial cysts, intraepithelial neoplasias, anogenital, oro-laryngeal and -pharyngeal papillomas, keratoacanthomas, and other types of hyperkeratoses. Their involvement in the etiology of certain major human cancers is of particular interest.

Cervical cancer represents one of the most frequent forms of malignancy in women,[27] and the connection between infection with specific HPV types and the development of this type of cancer is based on the observation that over 90% of cervical cancers contain the DNA of HPV viruses.[28]

More than 20 HPV types (such as types 16, 18, 31, 33, 35, and 39) selectively infect the genital epithelium and are related with squamous cell carcinoma of the genital tract.[29] Specific lesions caused by certain HPV types are shown in TABLE 1. HPV types are classified into "low-risk HPV" and "high-risk HPV" viruses. HPV6 and HPV-11 belong to low-risk types related with nonmalignant lesions such as condyloma acuminatum, whereas types 16 and 18 belong to high-risk HPVs and are associated with lesions that proceed to higher grade neoplasias and contribute to the formation of the majority of cervical cancers.[30]

The DNA molecule of these viruses contains the early ORF E1, E2, E4, E5, E6, and E7 as well as the late ORF L1 and L2. The proteins coded by the E6 and E7 ORFs of high-risk HPVs are small nuclear proteins with transforming activity. The E7 protein of HPV16 is a 98 amino acid nuclear phosphoprotein that binds to DNA as a zinc-binding protein.[31] E6 proteins of high-risk HPVs consist of 150 amino acids, bind to DNA, and are evolutionarily related to the E7 protein. These proteins probably evolved by gene duplication. The E6 protein of high-risk HPVs binds to cellular p53.[32] This binding promotes the degradation of p53m, mediated by the cellular ubiquitin proteolysis system.[33] p53 acts as a transcriptional activator by binding to specific DNA sequences and is required for the growth arrest following cellular DNA damage.[34] On the other hand, E6 proteins of low-risk HPVs cannot bind and degrade p53. The interaction between E6 and p53 is an important step in the creation and progression of the majority of cervical lesion.

The E7 protein, coded by high-risk HPVs, forms complexes with the retinoblastoma susceptibility protein pRB and with other proteins of the RB family such as the p107 and p130.[35] The E7 protein specifically binds the unphosphorylated form of RB, which is present in the G0 and G1 stages of the cell cycle and is found tightly tethered to the cell nucleus. E7 expression results in the activation of genes that allow entry into or progression through the cell cycle. It is interesting that E7 proteins coded by HPV-8 cannot bind to the RB protein.[36]

It has been suggested that the presence of HPV in tumors constitutes a prognostic marker of disease severity in cervical cancer. The presence of high-risk HPV-18 is equated with rapid progression through early disease stages, possibly resulting in a more aggressive clinical course. Patients with tumors containing HPV-18 and -33 have a significantly poorer prognosis than patients with tumors containing other types of HPV DNA,[37] whereas the presence of antibodies against HPV-16 E7 protein has been correlated with worse prognosis,[38] implying a prognostic significance for HPV typing. The absence of HPV from the tumor confers a worse prognosis than if any viral types were present.

The importance of additional factors in cervical carcinogenesis is emphasized. Multiple infections with other viruses such as CMV and HSV[39] might act as cofactors. Oncogene activation, such as the *ras* family, may also act as an additional cofactor, leading to cervical carcinogenesis.[40] Moreover, hormonal factors, such as oral contraceptives and high parity, appear to confer an additional risk, increasing the progression from chronic HPV infection to cancer.[41]

REFERENCES

1. Kiaris, H. & D.A. Spandidos. 1995. Mutations of ras genes in human tumours (Review). Int. J. Oncol. **7:** 413–421.
2. Sherman, M.E. *et al.* 1995. Endometrial cancer chemo-prevention: implications of diverse pathways of carcinogenesis. J. Cell. Biochem. Suppl. **23:** 160–164.
3. Mok, S.C. *et al.* 1993. Mutation of K-*ras* proto-oncogene in human ovarian epithelial tumors of borderline malignancy. Cancer Res. **53:** 1489–1492.
4. Bechuck, A. 1995. Biomarkers in the ovary. J. Cell. Biochem. Suppl. **23:** 223–226.
5. Khleif, S.N. *et al.* 1996. Inhibition of cyclin D-CDK4/CDK6 activity is associated with an E2F-mediated induction of cyclin kinase inhibitor activity. Proc. Natl. Acad. Sci. USA **93:** 4350–4354.
6. Kim, Y.T. *et al.* 1998. Underexpression of cyclin-dependent kinase (CDK) inhibitors in cervical carcinoma. Gynecol. Oncol. **71:** 38–45.
7. Sano, T. *et al.* 1998. Immunohistochemical overexpression of p16 protein associated with intact retinoblastoma protein expression in cervical cancer and cervical intraepithelial neoplasia. Pathol. Int. **48:** 580–585.
8. Blom, R. *et al.* 1998. Leiomyosarcoma of the uterus: a clinicopathologic, DNA flow cytometric, p53, and mdm-2 analysis of 49 cases. Gynecol. Oncol. **68:** 54–61.
9. Lu, X. *et al.* 1998. Expression of p21WAF1/CIP1 in adenocarcinoma of the uterine cervix: a possible immunohistochemical marker of a favorable prognosis. Cancer **82:** 2409–2417.

10. Zachos, G. *et al.* 1998. Transcriptional regulation of the c-H-*ras*1 gene by the P53 protein is implicated in the development of human endometrial and ovarian tumours. Oncogene **16:** 3013–3017.
11. Paterson, J.W. 1998. BRCA1: a review of structure and putative functions. Dis. Markers **13:** 261–274.
12. Rice, J.C. *et al.* 1998. Aberrant methylation of the BRCA1 CpG island promoter is associated with decreased BRCA1 mRNA in sporadic breast cancer cells. Oncogene **17:** 1807–1812.
13. Presneau, N. *et al.* 1998. New mechanism of BRCA-1 mutation by deletion/insertion at the same nucleotide position in three unrelated French breast/ovarian cancer families. Hum. Genet. **103:** 334–339.
14. Ionov, Y. *et al.* 1993. Ubiquitous somatic mutations in simple repeated sequences reveal a new mechanism for colonic carcinogenesis. Nature **363:** 558–561.
15. Lawrence, A. *et al.* 1994. Microsatellite instabity: marker of a mutator phenotype in cancer. Cancer Res. **54:** 5059–5063.
16. Arzimanoglou, I. *et al.* 1998. Microsatellite instability in human solid tumors. Cancer **82:** 1808–1820.
17. Parsons, R. *et al.* 1995. Microsatellite instability and mutations of the transforming growth factor β type II receptor gene in colorectal cancer. Cancer Res. **55:** 5548–5550.
18. Souza, R.F. *et al.* 1996. Microsatellite instability in the insuline–like growth factor II receptor gene in gastrointestinal tumors. Nat. Genet. **14:** 255–257.
19. Katabucchi, H. *et al.* 1995. Mutations in DNA mismatch repair genes are not responsible for microsatellite instablity in most sporadic endometrial carcinomas. Cancer Res. **55:** 5556–5560.
20. Fujita, M. *et al.* 1995. Microsatellite instability and alterations of the *HMSH2* gene in human ovarian cancer. Int. J. Cancer **64:** 361–366.
21. Kamik, P. *et al.* 1995. Microsatellite instability at a single locus (D11S988) on chromosome 11p15.5 is elevated in mammary tumorigenesis. Hum. Mol. Genet. **4:** 1889–1894.
22. Muta, H. *et al.* 1996. Clinical implications of microsatellite instability in colorectal cancers. Cancer **77:** 265–270.
23. Paulson, T.G. *et al.* 1996. Microsatellite instability correlates with reduced survival and poor disease prognosis in breast cancer. Cancer Res. **56:** 4021–4026.
24. Tangir, J. *et al.* 1996. Frequent microsatellite instability in epithelial borderline ovarian tumors. Cancer Res. **56:** 2501–2505.
25. Shenson, D.L. *et al.* 1995. Loss of heterogygosity and genomic instability in synchronous endometrioid tumors of the endometrium. Cancer **76:** 650–657.
26. zur Hausen, H. 1991. Viruses in human cancers. Science **254:** 1167–1173.
27. Parkin, D.M. *et al.* 1988. Estimates of the worldwide frequency of sixteen major cancers in 1980. Int. J. Cancer **41:** 184–197.
28. zur Hausen, H. 1991. Human papillomaviruses in the pathogenesis of anogenital cancers. Virology **184:** 9–13.
29. zur Hausen, H. & E.M. de Villiers. 1994. Human papillomavirus. Annu. Rev. Microbiol. **48:** 427–447.
30. zur Hausen, H. 1994. Disrupted dichotomous intracellular control of human papillomavirus infection in cancer of the cervix. Lancet **343:** 955–957.
31. Barbosa, M.S. *et al.* 1989. Papillomavirus polypeptides E6 and E7 are zinc-binding proteins. J. Virol. **63:** 1401–1407.
32. Scheffner, M. *et al.* 1993. The HPV-16 E6 and E6-AP complex functions as a ubiquitin-protein ligase in the ubiquitination of p53. Cell **75:** 495–505.
33. Vousden, K.H. 1991. Human papillomavirus transforming genes. Semin Virol **2:** 307–317.
34. Lechner, M.S. *et al.* 1992. Human papillomavirus E6 proteins bind p53 *in vivo* and abrogate p53-mediated repression of transcription. EMBO J. **11:** 5013–5020.
35. Davies, R. *et al.* 1993. HPV 16 E7 associates with a histone H1 kinase activity and p107 through sequences necessary for transformation. J. Virol. **67:** 2521–2528.
36. Iffner, T. *et al.* 1990. The E7 protein of human papillomavirus 8 is a nonphosphorylated protein of 17 kDa and can be generated by two different mechanisms. Virology **179:** 428–436.

37. HAGMAR, B. *et al.* 1995. Implications of human papillomavirus type for survival in cervical squamous cell carcinoma. Int. J. Gynecol. Cancer **5:** 341–345.
38. BAAY, M.F.D. *et al.* 1995. Antibodies to human papillomavirus type-16 E7 related to clinicopathological data in patients with cervical carcinoma. J. Clin. Pathol. **48:** 410–414.
39. PEI, X. *et al.* 1993. Co-transfection of HPV-18 and v-*fos* DNA induces tumorigenicity of primary human keratinocytes. Virology **196:** 855–860.
40. KOFFA, M. *et al.* 1994. Detection of *ras* gene mutations and HPV in lesions of the human female reproductive tract. Int. J. Oncol. **5:** 189–195.
41. MUNOR, N. 1994. The role of HPV in etiology of cervical cancer. Mutat. Res. **305:** 293–301.

The Hypothalamic–Pituitary–Thyroid Axis and the Female Reproductive System

ANTHONY G. DOUFAS AND GEORGE MASTORAKOS[a]

Endocrine Unit, Evgenidion Hospital, University of Athens Medical School, Athens, Greece

ABSTRACT: Increasing evidence derived from experimental and clinical studies suggests that the hypothalamic–pituitary–thyroid axis (HPT) and the hypothalamic–pitutitary–ovarian axis (HPO) are physiologically related and act together as a unified system in a number of pathological conditions. The suggestion that specific thyroid hormone receptors at the ovarian level might regulate reproductive function, as well as the suggested influence of estrogens at the higher levels of the HPT axis, seems to integrate the reciprocal relationship of these two major endocrine axes. Both hyper- and hypothyroidism may result in menstrual disturbances. In hyperthyroidism the most common manifestation is simple oligomenorrhea. Anovulatory cycles are very common. Increased bleeding may also occur, but it is rare. Hypothyroidism in girls can cause alterations in the pubertal process; this is usually a delay, but occasionally it can result in pseudoprecocious puberty. In mature women hypothyroidism usually is associated with abnormal menstrual cycles characterized mainly by polymenorrhea, especially anovulatory cycles, and an increase in fetal wastage.

INTRODUCTION

Physiological Aspects of the Thyroid–Reproductive Function Interplay

Thyroid hormone secretion and extrathyroidal hormone metabolism are the same in both men and nonpregnant women. Serum T_4, T_3, and TSH levels do not differ. Nevertheless, gender differences in the pattern of blood flow in the superior thyroid artery suggest an estrogen effect.[1]

Thyrotropin-Releasing Hormone (TRH) and the HPO Axis

The responses of both TSH and prolactin to a given dose of TRH are greater in women than in men, especially over the age of 40.[2–5] Furthermore, both responses are greater in women during the preovulatory compared to the luteal phase of the menstrual cycle.[6] Ramey *et al.*, however, found that TSH and prolactin responses to TRH were increased in women on oral contraceptive agents compared with controls.[7] On the other hand, Colon *et al.* have reported that in both phases of the cycle there is a significant increase of serum LH but not FSH following TRH administration.[8]

[a]Address for correspondence: Dr. George Mastorakos, 3, Neofytou Vamva St. 10674 Athens, Greece. Fax: 30-1-3636229.
e-mail: mastorak@mail.kapatel.gr

Thyrotropin (TSH) and the HPO Axis

Rasmussen *et al.* have found that during the menstrual cycle median serum TSH and thyroid volume increased. Serum thyroglobulin increased from 27 (day 2) to 32 mg/l (day 23, $p < 0.01$), and it correlated positively with thyroid volume ($r = 0.65$, $p < 0.02$).[9] The effect of estrogen on TSH secretion, however, is controversial. Contradictory results suggesting a stimulatory[7] and an inhibitory[2,10] effect have been obtained by different investigators.

Thyroxine, Triiodothyronine, Thyroxine-Binding Globulin, and the HPO Axis

Thyroid hormones seem to play a pivotal role of physiological significance on the generation and control of the seasonal reproductive cycles of ewes[11] and female American tree sparrows.[12] Thyroxine (T_4) takes part in an inhibitory regulation of the ovarian hormonal secretion and folliculogenesis in chorionic gonadotropin-primed, immature female rats.[13] It has been noted that small doses of thyroid hormones given to young female mice result in the early attainment of sexual maturity with an early opening of the vagina and onset of estrous cycle.[14] During the menstrual cycle, thyroid hormones levels fluctuate in relation to circulating estrogen levels.[15] There is no appreciable variation in radioactive iodine (RAI) uptake during the different phases of the menstrual cycle, however.

Estrogen-induced increases in pituitary total cellular RNA levels after ovariectomy in rats are dependent on protein synthesis, are gender-specific, are T_3-inhibited, and may be mediated by specific estrogen-induced changes in protein-DNA interactions.[16] The interaction of T_3 with gonadotropin hormones modulates follicular steroidogenesis *in vitro*, depending on the follicle size and cell type, probably by influencing aromatization processes in the follicle.[17] It seems that T_3 activates perch ovarian 3β-hydroxysteroid dehydrogenase/delta5-delta4-isomerase,[18] leading to a greater conversion of pregnenolone to progesterone.[19] Lariviere *et al.* found small changes in protein metabolism during the menstrual cycle in women, with an increase in oxidative leucine metabolism. The concomitant increase observed in circulating free T_3 raises the possibility that fluctuations in protein metabolism and thyroid hormone levels throughout the menstrual cycle are causaly related.[20] After the administration of oral contraceptives, the levels of reverse T_3 in the serum are increased, due to the increase in TBG.[7,21]

Dainat *et al.* have studied the ontogenesis of T_3 nuclear receptors in skeletal muscles in male and female chicks and found that the latter had significantly more T_3 nuclear receptors than the former.[22] Thyroid hormone receptor mRNA is expressed in both granulosa cells and ovarian stromal cells found in nonstimulated ovaries from normally cycling women.[23]

Although TBG production is stimulated by estrogen and inhibited by androgens, serum TBG concentrations are similar in men and women. Hyperestrogenism, either endogenous (caused by pregnancy, hydatidiform moles, or estrogen-producing tumors) or exogenous (due to the administration of estrogens), is associated with an increase in circulating levels of T_4-binding globulin (TBG) and a decrease in T_4-binding prealbumin (TBPA) concentrations in both women and men.[24,25] This phenomenon is due to an estrogen-induced increase of the sialic acid content of TBG. This change prolongs the half-life of TBG in the circulation, resulting in a higher plasma concentration with no change in the rate of TBG synthesis. The administration of estrogen increases the circulating level of TBG, probably due to decreased clearance of TBG rather than increased production.[26] Nevertheless, except for transient alterations in free T_4, a new steady-state level will be achieved with stable high T_4 and triiodothyronine (T_3) levels and T_4–TBG complexes, but normal levels of free T_4 and T_3. The administration of androgens, which lowers the concentration of serum TBG while increasing that of TBPA,[27] has no effect on free T_4.[28,29] In hypothyroid women on appropriate L-T_4 replacement therapy, however, androgen administration for breast cancer results in a rise in the serum free T_4 and a decrease in the serum thyroid-stimulating hormone (TSH) concentrations, requiring a lower dose of L-T_4.[30] This is due to the lack of thyroid adaptation to the decreased TBG induced by androgens. Certain progestins, such as norethindrone, that have androgenic potency will also result in a decrease in TBG and serum T_4 concentrations.[28]

Both choriocarcinomas and hydatidiform moles can be associated with the signs and symptoms of thyrotoxicosis.[31] The thyrotoxicosis in such instances appears to be due to increased secretion of T_4 secondary to thyroid stimulation from the high levels of human chorionic gonadotropin (hCG) especially asialo-variants of hCG.[32]

Fitko *et al.* have shown that ovaries from hyperthyroid rats were reduced in size and contained fewer LH/hCG receptors than control animals, whereas the latter had three times higher LH/hCG receptor concentrations than the ovaries from hypothyroid animals.[33]

Thyroid Gland, Iodine Environment, and the HPO Axis

Thyroid size, as measured by ultrasonography, varies during the menstrual cycle, being greatest at midcycle.[34] As expected, this increase correlates positively with serum thyroglobulin levels.[9] Thyroid cells contain estrogen receptors, but whether these receptors play a role in the higher incidence of papillary carcinoma in women compared with men is uncertain.[35] In areas with a low or moderate iodine intake, the thyroid gland enlarges during pregnancy because of the higher iodine requirements of pregnant women and the hypertrophic activity of chorionic gonadotropin.[36–39] Hegedus *et al.* found from the study of 11 healthy women that the mean thyroid gland volume in the second half of the menstrual cycle (24.4 ± 4.8 ml on day 23) was significantly larger than in the first (15.4 ± 3.1 ml on day 9).[40]

THYROTOXICOSIS AND THE FEMALE REPRODUCTIVE SYSTEM

Increased sex hormone-binding globulin (SHBG) concentration is characteristic of hyperthyroidism[41]—so much so that this globulin is used as a test of thyroid function, reflecting the tissue response to the thyroid hormones. Serum levels of estradiol and testosterone should thus be interpreted with this fact in mind because their total amounts are increased out of proportion to the free levels. Also, women with thyrotoxicosis have a decrease in the metabolic clearance rates of testosterone and of estradiol,[42–44] an increase in the $5\alpha/5\beta$-reduced metabolites in the urine, and an increase in catechol estrogens in the urine at the expense of estriol and other 16-hydroxylated estrogen metabolites.[45]

Southern *et al.* have found an increase in the peripheral aromatization of androgens to estrogens in some thyrotoxic women.[46] Other studies,[44] however, did not confirm these findings and suggested that any increase in the peripheral aromatization of androgens is likely to be due to an increase in the peripheral blood flow and and not to the direct effect of T_4 on the aromatase complex.[43,44,47]

One of the earliest clinical changes observed in thyrotoxicosis was the occurrence of amenorrhea, which was first reported in 1840.[48] Amenorrhea has been reported frequently since then, but a number of other changes in menstrual cycles have been noted, including anovulation, oligomenorrhea,[31] and menometrorrhagia, which is more common in hypothyroidism. Whether these changes are due to a direct action of T_4 on the ovary and uterus or on the pituitary and hypothalamus or both is uncertain. The effect of T_4 on fertility is less well established, although the disturbances in menstrual cycles will obviously disturb fertility. With therapy, the menstrual cycles return to their regular pattern for the individual.

In summary, thyrotoxicosis occurring in prepubertal girls may result in slightly delayed menarche. In adult women, the effects of thyrotoxicosis on the reproductive system are seen on the hypothalamic–pituitary axis with alterations in gonadotropin release and also in the circulating levels of SHBG, which alter steroid metabolism or biologic activity. These effects produce the variable clinical picture seen in women with thyrotoxicosis.

Experimental Data

There are few data on the effects of excess thyroid hormone on the development of the female reproductive tract. The administration of large doses of thyroxine (T_4) to the neonatal rat resulted in a delay in vaginal opening and the first estrous.[49] Because the period of administration was brief (5 days) and was followed by a period of hypothyroidism, whether the excess T_4 or the subsequent hypothyroidism caused the delay in sexual development is uncertain. In the adult female rat, administration of T_4 in high doses resulted in long periods of diestrous with few mature follicles of corpora lutea.[50] Cohen found in 1935 that pituitaries from hyperthyroid animals were more likely to cause precocious puberty after being implanted in immature females than pituitaries from control animals.[51] In contrast, the administration of excess thyroid hormone has been reported to cause an increase or no change in pituitary LH and a decrease in serum LH.[52] Thyroid hormone has been reported to synergize with FSH to stimulate differentiation of porcine granulosa cells.[53]

Because thyroid hormone receptors have been reported to be present in the uterus,[54] changes in the uterus could be expected after administration of thyroid hormone. Feeding thyroid hormone in excess to mice causes thickened endometria,[55] and Ruh *et al.* reported that T_4 decreased estradiol uptake and retention by the rat uterus.[56] Schultze and Noonan reported a reduced uterine response to estrogen in thyrotoxic rats.[57]

A marked excess of thyroid hormone would seem to be deleterious to pregnancy and has been reported to cause abortion and neonatal death,[58] perhaps through a direct effect on trophoblastic function.[59] However, a lesser degree of thyrotoxicosis was reported to help in the maintenance of implantation of delayed blastocysts and an increase in litter size.[57]

Hyperthyroidism and Physical Development

Children born with neonatal Graves' disease have no defects in the reproductive system that can be related to this disease. Physical development is normal, however, and skeletal growth is often accelerated without a modification of final height.[60] The delay in puberty may be related to the impact of thyrotoxicosis on body composition (i.e., decreased percentage of body fat), which is thought to be related to the onset of puberty and menarche.[61] Rarely, thyrotoxicosis may occur in children in association with polyostotic fibrous dysplasia, *café au lait* pigmentation, and precocious puberty (McCune-Albright syndrome).[62,63] Precosity has been described in one-third of the affected girls; and large, unilateral follicular cysts may be present and presumably are responsible for the sexual precocity of the gonadotropin-independent type. Thyrotoxicosis results from single or multiple thyroid adenomas.

Hyperthyroidism and Menstrual Cycle

Thyrotoxicosis occurring before puberty has been reported to delay sexual maturation and the onset of menses,[31] although Saxena did note that, in thyrotoxic girls, the mean age of menarche was slightly advanced over that of their control population without endocrine disease.[64] The association of thyrotoxicosis and precocity in this disorder appears to be coincidental.[65,66]

Although ovulatory menstrual cycles occur in women with thyrotoxicosis,[67] menstrual disturbances are common. Therefore, the possibility of pregnancy should be considered in an amenorrheic thyrotoxic woman. This is important because many of these women may receive treatment with radioactive iodine, which is contraindicated in pregnancy. Oligomenorrhea is the most common abnormality,[31] and it may progress to amenorrhea, first described in the classic study by von Basedow.[48] Polymenorrhea is distinctly less frequent, in comparison to its occurrence in hypothyroidism. The frequency of these menstrual disorders varies in different series. Benson and Dailey found that out of 221 hyperthyroid patients 58% had oligomenorrhea or amenorrhea and 5% polymenorrhea.[67] This is in general agreement with other older studies such as those of Goldsmith *et al.*[68] More recently, in India Joshi *et al.* found menstrual irregularities in 64.7% of hyperthyroid women, compared to 17.2% of healthy controls.[69] These irregularities sometimes preceded thyroid dysfunction. However, Krassas *et al.* found irregular cycles in only 21.5% out of 214 thyrotoxic patients. These discrepant results may be attributed to either genetic and other factors or to more delayed diagnosis in India than in Greece.[70] The weight loss and psychologic disturbances (primarily anxiety) seen in thyrotoxicosis may also contribute to sexual dysfunction.[71] Thyrotoxic women frequently present with increased LH, FSH, and estrogen levels[72]; and the gonadotropin response to gonadotropin-releasing hormone (GnRH) is increased,[73] although the mid-cycle LH peak may be reduced or absent.[72]

HYPOTHYROIDISM AND THE FEMALE REPRODUCTIVE SYSTEM

Production of SHBG is decreased in hypothyroidism. As a result, serum estradiol and testosterone concentrations are reduced, although free levels of these hormones remain normal. The metabolism of both androgens and estrogens is also altered in hypothyroidism. Androgen secretion is decreased, and the metabolic transformation of testosterone shifts toward androstenedione rather than androsterone, the reverse of that seen in hyperthyroidism.[43,45,74] With respect to estradiol and estrone, hypothyroidism favors metabolism of these steroids via 16α-hydroxylation over 2-oxygenation, resulting in increased formation of estriol at the expense of 2-hydroxyestrone and its derivative, 2-methohyestrone. The alterations in steroid metabolism disappear when the euthyroid state is restored.[43] Serum FSH and LH values are usually normal, but the midcycle FSH and LH surge may be blunted or absent. In postmenopausal women, serum FSH and LH concentrations may be somewhat lower than expected, and the response to GnRH may be reduced.[75]

The anovulation is reflected in the frequent finding of aproliferative endometrium on endometrial biopsy.[67] TRα-1 and TRβ-1 receptors have been found in follicular fluid.[76] Earlier work indicated that thyroxine enhanced the action of gonadotropins on luteinization and progestin secretion by cultured granulosa cells,[77] and it has been recently noted that in a group of infertile women, those with elevated TSH levels had a higher incidence of out-of-phase biopsies than women with normal TSH.[78] The defects in hemostasis reported in hypothyroidism, such as decreased levels of factors VII, VIII, IX, and XI, may also contribute to the pathogenesis of polymenorrhea.[79] Ovulation and conception can occur in mild hypothyroidism, but in the past those pregnancies that did occur were often associated with abortions in the first trimester, stillbirths, or prematurity.[31,80,81] Recent studies indicate these events may be less common but that gestational hypertension occurs often in pregnant women with untreated hypothyroidism.[82] Pregnancy occurring in women with myxedema has been reported to be uncommon,[81] but this is somewhat hard to document and may be the result of anovulation. The use of L-thyroxine is not helpful in treating euthyroid patients for infertility, menstrual irregularity, or the premenstrual syndrome.[83,84]

Some myxedematous women will present with amenorrhea and galactorrhea and elevated serum prolactin concentrations.[31] Thus, thyroid evaluation should be an essential part of the work-up in any person with galactorrhea. If hypothyroidism is the cause, the amenorrhea and galactorrhea and elevated serum prolactin will disappear promptly with thyroxine therapy.[85]

There is an increased incidence of Hashimoto's thyroiditis in individuals with Turner's syndrome,[86] and, although a chromosomal linkage between autoimmune disease and the X chromosome has been suggested, this has not been confirmed.[87] Inherited abnormalities in serum TBG are X-linked, and patients with Turner's syndrome may have low serum TBG values.[88]

Women with hypothyroidism have decreased metabolic clearance rates of androstenedione and estrone and increased peripheral aromatization.[89] The ratio of 5α/5β metabolites of androgens is decreased in hypothyroid women, and there is an increase in the excretion of estriol and a decrease in the excretion of 2-hydroxyestrone and its derivative 2-methoxyestrone.[45]

Experimental Data

In sheep, fetal hypothyroidism does not affect reproductive tract development but does result in prolonged gestation despite maternal euthyroidism.[90] However, in the rat, fetal hypothyroidism results in small ovaries deficient in lipid and cholesterol.[91] Thyroidectomy of sexually immature rats results in delayed vaginal opening and sexual maturation; smaller ovaries and follicles than in controls[58,92]; and uteri and vaginas that are not well developed.[93]

When adult female rats are rendered hypothyroid, their estrous cycles become irregular and their ovaries become atrophic.[94] There is an enhanced response to hCG with the development of large cystic ovaries in hypothyroid rats.[95] Hypothyroidism in hamsters and cows is associated with abnormal estrous cycles,[96,97] and in hypothyroid hens there is a decrease in egg production.[97] In the mature female rat, hypothyroidism apparently does not result in sterility but does interfere with gestation, especially in the first half of pregnancy,[98] with resorption of the embryo and subsequent reduction in litter size and an increase in stillbirths.[99]

In hypothyroid sheep, the uterus shows endometrial hyperplasia and smooth muscle hypertrophy, perhaps related to the prolonged estrous noted in hypothyroid ewes.[100] Ruh *et al.*[56] reported increased estradiol binding in uteri of hypothyroid rats, but Kirkland and coworkers[101] found a decrease in the uterine response to estrogen in hypothyroid rats. Hypothyroidism inhibits the photoperiod responses and seasonal breeding patterns in sheep and birds.[102,103]

Hypothyroidism and Physical Development

The reproductive tract appears to develop normally in cretins; thus, hypothyroidism during fetal life does not appear to affect the normal development of the reproductive tract. Hypothyroidism in prepubertal years generally leads to short stature and may lead to a delay in sexual maturity.[92]

Hypothyroidism and the Menstrual Cycle

An interesting syndrome described by Kendle[104] and Van Wyk and Grumbach[105] occurs not infrequently: it is characterized by precocious menstruation, galactorrhea, and sella enlargement in girls with juvenile hypothyroidism. The cause is thought to be an overlap in the pituitary production of TSH and gonadotropins, with the latter causing early ovarian secretion of estrogens and subsequent endometrial stimulation with vaginal bleeding. Prolactin levels are elevated, leading to galactorrhea. The estrogen and progesterone response of the ovary to human chorionic gonadotropin is increased, possibly from prolactin induction of ovarian LH receptors. In this way hyperprolactinemia may sensitize the ovaries to the low circulating gonadotropin levels present prepubertally. However, there is no pubertal increase in the adrenal production of androgen precursors, so that axillary and pubic hair are usually not apparent.[105] Therapy with thyroxine in proper dosage results in prompt alleviation of the symptoms.

In adult women, hypothyroidism results in changes in cycle length and amount of bleeding[31,106,107] and has been reported in association with the ovarian hyperstimulation syndrome.[108] In an Indian study, 68.2% of hypothyroid women had menstrual abnormalities, compared to 12.2% of healthy controls.[69] Menorrhagia is a frequent complaint and is probably due to estrogen breakthrough bleeding secondary to anovulation, which is frequent in severe hypothyroidism.[31]

Some investigators have reported a high incidence of thyroid hypofunction in women with premenstrual syndrome.[109–112] Most of the thyroid disease was subclinical hypothyroidism, defined as an augmented response of TSH to TRH. Many of the affected women were reported to have complete relief of premenstrual syndrome (PMS) symptoms with L-T_4 therapy. Questions have been raised, however, about patients selection, PMS diagnostic criteria, and the lack of well-defined controls.[113]

REFERENCES

1. CHAN, S.T., F. BROOK, A. AHUJA, *et al.* 1998. Alteration of thyroid blood flow during the normal menstrual cycle. Ultrasound Med. Biol. **24:** 15–20.
2. LEMARCHAND-BERAUD, T., G. RAPPOPORT, G. MAGRINI, *et al.* 1974. Influences of different physiological conditions on the gonadotropins and thyrotropin responses to LHRH and TRH. Horm. Metab. Res. **5**(Suppl.)**:** 170–179.
3. HAIGLER, E.D., JR., J.A. PITTMAN, JR., J.M. HERSHMAN & C.M. BAUGH. 1971. Direct evaluation of pituitary thyrotropin reserve utilizing synthetic thyrotropin releasing hormone. J. Clin. Endocrinol. Metab. **33:** 573–581.
4. SNYDER, P.J. & R.D. UTIGER. 1972. Response to thyrotropin releasing hormone (TRH) in normal man. J. Clin. Endocrinol. Metab. **34:** 380–385.
5. NOEL, G.L., R.C. DIMOND, L. WARTOFSKY, *et al.* 1974. Studies of prolactin and TSH secretion by continuous infusion of small amounts of thyrotropin-releasing hormone. J. Clin. Endocrinol. Metab. **39:** 6–17.
6. SANCHEZ-FRANCO, F., M.D. GARCIA, L. CACICEDO, *et al.* 1973. Influence of sex phase of menstrual cycle on thyrotropin (TSH) response to thyrotropin-releasing hormone. J. Clin. Endocrinol. Metab. **37:** 736–740.
7. RAMEY, J.N., G.N. BURROW, R.K. POLACKWICH & R.K. DONABEDIAN. 1975. The effect of oral contraceptive steroids on the response of thyroid-stimulating hormone to thyrotropin-releasing hormone. J. Clin. Endocrinol. Metab. **40:** 712–714.
8. COLON, J.M., J.B., LESSING, C. YAVETZ, *et al.* 1988. The effect of thyrotropin-releasing hormone stimulation on serum levels of gonadotropins in women during the follicular and luteal phases of the menstrual cycle. Fertil. Steril. **49:** 809–812.
9. RASMUSSEN, N.G., P.J. HORNES, L. HEGEDUS & U. FELDT-RASMUSSEN. 1989. Serum thyroglobulin during the menstrual cycle, during pregnancy, and post partum. Acta Endocrinol. (Copenhagen) **121:** 168–173.
10. GROSS, H.A., M.D. APPLEMAN & J.T. NICHOLOFF. 1971. Effect of biologically active steroids on thyroid function in man. J. Clin. Endocrinol. Metab. **73:** 242–248.
11. KARSCH, F.J., G.E. DAHL, T.M. HACHIGIAN & L.A. THRUN. 1995. Involvement of thyroid hormones in seasonal reproduction. J. Reprod. Fertil. Suppl. **49:** 409–422.
12. REINERT, B.D. & F.E. WILSON. 1996. The thyroid and the hypothalamus–pituitary–ovarian axis in American tree sparrows (*Spizella arborea*). Gen. Comp. Endocrinol. **103:** 60–70.
13. TAMURA, K., M. HATSUTA, G. WATANABE, *et al.* 1998. Inhibitory regulation of inhibin gene expression by thyroid hormone during ovarian development in immature rats. Biochem. Biophys. Res. Commun. **242:** 102–108.
14. ATALLA, F. & E.P. REINEKE. 1951. Influence of environmental temperature and thyroid status on reproductive organs of young female mice. Fed. Proc. **10:** 6–7.
15. BECK, R.P., D.M. FAWCETT & F. MORCOS. 1972. Thyroid function studies in different phases of the menstrual cycle and in women receiving norethindrone with or without estrogen. Am. J. Obstet. Gynecol. **112:** 369–373.
16. ZHU, Y.S., T. DELLOVADE & D.W. PFAFF. 1997. Gender-specific induction of pituitary RNA by estrogen and its modification by thyroid hormone. J. Neuroendocrinol. **9:** 395–403.
17. GREGORASZCZUK, E.L. & M. SKALKA. 1996. Thyroid hormone as a regulator of basal and human chorionic gonadotrophin-stimulated steroidogenesis by cultured porcine theca and granulosa cells isolated at different stages of the follicular phase. Reprod. Fertil. Dev. **8:** 961–967.
18. DATTA, M., R.J. NAGENDRA PRASAD & S. BHATTAHARYA. 1999. Thyroid hormone regulation of perch ovarian 3β-hydroxysteroid dehydrogenase/delta5-delta4-isomerase activity: involvement of a 52-kDa protein. Gen. Comp. Endocrinol. **113:** 212–220.

19. BHATTAHARYA, S., S. GUIN, A. BANDYOPADHYAY, *et al.* 1996. Thyroid hormone induces the generation of a novel putative protein in piscine ovarian follicle that stimulates the conversion of pregnenolone to progesterone. Eur. J. Endocrinol. **134:** 128–135.
20. LARIVIERE, F., R. MOUSSALLI & D.R. GARREL. 1994. Increased leucine flux and leucine oxidation during the luteal phase of the menstrual cycle in women. Am. J. Physiol. **267:** E422–E428.
21. PANSINI, F., P. BASSI, A.R. CAVALLINI, *et al.* 1987. Effect of hormonal contraception on serum reverse triiodothyronine levels. Gynecol. Obstet. Invest. **23:** 133–134.
22. DAINAT, J., C. BRESSOT, A. REBIERE & P. VIGNERON. 1986. Ontogenesis of triiodothyronine nuclear receptors in three skeletal muscles in male and female chicks. Gen. Comp. Endocrinol. **62:** 479–484.
23. WAKIM, A.M., W.R., PALJUG, K.M. JASNOSZ, *et al.* 1994. Thyroid hormone receptor messenger ribonucleic acid in human granulosa and ovarian stromal cells. Fertil. Steril. **62:** 531–534.
24. OPPENHEIMER, J.H. 1968. Role of plasma proteins in the binding distribution and metabolism of the thyroid hormones. N. Engl. J. Med. **278:** 1153–1162.
25. MAN, E.B., W.A. REID, A.E. HELHEGERS & W.E. JONES. 1969. Thyroid function in human pregnancy. III. Serum thyroxine-binding prealbumin (TBPA) and thyroxine-binding globulin (TBG) of pregnant women aged 14 through 43 years. Am. J. Obstet. Gynecol. **103:** 338–347.
26. AIN, K.B., Y. MORI & S. REFETOFF. 1987. Reduced clearance rate of thyroxine-binding globulin (TBG) with increased sialylation: a mechanism for estrogen-induced elevation of serum TBG concentration. J. Clin. Endocrinol. Metab. **65:** 689–696.
27. BRAVERMAN, L.E. & S.H. INGBAR. 1967. Effects of norethandrolone on the transport in serum and peripheral turnover of thyroxine. J. Clin. Endocrinol. Metab. **27:** 38–396.
28. BARTALENA, L. 1990. Recent achievements in studies on thyroid hormone-binding proteins. Endocrinol. Rev. **11:** 47–64.
29. MENDEL, C.M. 1989. The free hormone hypothesis: a physiologically based mathematical model. Endocrinol. Rev. **10:** 232–274.
30. ARAFAH, B.M. 1994. Decreased levothyroxine requirement in women with hypothyroidism during androgen therapy for breast cancer. Ann. Intern. Med. **121:** 247–251.
31. THOMAS, R. & R.L. REID. 1987. Thyroid disease and reproductive dysfunction: a review. Obstet. Gynecol. **70:** 789–798.
32. YAMAZAKI, K., K. SATO, K. SHIZUME, *et al.* 1995. Potent thyrotropic activity of human chorionic gonadotropin variants in terms of ^{125}I incorporation and *de novo* synthesized thyroid hormone release in human thyroid follicles. J. Clin. Endocrinol. Metab. **80:** 473–479.
33. FITKO, R. & B. SZLEZYNGIER. 1994. Role of thyroid hormone in controlling the concentration of luteinizing hormone/human chorionic gonadotropin receptors in rat ovaries. Eur. J. Endocrinol. **130:** 378–380.
34. DE REMIGIS, P., B. RAGGIUNTI, A. NEPAL, *et al.* 1990. Thyroid volume variation during the menstrual cycle in healthy subjects. *In* Chronobiology: Its Role in Clinical Medicine, General Biology, and Agriculture. D.K. Hayes, J.E. Pauly & R.J. Reiter, Eds.: 169. Wiley-Liss. New York.
35. JENKINS, E.P., S. ANDERSSON, J. IMPERATO-MCGINLEY, *et al.* 1992. Genetic and pharmacological evidence for more than one human steroid 5α-reductase. J. Clin. Invest. **89:** 293–300.
36. CROOKS, J., M.I. TULLOCH, A.C. TURNBULL, *et al.* 1967. Comparative incidence of goitre in pregnancy in Iceland and Scotland. Lancet **2:** 625–627.
37. BAUCH, K., W. MENG, F.E. ULRICH, *et al.* 1986. Thyroid status during pregnancy and postpartum in regions of iodine deficiency and endemic goiter. Endocrinol. Exp. **20:** 67–77.
38. GLINOER, D., P. DE NAYER, P. BOURDOUX, *et al.* 1990. Regulation of maternal thyroid during pregnancy.J. Clin. Endocrinol. Metab. **71:** 276–287.
39. GLINOER, D. & M. LEMONE. 1992. Goiter and pregnancy: a new insight into an old problem. Thyroid **2:** 65–70.
40. HEGEDUS, L., S. KARSTRUP & N. RASMUSSEN. 1986. Evidence of cyclic alterations of thyroid size during the menstrual cycle in healthy women. Am. J. Obstet. Gynecol. **155**(1): 142–145.

41. ROSNER, W. 1990. The functions of corticosteroid-binding globulin and sex hormone-binding globulin: recent advances. Endocrinol. Rev. **11:** 80–91.
42. RIDGWAY, E.C., C. LONGCOPE & F. MALOOF. 1975. Metabolic clearance and blood production rates of estradiol in hyperthyroidism. J. Clin. Endocrinol. Metab. **41:** 491–497.
43. GORDON, G.G. & A.L. SOUTHREN. 1977. Thyroid-hormone effects on steroid-hormone metabolism. Bull. N.Y. Acad. Med. **53:** 241–259.
44. RIDGWAY, E.C., F. MALLOF & C. LONGCOPE. 1982. Androgen and oestrogen dynamics in hyperthyroidism. J. Endocrinol. **95:** 105–115.
45. GALLAGHER, T.F., D.K. FUKUSHIMA, S. NOGUCHI, *et al.* 1966. Recent studies in steroid hormone metabolism in man. Recent Prog. Horm. Res. **22:** 283–303.
46. SOUTHREN, A.L., J. OLIVO, G.G. GORDON, *et al.* 1973. The conversion of androgens to estrogens in hyperthyroidism. J. Clin. Endocrinol. Metab. **38:** 207–214.
47. LONGCOPE, C. 1987. Peripheral aromatization: studies on controlling factors. Steroids **50:** 253–267.
48. VON BASEDOW, C.A. 1840. Exophthalmos durch hypertrophie des Zellgewebes in der Augenhohl. Wochenschrift Heilk. **6:** 197.
49. GELLERT, R.J., J.L. BAKKE & N.L. LAWRENCE. 1971. Delayed vaginal opening in the rat following pharmacologic doses of T_4 administered during the neonatal period. J. Lab. Clin. Med. **77:** 410–416.
50. LEATHEM, J.H. 1961. Nutritional effects on endocrine secretions. *In* Sex and Internal Secretions. W.C. Young, Ed.: 666. Williams & Wilkins. Baltimore.
51. COHEN, R.S. 1935. Effect of experimentally produced hyperthyroidism upon the reproductive and associated organs of the male rat. Am. J. Anat. **56:** 143–154.
52. HOWLAND, B.E. & E.A. IBRAHIM. 1973. Hyperthyroidism and gonadotropin secretion in male and female rats. Experientia **29:** 1398–1399.
53. MARUO, T., S. HIRAMATSU, T. OTANI, *et al.* 1992. Increase in the expression of thyroid hormone receptors in porcine granulosa cells early in follicular maturation. Acta. Endocrinol. **127:** 152–160.
54. EVANS, R.W., A.P. FARWELL & L.E. BRAVERMAN. 1983. Nuclear thyroid hormone receptors in the rat uterus. Endocrinology **113:** 1459–1463.
55. REINEKE, E.P. & F.A. SOLIMAN. 1953. Role of thyroid hormone in reproductive physiology in the female. Iowa State Col. J. Sci. **28:** 67.
56. RUH, M.F., T.S. RUH & H.M. KLITGAARD. 1970. Uptake and retention of estrogens by uteri from rats in various thyroid states. Proc. Soc. Biol. Med. **134:** 558–561.
57. SCHULTZE, A.B. & J. NOONAN. 1970. Thyroxine administration and reproduction in rats. J. Anim. Sci. **30:** 774–776.
58. LEATHEM, J.H. 1972. Role of the thyroid. *In* Reproductive Biology. H. Balin & S. Glasser, Eds.: 23. Excerpta Medica. Amsterdam.
59. MARUO, T., H. MATSUO & M. MOCHIZUKI. 1991. Thyroid hormone as a biological amplifier of differentiated trophoblast function in early pregnancy. Acta. Endocrinol. **125:** 58–66.
60. SCHLESINGER, S., M.H. MCGILLIVRAY & R.W. MUNSCHAUER. 1973. Acceleration of growth and bone maturation in childhood thyrotoxicosis. J. Pediatr. **83:** 233–236.
61. FRISCH, R.E. & J.W. MCARTHUR. 1974. Menstrual cycles: fatness as a determinant of minimum weight for height necessary for their maintenance or onset. Science **185:** 949–951.
62. DIGEORGE, A.M. 1975. Editorial: Albright syndrome: is it coming of age? J. Pediatr. **87:** 1018–1020.
63. MASTORAKOS, G., N.S. MITSIADES, A.G. DOUFAS & D.A. KOUTRAS. 1997. Hyperthyroidism in McCune-Albright syndrome with a review of thyroid abnormalities sixty years after the first report. Thyroid **7:** 433–439.
64. SAXENA, K.M., J.D. CRAWFORD & N.B. TALBOT. 1964. Childhood thyrotoxicosis: a long-term prospective. Br. Med. J. **4:** 1153–1158.
65. FEUILLAN, P., T. SHAWKER, S. ROSE, *et al.* 1990. Thyroid abnormalities in the McCune-Albright syndrome: ultrasonography and hormonal studies. J. Clin. Endocrinol. Metab. **71:** 1596–1601.
66. MARTIN, J.B. & S. REICHLIN. 1987. Clinical Neuroendocrinology. Davis. Philadelphia, PA.

67. BENSON, R.C. & M.E. DAILEY. 1955. Menstrual pattern in hyperthyroidism and subsequent post-therapy hypothyroidism. Surg. Gynaecol. Obstet. **100:** 19–26.
68. GOLDSMITH, R.E., S.H. STURGIS, J. LERMAN & J.B. STANBURY. 1952. The menstrual pattern of thyroid disease. J. Clin. Endocrinol. Metab. **18:** 846–855.
69. JOSCHI, J.V., S.D. BHANDARKAR, M. CHANDHA, *et al.* 1993. Menstrual irregularities and lactation failure may precede thyroid dysfunction of goitre. J. Postgrad. Med. **39:** 137–141.
70. KRASSAS, G.E., N. PONTIKIDES, TH. KALTSAS, *et al.* 1994. Menstrual disturbances in thyrotoxicosis. Clin. Endocrinol. **40:** 641–644.
71. ROGER, J. 1958. Menstruation and systemic disease. N. Engl. J. Med. **259:** 676–681.
72. AKANDE, E.O. & T.R. HOCKADAY. 1975. Plasma concentration of gonadotrophins, oesrtrogens and progesterone in thyrotoxic women. Br. J. Obstet. Gynaecol. **82:** 541–551.
73. ERFURTH, E.M. & P. HEDNER. 1987. Increased plasma gonadotropin levels in spontaneous hyperthyroidism reproduced by thyroxine but not by triiodothyronine administration to normal subjects. J. Clin. Endocrinol. Metab. **64:** 698–703.
74. GORDON, G.G., A.L. SOUTHREN, S. TOCHIMOTO, *et al.* 1969. Effect of hyperthyroidism and hypothyroidism on the metabolism of testosterone and androstenedione in man. J. Clin. Endocrinol. Metab. **29:** 164.
75. DISTILLER, L.A., J. SAGEL & J.E. MORLEY. 1975. Assessment of pituitary gonadotropin reserve using luteinizing hormone-releasing hormone (LRH) in states of altered thyroid function. J. Clin. Endocrinol. Metab. **40:** 512–515.
76. WAKIM, A.N., S.L. POLIZZOTO, M.L. BUFFO, *et al.* 1993. Thyroid hormones in human follicular fluid and thyroid hormone receptors in human granulosa cells. Fertil. Steril. **59:** 1187–1190.
77. CHANNING, C.P., V. TSAI & D. SACHS. 1976. Role of insulin, thyroxine and cortisol in luteinization of porcine granulosa cells grown in chemically defined media. Biol. Reprod. **15:** 235–247.
78. GERHARD, I., T. BECKER, W. EGGERT-KRUSE, *et al.* 1991. Thyroid and ovarian function in infertile woman. Hum. Reprod. **6:** 338–345.
79. ANSELL, J.E. 1991. The blood in hypothyroidism. *In* Werner & Ingbar's The Thyroid: A Fundamental and Clinical Text. 6th edit. L.E. Braverman & R.D. Utiger, Eds.: 1022–1026. Lippincott. New York.
80. DANIELS, G.H. 1995. Thyroid disease and pregnancy: A clinical overview. Endocrinol. Pract. **1:** 287–301.
81. DAVIS, L.E., K.J. LEVENO & F.G. CUNNINGHAM. 1988. Hypothyroidism complicating pregnancy. Obstet. Gynecol. **72:** 108–112.
82. LEUNG, A.S., L.K. MILLAR, P.P. KOONINGS, *et al.* 1993. Perinatal outcome in hypothyroid pregnancies. Obstet. Gynecol. **81:** 349–353.
83. NIKOLAI, T.F., G.M. MULLIGAN, R.K. GRIBBLE, *et al.* 1990. Thyroid function and treatment in premenstrual syndrome. J. Clin. Endocrinol. Metab. **70:** 1108–1113.
84. ROTI, E., R. MINELLI, E. GARDINI & L.E. BRAVERMAN. 1993. The use and misuse of thyroid hormone. Endocrinol. Rev. **14:** 401–423.
85. EDWARDS, C.R.W., I.A. FORSYTH & G.M. BESSER. 1971. Amenorrhea, galactorrhea and primary hypothyroidism with high circulating levels of prolactin. Br. Med. J. **3:** 462–464.
86. VAN CAMPENHOUT, J., J. VAN, A. ANTAKI & E. RASIO. 1973. Diabetes mellitus and thyroid autoimmunity in gonadal dysgenesis. Fertil. Steril. **24:** 1–9.
87. VALLOTTON, M.B. & A.P. FORBES. 1967. Autoimmunity in gonadal dysgenesis and Klinefelter's syndrome. Lancet **1:** 648–651.
88. REFETOFF, S. & H.A. SELENKOW. 1968. Familial thyroxine-binding globulin deficiency in a patient with Turner's syndrome (XO): genetic study of a kindred. N. Engl. J. Med. **278:** 1081–1087.
89. LONGCOPE, C., S. ABEND, L.E. BRAVERMAN & C.H. EMERSON. 1990. Androstenedione and estrone dynamics in hypothyroid women. J. Clin. Endocrinol. Metab. **70:** 90–907.
90. HOPKINS, P.S. & G.D. THORBURN. 1972. The effects of foetal thyrodectomy on the development of the ovine foetus. J. Endocrinol. **54:** 55.

91. Leathem, J.H. 1959. Extragonadal function in reproduction. *In* Recent Progress in the Endocrinology of Reproduction. C.W. Lloyd, Ed.: 179. Academic Press. New York.
92. Hayles, A.B. & M.D. Cloutire. 1972. Clinical hypothyroidism in the young—a second look. Med. Clin. N. Am. **56:** 871–884.
93. Scow, R.O. & M.E. Simpson. 1945. Thyroidectomy in the newborn rat. Anat. Rec. **91:** 209–226.
94. Ortega, E., E. Rodriguez & E. Ruiz. 1990. Activity of the hypothalamo–pituitary–ovarian axis in hypothyroid rats with or without triiodothyronine replacement. Life Sci. **46:** 391–395.
95. Takacs-Jarrett, M. & B.C. Bruot. 1994. Steroid secretion by follicles and cysts from the hypothyroid hCG-treated rat. Soc. Experimental. Biol. Med. **207:** 62–66.
96. Vriend, J., F.D. Bertalanffy & T.A. Ralcewicz. 1987. The effects of melatonin and hypothyroidism on estradiol and gonadotropin levels in female Syrian hamsters. Biol. Reprod. **36:** 719–728.
97. Maqsood, M. 1952. Thyroid functions in relation to reproduction of mammals and birds. Biol. Rev. **27:** 281–319.
98. Bonet, B. & E. Herrera. 1991. Maternal hypothyroidsm during the first half of gestation compromises normal catabolic adaptations of late gestation in the rat. Endocrinology **129:** 210–216.
99. Rao, P.M. & J.N. Panda. 1981. Uterine enzyme changes in thyroidectomized rats at parturition. J. Reprod. Fertil. **61:** 109–113.
100. Nesbitt, R.E., Jr., R.W. Abdul-Karim, J.T. Prior, *et al.* 1967. Study of the effect of experimentally induced endocrine insults upon pregnant and nonpregnant ewes. III. ACTH and propyl-thiouracil administration and the production of polycystic ovaries. Fertil. Steril. **18:** 739–758.
101. Kirkland, J.L., R.M. Gardner, V.R. Mukku, *et al.* 1981. Hormonal control of uterine growth: the effect of hypothyroidism on estrogen-stimulated cell division. Endocrinology **108:** 2346–2351.
102. Moenter, S.M., C.J.L. Woodfill & F.J. Karsch. 1991. Role of the thyroid gland in seasonal reproduction: thyroidectomy blocks seasonal suppression of reproductive neuroendocrine activity in ewes. Endocrinology **128:** 1337–1344.
103. Dawson, A. 1993. Thyroidectomy progressively renders the reproductive system of starlings (*Sturnus vulgaris*) unresponsive to changes in day length. J. Endocrinol. **139:** 51–55.
104. Kendle, F.W. 1905. Case of precocious puberty in a female cretin. Br. Med. J. **1:** 246.
105. Van Wyk, J. & M.M. Grumbach. 1960. Syndrome of precocious menstruation and gactorrhea in juvenile hypothyroidism: an example of hormonal overlap pituitary feedback. J. Pediatr. **57:** 416–435.
106. Wilansky, D.L. & B. Greisman. 1989. Early hypothyroidism in patients with menorrhagia. Am. J. Obstet. Gynecol. **160:** 673–677.
107. Higham, J.M. & R.W. Shaw. 1992. The effect of thyroxine replacement on menstrual blood loss in a hypothyroid patient. Br. J. Obstet. Gynecol. **99:** 695–696.
108. Rotmensch, S. & A. Scommegna. 1989. Spontaneous ovarian hyperstimulation syndrome associated with hypothyroidism. Am. J. Obstet. Gynecol. **160:** 122–1222.
109. Roy-Byrne, P.P., D.R. Rubinow, M.C. Hoban, *et al.* 1987. TSH and prolactin response to TRH in patients with premenstrual syndrome. Am. J. Psychiatr. **144:** 480–484.
110. Schmidt, P.J., R.A. Kahn & D.R. Rubinow. 1986. Thyroid function in premenstrual syndrome. N. Engl. J. Med. **317:** 1537–1538.
111. Brayshaw, N.D. & D.D. Brayshaw. 1986. Thyroid hypofunction in premenstrual syndrome. N. Engl. J. Med. **315:** 1486–1487.
112. Girdler, S.S., G.A. Pedersen & K.C. Light. 1995. Thyroid axis function during the menstrual cycle in women with premenstrual syndrome. Psychoneuroendocrinology. **20:** 395–403.
113. Casper, R.F., A. Patel-Christofer & Am. Powell. 1989. Thyrotropin and prolactin responses to thyrotropin-releasing hormone in premenstrual syndrome. J. Clin. Endocrinol. Metab. **68:** 608–612.

Thyroidopathies

DEMETRIOS A. KOUTRAS[a]

Athens University School of Medicine, Endocrine Unit, "Evgenidion" Hospital, Athens, Greece

ABSTRACT: Pregnancy affects thyroid physiology in many ways: (a) The renal iodide clearance rate is increased, hence iodine requirements increase. (b) The fetal requirements for thyroid hormones and iodide are an additional problem. (c) Serum thyroxine-binding globulin increases, thus producing an increase in the levels of total T_4 and T_3. (d) Chorionic gonadotropin has a thyroid-stimulating activity. This may be compensated for by a decrease in TSH, but in some cases gestational thyrotoxicosis occurs. (e) Thyroid autoimmunity usually subsides during pregnancy, but may rebound a few months after parturition, and postpartum thyroiditis may occur. Because maternal antithyroid autoantibodies cross the placenta readily, fetal and neonatal hyperthyroidism (or hypothyroidism) may develop. Pre-existing thyroid diseases are influenced. Nontoxic goiter increases in size. Iodine and/or thyroxine may be required. Graves' disease may remit. If present, antithyroid drugs should be given in small doses, and quite often they may be stopped altogether. Hypothyroid patients may require a larger T_4 dose.

INTRODUCTION

Pregnancy increases the iodine requirements and affects thyroid physiology in several ways. Pregnancy affects the presentation, diagnosis, evolution, and treatment of various thyroid diseases. Finally, some thyroid diseases occur only in association with a pregnancy. To discuss all these topics in some detail would require a book, or at least a monograph. Therefore, only a few salient points will be mentioned here.

THYROID PHYSIOLOGY IN PREGNANCY

Iodine Balance

In pregnancy the renal iodide clearance increases to about double the value in nonpregnant women, and so the plasma inorganic iodine (PII) falls accordingly.[1,2] This renal iodide leak is probably not harmful in countries with an adequate iodine intake, and may even be beneficial in countries with a very high one, such as the United States and Japan. However, in countries with a marginal iodine intake, iodine deficiency goiter may develop in the mother[3] and also in her progeny. More details can be found in the review by Glinoer.[4] In areas with a low iodine intake, frank hypothyroidism and even cretinism may occur. Even in areas with a mild iodine deficiency, the average newborn TSH level may be increased. This has been observed by

[a]Address for correspondence: Prof. Demetrios A. Koutras, 35, Vas. Sofias Avenue, GR-106 75 Athens, Greece.

our group in cooperation with that of Prof. Beckers[5] in Greece, and since then confirmed by many others in several countries.

The Feto–Placental Unit

As if the renal iodide loss were not enough, the feto–placental unit constitutes an additional burden to the mother, one that manifests itself in many ways:

- The fetus depends on the mother for its iodine supply and the building of its own iodine stores.
- The fetus depends on its mother for its supply of thyroid hormones. The thyroid hormones thyroxine (T_4) and triiodothyronine (T_3) cross the placenta to a small degree, but these small amounts are of crucial importance for fetal development, especially at the first half of the pregnancy when the fetus does not produce its own hormones. Endemic cretinism is attributed, to a large degree, to such a lack of maternal thyroid hormones.
- The placenta deiodinates and so neutralizes most of the maternal thyroid hormones presented to it, as reviewed by Glinoer.[4] This process may protect the fetus from an excessive concentration of thyroid hormones, but taxes the hormone-producing machinery of the maternal thyroid.

An Increase in the Thyroid Hormone-Binding Capacity of the Maternal Plasma

It is common knowledge that estrogens increase the plasma level of thyroxine-binding globulin (TBG). This occurs during estrogen administration and estrogen overproduction, as in pregnancy. The result is that the total levels of T_4 and T_3 are high, but the free levels (fT_4 and fT_3) normal, and so the woman remains euthyroid.

From a kinetic point of view, it may be deduced that at the initial phase, that of increasing TBG levels, the maternal thyroid must increase its hormone production so as to increase the plasma pool of total thyroid hormones. When this is achieved, a new steady state occurs, that is, normal thyroid hormone production and degradation, but high peripheral pool. After parturition, when estrogens are reduced and TBG falls, the maternal thyroid must decrease its hormone supply to achieve a normal plasma pool, until a new steady state is achieved, that of normal secretion, pool, and degradation. Of course, this sketchy model is modified by the other factors involved, such as placental deiodination of thyroid hormones, the action of hCG, and so forth.

TSH-Like Activity of hCG

Human chorionic gonadotrophin (hCG) has a TSH-like activity. It seems that pure hCG has only a weak thyrotrophic activity, but other variants, such as asialo variants, are more potent.[6,7] The TSH activity of hCG is anyway weak compared to TSH, but since large amounts of hCG circulate in the plasma, the overall effect may be substantial. The pituitary may compensate for this thyroid-stimulating effect of hCG by decreasing the secretion of TSH, but in some cases a true increase in the level of free thyroid hormones may occur, as discussed later.

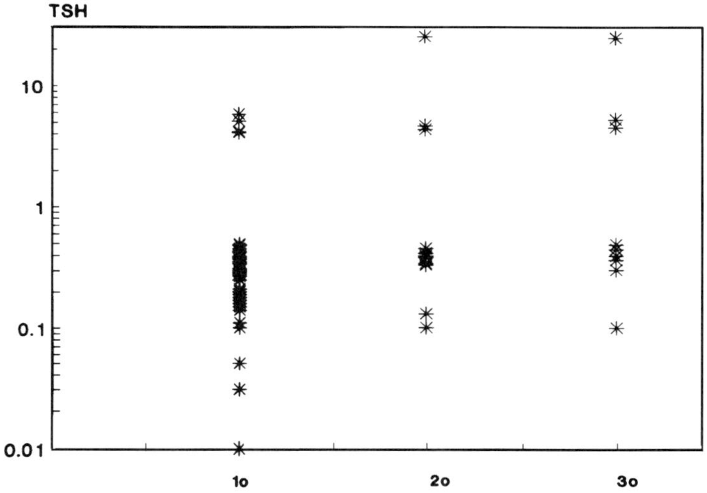

FIGURE 1. TSH values (mIU/l) in the three trimesters of pregnancy. The difference between the first and third trimester is almost significant ($p = 0.055$).

To better define this problem, we have done a cross-sectional study of pregnant women.[8] We studied a total of 411 pregnant women, 208 during the first trimester, 105 during the second, and 98 during the third. Their iodine intake was adequate even for pregnant women, with a mean ± SE urinary iodine:creatinine ratio of 284 ± 45 μg/g in the first trimester, 377 ± 66 in the second, and 301 ± 52 in the third.

The average TSH level (x ± SD) was 1.34 ± 0.76 mU/l in the first trimester, 1.48 ± 0.74 in the second, and 1.51 ± 0.73 in the third (FIG. 1). Out of 208 women in the first trimester, 48 (23%) had a low TSH (<0.4 μU/ml) and 4 (7%) a high one; of the 105 women in the second trimester, 14 (13%) had a low TSH and three (3%) a high one; whereas of 98 women in the third trimester, the corresponding figures were low, six (6%), and high, three (3%). Low TSH values were significantly more common during the first trimester ($\chi^2 = 14.92$; $p < 0.001$). The serum hCG was negatively correlated with the TSH level (FIG. 2) and positively to the fT_4 (FIG. 3) and the fT_3 (FIG. 4). Therefore, our findings are similar to those reported in the literature.

Immune Tolerance in Pregnancy

Pregnancy is associated with a degree of immune tolerance, which helps the mother to preserve the fetus and not reject it.[9] In this context, antithyroid autoantibodies (AAB) commonly decrease during pregnancy and rebound postpartum.[10–12] For this reason, autoimmune thyroid diseases frequently remit during pregnancy and exacerbate a few months after labor, as discussed later.

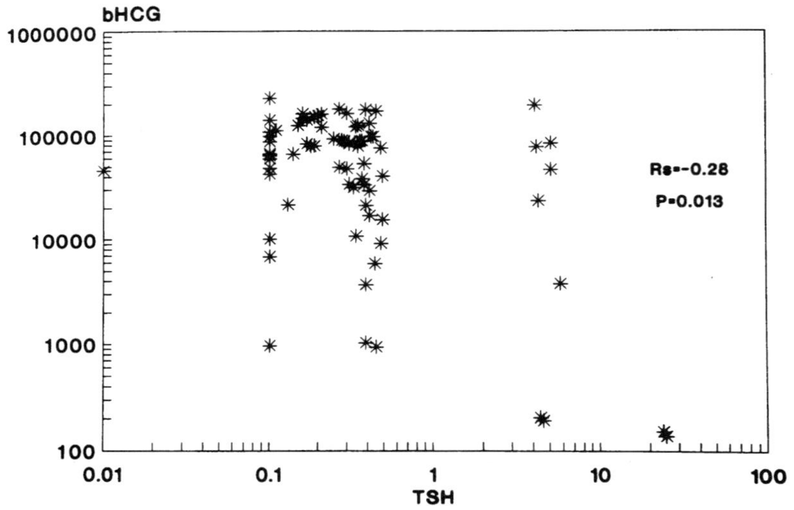

FIGURE 2. The relation between hCG (mIU/ml) and TSH (mIU/l). There is a significant negative correlation ($r = -0.28$; $p = 0.013$).

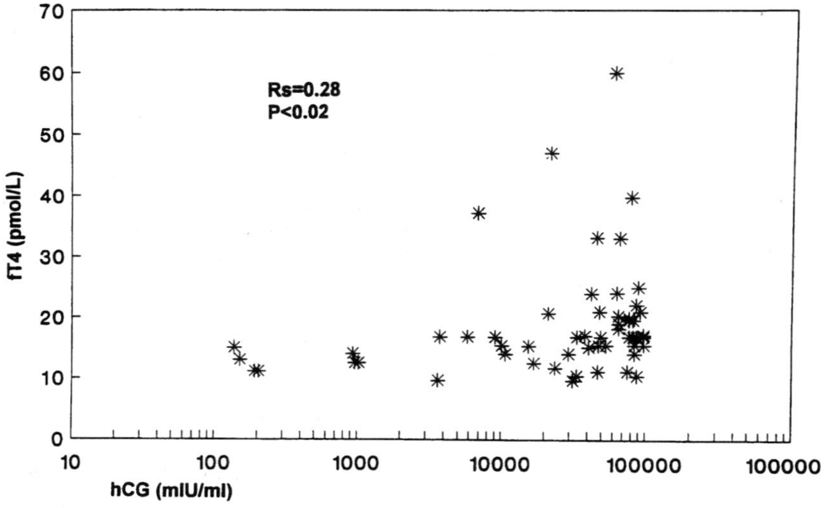

FIGURE 3. The relation between hCG and fT_4. There is a significant positive correlation ($r = 0.28$; $p < 0.02$).

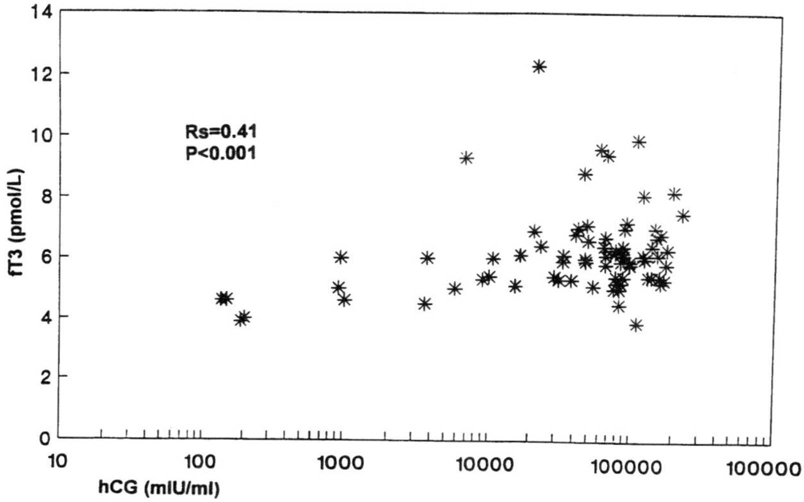

FIGURE 4. The relation between hCG and fT_3. There is a significant positive correlation ($r = 0.41$; $p = 0.001$).

DIAGNOSIS OF THYROID DISEASES IN PREGNANCY

Clinical diagnosis of thyroid diseases in pregnancy may be difficult. Tachycardia, sweating, and anxiety may be due to pregnancy itself rather than to hyperthyroidism; likewise, edema may simply be pregnancy-related, rather than due to hypothyroidism.

The main diagnostic difficulty in pregnancy is due to the increase in TBG and of the total thyroid hormone levels. An increase in total T_4 and total T_3 is a common finding in pregnancy and should by no means be taken as diagnostic of hyperthyroidism, as unfortunately happens from time to time. So, for diagnosing thyroid disease in pregnancy, the total levels of thyroid hormones should not be used. The physician must request estimations of the free levels (fT_4 and fT_3) or the indices: free thyroxine index (FTI); that is, $T_4 \times T_3U$ divided by the average normal T_3U value of the non-pregnant population. T_3U stands for T_3 uptake, that is, the *in vitro* uptake of T_3 by resin or some other substance. Similarly to the FTI, the FT_3I (free-T_3 index) may be calculated as $T_3 \times T_3U$ divided by the average normal T_3U value.

Determinations of the serum TSH levels in pregnancy remain a most valuable thyroid function test, in spite of a possible small decrease due to the presence of hCG.

COMMON THYROID DISEASES IN PREGNANCY

Nontoxic Goiter

As stated earlier in the discussion on iodine balance, pregnancy increases the iodine requirements and so induces or aggravates iodine-deficiency goiter. Chorionic gonadotropin also has a thyrotropic action. In ancient times, the visual detection of an increase in the goiter size in young women or pressure on a string tied round her neck were used as evidence of pregnancy. Recent, more sophisticated studies, using ultrasonograms, have amply confirmed these older observations, as reviewed by Glinoer[4] and Berghout and Wiersinga.[13] Not only does clinical goiter develop or enlarge during pregnancy, but also subclinical enlargements are detected by ultrasonography. In Belgium, Glinoer *et al.*[14] found an average increase of 18% initial size. These abnormalities may be prevented by an increase in the iodine supply to the mother with or without thyroxine.[15]

Established goiters in pregnancy should be treated with thyroxine administration. I advocate an aggressive approach in nonpregnant women in order to suppress the serum TSH level, but I am more conservative in pregnancy,[16] because suppressive thyroxine doses and the resulting iatrogenic hyperthyroidism may unduly tax the mother. In addition, in spite of the placental deiodination, some thyroxine may find its way to the fetus, and there is no guarantee that this may not be harmful. So, in pregnancy, it is better to aim at low-normal serum TSH values rather than to a complete suppression, for the purpose of preventing further growth of the goiter rather than achieving its eradication, which may be postponed for after parturition.

Autoimmune Graves' Hyperthyroidism

This type of hyperthyroidism is the most common one, especially in young women. It is due to autoantibodies against the TSH receptor. As an autoimmune disease, it may remit during pregnancy, and recur some time later. Active hyperthyroidism is associated with decreased fertility, and if pregnancy does occur, it is associated with several complications for both the mother (toxemia and miscarriage) and the fetus (congenital abnormalities).[17]

There is now no doubt whatsoever that a pregnant woman with Graves' disease should be treated. Radioiodine is completely contraindicated in pregnancy, because it readily crosses the placenta, and surgery should preferably be postponed. This leaves antithyroid drugs (ATDs), which are the treatment of choice.[18] Many years ago physicians were reluctant to use ATDs in pregnancy, because they cross the placenta and may result in goiter and hypothyroidism in the fetus. Now it is realized that with proper dosage these side effects are negligible,[18–20] and in any case the outcome is better with than without ATDs. Furthermore, the fact that they are crossing the placenta has also its beneficial aspect: ATDs protect the fetus from fetal Graves' disease due to the transplacental transfer of the maternal thyroid-stimulating autoantibodies, as discussed later.

ATDs should be given in as low a dose as possible, aiming at a high-normal maternal serum free thyroxine level (or FTI). In non-pregnant persons ATDs are commonly given with thyroid hormones (T_4 or T_3), in order to obtain smoother control. In pregnancy thyroid hormones should not be given together with ATDs. They cross the placenta at a smaller rate than ATDs, and so they cannot counteract their antithyroid action to the fetus. Furthermore, if they are omitted, hyperthyroidism may be controlled with a smaller dose of ATD. The proper treatment, then, is ATD at the lowest possible dose without thyroid hormones. Because thyroid hormones are not given and because the disease activity fluctuates in pregnancy, the woman should be examined frequently, every one or two months.

The three ATDs commonly used are methimazole, carbimazole (readily converted to methimazole after ingestion), and propylthiouracil. It has been stated that in pregnancy propylthiouracil is preferable, because it crosses the placenta to a smaller degree, a fact not confirmed by all authors, and because methimazole may induce aplasia cutis in the newborn. Nowadays, many endocrinologists consider that methimazole and propylthiouracil can both be recommended, without a clear advantage of one over the other.[21]

Nodular Toxic Goiter

Adequate data do not exist on nodular toxic goiter in pregnancy. One would expect that, since the plasma inorganic iodine falls, this condition should be ameliorated. Anyway, management should be as for Graves' disease: antithyroid drugs and after parturition probably thyroidectomy.

Hypothyroidism

Anovulation is common in overt hypothyroidism.[22] Hypothyroid women who nevertheless become pregnant have an increased risk of obstetricial complications[4] and also of a poor neonatal outcome, such as low birthweight, and also decreased (or impaired) mental capacity.[23] These complications of hypothyroidism may largely be prevented by adequate treatment with thyroxine.[24]

Thyroxine should be given, as usual, in doses that will normalize serum TSH. Pregnant women commonly, but not always, require a larger dose than nonpregnant women. According to Kaplan,[25] pregnant hypothyroid women needed an increase in their before-pregnancy thyroxine requirements of 52 μg/day if the hypothyroidism was due to total thyroidectomy and/or ^{131}I treatment, but only of 28 μg/day if their hypothyroidism was due to Hashimoto's thyroiditis, probably because in the latter there was some residual endogenous thyroxine secretion.

"Euthyroid" Autoimmune Disease

Many persons test positive for thyroid autoantibodies without other clinical evidence of thyroid disease. This serologic condition correlates (though not always) with the histological diagnosis of "focal thyroiditis." If the thyroid is also enlarged, the condition can be called autoimmune or Hashimoto's thyroiditis.

Focal or euthyroid Hashimoto's thyroiditis may be something more than an innocent laboratory finding. Even before the advent of sensitive indices of thyroid function, we had found that these persons have on average a pattern of iodine metabolism similar but milder than that found in Hashimoto's thyroiditis.[26] Thirty years later Vanderpump *et al.*[27] found that such persons have an eightfold increased chance to develop overt hypothyroidism. This occurs quite commonly in pregnancy.[28] The same women also have an increased risk of spontaneous abortion. Stagnaro-Green *et al.*[29] found a rate of 17%, compared to 8.4% for AAB negative women. Other authors found an even greater difference. Furthermore, these women are at an increased risk of developing postpartum thyroiditis, as discussed later. Finally, Pop *et al.*[30] reported that the offspring of TPOAb-positive mothers have on average a 10.5 point decrement in their IQs. This interesting and disturbing finding should, of course, receive further confirmation.

Thyroid Nodules and Neoplasms

Because the use of isotopes is contraindicated in pregnancy, thyroid nodules should be investigated by measuring the serum levels of fT_4, fT_3, and TSH by ultranosograms and, if necessary, by a fine-needle aspiration and biopsy. Even if a malignancy is discovered, definite surgical treatment can be deferred until after the end of the pregnancy.[31]

THYROID DISEASES PARTICULAR TO PREGNANCY

Gestational Thyrotoxicosis

As stated before, chorionic gonadotrophin has a TSH-like activity, and during the first trimester when its concentration is highest this may lead to a decrease in serum TSH and an increase in the level of thyroid hormones. Various series suggest an average frequency of about 18% of decreased TSH (subclinical hyperthyroidism) and, according to Glinoer,[4] of these some 2.4% also have high serum free thyroid hormone levels, that is, overt hyperthyroidism. In our own series,[8] 31 women out of 208 (14.9%) had a low TSH (<0.3 μU/ml) (FIG. 1), and of these 11 (35.5%), that is, 5.3% of the total, high serum fT_4 and/or fT_3 as well.

Gestational thyrotoxicosis is frequently associated with hyperemesis gravidarum. In general it is usually a mild and self-limiting disease, which subsides spontaneously in a few weeks without specific treatment. If necessary, small doses of ATD may be given for a few weeks.

Fetal and Neonatal Hyperthyroidism

Graves' disease is due to autoantibodies, which bind to the TSH receptor (thyrotrophin receptor antibodies, TRAb) and so lead to thyroid hyperfunction. These autoantibodies cross the placenta and can stimulate the thyroid gland of the fetus after it is mature enough to function, that is, the second trimester of pregnancy and later. This results in fetal Graves' disease.

Fetal hyperthyroidism is characterized by tachycardia, accelerated bone maturation, and so forth, leading to spontaneous abortion, premature birth, and birth defects, among other problems.[32] The diagnosis of fetal Grave's disease rests on the presence of fetal tachycardia (>160/min), accelerated bone maturation, and especially a very high TRAb level in the mother.[33]

Fetal Graves' disease can be treated by giving antithyroid drugs (ATD) to the mother. These treat not only the maternal hyperthyroidism, but also the fetus, since they cross the placenta. ATD may also be given when the mother has Graves' disease treated by thyroid ablation and is now euthyroid on thyroid hormones.[34] In this case, ATD drugs, although useless for the mother, may control fetal thyroid function.

Neonatal Graves' disease is the persistance of the fetal disease. It is due to the maternal TRAb that persist in the fetal circulation even after birth. Tachycardia, high levels of thyroid hormones, and other symptoms are present; but the diagnosis is mainly based on the mother having a history of high TRAb levels. Neonatal Graves' disease is self-limited and lasts only until the maternal TRAb are metabolized. Meanwhile, it can be treated with beta-blockers and ATD.

Fetal and Neonatal Hypothyroidism

Fetal and neonatal hypothyroidism is usually due to a defect in the fetus itself, such as aplasia or dyshormonogenesis, or to iodine deficiency and antithyroid-goitrogenic drugs, including iodine. There is, however, a special type of transient neonatal (and fetal) hypothyroidism, due to the transplancental transfer of maternal TSH receptor-blocking antibodies.

Systematic screening has shown that about 1:4000 neonates has congenital hypothyroidism of some kind or another. This should be treated as soon as possible, in order to avoid or minimize permanent brain damage. There have been attempts to treat fetal hypothyroidism *in utero*, either by intra-amniotic injection of thyroxine[35,36] or by giving the mother TRIAC (tri-iodo-thyro-acetic acid) orally. This thyromimetic substance crosses the placenta more readily than thyroxine or T_3.[37]

Molar Pregnancy and Choriocarcinoma

Molar pregnancy and choriocarcinoma are associated with high levels of hCG, and therefore not only with biochemical but also with clinical hyperthyroidism.[38–40] This hyperthyroidism is cured when the primary condition is cured.

Postpartum Thyroiditis

It was been stated above that during pregnancy thyroid autoimmunity subsides and then rebounds a few months after parturition. This results in so-called postpartum thyroiditis (PPT). More than 40 years ago, Skillern *et al.*[41] reported a goiter increase in a case of Hashimoto's thyroiditis after birth. This condition, however, has been widely known through the work of Amino *et al.*,[42,43] Ginsberg and Walfish,[44] Jansson *et al.*,[12] Nikolai *et al.*,[45] and many others. Since then, this subject has been studied extensively, and reviewed by many, for instance, Gerstein,[46] Smallridge,[47] Lazarus *et al.*[48]

Briefly, it is estimated that about 10% of pregnant women test positive for TPOAb (thyroid-peroxidase antibodies), and half of these, that is, about 5% of the total, develop PPT.[45,46,49,50] In the series of Kuijpens *et al.*,[51] 10.7% of pregnant women were positive for TPOAb, and altogether 5.2% developed PPT. However, only two-thirds of the PPT patients were TPOAb positive. These authors consider cell-mediated immunity an important mechanism for the development of PPT. The frequency of PPT is increased in mothers with insulin-dependent diabetes mellitus.[52] Postpartum thyroiditis has the tendency to recur after another pregnancy, and there is also an increased probability for the appearance of another thyroid disease.

Postpartum thyroiditis is considered a destructive form of autoimmune thyroiditis: the thyroidal iodide (or pertechnetate) uptake is usually very low. Clinically there is goiter, usually hard and non-tender, and either hyperthyroidism or hypothyroidism or hyperthyroidism followed by hypothyroidism. The disease commonly subsides in a few weeks or months, but in several cases permanent hypothyroidism remains. Roti *et al.*[49] in Italy found that 6.4% of 372 women presented with hypothyroidism and 1.8% with hyperthyroidism.

Diagnosis is easy if the disease is suspected and can be confirmed by a low thyroidal radioiodine uptake. Treatment with either beta-blockers or thyroxine, depending on the metabolic abnormality present, is required in severe and persisting cases, sometimes for life in the case of persistent hypothyroidism.

REFERENCES

1. Aboul-Khair, S.A., J. Crooks, A.C. Turnbull & F.E. Hytten. 1964. Physiological changes in thyroid function during pregnancy. Clin. Sci. **27:** 195–207.
2. Koutras, D.A., A.D. Pharmakiotis, N. Koliopoulos, *et al.* 1978. The plasma inorganic iodine and the pituitary–thyroid axis in pregnancy. J. Endocrinol. Invest. **1:** 227–231.
3. Crooks, J., M.I. Tulloch, A.C. Turnbull, *et al.* 1967. Comparative incidence of goitre in pregnancy in Iceland and Scotland. Lancet **2:** 625–627.
4. Glinoer, D. 1997. The regulation of thyroid function in pregnancy: pathways of endocrine adaptation from physiology to pathology. Endocrinol. Rev. **18:** 404–433.
5. Beckers, C., A. Cornette, A. Georgoulis, *et al.* 1981. The effect of mild iodine deficiency on neonatal thyroid function. Clin. Endocrinol. **14:** 295–299.
6. Tsuruta, E., H. Tada, H. Tamaki, *et al.* 1995. Pathogenic role of asialo human chorionic gonadotropin in gestational thyrotoxicosis. J. Clin. Endocrinol. Metab. **80:** 350–355.
7. Yamazaki K., K. Sato, K. Shizume, *et al.* 1995. Potent thyrotropic activity of human chorionic gonadotropin variants in terms of ^{125}I incorporation and *de novo* synthesized thyroid hormone release in human thyroid follicle. J. Clin. Endocrinol. Metab. **80:** 473–479.
8. Kostaras, G., M. Alevizaki, D.A. Koutras, *et al.* 1998. Data to be published.
9. Gleicher, N., G. Deppe & C.J. Cohen. 1979. Common aspects of immunologic tolerance in pregnancy and malignancy. Obstet. Gynecol. **54:** 335–342.
10. Amino, N., R. Kuro, O. Tenizawa, *et al.* 1978. Changes of serum anti-thyroid antibodies during and after pregnancy in autoimmune thyroid diseases. Clin. Exp. Immunol. **31:** 30–37.
11. Amino, N., H. Tada & Y. Hidaka. 1996. Autoimmune thyroid disease and pregnancy. J. Endocrinol. Invest. **19:** 59–70.
12. Jansson, R., S. Bernander, A. Karlsson, *et al.* 1984. Autoimmune thyroid dysfunction in the postpartum period. J. Clin. Endocrinol. Metab. **58:** 681–687.
13. Berghout, A. & W. Wiersinga. 1998. Thyroid size and thyroid function during pregnancy: an analysis. Eur. J. Endocrinol. **138:** 536–542.
14. Glinoer, D., P. de Nayer, P. Bourdoux, *et al.* 1990. Regulation of maternal thyroid during pregnancy. J. Clin. Endocrinol. Metab. **71:** 276–287.
15. Glinoer, D., P. de Nayer, F. Delange, *et al.* 1995. A randomized trial for the treatment of mild iodine deficiency during pregnancy: maternal and neonatal effects. J. Clin. Endocrinol. Metab. **80:** 258–269.
16. Koutras, D.A. 1991. Prevention and treatment of nontoxic goiter during pregnancy. *In* The Thyroid and Pregnancy. C. Beckers & D. Reinwein, Eds.: 125–130. [International Merck Symposium in Brussels, Jan 31–Feb 2, 1991.] Schattauer. Stuttgart/New York.
17. Momotani, N., K. Ito & N. Hamada. 1986. Maternal hyperthyroidism and congenital malformation in the offspring. Clin. Endocrinol. **20:** 695–700.
18. Burrow, G.N. 1985. The management of thyrotoxicosis in pregnancy. N. Engl. J. Med. **313:** 562–565.
19. Burrow, G.N., C. Bartsokas, E.H. Klatskin, *et al.* 1968. Children exposed in utero to propylthiouracil: subsequent intellectual and physical development. Am. J. Dis. Child. **116:** 161–165.
20. Burrow, G.N., E.H. Klatskin & M. Genel. 1978. Intellectual development in children whose mothers received propylthiouracil during pregnancy. Yale J. Biol. Med. **51:** 151–156.

21. MOMOTANI, N., J.Y. NOH, N. ISHIKAWA & K. ITO. 1997. Effects of propylthiouracil and methimazole on fetal thyroid status in mothers with Graves' hyperthyroidism. J. Clin. Endocrinol. Metab. **82:** 3633–3636.
22. THOMAS, R. & R.L. REIDL. 1987. Thyroid disease and reproductive dysfunction: a review. Obstet. Gynecol. **70:** 789–798.
23. LEUNG, A.S., L.K. MILLAR, P.P. KOONINGS, *et al.* 1993. Perinatal outcome in hypothyroid pregnancies. Obstet. Gynecol. **81:** 349–353.
24. MONTORO, M., J.V. COLLEA, S.D. FRASIER & J.H. MESTMAN. 1981. Successful outcome of pregnancy in women with hypothyroidism. Ann. Intern. Med. **94:** 31–34.
25. KAPLAN, M.M. 1992. Monitoring thyroxine treatment during pregnancy. Thyroid **2:** 147–152.
26. BUCHANAN, W.W., R. MCG. HARDEN, D.A. KOUTRAS & K.G. GRAY. 1965. Abnormalities of iodine metabolism in patients with complement-fixing antimicrosomal thyroid autoantibodies, but not clinical evidence of thyroid disease: a sub-clinical form of Hashimoto's thyroiditis. J. Clin. Endocrinol. Metab. **25:** 301–306.
27. VANDERPUMP, M.P.J., W.M.G. TUNBRIDGE, J.M. FRENCH, *et al.* 1995. The incidence of thyroid disorders in the community: a twenty-year follow-up of the Whickham survey. Clin. Endocrinol. **43:** 55–68.
28. GLINOER, D., M. FERNANDEZ SOTO, P. BOURDOUX, *et al.* 1991. Pregnancy in patients with mild thyroid abnormalities: maternal and neonatal repercussions. J. Clin. Endocrinol. Metab. **73:** 421–427.
29. STAGNARO-GREEN, A., S.H. ROMAN, R.H. COBIN, *et al.* 1990. Detection of at-risk pregnancy by means of highly sensitive assays for thyroid autoantibodies. JAMA **264:** 1422–1425.
30. POP, V.J., E. DE VRIES, A.L. VAN BAAR, *et al.* 1995. Maternal thyroid peroxidase antibodies during pregnancy: a marker of impaired child development? J. Clin. Endocrinol. Metab. **80:** 3561–3566.
31. MOOSA, M. & E.L. MAZZAFERRI. 1997. Outcome of differentiated thyroid cancer diagnosed in pregnant women. J. Clin. Endocrinol. Metab. **82:** 2862–2866.
32. PERELMAN, A.H. & R.D. CLEMONS. 1992. The fetus in maternal hyperthyroidism. Thyroid **2:** 225–228.
33. MCKENZIE, J.M. & M. ZAKARIJA. 1992. Fetal and neonatal hypothyroidism due to maternal TSH receptor antibodies. Thyroid **2:** 155–159.
34. COVE, D.H. & P. JOHNSTON. 1985. Fetal hyperthyroidism: experience of treatment in four siblings. Lancet **1:** 430–432.
35. PERELMAN, A.H., R.L. JOHNSON, R.D. CLEMONS, *et al.* 1990. Intrauterine diagnosis and treatment of fetal goitrous hypothyroidism. J. Clin. Endocrinol. Metab. **71:** 618–621.
36. DAVIDSON, K.M., D.S. RICHARDS, D.A. SCHATZ & D.A. FISHER. 1991. Successful in utero treatment of fetal goiter and hypothyroidism. N. Engl. J. Med. **324:** 543–546.
37. CORTELAZZI, D., A.M. BAGGIANI, A.M. MARCONI, *et al.* 1994. Treatment of fetal hypothyroidism by triac administration to the mother. J. Endocrinol. Invest. **17:** 144.
38. HERSHMAN, J.M. & H.P. HIGGINS. 1971. Hydatiform mole—a cause of clinical hyperthyroidism. N. Engl. J. Med. **284:** 573–577.
39. KENIMER, J.C., J.M. HERSHMAN & H.P. HIGGINS. 1975. The thyrotropin in hydatiform moles is human chorionic gonadotrophin. J. Clin. Endocrinol. Metab. **40:** 482–491.
40. KENNEDY, R.L., E. SHERIDAN, J. DOUNE, *et al.* 1990. Thyroid function in choriocarcinoma: demonstration of a thyroid stimulating activity in serum using FRTL-5 and human thyroid cells. Clin. Endocrinol. **33:** 227–237.
41. SKILLERN, P.G., G. CRILE, E.P. MCCULLOUGH, *et al.* 1956. Struma lymphomatosa: primary thyroid failure with compensatory thyroid enlargement. J. Clin. Endocrinol. Metab. **16:** 35–39.
42. AMINO, N., K. MIYAI, T. ONISHI, *et al.* 1976. Transient hypothyroidism after delivery in autoimmune thyroiditis. J. Clin. Endocrinol. Metab. **42:** 296–301.
43. AMINO, N., H. MORI, Y. IWARANI, *et al.* 1982. High prevalence of transient post-partum thyrotoxicosis and hypothyroidism. N. Engl. J. Med. **306:** 849–852.
44. GINSBERG, J. & P.G. WALFISH. 1997. Postpartum transient thyrotoxicosis with painless thyroitidis. Lancet **1:** 1125–1128.

45. NIKOLAI, T.F., S.L. TURNEY & R.C. ROBERTS. 1987. Postpartum lymphocytic thyroiditis. Arch. Intern. Med. **147:** 221–222.
46. GERSTEIN, H.C. 1990. How common is postpartum thyroiditis? A methodologic overview of the literature. Arch. Intern. Med. **150:** 1397–1400.
47. SMALLRIDGE, R.C. 1996. Postpartum thyroid dysfunction: a frequently undiagnosed endocrine disorder. Endocrinologist **6:** 44–50.
48. LAZARUS, J.H., R. HALL, S. OTHMAN, *et al.* 1996. The clinical spectrum of postpartum thyroid disease. Q. J. Med. **8:** 429–435.
49. ROTI, E., L. BIANCONI, E. GARDINI, *et al.* 1991. Postpartum thyroid dysfunction in an Italian population residing in an area of mild iodine deficiency. J. Endocrinol. Invest. **14:** 669–674.
50. STAGNARO-GREEN, A., S.H. ROMAN, R.H. COBIN, *et al.* 1992. A prospective study of lymphocyte-initiated immunosuppression in normal pregnancy: evidence of a T-cell etiology for postpartum thyroid dysfunction. J. Clin. Endocrinol. Metab. **74:** 645–653.
51. KUIJPENS, J.L., M. DE HAAN-MEULMAN, H.L. VADER, *et al.* 1998. Cell-mediated immunity and postpartum thyroid dysfunction: a possibility for the prediction of disease? J. Clin. Endocrinol. Metab. **83:** 1959–1966.
52. ALVAREZ-MOURHANY, M., S.H. ROMAN, A.J. DREXLER, *et al.* 1994. Long-term prospective study of postpartum thyroid dysfunction in women with insulin-dependent diabetes mellitus. J. Clin. Endocrinol. Metab. **79:** 10–16.

Placental Corticotropin-Releasing Factor

An Update

M. FADALTI,[a] I. PEZZANI,[a] L. COBELLIS,[a] F. SPRINGOLO,[a] M.M. PETROVEC,[a]
G. AMBROSINI,[b] F.M. REIS,[a] AND F. PETRAGLIA[a,c]

[a]*Department of Surgical Sciences, Obstetrics and Gynecology, University of Udine, Udine, Italy*

[b]*Department of Surgical Sciences, University of Sassari, Sassari, Italy*

ABSTRACT: Corticotropin-releasing factor (CRF) produced in placenta has paracrine effects within placenta, decidua, and myometrium and endocrine effects on mother and fetus. CRF is a potent local regulator of myometrial contractility and of prostaglandin release, Recently, urocortin, a new member of the CRF family, has been localized in human placenta and membranes. Urocortin mimics some of the local effects of CRF in intrauterine tissues, that is, increase of adrenocorticotrophic hormone (ACTH) and prostagiandin release and myometrial contractility. A local CRF-BP modulates the paracrine effects of CRF and urocortin. The various CRF receptor subtypes are well distributed in placenta and membranes. CRH also acts on placental blood vasculature and has an action on fetal adrenal gland to stimulate the productlon of the steroid DHEA-S. In nonpregnant women, plasma CRF levels are low; they become higher during the first and second trimesters of pregnancy. A clear increase is evident at term and when CRF-BP levels decrease. Women with preterm labor show high CRF and low CRF-BP levels, supporting an involvement of this pathway in mechanism of parturition.

INTRODUCTION

It is well established that labor and delivery are associated with a major stressful condition and with a complex neuroendocrine and behavioral adaptation. In the physiology of normal parturition, there is an important increase of corticotropin-releasing factor (CRF) levels in maternal and fetal plasma, amniotic fluid, and local tissues. Human placenta produces and represents the main source of this stress-related peptide during human gestation.

PLACENTAL CRF: PRODUCTION, RECEPTORS, AND SECRETION

CRF, a neuropeptide initially discovered in the paraventricular nucleus of the hypothalamus, was detected in the extracts of human placentas obtained at term from spontaneous deliveries.[1] Placental CRF content and mRNA is higher at term than at

[c]Address for correspondence: Prof. Felice Petraglia, Chair of Obstetrics and Gynecology, University of Udine, Piazz. le S. Maria della Misericordia, 33100 Udine, Italy. Phone:++39/0432/559635; fax:++39/0432/559641.
Felice.Petraglia@DSC.uniud.it

early gestation.[2,3] CRF is located in the cytotrophoblast, in the syncytiotrophoblast, and intermediate trophoblast of placenta at term.[4] CRF is also present in fetal membranes: in epithelial cells and in some cells in the subepithelial layer of amnion, in the reticular layer of the chorion, and in decidual stromal cells.[5] CRF mRNA expression in decidual cells has been shown during pregnancy, with the highest levels at term.[6] CRF is also produced by endometrial cells: the addition of CRF in cell cultures increases PRL release, inducing the process of decidualization.[7]

CRF receptor subtypes Rlα and Rc are present in human fetal membranes.[8] Syncytiotrophoblast and amniotic epithelium cells are the ones expressing CRF Rlα and Rc receptor mRNA. CRF receptors have been also described in human myometrium and in decidua. In particular, recent findings show the presence in pregnant myometrium of subtypes lα, lβ, 2α, and the variant C, whereas only the lα and lβ receptors are detectable in nonpregnant myometrium.[9]

It is known that glucocorticoids act on adrenocorticotrophic hormone (ACTH) secretion, but there is a difference between pituitary and placental cells. In fact, although glucocorticoids exert negative feedback on ACTH secretion from pituitary cells, they have a positive effect on CRF from amnion, chorion, and decidual placental cells.[10] Also, progesterone and nitric oxide can regulate CRF production: these products inhibit CRF output from amnion, chorion, decidua, and placental cells and decrease levels of CRF mRNA in human placental tissues in culture.[11] Cytokines regulate secretion of CRF from placental cells; these include IL-1 and NPY; neurotransmitters such as acetylcholine and noradrenaline; and peptides such as vasopressin, angiotensin 11, and oxytocin. These can enhance the accumulation of CRF in culture medium from placental tissues.[4]

PLACENTAL CRF: LOCAL EFFECTS

The addition of CRF to cultured trophoblastic cells stimulates ACTH secretion. A CRF antagonist inhibits the CRF-induced ACTH release.[4] Several other local effects for CRF have been described. CRF is also a potent local regulator of myometrial contractility and of prostaglandin release. In fact, the addition of CRF in cultures of human placenta, decidua, or amnion at term increases the release of PGE_2 and $PGF_{2\alpha}$.[12] Indeed, the incubation of human myometrial strips with CRF increases the contractile activity; this effect has been shown to be synergistic with oxytocin or prostaglandin and mediated by an increase in intracellular AMPc.[13] Altough CRF has no direct inotropic effect on the myometrium, it exerts priming and potentiating effects with oxytocin when they are administered together.[14] The human myometrium expresses a specific receptor for CRF that changes to a high-affinity state as term approaches[15]; oxytocin plays a pivotal role with this tissue at the onset of labor by stimulating myometrial contractility (FIG. 1).

Placental CRF secreted into the fetal compartment may support labor by stimulating fetal–pituitary secretion of ACTH and by direct action on fetal adrenal gland to stimulate the production of the steroid DHEA-S.[16] CRF also has a role in the immune response to stress: it is produced in peripheral inflammatory sites, and CRF binding sites are present on blood lymphocytes and monocyte. CRF may modulate cytokine production in cultured human peripheral mononuclear cells from healthy

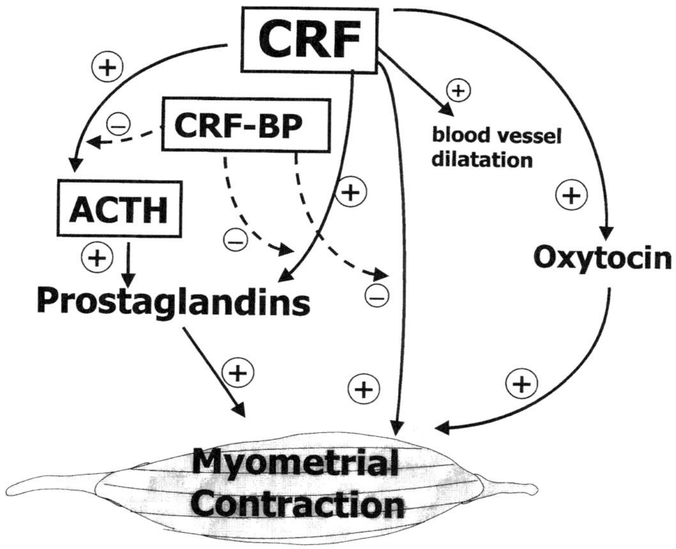

FIGURE 1. Paracrine effects of placental CRF on the control of myometrial contraction and modulation of CRF effects by CRF-BP.

subjects. Interferon-γ (IFNγ) release is depressed in a dose-dependent manner by CRF addition to medium, whereas interleukin-6 (IL-6) release increases without an evident CRF dose correlation. No significant effect was observed on human lymphocyte proliferation.[17]

CRF IN BIOLOGICAL FLUIDS

In nonpregnant women plasma CRF level is low (<10 pg/ml). Higher concentrations are present in the first and second trimesters of pregnancy.[18] After the second trimester, CRF levels rise steadily until about 35 weeks, and then increase more rapidly near term.[19] An analogue trend of CRF concentration has been shown in placenta: the CRF mRNA levels progressively increase from 8 to 9 weeks, through a midrange at 18 to 31 weeks of gestation, until the maximum at 39 to 40 weeks. CRF is also measurable in fetal circulation and amniotic fluid. In umbilical cord blood CRF levels are 20-fold lower than in maternal circulation.[20]

Amniotic fluid CRF concentrations are lower than in maternal and fetal serum and increase during the third trimester, reaching high values at term.[21] Amniotic CRF levels at 16–18 weeks are similar to those of maternal plasma. At term, amniotic CRF concentrations are similar to those of cord plasma, but are 100 times lower than those of the corresponding maternal plasma.

PLACENTAL CRF: PARTURITION

At the beginning of labor, CRF levels increase, reaching a maximum at the most advanced stages of cervical dilation. In the case of elective cesarean section, CRF levels during surgery were not significantly different from those before surgery.[22] Also, the accumulation in tissues of patients in spontaneous labor at term was consistenly higher than that obtained from patients at elective cesarean section at term in the absence of labor. In the case of spontaneous labor and elective cesarean section, maternal plasma CRF concentrations decreased to half of the predelivery values by 20–30 minutes.[23] By 1–5 days postpartum, the CRF levels are similar to those of nonpregnant women, suggesting that the placenta and the intrauterine tissues are the principal source of CRF in pregnancy. At labor, no significant differences were observed at the different stages of cervical dilation. At cesarean section, CRF levels in amniotic fluid were similar to those found in pregnancy.[22]

PLACENTAL CRF: GESTATIONAL DISEASES

In preterm labor, it was demonstrated that maternal plasma CRF levels were higher than normal pregnancy. One study evaluated maternal serum CRF levels during the latter half of pregnancy as well as their indication of the potential for spotaneous preterm delivery.[24] The gestational age-specific levels were increased for preterm premature rupture of membranes compared with the term values for the 24 to 32 weeks of gestation grouping, but the differences were not statistically significant.[25] On the other hand, McLean *et al.* have demonstrated that CRF levels were significantly higher in women delivering preterm and this elevation was evident from the second trimester of pregnancy. During early pregnancy a "placental clock," such as maternal placental CRF, may be a biological marker of preterm delivery. Women between 28 and 36 weeks of gestation with preterm labor who subsequently delivered within 24 hours have CRF levels significantly higher than do normal subjects.[26] Moreover, another study demonstrated that CRF levels in patients who delivered within 7 days are higher than in those contuining until term.[27]

THE ROLE OF CRF-BP

The presence of a CRF-binding protein explains why high levels of CRF in the third trimester of pregnancy do not cause an increase in ACTH during this period and consequently prevent the activation of the pituitary–adrenal axis during pregnancy.[28] The major site of production for circulating CRF-BP is the liver, but other sites, such as placenta, fetal membranes, and decidua have also beeen identified. In placenta, CRF-BP mRNA is expressed in the syncytial layer, whereas rare, positively hybridized cells were observed within the cytotrophoblast and mesenchymal cells.[29]

The concentrations of CRF-BP remain stable in nonpregnant women and during gestation until 25 weeks of pregnancy. Plasma concentration decreased slightly between 25 and 30 weeks, then rapidly at 4–6 weeks before labor at term. Thus, a reciprocal change in concentration of CRF and CRF-BP in maternal plasma was observed and suggests that a rise in CRF results in decreased CRF-BP levels.[30]

Maternal CRF-BP serum levels are low in patients with preterm labor and preeclampsia in the presence of high CRF levels, which supports the relevance of the CRF/CRF-BP system in the maintenance of gestational homeostasis.[31] A similar pattern is also present in patients in labor at term; the low level of CRF-BP correlates with the increase in maternal CRF. Thus, CRF-BP reverses the CRF-induced ACTH release and reduces the prostaglandin release from decidual cells as well as the myometrial contractility activated by CRF. Thus, CRF-BP probably acts in the fetal circulation to impede the maturation of the HPA axis and, consequently, activates the adaptative responses to stress.[32]

REFERENCES

1. Shibasaki, T., E. Odagiri, K. Shizume & N. Ling. 1982. Corticotropin releasing factor-like activity in human placenta extracts. J. Clin. Endocrinol. Metab. **55:** 384–386.
2. Frim, D.M., R.L. Emanuel, B.G. Robinson, *et al.* 1978. Characterization and gestational regulation of corticotropin releasing hormone messenger RNA in human placenta. J. Clin. Invest. **82:** 287–292.
3. Saijonama, O., T. Laatikainen & T. Whaistrom. 1988. Corticotropin releasing factor in human placenta: localization, concentration and release in vitro. Placenta **9:** 373–385.
4. Petraglia, F., P.E. Sawchenko, J. Rivier & W. Vale. 1987. Evidence for local stimulation of ACTH secretion by corricotropin releasing factor in human placenta. Nature **328:** 717–719.
5. Riley, S.C., J.C. Walton, J.M. Herlick & J.R.G. Challis. 1991. The localization and distribution of corticotropin releasing hormone in the human placenta and fetal membranes throughout gestation. J. Clin. Endocrinol. Metab. **72:** 1001–1007.
6. Petraglia, F., S. Tabanelli, M.C. Galassi, *et al.* 1992. Human decidua and in vitro decidualized endometrial stromal cells at term contain immunoreactive corticotropin releasing factor and CRF messenger ribonucleic acid. J. Clin. Endocrinol. Metab. **74:** 1427–1431.
7. Ferrari, A., F. Petraglia & E. Gurpide. 1995. CRF decidualizes human endometrial stromal cells in vitro. Interaction with progestin. Steroid Biochem. Molec. Biol. **54:** 251–255.
8. Karteris, E., D. Grammatopulos, Y. Dai, *et al.* 1998. The human placenta and fetal membranes express the corticotropin releasing hormone receptor 1α and the CRH-C variant receptor. J. Clin. Endocrinol. Metab. **83:** 1376–1379.
9. Grammatopoulos, D., Y. Dal, J. Chen, *et al.* 1998. Human corticotropin releasing hormone receptor: differences in subtype expression between pregnant and nonpregnant myometria. J. Clin. Endocrinol. Metab. **83:** 2539–2544.
10. Jones, S.A. & J.R.G. Challis. 1990. Steroid, corticotropin releasing hormone, ACTH and prostaglandin interaction in the amnion and placenta of early pregnancy in man. J. Endocrinol. **125:** 153–159.
11. Sun, K., R. Smith & P.J. Robinson. 1994. Basal and KCL stimulated corticotropin releasing hormone release from human placenta syncytiotrophoblasts is inhibited by sodium nitroprussiate. J. Clin. Endocrinol. Metab. **79:** 519–524.
12. Jones, S.A. & J.R.G. Challis. 1989. Local stimulation of prostaglandin production by corticotropin releasing hormone in human fetal membranes and placenta. Biochem. Biophys. Res. Commun. **159:** 192–199.
13. Quartero, H.W.P., W.A. Noort, C.H. Fry & J.N.C. Keirse. 1991. Role of prostaglandins and leukotrienes in the synergistic effect of oxytocin and corticotropin releasing hormone on the contraction force in human gestational myometrium. Prostaglandins **42:** 137–150.
14. Quartero, H.V.P. & C.H. Fry. 1989. Placental corticotropin releasing factor may modulate human parturition. Placenta **10:** 439–443.

15. HILLHOUSE, E.W., D. GRAMATOPULOS, N.G.N. MILTON & H.V.P. QUARTERO. 1993. The identification of a human myometrial corticotropin releasing hormone receptor that increases in affinity during pregnancy. J. Clin. Endocrinol. Metab. **76:** 736–741.
16. SMITH, R., S. MESIANO, E.C. CHAN, *et al.* 1998. CRH directy and preferentially stimulates DHEA-S secretion by human fetal adrenal cortical cells. J. Clin. Endocrinol. Metab. **83:** 2916–2920.
17. ANGIONI, S., F. PETRAGLIA, A. GAILINELLI, *et al.* 1993. Corticotropin releasing hormone modulates cytokines release in cultured human peripheral blood mononuclear cells. Life Sci. **53:** 1735–1742.
18. SASAKI, A., S. LIOTTA, M.J. LUCKEJ, *et al.* 1984. Immunoreactive corticotropin releasing factor is present in human plasma during the third trimester of pregnancy. J. Clin. Endocrinol. Metab. **59:** 812–814.
19. CAMPBELL, E.A., E.A. LINTON, C.D.A. WOLFE, *et al.* 1987. Plasma corticotropin releasing hormone concentrations during pregnancy and.parturition. J. Clin. Endocrinol. Metab. **63:** 1054–1059.
20. GOLAND, R.S., S.L. WARDLAW, M. BLUM, *et al.* 1988. Biologically active corticotrophin releasing hormone in maternal and fetal plasma during pregnancy. Am. J. Obstet. Gynecol. **159:** 884–890.
21. SASAKI, A., O. SHINKAWA & K. YOSHINAGA. 1990. Immunoreactive corticotropin releasing hormone in amniotic fluid. Am. J. Obstet. Gynecol. **162:** 194–198.
22. PETRAGLIA, F., L. GIARDINO, G. COUKOS, *et al.* 1990. Corticotropin releasing factor and parturition: plasma and amniotic fluid levels and placental binding sites. Obstet. Gynecol. **75:** 784–789.
23. LAATIKAINEN, T., T. VIRTANEN, I. RAISANEN & K. SAIMINEN. 1987. Immunoreactive corticotropin releasing factor and corticotrophin in plasma during pregnancy, labor and puerperium. Neuropeptides **10:** 343–353.
24. BERKOWITZ, G.S., R.H. LAPINSKI, C.J. LOCKWOOD, *et al.* 1996. Corticotropin releasing factor and its binding protein: maternal serum levels in term and preterm deliveries. Am. J. Obstet. Gynecol. **174:** 1477–1483.
25. MCLEAN, M., A. BISITS, J. DAVIES, *et al.* 1995. A placental clock controlling the length of human pregnancy. Nat. Med. **1:** 460–463.
26. KOREBRITS, C., M.M. RAMIREZ, L. WATSON, *et al.* 1998. Maternal corticotropin releasing hormone is increased with impending preterm birth. J. Clin. Endocrinol. Metab. **83:** 1585–1591.
27. BISITS, A., G. MADSEN, M. MCLEAN, *et al.* 1998. Corticotropin releasing hormone: a biochemical predictor of preterm delivery in a pilot randomized trial of the treatment of preterm labor. Am. J. Obstet. Gynecol. **178:** 862–866.
28. LINTON, E.A., C.D.A. WOLFE, D.P. BEHAN & P.J. LOWRY. 1988. A specific carrier substance for human corticotrophin releasing factor in late gestational maternal plasma which could mask the ACTH releasing activity. Clin. Endocrinol. **28:** 315–324.
29. PETRAGLIA, F., E. POTTER, V. CAMERUN, *et al.* 1993. Corticotropin releasing factor binding protein is produced by human placenta and intrauterine tissues. J. Clin. Endocrinol. Metab. **77:** 919–924.
30. CHALLIS, J.R.G., S.G. MATTHEWS, C.V. MEIR & M.M. RAMIREZ. 1995. Current topic: the placental corticotropin releasing hormone–adrenocorticotrophin axis. Placenta **16:** 481–502.
31. MCLEAN, M., A. BISITS, J. DAVIES, *et al.* 1995. A placental clock controlling the length of human pregnancy. Nat. Med. **1:** 460–463.
32. PETRAGLIA, F., P. FLORIO, T. SIMONCINI, *et al.* 1997. Cord plasma corticotropin releasing factor binding protein in term and preterm labor. Placenta **18:** 115–119.

Maternal Hypothalamic–Pituitary–Adrenal Axis in Pregnancy and the Postpartum Period

Postpartum-Related Disorders

G. MASTORAKOS[a] AND I. ILIAS

Endocrine Unit, "Evgenidion" Hospital, University of Athens, GR-11528, Athens, Greece

ABSTRACT: During pregnancy, placenta-derived CRH increases exponentially in the plasma. Circulating levels of CRH-binding protein decrease considerably in the last trimester of pregnancy, resulting in further elevation of bioavailable plasma CRH. The adrenal glands during pregnancy gradually become hypertrophic because of the increase in ACTH, which parallels that of CRH. Thus, pregnancy is a transient period of relative hypercortisolism. The activation of the hypothalamic–pituitary–adrenal axis during pregnancy has been proposed to function as a biological clock. In this model, the placenta is perceived as a stress-sensitive organ and placental CRH as a timing starter, determining a preterm, term, or postterm labor. During pregnancy, as well as during the immediate postpartum period, the hypothalamic maternal CRH secretion is suppressed, because of the circulating levels of cortisol. Hypothalamic CRH secretion normalizes within 12 weeks. This transient postpartum maternal hypothalamic CRH suppression, together with the steroid withdrawal that follows parturition, might be causally related to the mood disorders and the vulnerability to autoimmune diseases such as thyroiditis or rheumatoid arthritis often observed during the postpartum period.

INTRODUCTION: THE HYPOTHALAMIC–PITUITARY–ADRENAL AXIS

The hypothalamic–pituitary–adrenal (HPA) axis plays a major role in the stress response of vertebrates, together with the arousal and the autonomic nervous systems (locus ceruleus–norepinephrine system).[1,2] The principal modulators of the HPA axis are corticotropin-releasing hormone (CRH) and arginine-vasopressin (AVP) (FIG.1). Corticotropin-releasing hormone is a 41 amino acid long peptide found in brain cells, secreted principally by the parvicellular neurons of the paraventricular hypothalamic nuclei; the latter, by means of projecting fibers to the pituitary median eminence, release CRH into the hypophyseal portal circulation. Serotonin and acetylcholine stimulate the release of CRH from the hypothalamic nuclei, while norepinephrine and γ-aminobutyric acid inhibit it. Corticotropin-releasing hormone is not exclusively produced in the central nervous system, since its presence has also been demonstrated at peripheral inflammatory sites such as the synovial fluid and tissue in patients suffering from osteoarthritis and rheumatoid arthritis.[3] In these lo-

[a]Address for correspondence: George Mastorakos, M.D., D.Sc., Endocrine Unit, "Evgenidion" Hospital, University of Athens, 20 Papadiamantopoulou Street, GR-11528, Athens, Greece. Fax: +301+3636229.
e-mail: mastorak@mail.kapatel.gr

calizations, CRH acts as a proinflammatory cytokine through mechanisms that are only partially known, one being the degranulation of mast cells.[4] Corticotropin-releasing hormone secretion varies with age and reproductive function[5] (FIG. 2).

Adrenocorticotropic hormone (ACTH) is synthesized by the anterior pituitary corticotroph cells and is released after stimulation of the corticotrophs by CRH, via the activation of the adenylate cyclase–cyclic AMP system that opens voltage-gated calcium channels. Arginine-vasopressin is also a potent ACTH-releasing hormone. Its action is mediated via the inositol triphosphate system that opens receptor-gated calcium channels. The binding of ACTH to high-affinity membrane receptors on the adrenal cell activates the adenylate cyclase system, resulting in a net increase of cholesterol transport into the cell and, through the action of mitochondrial cholesterol ester hydroxylase, in pregnenolone synthesis. Pregnenolone is further metabolized in the smooth endoplasmic reticulum to cortisol after 11-hydroxylation. Cortisol is the main glucocorticoid in humans.[6]

Cortisol production follows, within minutes, the ACTH circadian rhythm, which is superimposed on the episodic secretion of ACTH. Cortisol also controls its own secretion by a fast negative-feedback, inhibiting ACTH secretion, and a delayed negative feedback, suppressing CRH and ACTH production.[6]

THE HYPOTHALAMIC–PITUITARY–ADRENAL AXIS AND THE FEMALE REPRODUCTIVE SYSTEM

There is a bidirectional interaction between the stress system (HPA axis and locus ceruleus–norepinephrine system) and the female reproductive system.[5]

Corticotropin inhibits the secretion of gonadotropin hormone-releasing hormone (GnRH) from the arcuate nuclei of the hypothalamus. Glucocorticoids inhibit both GnRH secretion and render resistant to sex hormones the tissues that are normally sensitive to them[7,8] (FIG. 1). The promoter area of the human CRH gene has been shown to have half estrogen-responsive elements, and estrogens have been shown to directly regulate the expression of the human CRH gene.[9] The observed relative hypercortisolism of women, as compared to men, can be attributed to this. Thus, a disregulated HPA response to stressors would facilitate the appearance of autoimmune phenomena more readily in women, since there exists a reciprocal relationship between the HPA axis and the immune/inflammatory reaction.[10]

Fundamental ovarian functions, such as ovulation and luteolysis, represent, in fact, aseptic inflammations. Also, the presence of CRH at peripheral sites other than the neural tissue[3] has been demonstrated in the rat and human testicular Leydig cell, where it inhibits the biosynthesis of testosterone in an autocrine function.[11–13] Because the theca cell of the ovary is the ontogenic and functional equivalent of the Leydig cell and CRH has been shown to act as a proinflammatory cytokine, research was focused on the ovaries for the presence of CRH. Thus, it was demonstrated that this molecule is present in the theca and stromal cells as well as in cells of the corpora lutea of rat ovaries.[14] Corticotropin-releasing hormone has been found in analogous locations in normal human ovaries and to a lesser degree in polycystic human ovaries.[15]

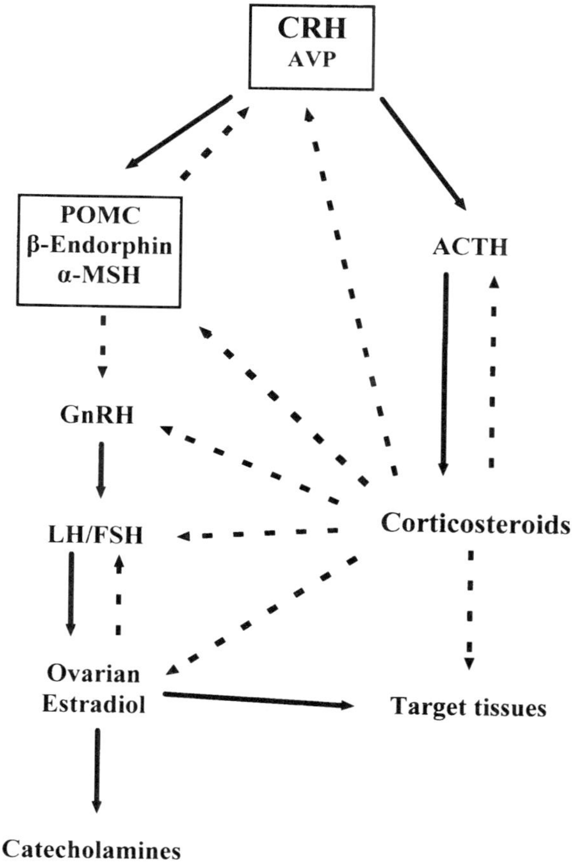

FIGURE 1. Interactions of the hypothalamic–pituitary–adrenal (HPA) axis with the female reproductive system. Stress generally inhibits the female reproductive system through the HPA axis. CRH, corticotropin-releasing hormone; AVP, arginine vasopressin; ACTH, adrenocorticotropin; POMC, proopiomelanocortin; α-MSH, melanocyte-stimulating hormone; GnRH, gonadotropin-releasing hormone; LH, luteinizing hormone; FSH, follicle-stimulating hormone; *solid arrows*: stimulation; *dashed arrows*: inhibition (adapted from Chrousos *et al.*[5]).

A regulatory role for CRH has been proposed in ovulation and luteolysis (based on its proinflammatory properties) as well as in steroid biosynthesis (based on autocrine and paracrine regulatory functions).[14,15] In fact, CRH has been shown to exert a CRH- and IL-1-receptor–mediated inhibitory effect on ovarian steroidogenesis of granulosa lutein cells. Thus, it might be actively involved in the still-enigmatic process of follicular atresia and luteolysis.[16]

The CRH gene is expressed in the endometrium.[19,20] The myometrium contains specific CRH receptors[17]; the cytoplasm of the glandular epithelial cells of the endometrium has been recently shown to contain CRH during the proliferative as well as the secretory phases of the menstrual cycle,[18–20] and a role for CRH in menstrual shedding and implantation of the blastocyst has been speculated.[20]

THE MATERNAL HPA AXIS DURING AND AFTER PREGNANCY

During pregnancy, the plasma level of circulating immunoreactive CRH increases exponentially up to a thousand times its nonpregnant values[21,22] (FIG. 2), the increase beginning from the 8*th* to 10*th* week of gestation[23,24]; however, this increase is not of hypothalamic origin, but the result of CRH production by the placenta, decidua, and fetal membranes.[18,25,26] Recently, the two subtypes of CRH receptor have been distinguished in the placenta.[27,28] Pregnant and nonpregnant women alike express CRH receptor mRNA and protein in uterine smooth muscle.[17,29,30] In twin gestations maternal plasma levels are significantly higher than in singletons.[31] Placental CRH does not exhibit a circadian rhythm.[32,33] Unique to humans, is the presence in plasma and amniotic fluid, of a CRH-binding protein (CRHbp).[34] Corticotropin-releasing hormone is bound with high affinity to CRHbp, considered to reduce the bioactivity of circulating CRH.[35,36] The CRHbp plasma concentrations in pregnant women remain similar to levels of nonpregnant women until the third trimester of pregnancy. At that time its values fall to roughly one-third the levels of earlier pregnancy or those of the nonpregnant state.[37] Amniotic fluid CRHbp levels also fall approaching term.[35] The unbound fraction of CRH stimulates the maternal ACTH secretion, leading to the relative hypercortisolism of pregnancy. The placental blood flow may be regulated by CRH, since this molecule has been shown to induce vasodilation in the uterine arteries.[38] Studies have failed to show overt circadian relations between plasma CRH and ACTH or cortisol levels during the third trimester of pregnancy.[32,39,40]

The mother's anterior pituitary gland hormones have little influence on pregnancy after implantation has occurred, though the gland enlarges (mainly due to hyperplasia of the lactotrophs) by about one-third; also normal neuroendocrine regulatory mechanisms remain intact.[41] The circadian rhythm of ACTH plasma levels is maintained during pregnancy.[32] Pituitary ACTH secretion and plasma ACTH levels rise during pregnancy—remaining, though, within normal limits—following in parallel the rise of plasma free and total cortisol levels.[42] This rise in ACTH levels is due to circulating unbound placental CRH, whereas the maintenance of its circadian rhythmicity is probably due to AVP secreted by the parvicellular paraventricular nuclei.[32] Corticotropin concentration in amniotic fluid rises during pregnancy, peaking at the beginning of the third trimester and then showing a decline.[43]

The adrenal glands during pregnancy gradually become hypertrophic. Pregnancy is a transient, but physiologic, period of relative hypercortisolism for the normal woman; total and free plasma cortisol steadily rise, peaking during the third trimester at about two and three times nonpregnant values, respectively (FIG. 3). These levels are comparable to those observed in Cushing's disease, severe depression, anorexia nervosa, and in athletes doing strenuous exercise.[10,41,44,45] A mechanism involved in the induction of this relative hypercortisolism is the doubling of corticosteroid-binding globulin (CBG) levels, attributed to the increased estrogen ones dur-

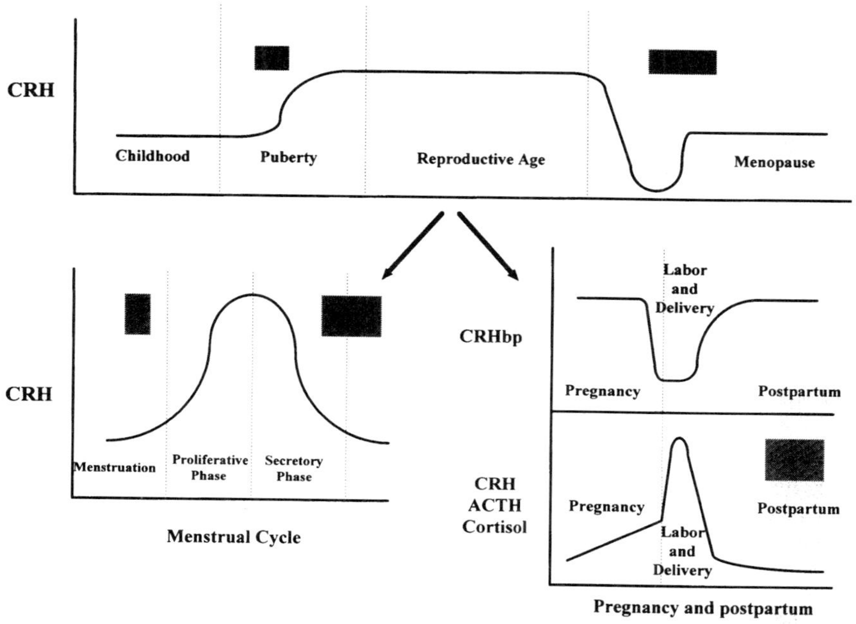

FIGURE 2. Heuristic representations of lifetime changes in the hypothalamic–pituitary–adrenal (HPA) axis of women. Changes in the reproductive system during puberty, the menstrual cycle, pregnancy, the postpartum period, and menopause are associated with changes in the HPA axis, as shown by changes in secretion. Shaded areas denote periods of vulnerability to mood disorders and autoimmune diseases (adapted from Chrousos *et al.*[5]).

ing pregnancy.[41] Increased CBG levels result in low catabolism of cortisol by the liver. Thus the plasma half-life of this hormone is actually doubled. To a lesser but not negligible degree cortisol production in the adrenal zona fasciculata is also increased, because of the relatively increased ACTH secretion. The diurnal variation of plasma cortisol levels is maintained in pregnancy,[45,46] whereas the existence of further longer-duration cycles has been suggested.[47] During pregnancy, amniotic fluid cortisol levels follow the plasma levels of this hormone.[48]

The activation of the HPA axis during parturition has been observed in primates[49]; CRH increase is a prominent finding, but the overall effect of the HPA axis on the mechanisms of parturition is yet difficult to ascertain, and interprimate differences exist.[49] In humans, maternal plasma CRH, ACTH, and cortisol levels increase during normal labor and drop at about four days postpartum. Maternal ACTH and cortisol levels at this stage, however, are not correlated.[50,51] Moreover, maternal ACTH levels are not correlated with parity, weight of the newborn, or duration of the delivery.[51]

The activation of the HPA axis during pregnancy has been proposed to function as a biological clock, timing from the early stages of gestation.[52] In this model, placental CRH is the timing starter, determining the course of pregnancy and culminat-

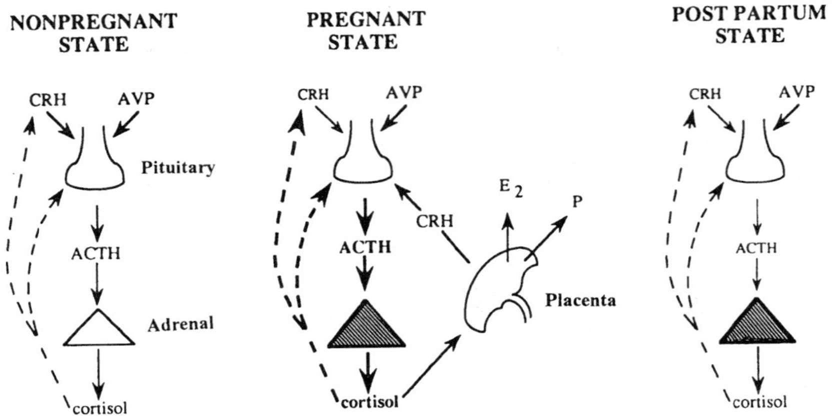

FIGURE 3. Comparative schematic representation of the HPA axis in the nonpregnant, pregnant, and postpartum state. CRH, corticotropin releasing hormone; AVP, arginine vasopressin; ACTH, adrenocorticotropin; E_2, estradiol; P, progesterone; shaded areas represent relative hypertrophy of the adrenals.

ing, accordingly, to a preterm, term, or postterm labor.[52] Moreover, in the same model, a direct effect on the triggering of parturition has been proposed, taking into account the course of maternal CRH levels and the increase of its unbound fraction by the third trimester of pregnancy.[53]

The maternal hormonal environment influences the mother's psychological status and the mother–infant relationship/bonding; to this the activation of the HPA axis seems to play a role. Primiparous women with uneventful pregnancies that deliver spontaneously vaginally, show elevated ACTH levels when their labor is not progressing satisfactorily.[54] Among first-time mothers, those with higher plasma cortisol levels recognize, in the early postpartum period, their own infant's odors more easily and are more attracted to them than women with low plasma cortisol levels.[55]

During the postpartum period, maternal plasma cortisol levels start a progressive decrease to normality. The HPA axis during the postpartum period gradually finds its prepregnant dynamic equilibrium. In the immediate postpartum period, the maternal HPA axis is mildly suppressed, in a way analogous to post-cure Cushing's syndrome.[56] Stimulation testing of the HPA axis presents evidence that hypothalamic CRH secretion is transiently suppressed at three and six weeks postpartum, normalizing at 12 weeks.[57] Despite the suppressed ACTH responses, total plasma cortisol levels are within normal range in postpartum women, probably because of the elevated CBG concentrations and because the adrenal glands are hypertrophic, and hence hyperresponsive to ACTH[5] (FIG. 3). In healthy lactating women, the HPA stress responses are blunted, as exemplified by attenuated plasma ACTH and cortisol responses to treadmill exercise.[58] In these women estrogen levels were lower and prolactin levels were higher compared to nonlactating women. Although the causal mechanism of this HPA axis response attenuation has yet to be elucidated, the role of estrogen levels should be taken into consideration, since half of the estrogen response elements have been found on the promoter region of the human CRH gene.[59] Also, in animal studies prolactin was shown to suppress HPA responses to stress.[60,61]

THE HPA AXIS IN PREGNANCY AND THE POSTPARTUM PERIOD: PATHOPHYSIOLOGIC CONSIDERATIONS

The placenta is a stress-sensitive organ[62–64]; placental CRH secretion is stimulated by adrenal cortisol.[65] Thus, during pregnancy an amplification of the stress response via the placenta has been suggested, whereas a desensitization of the anterior pituitary to hypothalamic CRH has been postulated.[66] The HPA axis is enmeshed in the response of pregnant women to psychosocial stress; higher plasma levels of ACTH and cortisol have been measured in such cases.[62] Because prenatal maternal stress is associated with premature birth,[50,67] and the latter is also associated with elevated maternal plasma CRH,[68] it can be assumed that the timing of birth is modified via the HPA axis.[52,53] Women suffering from pregnancy-induced hypertension present, at any stage of gestation from the 10th week and onwards, higher plasma CRH levels compared to healthy pregnant women.[69] Placental CRH secretion can be triggered by anoxia, inflammatory cytokines, and several prostaglandins, as well as by corticosteroids.[5] Preeclampsia- or eclampsia-induced anoxia, increased levels of circulating cytokines (as a result of infection or inflammation), and increased levels of corticosteriods (following physical or emotional stress) can promote CRH secretion and culminate in premature labor (FIG. 4). The measurement of maternal plasma CRH has been included in a proposed panel of markers of preterm labor,[53] and CRH receptor antagonists are under development as agents delaying premature labor and delivery.[70]

Almost half of postpartum women develop a short-lived dysthymic disorder, called the "postpartum blues," and epidemiological studies have shown consistently that the prevalence of nonpsychotic major depressive disorder in the first months after delivery is about 10%.[71–73] Mood disorders after pregnancy can last up to a year postpartum.[71,72] Women who have postpartum "blues" or postpartum depression show more blunted ACTH responses to ovine CRH stimulation testing than euthymic women in postpartum. Thus, the gradual recuperation of the HPA axis in the postpartum may be implicated in the mood disorders of that time period.[57] Similar disorders are observed after surgical cure in patients with Cushing's syndrome, in which atypical depression resolves earlier than the return of the HPA to normality.[74] Estrogen administered at high doses during the postpartum period has a marked antidepressant effect, and a possible explanation for this is that it may act to reestablish normal CRH and norepinephrine responses to stressors.[5,75]

During pregnancy cell-mediated immune function and Th1 cytokine production (e.g., IL-12, interferon-γ) are suppressed, and humoral immunity and Th2 cytokine production (e.g., IL-4, IL-10) are enhanced.[76] These cytokine patterns reverse in the postpartum period.[76] Thus, opposite Th1/Th2 cytokine profiles characterize pregnancy and the postpartum period.[75] Convincing evidence exists to indicate that changes in the production of cortisol (as well as in progesterone and estrogen) play major roles in modulating the balance between Th1 and Th2 cytokines.[75] Rheumatoid arthritis often remits during pregnancy and flares or develops initially in the

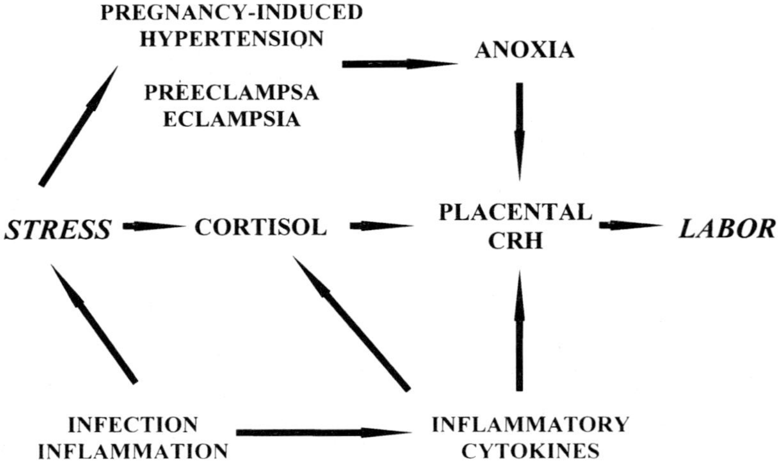

FIGURE 4. Model of premature labor mediated by placental corticotropin-releasing hormone (CRH) secretion. Anoxia caused by preeclampsia or eclampsia, increased levels of circulating cytokines, as a result of infection or inflammation, and increased levels of corticosteriods, following physical or emotional stress, can promote CRH secretion and culminate in premature labor (adapted from Chrousos *et al.*[5]).

postpartum period.[76–78] Also, thyroiditis occurs overall in 4 to 9% of women in the postpartum period.[79–81] The increased postpartum vulnerability to such autoimmune diseases could be attributed to the steroid withdrawal syndrome, the suppressed hypothalamic CRH secretion (FIG. 2), and the subsequent changes in cytokine profiles. In an analogous way patients with Cushing's syndrome present a post-cure vulnerability to such diseases.[82,83]

REFERENCES

1. CHROUSOS, G.P. *et al.*, Eds. 1988. Mechanisms of Physical and Emotional Stress. Advances in Experimental Medicine and Biology. Vol. 245. Plenum Press. New York.
2. CHROUSOS, G.P. *et al.* 1992. The concepts of stress and stress system disorders: overview of physical and behavioral homeostasis. JAMA **267:** 1244–1252.
3. CROFFORD, L.J. *et al.* 1993. Corticotropin releasing hormone in synovial fluids and tissues of patients with rheumatoid arthritis and osteoarthritis. J. Immunol. **151:** 1–10.
4. THEOHARIDES, T.C. *et al.* 1998. Corticotropin-releasing hormone induces skin mast cell degranulation and increased vascular permeability, a possible explanation for its proinflammatory effects. Endocrinology **139:** 403-413.
5. CHROUSOS, G.P. *et al.* 1998. Interactions between the hypothalamic–pituitary–adrenal axis and the female reproductive system: clinical implications. Ann. Intern. Med **129:** 229–240.
6. ARON, D.C. *et al.* 1994. Glucocorticoids and adrenal androgens. *In* Basic and Clinical Endocrinology. F.S. Greenspan & J.D. Baxter, Eds.: 307-346. Prentice-Hall. Connecticut.

7. Rabin, D. *et al.* 1988. Stress and reproduction: interactions between the stress and reproductive axis. In Mechanisms of Physical and Emotional Stress. G.P. Chrousos, D.L. Loriaux & P.W. Gold, Eds.: 377–387. Plenum Press. New York.
8. Rivier, C. *et al.* 1986. Stress-induced inhibition of reproductive function: role of endogenous corticotropin releasing factor. Science **231:** 607–609.
9. Vamvakopoulos, N.C. *et al.* 1993. Evidence of direct estrogen regulation of human corticotropin releasing hormone gene expression: potential implications for the sexual dimorphism of the stress response and immune/inflammatory reaction. J. Clin. Invest. **92:** 1896–1902.
10. Magiakou, M.A. *et al.* 1997. The hypothalamic–pituitary–adrenal axis and the female reproductive system. Ann. N.Y. Acad. Sci. **816:** 42–56.
11. Audhya, T. *et al.* 1989. Structural characterization and localization of corticotropin releasing factor in the testis. Biochem. Biophys. Acta **995:** 10–16.
12. Ulisse, S. *et al.* 1989. Corticotropin releasing factor receptors and actions in rat Leydig cells. J. Biol. Chem. **264:** 2156–2163.
13. Fabri, A. *et al.* 1990. Corticotropin releasing factor is produced by the rat Leydig cells and has a major antireproductive role in the testis. Endocrinology **127:** 1541–1543.
14. Mastorakos, G. *et al.* 1993. Immunoreactive corticotropin releasing hormone and its binding sites in the rat ovary. J. Clin. Invest. **92:** 961-968.
15. Mastorakos, G. *et al.* 1994. Presence of immunoreactive corticotropin releasing hormone in normal and polycystic human ovaries. J. Clin. Endocrinol. Metab. **79:** 1191–1197.
16. Ghizzoni, L. *et al.* 1997. Corticotropin-releasing hormone (CRH) inhibits steroid biosynthesis by cultured human granulosa-lutein cells in a CRH and interelukin-1 receptor-mediated fashion. Endocrinology **138:** 4806–4811.
17. Rodriguez-Linares, B. *et al.* 1998. Expression of corticotropin-releasing hormone receptor mRNA and protein in the human myometrium. J. Endocrinol. **156:** 15–21.
18. Petraglia, F. *et al.* 1992. Human decidua and in vitro decidualized endometrial stromal cells at term contain immunoreactive corticotropin-releasing factor (CRF) and CRF messenger ribonucleic acid. J. Clin. Endocrinol. Metab. **74:** 1427–1431.
19. Makrigannakis, A. *et al.* 1995. The corticotropin releasing hormone in normal and tumoral epithelial cells of human endometrium. J. Clin. Endocrinol. Metab. **80:** 185–189.
20. Mastorakos, G. *et al.* 1996. Presence of immunoreactive corticotropin releasing hormone in human endometrium. J. Clin. Endocrinol. Metab. **81:** 1046–1050.
21. Nolten, W.E. *et al.* 1980. Diurnal patterns and regulation of cortisol secretion in pregnancy. J. Clin. Endocrinol. Metab. **51:** 466–472.
22. Goland, R.S. *et al.* 1998. Biologically active corticotropin-releasing hormone in maternal and fetal plasma during pregnancy. Am. J. Obstet. Gynecol. **159:** 884–890.
23. Goland. R.S. *et al.* 1986. High levels of corticotropin releasing hormone immunoreactivity in maternal and fetal plasma during pregnancy. J. Clin. Endocrinol. Metab. **63:** 1199–1203.
24. Riley, S.C. *et al.* 1991. Corticotropin-releasing hormone production by the placenta and fetal membranes. Placenta. **12:** 105–119.
25. Grino, M. *et al.* 1987. The corticotropin releasing hormone gene is expressed in human placenta. Biochem. Biophys. Res. Commun. **148:** 1208–1214.
26. Sasaki, A. *et al.* 1987. Immunoreactive corticotropin-releasing hormone in human plasma during pregnancy, labor, and delivery. J. Clin. Endocrinol. Metab. **64:** 224–229.
27. Saeed, B.O. *et al.* 1997. Characterization of corticotropin-releasing hormone binding sites in the human placenta. J. Recept. Signal. Transduct. Res. **17:** 647–666.
28. Karteris, E. *et al.* 1998 The human placenta and fetal membranes express the corticotropin-releasing hormone receptor 1alpha (CRH-1alpha) and the CRH-C variant receptor. J. Clin. Endocrinol. Metab. **83:**1376–1379.
29. Grammatopoulos, D. *et al.* 1996. The biological activity of the corticotropin-releasing hormone receptor–adenylate cyclase complex in human myometrium is reduced at the end of pregnancy. J. Clin. Endocrinol. Metab. **81:** 745–751.
30. Zoumakis. E. *et al.* 1997. Endometrial corticotropin-releasing hormone. Its potential autocrine and paracrine actions. Ann. N.Y. Acad. Sci. **828:** 84–94.

31. WARREN, W.B. *et al.* 1990. Elevated maternal plasma corticotropin releasing hormone levels in twin gestation. J. Perinat. Med. **18:** 39–44.
32. MAGIAKOU, M.A. *et al.* 1996. Placental CRH secretion and the maternal hypothalamic–pituitary–adrenal axis in human pregnancy. Clin. Endocrinol. (Oxford) **44:** 419–428.
33. WADHWA, P.D. *et al.* 1997. Placental CRH modulates maternal pituitary–adrenal function in normal pregnancy. Ann. N.Y. Acad. Sci. **814:** 276–281.
34. SUDA, T. *et al.* 1991. Presence of CRH-binding protein in amniotic fluid and in umbilical cord plasma Acta Endocrinol. (Copenhagen) **125:** 165–169.
35. ORTH, D.N. *et al.* 1987. Specific high-affinity binding protein for human corticotropin-releasing hormone in normal human plasma. Biochem. Biophys. Res. Commun. **143:** 411–417.
36. SUDA, T. *et al.* 1988. Characterization of corticotropin-releasing hormone binding protein in human plasma by chemical cross-linking and its binding during pregnancy. J. Clin. Endocrinol. Metab. **67:** 1278–1283.
37. LINTON, E.A. *et al.* 1993. Corticotropin-releasing hormone-binding protein (CRH-BP): Plasma levels decrease during the third trimester of normal human pregnancy. J. Clin. Endocrinol. Metab. **76:** 260–262.
38. CLIFTON, V.L. *et al.* 1994. Corticotropin-releasing-hormone-induced vasodilation in the human fetal placental circulation. J. Clin. Endocrinol. Metab. **79:** 666–669.
39. JESKE, W.P. *et al.* 1989. Plasma GHRH, CRH, ACTH, β-endorphin, human placental lactogen, GH and cortisol concentrations at the third trimester of pregnancy. Acta Endocrinol. **120:** 785–789.
40. SCHULTE, H.M. *et al.* 1990. The corticotropin-releasing hormone test in late pregnancy: lack of adreenocorticotropin and cortisol response. Clin. Endocrinol. (Oxford) **33:** 99–106.
41. MARTIN, M.C. *et al.* 1994. The endocrinology of pregnancy. *In* Basic and Clinical Endocrinology. F.S. Greenspan & J. D. Baxter, Eds.: 525–550. Prentice-Hall. Connecticut.
42. LAATIKANEN, T. *et al.* 1987. Immunoreactive corticotropin releasing factor and corticotropin in plasma during pregnancy, labor and puerperium. Neuropeptides **10:** 343–353.
43. TUIMALA, R. *et al.* 1976. ACTH levels in amniotic fluid during pregnancy. Br. J. Obstet. Gynaecol. **83:** 853–856.
44. ROSENTHAL, H.E. *et al.* 1969. Transcortin: a cortocosteroid-binding protein of plasma. X. Cortisol and progesterone interplay and unbound levels of these steroids in pregnancy. J. Clin. Endocrinol. Metab. **29:** 352–367.
45. ABOU-SAMRA, A.B. *et al.* 1984. Increased plasma concentrations of N-terminal α-lipoprotein and unbound cortisol during pregnancy. Clin. Endocrinol. (Oxford) **20:** 221–228.
46. LINDHOLM, J. *et al.* 1973. Plasma and urinary cortisol in pregnancy and during estrogen-gestagen treatment. Scand. J. Clin. Lab. Invest. **31:** 119–122
47. PAABY, P.A. *et al.* 1990. A monthly cycle in the adrenocortical function during third-trimester pregnancy. Acta Endocrinol. **122:** 617–622.
48. OHANA, E. *et al.* 1996. Maternal plasma and amniotic fluid cortisol and progesterone concentrations between women with and without term labor. A comparison. J. Reprod. Med. **41:** 80–86.
49. GIUSSANI, D.A. *et al.* 1998. Changes in fetal plasma corticotropin-releasing hormone during androstenedione-induced labor in the rhesus monkey: lack of an effect on the fetal hypothalamo–pituitary–adrenal axis. Endocrinology **139:** 2803–2810.
50. KOREBRITS, C. *et al.* 1998. Maternal corticotropin-releasing hormone is increased with impending preterm birth. J. Clin. Endocrinol. Metab. **83:** 1585–1591.
51. BERGANT, A.M. *et al.* 1998. Childbirth as a biological model for stress? Associations with endocrine and obstetric factors. Gynecol. Obstet. Invest. **45:** 181–185.
52. MCLEAN, M. *et al.* 1995. A placental clock controlling the length of human pregnancy. Nat. Med. **1:** 460–463.
53. KEELAN, J.A. *et al.* 1997. The molecular mechanisms of term and preterm labor: recent progress and clinical implications. Clin. Obstet. Gynecol. **40:** 460–478.
54. FLORIDO, J. *et al.* 1997. Plasma concentrations of β-endorphin and adrenocorticotropic hormone in women with and without childbirth preparation. Eur. J. Obstet. Gynecol. Reprod. Biol. **73:** 121–125.

55. FLEMING, A.S. *et al.* 1997. Cortisol, hedonics, and maternal responsiveness in human mothers. Horm. Behav. **32:** 85–98.
56. GOMEZ, M.T. *et al.* 1993. The pituitary corticotroph is not the rate limiting step in the postoperative recovery of the hypothalamic–pituitary–adrenal axis in patients with Cushing syndrome. J. Clin. Endocrinol. Metab. **77:** 173–177.
57. MAGIAKOU, M.A. *et al.* 1996. Hypothalamic CRH suppression during the postpartum period: implications for the increase of psychiatric manifestations in this period. J. Clin. Endocrinol. Metab. **81:** 1912–1917.
58. ALTEMUS, M. *et al.* 1995. Suppression of hypothalamic–pituitary–adrenal axis responses to stress in lacating women. J. Clin. Endocrinol. Metab. **80:** 2954–2959.
59. VAMVAKOPOULOS, N.C. *et al.* 1993. Structural organization of the 5' flanking region of the human corticotropin releasing hormone gene. DNA Seq. **4:** 197–206.
60. SCLEIN, P.A. *et al.* 1974. The role of prolactin in the depressed or "buffered" adrenocorticostroid response in the rat. J. Endocrinol. **62:** 93–99.
61. ENDROCZI, E. *et al.* 1972. Pituitary adrenal responses of lactating rats and the effect of prolactin administration. Hormones **3:** 267.
62. SANDMAN, C.A. *et al.* 1997. Maternal stress, HPA activity, and fetal/infant outcome. Ann. N.Y. Acad. Sci. **814:** 266–275.
63. JONES, S.A. *et al.* 1989. Steroids modulate corticotropin releasing hormonee production in human fetal membranes and placenta. J. Clin. Endocrinol. Metab. **68:** 825–830.
64. PETRAGLIA, F.L. *et al.* 1995. Maternal plasma and placental immunoreactive corticotropin-releasing factor concentrations in infection-associated term and pre-term delivery. Placenta **16:** 157–164.
65. KARALIS, K. *et al.* 1995. Regulation of placental corticotropin-releasing hormone by steroids. Possible implications in labor initiation. Ann. N.Y. Acad. Sci. **771:** 551–555.
66. MAJZOUB, J.A. *et al.* 1999. Placental corticotropin-releasing hormone: function and regulation. Am. J. Obstet. Gynecol. **180:** S242–246.
67. HEDEGAARD, M. *et al.* 1993. Psychological distress in pregnancy and preterm delivery. Br. Med. J. **307:** 234–239.
68. KURKI, T. *et al.* 1991. Maternal plasma corticotropin-releasing hormone—elevated in preterm labour but unaffected by indomethacin or nylidrin. Br. J. Obstet. Gynaecol. **98:** 685–691.
69. WEBSTER, E.L. *et al.* 1996. In vivo and in vitro characterization of antalarmin, a nonapeptide corticotropin-releasing hormone (CRH) receptor antagonist: suppression of pituitary ACTH release and peripheral inflammation. Endocrinology **137:** 5747–5750.
70. LIAPI, C.A. *et al.* 1996. Corticotropin-releasing hormone levels in pregnancy-induced hypertension. Eur. J. Obstet. Gynecol. Reprod. Biol. **68:** 109–114.
71. COPPER, P.J. *et al.* 1998. Postnatal depression. Br. Med. J. **316:** 1884–1886.
72. O'HARA, M.W. 1997. The nature of postpartum depressive disorders. *In* Postpartum Depression and Child Development. L. Murray & P.J. Cooper, Eds.: 3–37. Guilford. New York.
73. NONACS, R. *et al.* 1998. Postpartum mood disorders: diagnosis and treatment guidelines. J. Clin. Psychiatry **59**(Suppl. **2**)**:** 34–40.
74. AVGERINOS, P.C. *et al.* 1987. The corticotropin releasing hormone test in the postoperative evaluation of patients with Cushing's syndrome. J. Clin. Endocrinol. Metab. **65:** 906–913.
75. GREGOIRE, A.J. *et al.* 1996. Transdermal oestrogen for treatment of severe postnatal depression. Lancet **347:** 930–933.
76. WILDER, R.L. 1998. Hormones, pregnancy, and autoimmune diseases. Ann. N.Y. Acad. Sci. **840:** 45–50.
77. ELENKOV, I.J. *et al.* 1997. Does differential neuroendocrine control of cytokine production govern the expression of autoimmune diseases in pregnancy and the postpartum period? Mol. Med. Today **3:** 379–383.
78. LANSINK, M. *et al.* 1993. The onset of rheumatoid arthritis in relation to pregnancy and childbirth. Clin. Exp. Rheumatol. **11:** 171–174.
79. VARGAS, M.T. *et al.* 1988. Antithyroid microsomal autoantibodies and HLA-DR5 are associated with postpartum thyroid dysfunction: evidence supporting an autoimmune pathogenesis. J. Clin. Endocrinol. Metab. **67:** 327–333.

80. STAGNARO-GREEN, A. 1993. Postpartum thyroiditis: prevalence, etiology and clinical implications. Thyroid Today **16:** 1–11.
81. GERSTEIN, H.C. 1990. How common is postpartum thyroiditis? A methodologic review of the literature. Arch. Intern. Med. **150:** 1397–1400.
82. CHROUSOS, G.P. 1995. The hypothalamic–pituitary–adrenal axis and immune-mediated inflammation. N. Engl. J. Med. **332:** 1309–1315.
83. STRATAKIS, C.A. *et al.* 1997. Thyroid function in children with Cushing's disease before and after transsphenoidal surgery. J. Pediatr. **131:** 905–909.

Clinical Implications of the Ovarian/Endometrial Renin–Angiotensin–Aldosterone System

E. HASSAN,[a] G. CREATSAS, G. MASTORAKOS, AND S. MICHALAS

1st and 2nd Departments of Obstetrics and Gynecology, University of Athens, Athens, Greece

Abstract: New organ-specific functions of angiotensin II have recently been described: the importance of its role in the regulation of secretory epithelial function in many tissues including components of the reproductive tract has been documented. The source of angiotensin II in these tissues is the reproductive tract itself, and there is considerable evidence to suggest a distinct renin–angiotensin–aldosterone system in the ovary and uterus. Two main subtypes of angiotensin II receptors are recognized as angiotensin-receptor I and II, according to their sensitivity to the angiotensin II antagonists. However, the presence of angiotensin II receptors in the male and female reproductive tract suggests a multiplicity of roles that are unrelated to their primary functions or to each other. The renin–angiotensin–aldosterone system is a major determinant of sodium balance in pregnancy. More recently RT-PCR methods have revealed angiotensinogen transcription in the smooth muscle of spiral anteries of the decidua; a specific allele of this gene may be associated with hypertension in pregnancy as well as in pre-eclampsia. We investigated the evolution of plasma renin activity and aldosterone levels during normal and hypertensive pregnancy. Both were found to increase progressively during all three trimesters of normotensive pregnancy. Plasma renin activity in hypertensive women remained unchanged during all three trimesters of pregnancy. Plasma aldosterone levels in hypertensive women increased progressively during all three trimesters of pregnancy. However, plasma aldosterone levels remained significantly lower than the ones of normotensive pregnant women. These increased aldosterone levels were noticed despite unchanged renin levels. Further clinical studies investigating the renin–angiotensin–aldosterone system in the pathogenesis of pregnancy hypertension are needed. A renin-independent role of aldosterone in this pathological entity is suggested.

INTRODUCTION

The renin–angiotensin system is a hormonal system that plays a major role in the regulation of sodium excretion. Its activation results in extremely potent vasoconstriction. On the other hand, this system also plays a major functional role in the genital tract. This system is of considerable interest and importance in many studies of reproduction. Renin acts locally in the tissues of the genital tract as a tissue hormone

[a]Address for correspondence: Elsheikh Hassan, M.D., Pindarou 1A, 145 78 Ekali, Greece. Phone: +30-944-391699; fax: +30-1-6229966.

through modification or stimulation of other, locally acting, vasoconstrictor and vasodilator hormone.

Renin is an aspartyl protease that is capable of cleaving its hepatic substrate, angiotensinogen, to form angiotensin I, a decapeptide. The latter is in turn converted to angiotensin II by angiotensin-converting enzymes. Angiotensin II is thus viewed as the main active peptide in the renin–angiotensin–aldosterone system. Most of the physiological functions of angiotensin II are believed to be mediated by the angiotensin I receptor through the activation of phosphoinositide/calcium pathway, tyrosine phosphorylation pathway, or the inhibition of adenylate cyclase activity.[1,2] Angiotensin II, a key regulator of cardiovascular homeostasis, is involved in various biological functions, such as hormone secretion, neuronal activities, and tissue growth.[1] Although traditionally viewed in the context of fluid and electrolyte economy, the renin–aldosterone system has now been observed in a variety of tissues, and it is subservient to the special needs of the tissues in question. Over the past few years, evidence has mounted to suggest the existence of an intrinsic ovarian renin–aldosterone system, and its role in reproduction is currently being explored.

After cleavage from its precursor prorenin by the juxtaglomerular cells of the kidney, renin is secreted into the blood. Decapeptide angiotensin I is then yielded from active renin in turn by cleaving of the α_2 globulin angiotensinogen.[1–3] The active octapeptide hormone angiotensin II is formed by the angiotensin-converting enzyme, which cleaves two amino acids from the carboxyl terminus; this action is shared by chymase, which may occur in the reproductive tract.[4] The presence of angiotensin-converting enzyme was identified in the rat ovary.[2] The basal ovarian angiotensin-converting enzyme activity in fertile women is relatively high; it is about threefold greater than that in human veins and heart auricle tissues and similar to that in human arteries. In the follicular fluid of gonadotropin-stimulated women, renin-like activity was reported to be 10-fold greater than that in the plasma, and follicular aspirates from human-stimulated ovarian follicles were shown to contain 14 times greater angiotensin II immunoreactivity than plasma angiotensin II concentrations.[5,6]

RECEPTORS

Angiotensin II receptors have been identified and characterized. Their expression varies with animal species and the developmental stage of the ovarian follicle.[1,2] The main subtypes of angiotensin II receptors are recognized as angiotensin receptor subtypes 1 and 2, according to their sensitivity to angiotensin II antagonists.[5,6] The literature suggests that more receptor subtypes may exist.[7–10] These two receptor subtypes vary significantly in tissue distribution: in the adrenal glands, most of those in the glomerulosa are subtype 1, whereas those in the medulla are mainly subtype 2.[11] The nonpregnant human uterus contains mainly subtype 2 receptors, whereas the rat uterus contains both subtypes.[12] Although both receptors are present in the rat brain, subtype 2 receptor concentration is particularly high in newborn, neonatal, and young animals.[13] Subtype 2 receptors are expressed in the rat and bovine ovary,[14,15] whereas other tissues contain both receptor subtypes in varying proportions.[16] Ovariectomy and progesterone treatment cause a progressive decrease in receptor concentration, whereas estrogen treatment progressively increases them.[7]

Receptor binding studies and Northern blot analyses revealed that the human myometrium abundantly expresses angiotensin II receptors and that more than 90% of the angiotensin II receptors in the human myometrial tissue consist of the angiotensin II-subtype 2 receptor.[16] Because angiotensin II-subtype 2 receptors do not mediate contractile responses, their presence may contribute to the attenuated responses to angiotensin II by the uteroplacental and cerebral vasculature.[17] Myometrium is a nonvascular smooth muscle that expresses angiotensin receptors. In nonpregnant women, myometrium expresses predominantly the angiotensin II-subtype 2 receptor regulated as in vascular smooth muscle. Pregnancy causes significant changes in the receptor concentration in the rat uterus; an initial threefold increase during the first half of pregnancy is followed by a decrease to below nonpregnant levels. These changes occur mainly in the implantation area, and they may be related to the decidualization process.[7] Total angiotensin receptor number in myometrium fell by 92% in pregnancy, whereas that in uterine artery remained unchanged, demonstrating differences in receptor regulation in vascular and nonvascular smooth muscle in gravid women.[14] The physiological role of the myometrial angiotensin II receptor remains unknown. It is possible that the decrease of their number in the myometrium during pregnancy results in a relative increase of the angiotensin I receptor number, and cosequently contributes to the increased uterine sensitivity to angiotensin II.[6]

REPRODUCTIVE TRACT

The importance of angiotensin II has been documented in relation to its action in normal mammalian electrolyte homeostasis and hemodynamics as well as in cardiovascular disease in humans.[17–19] However, the presence of angiotensin II receptors in such a wide variety of tissues suggests a multiplicity of roles that are unrelated to these primary functions, or to each other.[20,21] Immunohistochemical studies localized renin and angiotensin II to thecal cells, corpus luteum, and luteinized granulosa cells of human ovaries.[15] Abundant evidence indicates that numerous tissues receive angiotensin II from local paracrine sources; local renin–angiotensin–aldosterone systems have been found in the reproductive tract, as well as in other organs.[22–27] There is also evidence indicating a primary, direct role for angiotensin II in ovarian steroidogenesis and ovulation. This evidence depends on the identification of this system in specific tissue locations, including angiotensinogen, renin, angiotensin-converting enzyme, and/or the mRNA that codes for them, as well as angiotensin I and II themselves in the reproductive tract.

Several roles of angiotensin II in mammalian ovarian function have been suggested. The effects are presumably species-specific and cycle stage–specific as the expression of angiotensin II receptor varies with species and stage follicular development.[27] Both the corpus luteum of cycling ovaries and the corpus luteum of pregnancy show heavy immunostaining for renin and angiotensin II. Thus, the increased activity of the ovarian renin–angiotensin system, which appears to be triggered by the preovulatory rise of LH, persists during the life span of the corpus luteum.[1,3]

Male

Components of the renin–angiotensin–aldosterone system have been found throughout the male reproductive tract in various species; prorenin mRNA and mRNA coding for angiotensinogen have been identified in rat and mouse testes,[25,28–30] and renin has been identified in the Leydig cell of both the human and rat testes.[25,28,31,32] Testicular renin is reduced by hypophysectomy in rats and increased during human chorionic gonadotropin treatment.[33] This demonstrates its independence from the circulating renin–angiotensin–aldosterone system. Prorenin was also found in the male reproductive tract. Prorenin may be secreted by the testes into both circulation and human seminal fluid.[1,34,35]

Female

In the female reproductive system, prorenin and renin have been found in the ovary and the uterus and both are a major source of prorenin in the plasma. Angiotensin I and II receptors were found in the fallopian tubes.[36,37] Relatively high levels of prorenin, renin-like activity, and angiotensin II have been found in human follicular fluid as compared with plasma, implicating the ovary as a source of these hormones.[17] Circulating levels of prorenin have been reported to change cyclically during the human menstrual cycle. Prorenin concentrations were found to be the highest in both the ovary and uterus during the luteotropic hormone surge, in pregnancy and after human chorionic gonadotropin treatment.[1,2,38,39] Even though plasma prorenin is correlated with the number of ovarian follicles and with plasma estradiol and progesterone levels in stimulated cycles,[38,39] it is not increased during pregnancy in women who, due to ovarian failure, conceived using donated eggs.[39,40] Uptake from the circulation may be responsible for the increased levels of both prorenin and renin in the myometrium during pregnancy.[41,42]

Correlation between active renin concentration and oocyte maturity is still controversial.[43,44] Angiotensinogen may be present in human follicular fluid, but its concentration (similar or lower to that in the plasma), may suggest its derivation from the circulation.[40,45] Also, in a group of premenopausal and postmenopausal women, the ovarian angiotensin converting enzyme has been shown to increase with age.[46] Immunoreactive angiotensin II has been found to be higher in the follicular fluid than in the plasma, and as with renin activity, it is significantly increased in gonadotropin-stimulated cycles.[44,47,48]

The angiotensin subtype II receptors occur in the granulosa and theca interna cells in rats while they are the most abundant angiotensin receptors in the human ovary.[14,49–51] Angiotensin II may play a role in the stimulation of ovarian estrogen production.[49,52,53] Both stimulatory and inhibitory effects of angiotensin II on steroidegenesis have been reported, but there are differences in the response to different steroids[54] or their cellular sites of formation. It has been reported that in bovine ovaries, follicular fluid concentrations of prorenin correlate negatively with estrogen but positively with progesterone, although follicular wall renin and prorenin correlate positively with both steroids.[55] Such variability may reflect differences in response that depend on the stage of the ovarian cycle or the state of differentiation or maturation of the various follicular cell types. It has been also reported that estrogens regulate angiotensin-converting enzyme activity and the number of angiotensin receptors in the female rat anterior pituitary. In human and rats, estrogen produces a rapid and persistent increase in the plasma renin substrate, angiotensinogen. In addition, estrogen administration stimulates the hepatic synthesis of plasma renin substrate.[46]

Although much remains to be learned, there is little doubt that the activity of the ovarian renin–angiotensin–aldosterone system fluctuates in the course of the normal menstrual cycle, reaching a peak at approximately midcycle; similarly, angiotensin II receptors display cyclical variation. It has been proposed that the high preovulatory levels of angiotensin II in follicular fluid may be involved, either directly or through other ovarian regulators, in oocyte maturation. It has also been suggested that angiotensin II may play a part in the formation of the corpus luteum and in the regulation of steroid secretion by luteal cell.[52,55] The role of angiotensin II in ovulation also remains unclear. Some reports suggest that it has no effect,[56,57] while others show that it stimulates ovulation in the rabbit.[58] It was also noted that the angiotensin II antagonist, saralasin, inhibited ovulation in perfused rat ovaries, whereas converting enzyme inhibitors did not.[57,59,60]

The role of angiotensin II in follicular atresia has been documented.[53] High concentrations of subtype II receptor of angiotensin II and prorenin were found in atretic follicles.[61] Renin and angiotensin II were noticed in granulosa cells of the atretic follicles, but only in theca cells of developing follicles.[62] The renin–angiotensin–aldosterone system may play a role in the pathogenesis of polycystic ovary syndrome. Polycystic ovaries show an increased expression of renin and angiotensin II in theca, granulosa, and stromal cells.[63]

PREGNANCY

Pregnancy is associated with substantial alterations in the hormonal milieu. The renin–angiotensin–aldosterone system is a major determinant of sodium balance in pregnancy,[64,65] as opposed to the natriuretic effects of progesterone, arginine vasopressin,[66,67] atrial natriuretic factor,[68] prostaglandins,[69] and other factors related to filtered sodium. The net result of this interplay between sodium regulatory factors is gradual sodium retention of approximately 900 mmol by the end of gestation[70] with attendant plasma volume expansion.[71] Although the components of this system are markedly stimulated as compared to the nonpregnant state, both renin and aldosterone respond physiologically to these new "set points" during normotensive pregnancy.[65] Furthermore, the interrelations between sodium balance and this system are changed as pregnancy progresses. Therefore, in the past, this system has been often implicated in pregnancy hypertension.

PREGNANCY HYPERTENSION

More recently, radiologic technology–polymerase chain reaction (RT-PCR) methods have revealed angiotensinogen transcription in the smooth muscle of spiral arteries of the decidua; a specific allele of this gene may be associated with hypertension in pregnancy as well as in pre-eclampsia.[72] Hypertension complicates 5–10% of all pregnancies; hypertensive disorders remain one of the leading causes of

TABLE 1. Aldosterone and plasma renin activity levels during normal and hypertensive pregnancy

	Gestational week					
	11–19		20–29		30–37	
	A	B	A	B	A	B
Aldosterone	520±175.4	140±50.5	811±227.0	214±73.5	888±123.2	462±253.1
(pg/ml)	$p < 0.01$		$p < 0.001$		$p < 0.001$	
Plasma renin activity	8.3±4.10	5.2±1.31	10.1±2.58	42.±0.91	15.7±5.16	4.7±1.33
(ng/ml/hr)	$p < 0.10$ N.S.		$p < 0.01$		$p < 0.001$	

NOTE: A, normotensive; B, hypertensive. The comparisons are between normotensive and hypertensive subjects.

maternal mortality and perinatal death in developed countries.[73] Pregnancy-induced hypertension (PIH) is a multisystem disorder, and its primary pathology remains unclear. During a normal pregnancy, blood pressure usually decreases by the second trimester, and in some cases this decrease may mask the presence of chronic hypertension. The major maternal hazard is that of eclampsia or grand mal seizures resulting from the profound cerebral effects of PIH[73]; hazards to the fetus mainly result from the decreased placental perfusion that is typical of this vasospastic disorder. To date, no biochemical markers have been found sensitive and/or specific enough to screen or prognose PIH.

To examine the involvement of the renin–angiotensin–aldosterone system in the pathogenesis of hypertension in pregnancy, we investigated the evolution of plasma renin activity and aldosterone levels during normal and hypertensive pregnancy in 71 pregnant (43 normotensive, 28 hypertensive) and 24 nonpregnant (12 normotensive, 12 hypertensive) women, aged 19–43 years (mean ± SD 28 ± 2.8). Plasma renin activity and aldosterone levels were determined by radioimmunoassay (RIA).

Renin–Aldosterone Levels in Normotensives during Pregnancy

Plasma renin activity and aldosterone levels were found to increase progressively during all three trimesters of normotensive pregnancy (TABLE 1); both were higher than in normotensive nonpregnant women.

Renin–Aldosterone Levels in Hypertensives during Pregnancy

In all three trimesters of pregnancy, plasma renin activity in hypertensive women remained unchanged (FIG. 1); the levels of this hormone were higher than those of hypertensive nonpregnant women and lower than those of pregnant normotensive women.

Plasma aldosterone levels in hypertensive women increased progressively during all three trimesters of pregnancy (FIG. 2); they were lower during the first and higher during the second and third trimester, as compared to hypertensive nonpregnant women. However, plasma aldosterone levels remained significantly lower than those of normotensive pregnant women during all three trimesters of pregnancy. The age and the parity of the woman did not affect plasma renin activity or the aldosterone level. In addition, the fluctuation of plasma renin activity and aldosterone levels bore

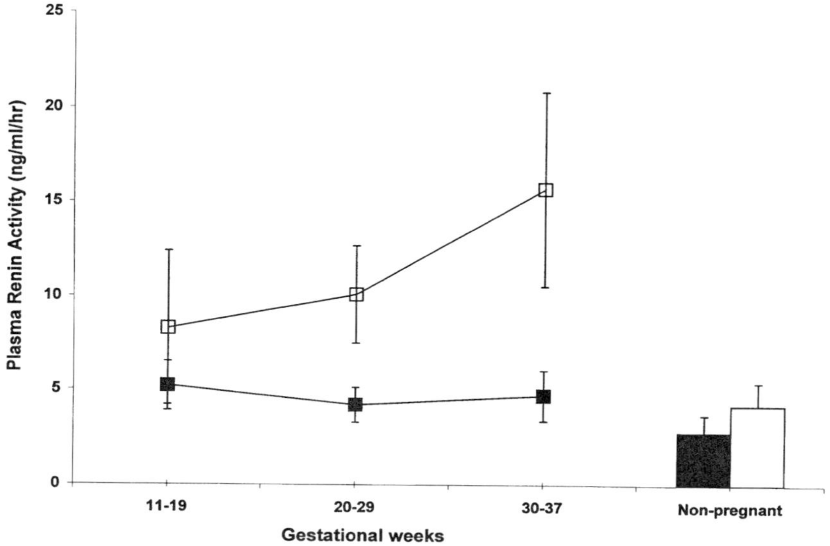

FIGURE 1. Plasma renin activity levels during normal (white squares) and hypertensive (black squares) pregnancy and in normotensive (white bar) and hypertensive (black bar) nonpregnant women.

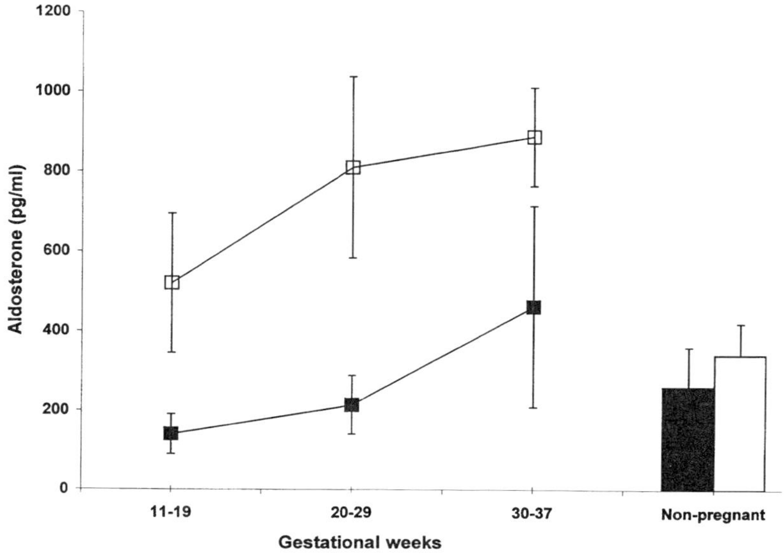

FIGURE 2. Aldosterone plasma levels during normal (white squares) and hypertensive (black squares) pregnancy and in normotensive (white bar) and hypertensive (black bar) nonpregnant women.

no relationship to the severity of hypertension. It is noteworthy that in hypertensive pregnancies aldosterone levels increase significantly during the third trimester despite unchanged renin levels. Thus, we have suggested that aldosterone biology seems to be involved directly and/or indirectly with the etiology of PIH.

It is difficult to characterize the renin–aldosterone system in hypertensives during pregnancy because longitudinal follow-up of these patients is missing. It is equally difficult to interpret renin and aldosterone levels in pre-eclampsia because of differences in the definition of the latter, such as parity, degree of proteinuria, and early or late onset of the disease. Also, it might depend on differences in assay techniques and collection of blood samples, which may be affected by bed rest, sodium intake, or labor.

In the majority of studies, renin and aldosterone are both decreased in pre-eclampsia compared to normotensive pregnancy.[66,67] Our data confirmed this, although it indicated a disruption of the renin–aldosterone system during the third trimester of pregnancy where aldosterone increased despite unchanged renin levels. Moreover, components of the renin–aldosterone system have not yet been correlated with the development of PIH.[74,75] Available evidence suggests a secondary involvement of the renin–aldosterone system in pre-eclampsia, the effects of the renin–aldosterone system being a consequence to impaired production of vasodilating prostaglandins. Suppressed plasma renin levels in women with PIH suggest that in this disorder the effective plasma volume may be expanded. However, this does not concur with the observation that plasma volume is lower in pre-eclampsia compared with normal pregnancy.[76] A possible explanation for this apparent inconsistency is that the measured decrease in plasma renin levels in PIH does not truly reflect hypervolemia or overfilling, but rather increased vasoconstriction. Alternatively, plasma atrial natriuretic factor may be increased in PIH by mechanisms other than volume expansion, which may still directly inhibit renin.[77,78] Furthermore, the renin–aldosterone system in both normotensives and hypertensives during pregnancy may respond to physiologic signals such as changes in blood pressure, volume status, and alterations in placental hormones such as estradiol and progesterone.

CONCLUSION

Angiotensin II plays critical roles in fertility and production of a fertilized ovum.[79,80] Its presence in the semen and the follicular fluid, as well as its production along the length of the reproductive tract in both sexes, justify these roles. Much attention is focused on the sperm itself; the ubiquitous presence of angiotensin receptors within the genital tract confers a role to this hormone in motility, acrosome reaction, and sperm binding both to the fallopian tube epithelium and to the ovum, as well as in sperm viability.[81] In the female genital tract, angiotensin II is also involved with oocyte maturation, ovulation, and follicular atresia,[20,82] as well as, potentially, ovum transport and support within the reproductive tract. These functions also raise the possibility of new therapeutic approaches both for improving fertility and for reducing it as well. There is enhanced activity of the renin–aldosterone system in normotensive pregnancies, reflected by increased circulating levels of plasma renin activity and aldosterone which may be important in maintaining vascular tone.

In hypertensive pregnancies the renin–aldosterone system is found to be suppressed as reflected by decreased levels of aldosterone and plasma renin activity as compared to normotensive pregnancy. Further clinical studies investigating the renin–angiotensin–aldosterone system in the pathogenesis of PIH are needed. A renin-independent role of aldosterone in this pathological entity is suggested.

REFERENCES

1. Sealey, J.E. & S. Rubattu. 1989. Prorenin and renin as separate mediators of tissue and circulating systems. Am. J. Hypertens. **2:** 358–366.
2. Ganong, W.F. 1995. Reproduction and the renin–angiotensin system. Neurosci. Biobehav. Rev. **19:** 241–250.
3. Sealey, J.E. *et al.* 1996. Specific prorenin/renin binding (probp)—identification and characterization of a novel membrane site. Am. J. Hyperptens. **9:** 491–502.
4. Urata, H. *et al.* 1994. Widespread tissue distribution of human chymase. J. Hypertens. **12:** S17–S22.
5. Wong, P.C. *et al.* 1990. Functional studies of nonpeptide angiotensin II receptor subtype-specific ligands: DuP 753(AII-1) and PD123177 (AII-2). J. Pharmacol. Exp. Ther. **255:** 584–92.
6. Smith, R.D. *et al.* 1992. Analysis of angiotensin II receptor antagonists. Annu. Rev. Pharmacol. Toxicol. **58:** 1883–1888.
7. Vinson, G.P. *et al.* 1995. The distribution of angiotensin II type 1 receptors, and the tissue renin–angiotensin systems. Mol. Med. Today **1:** 35–39.
8. Chaki, S. & T. Inagami. 1992. Identification and characterisation of a new binding site for angiotensin II in mouse neuroblastoma neuro-2A cells. Biochem. Biophys. Res. Commun. **182:** 388–390.
9. Tsutsumi, K. *et al.* 1992. Heterogeneity of angiotensin II AT2 receptors in the rat brain. Mol. Pharmacol. **41:** 290–297.
10. Song, K. *et al.* 1992. Nephrectomy and a newly identified binding site for angiotensin II in the rat adrenal cortex. Life Sci. **51:** 165–170.
11. Balla, T. *et al.* 1991. Angiotensin II receptor subtypes and biological responses in the adrenal cortex and medulla. Mol. Pharmacol. **40:** 401–406.
12. Tsutsumi, K. & J.M. Saavedra. 1991. Characterization and development of angiotensin II receptor subtypes (AT1 and AT2) in rat brain. Am. J. Physiol. **261:** R209–216.
13. Millan, M.A. *et al.* 1991. Differential distribution of AT1 and AT2 receptor subtypes in the rat brain during development. Proc. Soc. Natl. Acad. Sci. USA **88:** 1440–1444.
14. Pucell, A.G. *et al.* 1991. Biochemical properties of the ovarian granulosa-cell type-2-angiotensin-II receptor. Endocrinology **128:** 1947–1959.
15. Aiyar, N. *et al.* 1993 Characterization of bovine ovary angiotensin II receptors using subtype selective antagonists. Pharmacology **46:** 1–8.
16. Montiel, M. *et al.* 1993. Angiotensin II receptor isoforms in the rat adrenal gland: studies with the selective subtype antagonists DuP 753 and CGP42112A. J. Mol. Endocrinol. **11:** 69–75.
17. Peach, M.T. 1977. Renin–angiotensin system: biochemistry and mechanism of action. Physiol. Rev. **57:** 363–370.
18. Jeunemaitre, X. *et al.* 1992. Molecular basis of human hypertension: role of angiotensinogen. Cell **71:** 169–180.
19. Cambien, F. *et al.* 1991. Deletion polymorphism in the gene for angiotensin-converting enzyme is potent risk factor for myocardial infarction. Nature **359:** 641–644.
20. Vinson, G.P. *et al.* 1997. Tissue renin–angiotensin systems and reproduction. Hum. Reprod. **12:** 651–662.
21. Smits, J.F.M. *et al.* 1998. Should we aim at tissue renin–angiotensin systems? Pharm. World Sci. **20:** 93–99.

22. SOUBRIER, F. & P. CORVOL. 1990. Clinical implications of the molecular biology of the renin–angiotensin system. Eur. Heart J. **11**(Suppl D)**:** 3–10.
23. MULROW, P.J. 1992. Adrenal renin: regulation and function. Front. Neuroendocrinol. **13:** 47–60.
24. DOSTAL, D.E. *et al.* 1992. Intracardiac detection of angiotensin and renin: a localised renin–angiotensin system in neonatal heart. Am. J. Physiol. **263:** C838–850.
25. DESCHEPPER, C.F. *et al.* 1986. Analysis by immunocytochemistry and in situ hybridisation of renin and its mRNA in kidney, testis, adrenal, and pituitary of the rat. Proc. Soc. Natl. Acad. Sci. USA **83:** 7552–7556.
26. PHILIPS, M.I. *et al.* 1994. Levels of angiotensin and molecular biology of the tissue renin angiotensin systems. Regul. Pept. **43:** 1–20.
27. HAGEMANN, A. *et al.* 1993. The uteroplacental renin–angiotensin system—a review. Exp. Clin. Endocrinol. **102:** 252–261.
28. DZAU, V.J. *et al.* 1987. A comparative study of the distributions of renin and angiotensin messenger ribonucleic acids in rat and mouse. Endocrinology **120:** 2334–2338.
29. DZAU, V.J. *et al.* 1987. Tissue-specific regulation of renin expression in the mouse. Hypertension **9:** 1136–1141.
30. HELLMAN, W. *et al.* 1988. Angiotensinogen gene expression in extrahepatic rat tissues: application of a solution hybridization assay. Naunyn-Schmiedeberg's Arch. Pharmacol. **338:** 327–331.
31. PANDEY, K.N. *et al.* 1984. Evidence for intracellular formation of angiotensins—coexistence of renin and angiotensin-converting enzyme in Leydig cells of rat testis. Biochem. Biophys. Res. Commun. **122:** 1337–1343.
32. NARUSE, K. *et al.* 1985. Immunohistochemical evidence for renin in human endocrine tissues. J. Clin. Endocrinol. Metab. **61:** 172–177.
33. NARUSE, M. *et al.* 1984. Gonadotropin-dependent renin in rat testes. Proc. Soc. Exp. Biol. Med. **177:** 337–342.
34. OKUYAMA, A. *et al.* 1988. Induction of the renin–angiotensin system in human testis in vivo. Arch. Androl. **21:** 29–35.
35. MUKHOPADHYAY, A.K. *et al.* 1995. Human seminal fluid contains significant quantities of protenin—its correlation with the sperm density. Mol. Cell. Endocrinol. **109:** 219–224.
36. SARIDOGAN, E. *et al.* 1996. Angiotensin II receptors and angiotensin II stimulation of ciliary activity in human fallopian tube. J. Clin. Endocrinol. Metab. **81:** 2719–2725.
37. JOHNSON, M.C. *et al.* 1998. Presence of angiotensin II and expression of angiotensin II type-2 receptor in human fallopian tube. Fertil. Steril. **70:** 740–746.
38. ITSKOVITZ, J. & J.E. SEALEY. 1987. Ovarian prorenin–renin–angiotensin system. Obstet. Gynecol, Surv. **42:** 545–551.
39. SEALEY, J.E. *et al.* 1987. Ovarian prorenin. Clin. Exp. Hypertens. A**9:** 1435–1454.
40. DERKX, F.H. *et al.* 1987. High concentrations of immunoreactive renin, prorenin and enzymatically-active renin in human ovarian follicular fluid. Br. J. Obstet. Gynaecol. **94:** 4–9.
41. WARREN, A.Y. *et al.* 1982. Production of active and inactive renin by cultured explants from the human female genital tract. Br. J. Obstet. Gynaecol. **89:** 628–632.
42. NIELSEN, A.H. *et al.* 1995. The tissue renin–angiotensin system in the female reproductive tissues. *In* Tissue Renin–Angiotensin Systems. A.K. Mukhopadhyay & M.K. Raizada, Eds.: 253–268. Plenum. New York/London.
43. PAULSON, R.J. *et al.* 1989. Ovarian renin production in vitro and in vivo: characterization and clinical correlation. Fertil. Steril. **51:** 634–638.
44. SATO, Y. 1991. Renin- and angiotensin-like immunoactivities in human follicular fluid in in vitro fertilization. Horm. Res. **35(Suppl 1):** 47–49.
45. GLORIOSO, N. *et al.* 1986. Prorenin in high concentrations in human ovarian follicular fluid. Science **233:** 1422–1424.
46. ERMAN, A. *et al.* 1996. Ovarian angiotensin-converting enzyme activity in humans: relationship to estradiol, age, and uterine pathology. J. Clin. Endocrinol. Metab. **81:** 1104–1107.

47. CULLER, M.D. *et al.* 1986. Angiotensin-II-like immunoreactivity in human ovarian follicular-fluid. J. Clin. Endocrinol. Metab. **62:** 613–615.
48. LIGHTMAN, A. *et al.* 1987. The ovarian renin–agniostenin system: renin-like activity and angiotensin II/III immunoreactivity in gonadotropin-stimulated and unstimulated human follicular fluid. Am. J. Obstet. Gynecol. **156:** 808–816.
49. SPETH, R.C. *et al.* 1988. Distribution of angiotensin-converting enzyme and angiotensin II–receptor binding sites in the rat ovary. Biol. Reprod. **38:** 695–702.
50. SPETH, R.C. *et al.* 1986. Identification of angiotensin-II receptors in the rat ovary. Eur. J. Pharmacol. **130:** 351–352.
51. OBERMULLER, N. *et al.* 1998. Localization of the mRNA for the angiotensin II receptor subtype 2 (AT2) in follicular granulosa cells of the rat ovary by nonradioactive in situ hybridization. J. Hisotchem. Cytochem. **46:** 865–870.
52. BUMPUS, F.M. *et al.* 1998. Angiotensin II: an intraovarian regulatory peptide. Am. J. Med. Sci. **295:** 406–408.
53. NEMETH, G. *et al.* 1994. The basis and evidence of a role for the ovarian renin–angiotensin system in health and disease. J. Soc. Gynecol. Invest. **1:** 118–127.
54. KUJI, N. *et al.* 1996. Involvement of angiotensin II in the process of gonadotropin-induced ovulation in rabbits. Biol. Reprod. **55:** 984–991.
55. HAGEMANN, A. *et al.* 1997. Relationship between follicular fluid steroids and tissue renin concentrations and secretion rates in bovine ovaries. Exp. Clin. Endocrinol. **105:** 271–276.
56. DAUD, A.I. *et al.* 1989. Angiotensin-II does it have a direct obligate role in ovulation. Science **245:** 870–871.
57. DAUD, A.I. *et al.* 1990. Characterization of angiotensin I converting enzyme (ACE)-containing follicles in the rat ovary during the estrous cycle and effects of ACE inhibitor on ovulation. Endocrinology **126:** 2927–2935.
58. YOSHIMURA, Y. *et al.* 1993. Locally produced angiotensin-II induces ovulation by stimulating prostaglandin production in in-vitro perfused rabbit ovaries. Endocrinology **133:** 1609–1616.
59. PETERSON, C.M. *et al.* 1993. The angiotensin II antagonist saralasin inhibits ovulation in the perfused rat ovary. Am. J. Obstet. Gynecol. **168:** 242–245.
60. PETERSON, C.M. *et al.* 1993. Angiotensin-converting enzyme inhibitors have no effect on ovulation and ovarian steroidogenesis in the perfused rat ovary. Reprod. Toxicol. **7:** 131–135.
61. DAUD, A.I. *et al.* 1988. Evidence for selective expression of angiotensin-II receptors on atretic follicles in the rat ovary and autoradiographic study. Endocrinology **122:** 2727–2734.
62. MUKHOPADHYAY, A.K. *et al.* 1991. The relationship between prorenin levels in follicular-fluid and follicular atresia in bovine ovaries. Endocrinology **129:** 2367–2375.
63. PALUMBO, A. *et al.* 1993. Immunohistochemical localization of renin and angiotensin in the ovary—comparison between normal women and patients with histologically proven polycystic ovarian disease. Fertil. Steril. **60:** 280–284.
64. AUGUST, P. *et al.* 1990. Longitudinal study of the renin–angiotensin–aldosterone system in hypertensive pregnant women: deviations related to the development of superimposed preeclampsia. Am. J. Obstet. Gynecol. **163:** 1612–1625.
65. BROWN, M. *et al.* 1988. Sodium–renin–aldosterone relations in normal and hypertensive pregnancy. Br. J. Obstet. Gynecol. **95:** 1237–1246.
66. BROWN, M. & E. GALLERY. 1986. Sodium excretion in pregnancy: a role for arginine vasopressin. Am. J. Obstet. Gynecol. **154:** 914–919.
67. BROWN, M. *et al.* 1987. Progressive resetting of sodium–renin–aldosterone relationships in human pregnancy. Clin. Exp. Hypertens. **5:** 349–374.
68. BEERENDONK, C.C.M. *et al.* 1996. The influence of dietary-sodium restriction on renal and ovarian renin and prorenin production during ovarian stimulation. Hum. Reprod. **11:** 956–961.
69. LEWIS, P. *et al.* 1980. Prostacyclin in pregnancy. Br. Med. J. **280:** 1581–1582.
70. CHESLY, L. 1978. Hypertensive Disorders in Pregnancy. Appleton Century Crofts. New York. p. 190.

71. GALLERY, E. *et al.* 1979. Plasma volume contraction: a significant factor in both pregnancy-associated hypertension (preeclampsia) and chronic hypertension in pregnancy. Q. J. Med. **48:** 593–602.
72. MORGAN, T. *et al.* 1997. Angiotensinogen T235 expression is elevated in decidual spiral arteries. J. Clin. Invest. **100:** 1406–1415.
73. ALES, K.L. *et al.* 1989. Early prediction of antepartum hypertension. Obstet. Gynecol. **73:** 928–933.
74. BROUGHTON-PIPKIN, F. *et al.* 1983. Renin and aldosterone concentration in pregnant essential hypertension—a prospective study. Clin. Exp. Hypertens. **B2**(2)**:** 255–269.
75. GALLERY, E. *et al.* 1980. Plasma renin activity in normal human pregnancy and in pregnancy associated hypertension with reference to cryoactivation. Clin. Sci. **59:** 49–53.
76. CHESLY, L.C. 1972. Plasma and red cell volumes during pregnancy. Am. J. Obstet. Gynecol. **112:** 440–449.
77. ATLAS, S.A. & J.H. LARAGH. 1990. Atrial natriuretic factor and its involvement in hypertensive disorders. *In* Hypertension Pathophysiology, Diagnosis and Management. J. H. Laragh & B.M. Brenner, Eds.: 861–885. Raven Press. New York.
78. BROCHU, M. *et al.* 1997. Effects of gestation on enzymes controlling aldosterone synthesis in the rat adrenal. Endocrinology **138**(6)**:** 2354–2358.
79. VINSON, G. *et al.* 1998. The renin–angiotensin system in the reproductive tract. Gynecol. Endocrinol. **12**(2)**:** 10.
80. VINSON, G. *et al.* 1999. Renin–angiotensin system and reproduction. Gynecol. Endocrinol. **13:** 56–70.
81. GROVE, K.L. *et al.* 1997 Angiotensin II as a semen extender component increases retention of spermatoza within the uterus of the heifer. Reprod. Fertil. Dev. **9:** 545–549.
82. YOSHIMURA, Y. 1997 The ovarian renin–angiotensin system in reproductive physiology. Front. Neuroendocrinol. **18:** 247–291.

Reproductive Health in Female Patients with β-Thalassemia Major

ANTHI A. PROTONOTARIOU[a] AND GEORGE J. TOLIS

Division of Endocrinology, Hippokratio General Hospital, 108 Vas. Sofias Avenue, 115 27 Athens, Greece

GONADAL DYSFUNCTION

Modern therapeutic approaches of β-thalassemia major—consisting of early and intensive blood transfusion protocols (in order to keep Hb level above 10 gr/dl) and regular iron chelation—have significantly increased the average lifespan and improved the quality of life of β-thalassemia (β-thal) patients. Consequently, issues such as normal sexual maturation, attainment of reproductive capacity, and creation of a family are now becoming of great importance for β-thal women.

Multiple endocrine abnormalities develop during the course of β-thal major, attributable mainly to iron overload: growth retardation or failure, pubertal delay or failure, primary or secondary amenorrhea and infertility, diabetes mellitus, thyroid dysfunction, hypoparathyroidism, and metabolic bone disease. With the exception of growth retardation, hypothalamic–pituitary–gonadal (HPG) axis dysfunction represents the commonest disorder of the endocrine system.

The etiology of the HPG axis altered functionality is multifactorial involving physical and psychological stress, concurrent infections, liver–spleen involvement, nutritional deviation, and damage of the gonadostat by chronic iron deposition. Studies of gonadotropin pulsatility (frequency and amplitude) reveals abnormalities even in cycling β-thal women. When, later on, secondary amenorrhea occurs, demonstration of a blunted gonadotropin response to single or multiple doses of GnRH stongly indicates pituitary gonadotrope failure.[1] Histological data are supportive of this notion.[2] The selective damage of gonadotrops among all pituitary cells is possibly explained by the expression of transferrin receptors in these cells.[3] Iron can also directly harm the ovaries, as is true for other endocrine targets, that is, thyroid and pancreas. The poor gonadal response to exogenous gonadotropin administration and the report of a pregnancy achieved with *donor* oocytes—after many unsuccessful IVF efforts—are consistent with the above.[4–7]

The spectrum of clinical presentation of HPG axis dysfunction in β-thal patients includes pubertal failure or delay, failure of menstruation despite the spontaneous onset of puberty and development of secondary amenorrhea after a period of regular menstruation.

[a]Address for correspondence: Phone and fax: 01-7786889.
gtolis@atlas.uoa.gr

Delayed puberty onset or absence of pubertal development, apart from being mainly due to malfunctioning of HPG axis, has been also attributed to abnormal conversion of steroid hormones to their active metabolites[8] and to defective hepatic biosynthesis of IGF1. Depressed serum IGF1 activity is correlated with the extent of iron overload, suggesting that there may be a specific inhibitory effect of iron on somatomedin production or a direct stimulation of degradation mechanisms.[9,10] So, defective growth and lack of pubertal development are probably closely related.[11,12]

Moreover, patients with β-thal have low baseline and stimulated (after prolonged ACTH infusion) levels of the adrenal adrogens DHEA and DHEA-S. The role of adrenal function in the initiation and control of puberty, as well as the extent to which low adrenal adrogen levels contribute to the delayed onset of puberty in β-thal patients, have not yet been clarified.

The role of chronic anemia in the delay of sexual maturation was envisaged when β-thal patients with Hb levels less than 7 gr/dl (5.4–6.3 gr/dl) entered puberty only after a higher Hb level was achieved and maintained with transfusion regimen improvement.[13]

Hypogonadotropic hypogonadism is manifested in up to 40% of β-thal patients, and this percentage increases dramatically with advancing age. Primary amenorrhea occurs in 42.9–81% of β-thal women, and secondary amenorrhea follows in almost all patients within 1 month to 15 years after menarche with an average time of 3.8 years.[1,4,13,14] The derangement of the HPG axis seems to progress in an irreversible manner, with no reports of spontaneous remission to menstrual function after development of secondary amenorrhea. The variable degree of gonadal dysfunction among β-thal patients is possibly attributed to differences in individual susceptibility and in particular if toxic substances, such as iron, are accumulated at an early age.[15]

A 10-year study of 15 menstruating β-thal women enabled investigation of the progressive deterioration of HPG axis functionality.[1] At the beginning of the study, both patients and control subjects had regular ovulatory menstrual cycles. The patients experienced menarche at an age of 14.2 ± 0.22 years, two years later than the control group (12.2 ± 0.2 years). During the period of follow-up, the entire population of β-thal patients became amenorrheic. Patients were evaluated using an ultradian profile of LH and FSH levels and a GnRH stimulation test during follicular and luteal phases of their cycle and at 12 to 14 months, as well as 5 to 6 years following the onset of anemorrhea. During menstrual cycles basal gonadotropin levels were not different from the control group, but reduced gonadotrope responsiveness to GnRH as well as LH pulse defects—regarding peak amplitude and frequency—were noted. Progressive deterioration of the HPG axis function resulted in LH α–pulsatility in the majority of patients and dramatic decrease of pituitary gonadotrope reserves by the end of the follow-up period.

In conclusion, despite improved medical treatment of β-thal patients, delayed sexual development, amenorrhea, anovulation, and infertility remain usual events, although pubertal failure and infertility are no longer either universal or inevitable. Reports of spontaneous pubertal development and successful reproduction are increasing. Early and strict control of iron concentration is at the present the best option for normal sexual maturation and prevention of endocrine damage in β-thal patients. Early recognition and treatment of endocrine abnormalities is also important to prevent late complications and increase the chances of successful reproduction.

PREGNANCY

Up to the end of 1980s, there were only a few reports of pregnancies in patients with β-thal. The small number of pregnancies, most of which were in women with thalassemia intermedia, was the consequence of shortened life expectancy and reduced fertility resulting from dysfunction of the HPG axis. This was the case especially in older patients treated before the hypertransfusion regimen in combination with early and intensive chelation therapy had been established. In the past few years the number of pregnancies (spontaneous or assisted) reported in the literature has significantly increased, reflecting the improvement of conventional therapy—especially in the management of iron overload—and the new approaches to assisted conception.

Earlier studies in a number of amenorrheic β-thal females were unable to demonstrate an adequate estradiol response to the administration of human menopausal gonadotropins, suggesting either ovarian dysfunction or insufficient quantities of gonadotropins used.[4–6] In 1989, however, a successful full-term pregnancy was achieved with the combination of ovulation induction and intrauterine insemination.[16] More recently, successful ovulation has been reported with a certain schedule of HMG and hCG.[17] Since then, results from a number of studies have been encouraging for the attainment of reproductive capacity and achievement of successful and safe pregnancies in β-thal patients.[18–24] Most of these reports include data concerning (a) spontaneous or induced ovulation, (b) method of conception, (c) pregnancy monitoring and management, (d) presence of medical and obstetric complications, (e) pregnancy outcomes, (f) method of delivery, and (g) evaluation of the subsequent state of health of the mothers and the babies. In β-thal patients screening for bloodborne viral infections was performed, as well as frequent hematological, cardiological, hepatological, and endocrine evaluation throughout pregnancy. In these reports the importance of careful assessment and monitoring of the patients' general condition to ensure an uneventful pregnancy and a successful outcome has been emphasized.

The study of 90 pregnancies in 62 β-thal patients (50 with thal major and 12 with thal intermedia) represents the largest number reported so far.[24] Most of the patients became pregnant around the age of 25 years. In the 16 β-thal major patients with primary and secondary amenorrhea, 17 pregnancies were achieved after ovulation induction (intercourse 10, insemination 3, IVF 4). In the remaining 34 β-thal major patients with normal menstrual function and in the 12 patients with thal intermedia, 66 pregnancies were achieved spontaneously and 7 following induction (insemination 3, IVF 4).

The 90 pregnancies—among which there were four twin and one triple—resulted in 69 full-term births, 12 preterm births, 7 miscarriages, and 2 stillbirths; 81 healthy babies were born. No severe obstetric complications were observed except for two patients with preeclampsia, in whom premature delivery followed cesarian section. The high incidence of cesarian section (32%) was mainly attributed to cephalopelvic dispoportion. A 28-year-old patient, who carried the triple pregnancy, developed severe cardiac failure, successfully treated while another patient had an uneventful episode of pericarditis. A small number (8.8%) of the patients developed secondary amenorrhea after delivery.

Despite the undeniable progress in obstetrics, the fact is that the pregnancy in β-thal patients is a high-risk one, necessitating careful monitoring. Both the mother and the fetus may face deleterious consequences. Cardiological abnormalities, such as arrhythmias and congestive heart failure due to severe anemia, chronic hypoxia, and myocardial hemosiderosis, can be aggravated during pregnancy as a result of alterations in the hemodynamic state. Expansion of plasma and total red cell volume with increase of cardiac output may potentially lead to cardiac failure. Therefore, cardiac function should be thoroughly evaluated when pregnancy is contemplated by the assessment of the left ventricular ejection fraction. Periodic evaluation of the cardiac function, as well as careful monitoring of the transfusion regime in order to avoid overload, should be carried out during pregnancy.

Chronic maternal anemia may result in fetal hypoxia predisposing to pregnancy loss, premature labor, and intrauterine growth retardation.[25,26] To maintain adequate fetal perfusion, maternal anemia should be carefully controlled, usually with more frequent blood transfusions particularly during the third trimester of pregnancy, to maintain Hb levels above 10 gr/dl.[16,26,27] Other complications have also been reported in pregnancies of β-thal women, such as aggravation of splenomegaly and hypersplenism due to the physiological increase in cardiac output and splenic congestion.[25,28] Preeclampsia and thrombophlebitis can occur in splenectomized patients, because of changes in the clotting system superimposed on the hematological effects of splenectomy.[16,28] In such patients a daily low-dose aspirin regime has been proposed and used as a preventive measure.[7]

Desferrioxamine treatment—in the current state of knowledge—should be withheld during pregnancy with resumption immediately after delivery. This policy is followed because of concerns about its potential teratogenetic effect (as reported in animal studies) and other toxic effects such as ocular damage and rickets-like bone alterations encountered in the human. Interestingly, seven women who received desferrioxamine for various periods of time during pregnancy, including the first trimester, gave birth to normal infants.[23,29]

Folate supplementation, at a dose of 5 mg daily, is recommended and has been shown to improve maternal Hb concentration by correcting a relative folate deficiency common in β-thal patients due to increased bone marrow activity.[30] Vitamin C has to be stopped, because it increases gastrointestinal iron absorption, which can precipitate cardiac failure during pregnancy.[15]

In conclusion, the thorough evaluation of cardiac function in combination with a low iron load and satisfactory endocrine and hepatic surveillance can envisage a successful pregnancy outcome in β-thal women with minimal adverse effects. The strong desire for motherhood expressed by many β-thal women has to be respected, yet the risk for their pregnancies should not be overlooked. It is the responsibility of the medical team (hematologist, cardiologist, endocrinologist, obstetrician) to properly select the best candidates on the basis of a preconceptually established optimum health status and, once pregnancy is achieved, to monitor it intensively.

REFERENCES

1. CHATERJEE, R., M. KATZ, T.F. COX & J.B. PORTER. 1993. Prospective study of the hypothalamic–pituitary axis in thalassaemic patients who developed secondary amenorrhea. Clin. Endocrinol. **39:** 287.

2. BERGERON, C. & K. KOVACS. 1978. Pituitary siderosis: a histologic, immunologic and ultrastructural study. Am. J. Pathol. **9:** 295.
3. ATKIN, S.L, H.E. BURNETT, M.C. WHITE & M. LOMBARD. 1993. Human gonadotrophin-secreting pituitary adenomas express the transferrin receptor in vitro. J. Endocrinol. **139**(Suppl.)**:** 121.
4. DE SANCTIS, V., C. VULLO, M. KATZ, *et al.* 1988. Hypothalamic–pituitary–gonadal axis in thalassaemic patients with secondary amenorrhea. Obstet. Gynecol. **72:** 643.
5. DE SANTIS, V., C. VULLO, M. KATZ, *et al.* 1988. Gonadal function in patients with β-thalassaemia major. J. Clin. Pathol. **41:** 133.
6. ALLEGRA, A., M. CAPRA, L. CUCCIA, *et al.* 1990. Hypogonadism in β-thalassemic adolescents: a characteristic pitiutary–gonadal impairement. The effectiveness of long-term iron chelation therapy. Gynecol. Endocrinol. **4:** 181.
7. REUBINOFF, B.E., A. SIMON, S. FRIEDLER, *et al.* 1994. Defective oocytes as a possible cause of infertility in a β-thal major patient. Hum. Reprod. **9:** 1143.
8. BAKER, H.W.G., H.K. BURGER & D.M. DE KRETSER. 1976. A study of the endocrine manifestations of hepatic cirrhosis. Q. J. Med. **45:** 145.
9. SAENGER, P., E. SCHWARTZ, A.L. MARKENSON, *et al.* 1980. Depressed serum somatomedin activity in β-thalassemia. J. Pediatr. **96:** 214.
10. HERINGTON, A.C., G.A. WERTHER, R.N. MATTHEWS & H.G. BURGER. 1981. Studies on the possible mechanism for deficiency of non-suppressible insulin-like activity in thalassemia major. J. Clin. Endocrinol. Metab. **52:** 393.
11. ROSENFIELD, R.L., R. FURLANETTO, R. SYKES & D. BOCK. 1983. The relationship of somatomedin C to puberty, pubertal growth and sex hormones. Pediatr. Res. **17** (Suppl. 171A)**:** 1.
12. CARA, J.F. & R.L. ROSENFIELD. 1988. Insulin-like growth factor I and insulin potentiate luteinizing hormone-induced androgen synthesis by rat ovarian thecal-interstitial cells. Endocrinology **123:** 733.
13. LANDAN, H., V. GROSS, I. DAGAN, *et al.* 1984. Growth and sexual development before and after sex steroid therapy in patients with thalassemia major. Arch. Intern. Med. **144:** 2341.
14. BRONSPIEGEL-WEINTROB, N., N.F. OLIVIERI, B. TYLER, *et al.* 1990. Effect of age at the start of iron chelation therapy on gonadal function in β-thalassemia major. N. Engl. J. Med. **323:** 713.
15. TOLIS, G., E. VLACHOPAPADOPOULOU & I. KARYDIS. 1996. Reproductive health in patients with β-thalassemia. Curr. Opin. Pediatr. **8:** 406.
16. MORDEL, N., A. BANKENFELD, A.N. GOLDFARB & E.A. RACHMILEWITZ. 1989. Successful full-term pregnancy in homozygous thalassemia major: case report and review of the literature. Obstet. Gynecol. **73:** 837.
17. DANESI, L., M. SCACCHI, A.M. MIRAGOLI, *et al.* 1994. Induction of follicle maturation and ovulation by gonadotropin administration in women with β-thalassemia. Eur. J. Endocrinol. **131:** 602.
18. JENSEN, C.E., S.M. TUCK & B. WONKE. 1995. Fertility in β-thalassemia major: a report of 16 pregnancies, preconceptual evaluation and a review of the literature. Br. J. Obstet. Gynecol. **102:** 625.
19. KUMAR, R.M., D.E. RIZK & A. KHURANNA. 1997. Beta-thalassemia and successful pregnancy. J. Reprod. Med. **42:** 294.
20. SERACCHIOLI, R., E. PORCU, C. COLOMBI, *et al.* 1994. Transfusion-dependent homozygous β-thalassemia major: successful twin pregnancy following in vitro fertilization and tubal embryo transfer. Hum. Reprod. **9:** 1964.
21. VEGRI, P., V. DE SANCTIS, E. GRECHI, *et al.* 1998. Preliminary observations about assisted reproduction in thalassemia. JPEM **11**(Suppl. 3)**:** 929.
22. KARAGIORGA-LAGANA, M. 1998. Fertility in thalassemia: the Greek experience. JPEM **11**(Suppl. 3)**:** 945.
23. TUCK, S.M., C.E. JENSEN, B. WONKE & A. YARDUMIAN. 1998. Pregnancy management and outcomes in women with thalassemia major. JPEM **11** (Suppl. 3)**:** 923.
24. SKORDIS, N., S. CHRISTOY, M. KOLIOY, *et al.* 1998. Fertility in female patients with thalassemia. JPEM **11**(Suppl. 3)**:** 935.
25. SAVONA-VENTURA, C. & F. BONELLO. 1994. Beta-thalassemia syndromes and pregnancy. Obstet. Gynecol. Surv. **49:** 129.

26. Tampakoudis, P., C. Tsatalas, M. Mamopoulos, *et al.* 1997. Transfusion-dependent homozygous β-thalassemia major: successful pregnancy in five cases. Eur. J. Obstet. Gynecol. Reprod. Biol. **74:** 127.
27. Naef, R.W. & J. Morrison. 1995. Transfusion therapy in pregnancy. Clin. Obstet. Gynecol. **38:** 547.
28. Savona Ventura, C.S. & E.S. Grech. 1991. Pregnancy complications in homozygous thalassemia patients. J. Obstet. Gynecol. **11:** 175.
29. Voskaridou, E., K. Konstantopoulos, D. Kyriakou & D. Loukopoulos. 1993. Desferrioxamine treatment during early pregnancy: absence of teratogenicity in two cases. Hematologica **78:** 183.
30. Leung, C.F., T.T. Lao & A.M.Z. Chang. 1989. Effect of folate supplementation on pregnant women with beta thalassemia minor. Eur. J. Gynecol. Reprod. Biol. **33:** 209.

Anemia in Pregnancy

S. SIFAKIS[a] AND G. PHARMAKIDES

Department of Obstetrics and Gynecology, University Hospital of Heraklion, University of Crete, Heraklion, Greece

ABSTRACT: Anemia is one of the most frequent complications related to pregnancy. Normal physiologic changes in pregnancy affect the hemoglobin (Hb), and there is a relative or absolute reduction in Hb concentration. The most common true anemias during pregnancy are iron deficiency anemia (approximately 75%) and folate deficiency megaloblastic anemia, which are more common in women who have inadequate diets and who are not receiving prenatal iron and folate supplements. Severe anemia may have adverse effects on the mother and the fetus. Anemia with hemoglobin levels less than 6 gr/dl is associated with poor pregnancy outcome. Prematurity, spontaneous abortions, low birth weight, and fetal deaths are complications of severe maternal anemia. Nevertheless, a mild to moderate iron deficiency does not appear to cause a significant effect on fetal hemoglobin concentration. An Hb level of 11 gr/dl in the late first trimester and also of 10 gr/dl in the second and third trimesters are suggested as lower limits for Hb concentration. In an iron-deficient state, iron supplementation must be given and follow-up is indicated to diagnose iron-unresponsive anemias.

INTRODUCTION

Anemia is one of the most frequent complications related to pregnancy. The word implies a decrease in the oxygen-carrying capacity of the blood and is best characterized by a reduction in hemoglobin concentration. This may be either relative or absolute. It is known that there is a larger increase in plasma volume relative to red cell mass in almost all pregnancies, and it accounts for "physiologic anemia." These alterations have been known for centuries, and the term "plethora gravidarum" from medieval ages indicates this condition. However, it is still an open question to what extent this "hydremia" is physiologic or pathologic.

There are two contrasting medical philosophies covering this problem. According to the first, it is preferable to prevent pregnant women from developing too low hemoglobin concentrations. According to another point of view the "physiologic anemia" is of great importance for normal fetal growth and should be passively observed. Moreover, the relationship between a successful outcome of pregnancy and this normal expansion in maternal plasma volume has been noted.[1] This controversy is reflected in the recommendations from the World Health Organization on the optimal hemoglobin (Hb) concentrations or hematocrit (Hct) level. Thus, in 1965 a WHO expert committee suggested that 10 gm/dl should be accepted as the lower limit of the physiologic adjustments made during pregnancy.[2] However, three years

[a]Address for correspondence: Stavros Sifakis, 22 Apolloniou Rodiou Str., 71305, Heraklion Crete, Greece. Phone: 0030 81 212915; fax: 0030 81 392759.

later another WHO scientific group recommended that when Hb values are lower than 11 gr/dl anemia should be considered to exist in pregnant women, and diets must be supplemented with medical iron.[3]

PHYSIOLOGIC BACKGROUND

The plasma volume starts to increase at about 6 weeks of pregnancy in a healthy woman.[4] This increase, which is disproportionately greater than the corresponding changes on the red cell mass, accounts for the physiologic fall in the Hb concentration during pregnancy. As a consequence, there is a significant reduction in arteriovenous oxygen extraction at the heart and an important increase of the oxygen-carrying capacity of the pregnant woman, despite the fall in the Hb level.

The increase in plasma volume is about 1,250 ml at term, a total increase of about 48% above the nonpregnant state. This is the result of an initial rapid rise, followed by a slower rise after the 30th week of pregnancy. Several studies demonstrate the positive correlation between the weight of the newborn and the increase in the plasma volume.[1,5–8] It seems that the increase in plasma volume is an indication of normal growth of the fetus and one of the hallmarks of a successful pregnancy.

As regards the red cell mass, it also increases although, in contrast to the plasma volume, it does so more slowly. The total increase is about 18% or 250 ml at term. After stimulation with iron supplements, however, the red cell mass may reach 400 ml—a total increase of about 30% compared with the nonpregnant state. Similar to the plasma volume, the increased red cell mass is linked to fetal growth, although probably to a lesser degree.

CAUSES OF ANEMIA IN PREGNANCY

Because of the normal physiologic changes in pregnancy that affect the hematocrit and certain other parameters, such as hemoglobin, reticulocytes, plasma ferritin, and unsaturated iron-binding capacity, diagnosing true anemia, as well as determining the etiology of anemia, is challenging. The most common anemias are iron-deficiency anemia and folate deficiency megaloblastic anemia. These anemias are more common in women who have inadequate diets and who are not receiving prenatal iron and folate supplements. Other less common causes of acquired anemia in pregnancy are aplastic anemia and hemolytic anemia. In addition, anemias such as thalassemia and sickle cell disease can have an impact on the health of the mother and fetus.

As was stated above, the most frequent causes of true or absolute anemia are nutritional deficiencies. Frequently, these deficiencies are multiple, and the clinical presentation may be complicated by attendant infections, generally poor nutrition, or hereditary disorders such as hemoglobinopathies.[9,10] However, the fundamental sources of nutritional anemia embody insufficient intake, inadequate absorption, increased losses, expanded requirements, and insufficient utilization of hemopoietic nutrients. Approximately 75% of all anemias diagnosed during pregnancy are due to iron deficiency. Significant deficiency of iron leads to characteristic hypochromic, microcytic erythrocytes on the peripheral blood smear. Other causes of hypochromic anemias, even rare, must be considered, including hemoglobinopathies, inflammatory processes, chemical toxicity, malignancy, and pyridoxine-responsive anemia. However the greater percentage of the remaining cases of anemia in pregnancy other than the iron-deficiency type consists of the megaloblastic anemia of pregnancy due to folic acid deficiency and, to a lesser extent, to vitamin B12 deficiency. Anemia caused by deficiencies of other vitamins or elements does not commonly occur in humans.

Nutritional anemia is not a broad-based problem in the populations of developed countries. It is nevertheless a problem for many individuals in these countries, and it is certainly a major health problem in poor, underdeveloped countries. Pregnant women as well as menstruating women and children make up the segment of the population in third-world countries—and even in the United States and Europe—that is affected by nutritional deficiency, sometimes accompanied by frank anemia.[11]

In conclusion, the investigation of acquired anemias during pregnancy is very important, considering that inadequate nutrition and nutritional deficiencies have an adverse impact on pregnancy outcome, without excluding *a priori* other, less common types of anemia.

MATERNAL EFFECTS OF ANEMIA

Obviously, severe anemia has adverse effects on the mother and the fetus. There is also evidence that less severe anemia is associated with poor pregnancy outcome. Major maternal complications directly related to anemia are not common in women with a hemoglobin level greater than 6 gr/dl. However, Hb levels even lower may lead to significant morbidity in pregnant women, such as infections, increased hospital stays, and other general health problems.[10]

A lot of symptoms and signs may accompany this clinical state, to a variable degree. The commonest of these are headache, fatigue, lethargy, paresthesia, and the clinical signs of tachycardia, tachypnea, pallor, glossitis, and cheilitis. In more severe cases, especially in pregnant women with hemoglobin levels less than 6 gr/dl, significant life-threatening problems secondary to high-output congestive heart failure and decreased oxygenation of tissues, including heart muscle may be encountered. Such conditions are rare as a result of nutritional deficiency anemias, at least in developed countries or when the pregnant woman receive iron supplementations. However, severe iron deficiency anemia or methemorragic anemia may be presented by complications of pregnancy, such as placenta previa or abruptio placenta, operative delivery and post partum hemorrhage.[12] These conditions if untreated by iron supplementation or blood transfusion may lead to severe complications.

EFFECTS ON THE FETUS

There are a lot of indications that severe maternal anemia in pregnancy is associated with poor pregnancy outcome and that the cause of this association has yet to be elucidated.[10] Moreover, what effects the maternal anemia has on the fetus are not well defined; however, several reports in the literature associate the reduction in hemoglobin level with prematurity, spontaneous abortions, low birth weight, and fetal deaths. Some authors believe that even a mild reduction in Hb level (8–11 gr/dl) may produce a predisposition to these conditions; in contrast, other authors support a direct relationship between anemia and fetal distress only when the maternal Hb levels re less than 6 gr/dl.[13]

It is important to know what effect the iron status of the mother has on the iron status of the fetus for definitive and correct conclusions about management. There are controversial opinions about this: some investigators found that levels of maternal iron exert little effect on that of the neonate at birth.[14] On the other hand, studies of cord blood serum iron levels have shown a direct relationship between maternal and fetal iron levels.[15] Additionally, when serum ferritin is used as an indicator of iron status, it was found that babies born to mothers who did not take iron supplements during pregnancy had reduced iron stores at birth.[16,17] Most authors agree that only severe anemia may have direct adverse effects on the fetus and neonate and that a mild to moderate maternal iron deficiency does not appear to cause a significant effect on fetal hemoglobin concentration.[15]

There are several reports that correlate the anemia during pregnancy with prematurity and low-birthweight infants, indicating a direct relationship between low birth weight and low maternal Hb level.[18–20] In a large epidemiologic study, it was shown that the risk of a preterm delivery was increased by 20% in pregnancies with Hb levels between 10 and 11 gr/dl and by 60% in pregnancies with Hb levels between 9 and 10 gr/dl. Below 9 gr/dl, the risk was more than doubled, tripled, and so on for each fall of 1 gr/dl.[21] In the same study, no correlation was found between maternal Hb levels and growth retardation. In another large epidemiologic study, perinatal mortality was found to be tripled when the maternal Hb levels fell below 8 gr/dl in comparison with Hb levels above 11 gr/dl.[22] In addition, Garn *et al.*[23] demonstrated an association between low maternal Hb levels and poor pregnancy outcomes such as prematurity, low birth weight, fetal death, and other medical abnormalities with increasing complication rates when there were lower maternal Hb concentrations. Nevertheless, all these reports are strong indications of an adverse effect of maternal anemia on fetal growth and pregnancy outcome. Nevertheless, it would be better, at least in cases of mild to moderate maternal anemia, to characterize these simply as possible risk factors rather than as an adequate evaluation indicating an obvious adverse impact on the fetus. Moreover, it is important to stress that low maternal Hb levels are often associated with other pathologic conditions, so it is difficult to be sure whether maternal anemia *per se* causes or even contributes directly to the increased mortality and morbidity rates. In other words, low Hb levels are often a secondary phenomenon caused by antecedent infections or chronic illnesses that in turn may lead to severe complications during pregnancy that do not fundamentally depend on the hematologic profile of the pregnant woman.

NORMAL VALUES AND LOWER LIMITS FOR HEMOGLOBIN LEVELS IN PREGNANT WOMEN

There are conflicting views on the optimal Hb concentrations during pregnancy. One of the reasons for this is that the prepregnant hematologic state of the woman is rarely known, and this, to a large extent, determines the hematologic reactions during pregnancy. Thus, one important parameter is the knowledge of normal nonpregnant Hb variation. Another point is the use of ±2 SD as limits for the variation of Hb levels during pregnancy. Finally, it is best to consider what is known about the physiological changes in plasma volume and in red cell mass during pregnancy that lead to physiological anemia.

In the nonpregnant state, Hb and Hct values are more indicative of the plasma volume than of the red cell mass in women. It is possible that individual factors influence the plasma volumes from consistently high to average or low.[4] There is also often a gradual transition from normal iron stores to slight or moderate iron deficiency anemia during which the symptoms are inconspicuous. Two-thirds or more of healthy women of reproductive age in several countries have been found to have scanty or absent iron stores.[24] This situation may have not consequences in a nonpregnant state but during pregnancy such women are at a variable risk of developing frank anemia.

The normal variations of Hb and Hct values in a nonpregnant state are wide. In one study, however, which is in close agreement with the results of many others,[25] young, healthy, nonpregnant women have the following values: Hb: 12.3 ± 0.9 gr/dl (range, 11.4–14.3 gr/dl); Hct: 38% ± 3 (range: 34–45%).

It is important to ask, however, what is the optimal (or normal) Hb level for pregnant women and what is the lower limit of normal variation? This is a very difficult problem for which there are lot of conflicting views and strong discrepancies. Nevertheless, there is fairly good agreement among several investigators that the lower limit of normal physiologic variation of Hb levels is about 10 gr/dl.[23,26,27] This lowest value occurs in weeks 25 and 26 with a mean Hb value of 11.4 gr/dl, making the lower (± 2 SD) limit 9.8 gr/dl,[26] a figure very close to the lower limits of 10 gr/dl and 10.4 gr/dl of two other reports.[23,27]

In the other trimesters of pregnancy, an Hb level of 11 gr/dl in the late first trimester and of 10 gr/dl in the third trimester are suggested as lower limits for Hb concentration. Koller *et al.* investigated the optimal Hb levels in iron-supplemented pregnant women and created a diagram based on the results of uncomplicated pregnancies resulting in healthy, normal neonates.[26] This pregnant population routinely used iron supplementation of 100 to 200 mg Fe per day (both doses have about the same effect on Hb levels).[28] According to the results of this study, it is remarkable that supplements had very little influence on the Hb levels before 25 weeks of gestation, although from that time on, these levels increased gradually compared with those of nonsupplemented women. Other authors supported that the difference at term between Hb levels in pregnant women with or without iron supplementation will be about 1 gr/dl.[29,30]

About of 3% pregnant women have Hb levels below the lower limit of 10 gr/dl in the second trimester,[26,31] whereas the corresponding number in the third trimester is 1%.[31] The decrease in Hb concentration is positively correlated with the prepregnancy Hb value.[24] The low values (10 to 11 gr/dl) often show no drop in value, however.[28] This may be explained by considering that these low values indeed represent iron deficiency anemia that reacts rapidly to iron supplementation with hemoglobin production, thus preventing a further drop in Hb concentration. It is remarkable that this "resistance" to further decrease in Hb levels also appears in pregnant women without iron supplementation. It may represent a physiologic "adaptation" to pregnancy in order to keep the Hb concentration at sufficient levels for placental perfusion.[24]Another explanation is that women with low prepregnancy Hb levels may have larger plasma volumes than the women with higher Hb levels, and as a consequence they do not experience the plasma expansion that appears at early stages of pregnancy.

COMMON TYPES OF ANEMIA IN PREGNANCY

Iron-Deficiency Anemia

The majority of all anemias diagnosed during pregnancy are characterized as iron-deficiency anemias. It is estimated that about 80% of pregnant women at term who do not use iron supplementation have hemoglobin concentrations less than 11 gr/dl.[13] The increased fetal need for iron as well as a number of other factors constitute the iron-deficiency profile of the pregnant woman and the need for supplementation. The factors contributing to that state include poor iron absorption during pregnancy, multiple gestations or successive gestations less than two years apart, adolescent pregnancy, and any associated chronic blood loss, as well as decreased amounts of total body iron before the pregnancy.

The most usual clinical symptoms of iron-deficiency anemia are lethargy and fatigue, although they are also seen in normal pregnancy. Other symptoms are headache, paresthesia, burning sensation of the tongue, and pica, which is the ingestion of substances with no dietary value and appears in severe cases of anemia after the twentieth week of gestation. Glossitis, pallor, and inflammation of the lips (cheilitis) are clinical signs of iron deficiency, whereas koilonychia and "spooning" nails are less common findings. In cases of severe anemia, retinal bleeding, conjunctivitis, tachypnea or tachycardia, and splenomegaly may be presented. Nevertheless, these signs are rarely seen in developed countries because of the rarity Hb levels of 5 or 6 gr/dl. Some authors support a correlation of iron-deficiency anemia with defects in cellular immunity and decreased defense to bacteria by white blood cells,[32] but it is not clear whether this immune depression associated with anemia, predisposes a person to infection.[33]

The laboratory evaluation of iron-deficiency anemia is quite difficult because of the physiologic hydremia of pregnancy and the subsequent changes in the values of the main hematologic parameters. Moreover, a differential diagnosis must be done between the hypochromic microcytic anemia of iron deficiency and other hypochromic anemias such as hemoglobinopathies or anemias induced by chemicals or inflammatory processes or malignancies. In these conditions the mean corpuscular volume (MCV) is often decreased, although it is the rule in iron-deficiency anemia.[34] The expected increase in the red blood cell mass after week 20 of gestation will not observed if iron stores are depleted. The serum iron levels decline as pregnancy advances for the reasons presented above. Values < 30 g/dl are usually diagnostic of iron deficiency, but the best indicator for this is the measurement of serum ferritin (normal values in pregnancy: 55–70 μg/l). Additionally, quite a good indication is the transferrin saturation, which in iron deficiency is $< 15\%$. Some authors consider the unsaturated iron-binding capacity (UIBC) an important marker of iron deficiency states, when it takes values > 400 μg/dl.[35] The earliest tissue indicator of an iron-deficient state is decreased iron stores in the bone marrow, but aspiration in pregnancy is usually not indicated.

Therapy of Iron-Deficiency Anemia and Iron Supplementation

Most clinicians advocate iron supplementation in pregnant women. Others believe that supplementation has no value when hemoglobin levels are equal to or greater than 10 gr/dl. They believe that there is no need for extra therapy, on the grounds that hemodilution during pregnancy is an important physiologic adaptation, important for adequate uteroplacental circulation.[36] In an iron-deficient state, however, iron supplementation must be given, and follow-up is indicated to diagnose iron-unresponsive anemias. Reticulocytosis is normally observed 10 days after the initiation of iron therapy. The increased demand for iron and the hemodilution during pregnancy may mask the response to iron supplementation. It is self-evident that other causes of anemia have been excluded. In these cases iron supplementation should continue throughout pregnancy, and it can be accomplished with a variety of agents. Oral preparations containing elemental salt are the most commonly employed, whereas ferous sulfate compounds are the least expensive and have been demonstrated to be efficacious for iron supplementation. It should be taken three or four times daily in a dosage of 30–60 mg for a conservative dosage to 200–300 mg per day in the iron-deficient state. Nausea, vomiting, diarrhea, and constipation are the most common side effects of the ingestion of oral iron. The sustained release capsules, iron compounds that are slowly absorbed, and syrups may reduce some of the intolerance and increase patient compliance. Patients with severe iron deficiency anemia who cannot tolerate oral administration or who demonstrate noncompliance with the oral administration of iron, can be treated with intramuscular (i.m.) or intravenous (i.v.) administration. Additionally, parenteral therapy is preferred when rapid replenishment of iron stores is necessary. However, the hematologic response to the i.m. or i.v. route of therapy is no more rapid than that of the response to oral iron, and adverse effects including fatal anaphylaxis can be observed due to immediate or delayed reactions to iron dextran. It is more likely to appear when oral iron and parenteral iron are given concomitantly; therefore, this combination is not indicated. A test dose is strongly recommended before the first parenteral administration. A formula for the dose of iron needed to restore hemoglobin is the following[37]:

$$\text{elemental iron (mg)} = 0.3 \times \text{weight (lbs)} \times 100 = \frac{\text{patient's Hb (gr/dl)} \times 100}{14.8}.$$

The side effects of such a route of iron administration include discomfort at the injection site, skin staining, malaise, and metallic taste. Moderate reactions of hyperpyrexia, lymphadenopathy, and phlebitis occur in 1–2% of patients, whereas anaphylaxis may occur in about 0.5% of them.

Folic Acid Deficiency Anemia

Folic acid deficiency causes a megaloblastic type of anemia that is second in occurrence as a cause for nutritional deficiency anemia of pregnancy after iron deficiency anemia. Folates and especially their derivative formyl FH_4 are necessary for appropriate DNA synthesis and amino acid production. Insufficient levels of folic acid may lead to the manifestations noted in megaloblastic anemia.[38] Folic acid must be provided in the diet: common sources are green vegetables, fruits (lemons, melons), and meats (liver, kidney). The absorption happens in the proximal jejunum.

The etiology of folic acid deficiency is variable and decreased intake is associated with poor nutrition and impaired absorption as well as increased folic acid requirements seen in pregnancy because of the increased demands of fetal growth and maternal erythropoiesis. Additionally, the higher levels of estrogen and progesterone during pregnancy seem to have an inhibitory effect on folate absorption The symptoms of folic acid deficiency are those of general anemia plus roughness of the skin and glossitis. The erythrocyte precursors are morphologically larger ("macrocytic"), and an abnormal nuclear–cytoplasmic appearance as well as normochromic and macrocytic findings are diagnostic criteria for megaloblastic anemia. MCH and MCHC are usually normal, whereas the large MCV is helpful in differentiation of this anemia from physiologic changes of pregnancy or iron-deficiency anemia. For MCV, the presence of increased serum iron and transferrin saturation are also helpful. Neutropenia and thrombocytopenia are the results of abnormal maturation in granulocytes and thrombocytes. A low serum level (<3 g/l) may occur early in folic acid deficiency.

The daily requirement in a nonpregnant state is at least 0.4 mg. In pregnancy or increased growth states, such as during infancy and adolescence, however, the requirements are increased to 0.8–1.0 mg.[39,40] It is possible that multiple gestations or short intervals between pregnancies increase folate requirements further. It has been reported that folate deficiency affects about 60 to 95% of untreated women at term.[13] However, true megaloblastic anemia due to folic acid deficiency is uncommon, although megaloblastic changes produced by this state are not uncommon. Half of the pregnant women with this type of anemia present before delivery with the remaining cases being detected puerperally. The majority of folic acid deficiencies during pregnancy appear in the third trimester.[13] Severe folic acid deficiency in experimental animals has been linked to an increased appearance of pregnancy abnormalities such as prematurity, fetal death, hypertension, placental abruption, or fetal malformations. A direct relationship of these outcomes with iron deficiency in humans has not been proven.[38] The fetus seems to have the ability to sustain stable hemoglobin and folate levels even in cases of obvious or severe maternal folate deficiency anemia. It is possible that the fetus removes folic acid from maternal circulation even in her deficit state. Thus, the infants in such cases are not anemic and appear unaffected. However, it has been found that megaloblastic anemia in pregnancy may be accompanied by smaller blood volume[40] and may be related to fetal growth retardation in some cases.[41] On the other hand, when there are no signs of anemia, the effects of folic acid deficiency are controversial or unclear. Nevertheless, the majority of physicians consider folate supplementation useful, especially for those at risk for developing deficiency states. Intake of 0.5 mg to 1 mg two or three times daily orally is generally adequate. A response to therapy within 48–72 hours can be expected as reticulocytes and platelets increase. A neutrophilic response can be observed within 2 weeks. If there are low serum iron levels, the existence of concomitant iron deficiency anemia is possible.[42] In these cases serum iron levels may be elevated and erythropoiesis will not be efficient.

Other Deficiency Anemias in Pregnancy

Hemic nutrients, trace elements, vitamins, and proteins are necessary for growth and maintenance of various bodily functions, especially for the hematologic system functions of the mother, fetus, and newborn. They are vital in facilitating the metabolism of amino acids, carbohydrotes, and fat and are therefore involved in anemias. The increased nutritional requirements during pregnancy commonly result in inadequate dietary intake. Nutritional anemia is not a very common problem in developed countries, except for iron-deficiency or folic acid deficiency anemia. However, anemia caused by deficiencies in a number of iron, folic acid, vitamins, and proteins may be an important problem in poor, underdeveloped countries.

Except for iron deficiency, which is responsible for the great majority of anemias diagnosed during pregnancy, deficiencies in some other minerals may account for some cases of anemias in rare cases. Severe phosphorus deficiency can cause hemolytic anemia because of adenosine triphosphate depletion in the red cells with subsequent osmotic fracture.[13] Moreover, severe copper deficiency has been characterized to iron supplementation.[43] Zinc deficiency has been noted in patients with sickle cell anemia and thalassemia. However, there is no evidence that this deficiency causes worsening of anemia.[44]

Of the water-soluble vitamins, folic acid deficiency accounts for a large pregnancy which is megaloblastic in type. Except for folic acid, vitamin B_{12} deficiency is clinically important because of its role in the metabolism of folate through the production of active FH4. When serum B_{12} levels are depressed during pregnancy, it may lead to a type of megaloblastic anemia which exists in common with folic acid–related anemia in 98% of megaloblastic anemias at pregnancy.[45] Other B complex vitamin–related anemias are almost never seen in pregnancy. Though rare, vitamin B_6 (pyridoxine) deficiency is noted during pregnancy by a decrease to about 75% of normal levels. A relationship between this deficiency and hypochromic microcytic anemia has been reported.[43] Another hypochromic-type anemia has been noted in 80% of pregnant women with ascorbic acid (vitamin C) deficiency (scurvy). The interaction of ascorbic acid and iron metabolism is regarded as the etiologic reason for this anemia.[13] Of the fat-soluble vitamins (A, D, E, K), vitamin A deficiency has been shown by some investigators to produce an anemia similar to iron-deficiency anemia.[43]

A mixed pattern of anemias has been associated with protein deficiency in pregnancy. The increasing needs of the mother and the demands from the fetus increase protein requirements from about 45 g in the nonpregnant state. Protein deficiency is not uncommon in a great part of the world, and anemia associated with kwashiorkor is a characteristic normochromic and hormocytic anemia[43] that is associated with decreased erythropoiesis and reduced iron intake.[46]

A variety of anemias are associated with chronic ingestion of alcohol. Alcohol decreases folate levels through a direct effect on folate metabolism, and poor dietary intake leading to nutritional deficiency is common in these pregnant women. Therefore alcohol-related anemia may present with microcytic red cells or normochromic and macrocytic cells, with an increased number of ring sideroblasts.[43]

HIGH MATERNAL HEMOGLOBIN AND THE FETUS

Significantly higher Hb levels have been found in pregnancies complicated by fetal growth retardation and perinatal distress.[47,48] A number of important reports have also demonstrated a correlation between high maternal Hb levels in the first and second trimester with pregnancy complications including low birth weight, preterm birth, pregnancy-induced hypertension, and intrauterine death of unknown cause.[27,49] Murphy *et al.* showed that the frequency of hypertension in primiparas ranged from 7% with Hb values under 10.5 gr/dl to 42% with Hb concentrations over 14.5 gr/dl.[27] Garn *et al.* found that fetal death was 2.6 times more frequent with maternal Hb levels around 14 gr/dl than when it was around 8 gr/dl.[23]

It is probably that the explanation for the development of these complications is the failure of the pregnancy to induce sufficient hemodilution, a major adjustment of normal pregnancy. This failure may be caused by faulty implantation or by inadequate genetic endownment. Moreover, a number of studies have shown that abnormally high maternal Hb levels probably impair the uteroplacental circulation by raising the whole-blood viscosity.[50,51] It is known that the major component of whole-blood viscosity is the concentration of Hb/Ht.[52]

Garn *et al.* found that Hb values of 11 gr/dl (Ht 34) for blacks and Hb 12 gr/dl (Ht 36) for whites are the optimum values for pregnant women, whereas Hb values of 13 gr/dl (Ht 41) are the upper border values for an optimal outcome.[23] A practical conclusion is that an Hb value of 13 gr/dl or higher in the second trimester should be a cause for concern.

REFERENCES

1. GOODLAND, R.D. *et al.* 1983. Clinical science of normal plasma volume expansion during pregnancy. Am. J. Obstet. Gynecol. **145:** 1001.
2. WORLD HEALTH ORGANIZATION. 1965. Nutrition in pregnancy and lactation. WHO Tech. Rep. Ser. 302.
3. WORLD HEALTH ORGANIZATION. 1968. Nutritional anemias. WHO Tech. Rep. Ser. 405.
4. LUND, C.J. *et al.* 1967. Blood volume during pregnancy. Significance of plasma red cell volumes. Am. J. Obstet. Gynecol. **98:** 393.
5. RETIEF, F.P. *et al.* 1967. P study of pregnancy anemia, blood volume changes correlatated with other parameters of haemopoietic efficiency. J. Obstet. Gynaecol. Br. Commonw. **74:** 683.
6. DUFFUS, G.M. *et al.* 1971. The relationship between baby weight and changes in maternal weight, total body water, plasma volume electrolytes and proteins, and urinary oestriol excretion. J. Obstet. Gynaecol. Br. Commonw. **78:** 97.
7. GIBSON, H.M. 1973. Plasma volume and glomerular filtration rate in pregnancy and their relation to differences in fetal growth. J. Obstet. Gynaecol. Br. Commonw. **80:** 1067.
8. PIRANI, B.B.K. *et al.* 1973. Plasma volume in normal first pregnancy. J. Obstet. Gynaecol. Br. Commonw. **80:** 884.
9. BAKER. S.J. 1983. Nutritional anemias. Part 2: Tropical Asia. Clin. Haematol. **10:** 843.
10. WILLIAMS, M.D. *et al.* 1992. Anemia in pregnancy. Med. Clin. N. Am. **76(3):** 631–647.
11. COOK, J.D. 1983. Nutritional anemia. Contemp. Nutr. **8:** 366.
12. FLESSA, H.C. 1974. Hemorrhagic disorders and pregnancy. Clin. Obstet. Gynecol. **17:** 236.
13. PRYOR, J. *et al.* 1990. *In* Hematologic Disorders in Maternal—Fetal Medicine. Wiley-Liss Inc. New York. pp. 93–111.
14. STURGEON, P. 1959. Studies of iron requirements in infants III. Influence of supplemental iron during normal pregnancy on mother and infant. B. The infant. Br. J. Haematol. **5:** 45.
15. WERNER, E.J. *et al.* 1983. Red cell disturbances in the feto–maternal unit. Semin. Perinatol. **3:** 139.
16. PUOLAKKA, J. *et al.* 1980. Evaluation by serum ferritin assay of the influence of maternal iron stores on the iron status of newborns and infants. Acta Obstet. Gynecol. Scand. [Suppl.] **95:** 53.

17. KANESHIGE, E. 1981. Serum ferritin as an assessment of iron stores and other hematologic parameters during pregnancy. Obstet. Gynecol. **57:** 238.
18. MCFEE, J.G. 1973. Anemia: a high risk complication of pregnancy. Clin. Obstet. Gynecol. **16:** 153.
19. KALTREIDER, D.F. *et al.* 1976. Patients at high risk for low birth weight deliveries. Am. J. Obstet. Gynecol. **124:** 251.
20. HIGGINS, A.C. e*t al.* 1982. Maternal hemoglobin changes and their relationship to infant birth weight in mothers receiving a program of nutritional assessment and rehabilitation. Nutr. Res. **2:** 641.
21. KALTREIDER, F. *et al.* 1980. Epidemiology of preterm delivery. Clin. Obstet. Gynecol. **23:** 17.
22. MEYER, M.B. *et al.* 1975. The interrelationship of maternal smoking and increased perinatal mortality with other risk factors. Analysis of the Ontario Perinatal Mortality Study, 1960–61. Am. J. Epidemiol. **100:** 443.
23. GARN, S.M. *et al.* 1981. Maternal hematologic levels and pregnancy outcomes. Semin. Perinatol. **5:** 155.
24. KOLLER, O. *et al.* 1990. Maternal hemoglobin concentrations and fetal health. *In* Hematologic Disorders in Maternal–Fetal Medicine.: 31–46. Wiley-Liss Inc. New York.
25. PUOLAKKA, J. 1980. Serum ferritin in the evaluation of iron status in young, healthy women. Acta Obstet. Gynecol. Scand. [Suppl.] **95:** 35.
26. KOLLER, O. *et al.* 1979. Fetal growth retardation associated with inadequate haemodilution in otherwise uncomplicated pregnancy. Acta Obstet. Gynecol. **58:** 9.
27. MURPHY, J.F. *et al.* 1986. Relation of haemoglobin levels in first and second trimester to outcome of pregnancy. Lancet **1:** 992.
28. SJÖSTEDT, J.E. *et al.* 1977. Oral iron prophylaxis during pregnancy. Acta Obstet. Gynecol. Scand. [Suppl.] **60:** 3.
29. ROMSLO, I. *et al.* 1983. Iron requirement in normal pregnancy as assessed by serum ferritin, serum transferrin saturation and erythrocyte protoporphyrin determination. Br. J. Obstet. Gynaecol. **90:** 101.
30. PUOLAKKA, J. *et al.* 1980. Serum ferritin as a measure of iron stores. Acta Obstet. Gynecol. Scand. [Suppl.] **95:** 43.
31. PRINTCHARD, J.A. 1973. Anemia in pregnancy—a reappraisal. Obstet. Gynecol. Surv. **28:** 769.
32. PRASAD, A.S. 1979. Leukocyte formation in iron deficiency anemia. Am. J. Clin. Nutr. **32:** 550.
33. PREMA, K. *et al.* 1982. Immune status of anaemic pregnant women. Br. J. Obstet. Gynaecol. **89:** 222.
34. FAIRBANKS, V.F. *et al.* 1983. Erythrocyte disorders—anemias related to disturbances of hemoglobin synthesis. *In* Hematology. W.J. Williams, E. Beutler, A.J. Erslev & M.A. Lichtman, Eds.: 466. McGraw-Hill. New York.
35. DZ. 1987. Hematologic Problems in Pregnancy. Medical Economics Books. Oradell, NJ.
36. KOLLER, O. 1982. Clinical significance of hemodilution during pregnancy. Obstet. Gynecol. Surv. **37:** 649.
37. PREMA, K. *et al.* 1982. The effect of intramuscular iron therapy in anaemic pregnant women. Indian J. Med. Res. **75:** 534.
38. BECK, W.S. 1983. Erythrocyte disorders—anemias related to disturbance of DNA synthesis (megaloblastic anemias). *In* Hematology. W.J. Williams, E. Beutler, A.J. Erslev & M.A. Lichtman, Eds.: 434. McGraw-Hill. New York.
39. FOOD AND NUTRITION BOARD, NATIONAL RESEARCH COUNCIL. 1980. Recommended Dietary Allowances. National Academy of Sciences. Washington, DC.
40. PRITCHARD J.A. & P.C. MCDONALD, Eds. 1980. Megaloblastic anemia. *In* Williams Obstetrics, 16th edit.: 717. Appleton-Century-Crofts. New York.
41. ROLSCHAUJ, J. *et al.* 1979. Folic acid supplement and intrauterine growth. Acta Obstet. Gynaecol. Scand. **58:** 343.
42. JOHAN, E. *et al.* 1981. Plasma and red blood cell folate during normal pregnancy. Acta Obstet. Gynaecol. Scand. **60:** 247.
43. OSKI, F.A. 1983. Anemia related to nutritional deficiencies other than vitamin B12 and folic acid. *In* Hematology. W.J. Williams, E. Beutler, A.J. Erslev & M.A. Lichtman, Eds.: 522. McGraw-Hill. New York.

44. WARTH, J.A. *et al.* 1981. Abnormal dark adaptation in sickle cell anemia. J. Lab. Clin. Med. **98:** 189.
45. MORRISON, J.C. *et al.* 1985. Anemia associated with pregnancy. *In* Gynecology and Obstetrics: Maternal and Fetal Medicine. R. Depp & D.A. Eschenbach, Eds.: 16. Harper Row. New York.
46. GRASSO, J.A. *et al.* 1980. Energy-dispersive X-ray analysis of mitochondria of sideroblastic anemia. Br. J. Haematol. **46:** 57.
47. SAGEN, N. *et al.* 1984. The predictive value of total estriol; HPL and Hb on perinatal outcome in severe pre-eclampsia. Acta Obstet. Gynecol. Scand. **63:** 603.
48. MAU, G. 1977. Hemoglobin changes during pregnancy and growth disturbances in neonate. J. Perinatol. Med. **5:** 172.
49. HUISMAN, A. & J.G. AARNOUDSE. 1986. Increased 2nd trimester hemoglobin concentration in pregnancies later complicated by hypertension and growth retardation. Acta Obstet. Gynecol. Scand. **65:** 605.
50. SIEKMANN, U. & L. HEILMANN. 1981. Die Bezieungen hämorheologischer parameter zu biochemischen daten bei risikoschwargerschaften. Arch. Gynäkol. **232:** 443.
51. BUCHAN, P.C. 1982. Pre-eclampsia—a hyperviscosity syndrome. Am. J. Obstet. Gynecol. **142:** 111.
52. BEGG, T.V. & D.B. HEARNS. 1966. Components in blood viscosity. The relative contributions of hematocrit, plasma fibrinogen and other proteins. Clin. Sci. **31:** 87.

Antenatal Assessment for the Detection of Fetal Asphyxia

An Evidence-Based Approach Using Indication-Specific Testing

ANTHONY M. VINTZILEOS[a]

Division of Maternal–Fetal Medicine, Department of Obstetrics, Gynecology and Reproductive Sciences, University of Medicine and Dentistry of New Jersey, Robert Wood Johnson Medical School/St. Peter's University Hospital, New Brunswick, New Jersey 08903, USA

ABSTRACT: One of the most important advances in perinatal health care is the use of antepartum fetal testing. Antepartum fetal testing methods may include inexpensive tests such as fetal kick counts or tests that can be quite expensive such as non-stress tests, fetal biophysical profiles, and Doppler assessments as well as invasive tests such as amniocentesis or cordocentesis. Clinical experience, combined with recent literature, suggest that there is no ideal test for all high-risk fetuses and that some antepartum fetal tests may be more appropriate than others, depending on the underlying pathophysiology or the indication for testing.[1] Because many different pathophysiological processes lead to fetal acidemia and *in-utero* death, indication-specific testing may be not only logical, but also cost-effective. In this article, specific guidelines of antepartum fetal testing are presented. These indication-specific guidelines are based on the underlying pathophysiological processes that place the fetus at risk and also on the need to use the fewest number of tests without compromising safety.

PATHOPHYSIOLOGICAL PROCESSES LEADING TO FETAL ASPHYXIA AND DEATH

Although fetal asphyxia is the common pathway leading to irreversible damage or death, there are many different pathophysiological processes that may place the fetus at risk. Once the at-risk fetus is identified by screening criteria (or tests), then specific testing schemes can be devised. The most common pathophysiological processes include decreased uteroplacental blood flow, decreased gas exchange at the trophoblastic membrane level (with normal blood flow), derangement of metabolic processes, fetal sepsis, fetal anemia, fetal heart failure, and umbilical cord accidents. Examples of conditions that could possibly be associated with reduced uteroplacental blood flow as the primary insult, include maternal chronic hypertension, pregnan-

[a]Address for correspondence: Anthony M. Vintzileos, M.D., Professor, Obstetrics, Gynecology and Reproductive Sciences, Director, Maternal–Fetal Medicine and Obstetrics, Robert Wood Johnson Medical School/University of Medicine and Dentistry of New Jersey, St. Peter's University Hospital, 254 Easton Avenue, MOB 4th Floor, New Brunswick, New Jersey 08903. Phone: 732-745-6673; fax: 732-249-5729.
vintziam@umdnj.edu

cy-induced hypertension, preeclampsia, maternal collagen, renal or vascular disease, or idiopathic intrauterine growth restriction (IUGR). In the presence of one or more of the above conditions, it is logical to use an initial test (or tests) that could differentiate between at-risk fetuses who need intensive biophysical surveillance and those who need little or no surveillance. Clinical experience, as well as the available literature,[2,3] strongly suggest that Doppler velocimetry, especially of the umbilical artery, can serve this purpose. Thus, it makes sense from the medical as well as the cost-effectiveness point of view to use Doppler velocimetry in all conditions that may be associated with reduced uteroplacental blood flow.

Examples of conditions that could possibly be associated with decreased gas exchange at the level of the trophoblastic membrane as the primary insult, rather than reduced blood flow, include post-dates and some cases of IUGR. In these settings, assessment of fetal growth by ultrasound, as well as amniotic fluid volume assessment, constitute the appropriate testing in detecting the at-risk fetuses who need further intensive biophysical surveillance.

An example of a metabolic process (or cause) leading to antepartum fetal distress is the presence of fetal hyperglycemia as seen in fetuses of diabetic mothers with uncontrolled blood sugars. Here, the best differentiator of at-risk fetuses who need intensive biophysical surveillance versus those who do not need further testing is the maternal blood sugar control. The presence of normal maternal blood sugars during the antepartum period combined with normal fetal growth and the absence of polyhydramnios call for little, if any, fetal surveillance. However, in the presence of high maternal blood sugars during the antepartum period, polyhydramnios, or accelerated fetal growth, the fetus is at risk for developing acidemia and therefore intensive biophysical surveillance is needed.

Examples of conditions that may possibly lead to fetal sepsis is the presence of intraamniotic infection that could be seen in patients with premature rupture of the membranes or preterm labor. Here, the tests of choice that can detect the fetuses at risk for sepsis are transabdominal amniocentesis (for rapid tests to rule out intraamniotic infection and culture) and frequent non-stress tests (NSTs) or fetal biophysical profiles.[4–6]

Some examples of conditions that could possibly lead to fetal anemia include maternal blood group immunization, feto–maternal hemorrhage or fetal parvovirus B19 infection. In these conditions, tests that should be used to differentiate between at risk fetuses who need intensive biophysical surveillance versus those who do not need such a surveillance include amniocentesis (for amniotic fluid bilirubin studies) and/or cordocentesis (to assess fetal hemoglobin levels).

Examples of conditions that could possibly lead to or are associated with fetal heart failure include persistent severe fetal tachyarrhythmias or bradyarrhythmias or the presence of nonimmune hydrops. In these conditions, surveillance for development of fetal heart failure or worsening fetal heart failure is indicated by serial ultrasounds. Only fetuses who become hydropic are at risk and, therefore, in need of further intensive biophysical surveillance.

Finally, some examples of conditions that possibly could lead to a cord accident are the presence of umbilical cord entanglement in monoamniotic twins, oligohydramnios, velamentous cord insertions, and funic presentations. Under these conditions, the at-risk fetuses are detected by the demonstration of umbilical cord

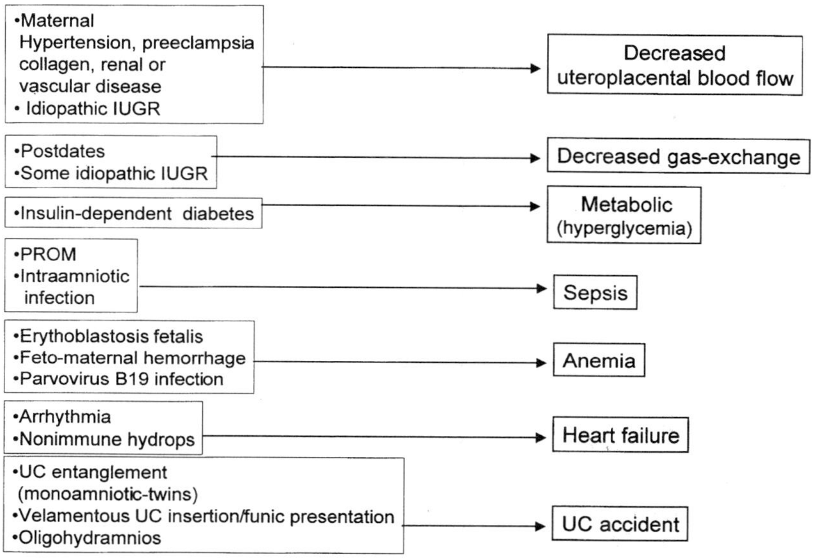

FIGURE 1. Illustration of the various maternal and fetal conditions linked to specific fetal pathophysiological processes. Abbreviations: abn, abnormal; AF, amniotic fluid; AFI, AF index; AFV, AF volume; Amnio, amniocentesis; CHF, congestive heart failure; CST, contraction stress test; Cx, cervix; echo, echocardiography; FHR, fetal heart rate; FBP, fetal biophysical profile; IAI, intraamniotic infection; IUGR, intrauterine growth restriction; nor, normal; NST, nonstress test; Oligo, oligohydramnios; Poly, polyhydramnios; PROM, premature rupture of membranes; PUBS, percutaneous umbilical blood sampling; R/O, rule out; VAS, vibroacustic stimulation; wks, weeks; UC, umbilical cord; U/S, ultrasound.

entanglement (in monoamniotic twins) or velamentous and/or funic presentation, which are best diagnosed by the use of color flow imaging.

The various high-risk conditions leading to specific fetal pathophysiological processes are shown in FIGURE 1. FIGURE 2 shows the pathways from the primary pathophysiological processes to asphyxia and death and depicts the appropriate screening tests (or criteria) according to the specific underlying pathophysiology. As illustrated in FIGURE 2, arrest of biophysical activities could be the result of either fetal adaptation or irreversible fetal damage. However, current techniques do not allow differentiation between fetuses who may be in the adaptation process versus those who are irreversibly damaged.

INDICATION-SPECIFIC (OR CONDITION-SPECIFIC) FETAL TESTING

The most common indications for fetal testing are post-dates, preexisting maternal vascular disease, diabetes (diet or insulin-controlled), suspected IUGR, maternal blood group immunization, multiple gestation, preeclampsia, premature rupture of the membranes or decreased fetal movement (decreased kick-counts). The selection

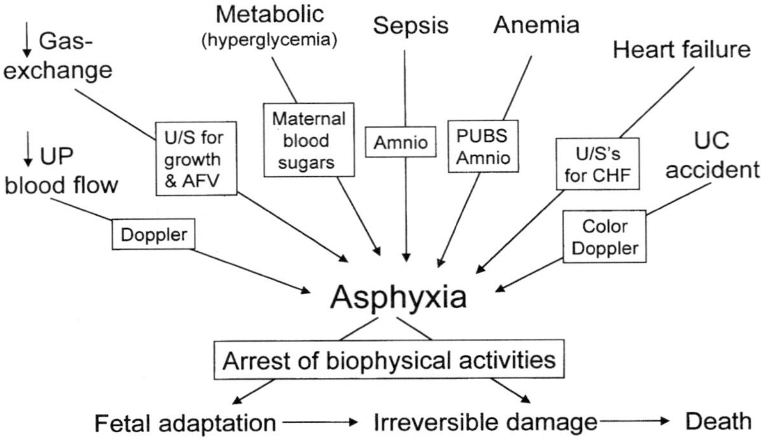

FIGURE 2. Illustration of the pathways to fetal asphyxia and death as well as the specific screening tests (or criteria) that should be used to identify at-risk fetuses according to the underlying pathophysiology. Abbreviations as in FIGURE 1.

of the appropriate test (or tests) for fetal testing should be dictated by the existing underlying pathophysiology and gestational age. The intelligent use of antepartum fetal tests should identify at-risk fetuses early enough to allow effective intervention and should also be cost effective. Our indication-specific protocols (or guidelines) were constructed on the basis of three basic principles:

(1) There is an initial application of screening tests or criteria (i.e., ultrasound fetal growth, Doppler velocimetry, or maternal historical factors) to detect at-risk fetuses. These screening tests or criteria are condition-specific, and they are selected on the basis of underling pathophysiological process;

(2) At-risk fetuses are followed with intensive biophysical surveillance, which includes either non-stress tests (NSTs) combined with amniotic fluid volume assessments (if the condition is associated with increased incidence of oligohydramnios, see FIG. 3) or NST only (if the condition is not associated with increased incidence of oligohydramnios, see FIG. 4); and

(3) Under some high-risk conditions, fetal testing is not recommended beyond a certain gestational age because of increased possibility of a false negative examination.

Based on the above three principles, the guidelines (or protocols) recommended for antepartum fetal testing are summarized in FIGURES 3–14. FIGURES 3 and 4 reflect generic indication-specific fetal surveillance schemes for fetuses at risk. The factor that determines the specific biophysical surveillance (FIG. 3 versus FIG. 4 protocol) is the possibility of oligohydramnios. When the primary indication for testing is post-dates, maternal hypertension, maternal renal or collagen disease, suspected IUGR, antiphospholipid syndrome, or diabetes mellitus classes D–T, and the fetus is judged to be at risk, the protocol of FIGURE 3 is followed. If the primary indication

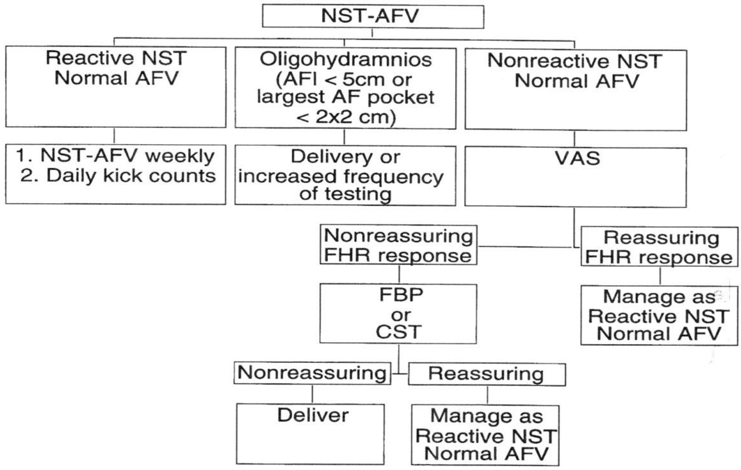

FIGURE 3. The antepartum fetal surveillance to be used in at-risk fetuses when the condition is associated with increased incidence of oligohydramnios (i.e., postdates, maternal hypertension, maternal renal or collagen disease, diabetes mellitus classes D-T, fetal growth restriction, antiphospholipid syndrome, and so forth). Abbreviations as in FIGURE 1.

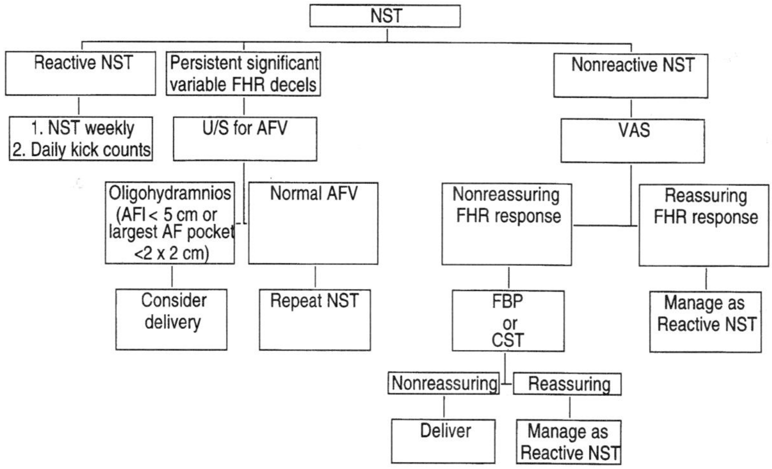

FIGURE 4. The antepartum fetal surveillance to be used with at-risk fetuses when the condition is not associated with increased incidence of oligohydramnios (i.e., diabetes classes A–C, suspected erythroblastosis fetalis, and so forth). Abbreviations as in FIGURE 1.

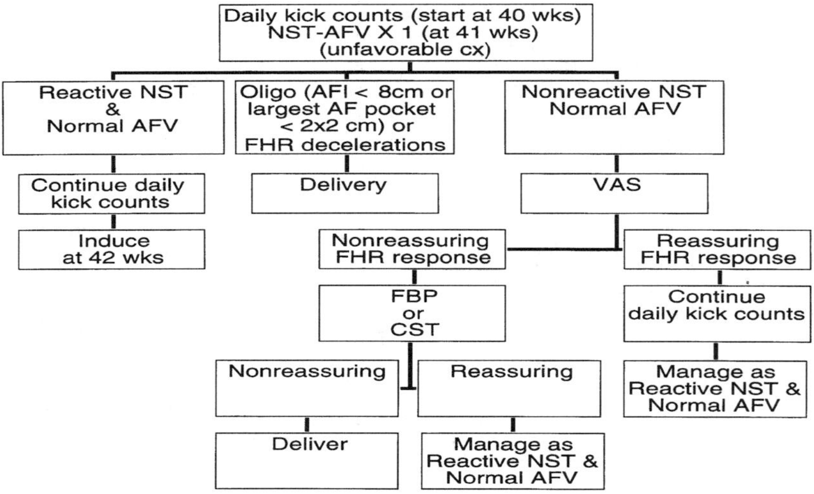

FIGURE 5. Antepartum fetal testing for postdates. Abbreviations as in FIGURE 1.

for testing is a condition that is not usually associated with oligohydramnios (e.g., maternal diabetes mellitus classes A–C, suspected maternal blood group sensitization, or any other condition with expected normal fluid), at-risk fetuses are followed with the protocol illustrated in FIGURE 4. In both protocols (FIG. 3 or 4) a nonreactive NST is always followed up by the least expensive test that is also safe, that is, fetal vibroacoustic stimulation. Fetal biophysical profiles or contractions stress tests, which are expensive tests, are used only in the minority of patients who continue to have a nonreactive NST after vibroacoustic stimulation.

FIGURES 5–14 reflect condition-specific fetal testing and include the screening tests (or screening criteria) to be used to differentiate between at-risk fetuses who need intensive biophysical surveillance versus those who need little, if any, surveillance. FIGURE 5 illustrates the suggested protocol for post-dates. Daily kick counts are started at 40 weeks. If the cervix is favorable for induction, there is no proof that fetal testing is better than induction of labor; thus, labor induction is recommended no later than 41 weeks. If the cervix is unfavorable, one-time testing by using NST-amniotic fluid volume assessment is appropriate. No pregnancies are allowed to go beyond 42 weeks regardless of testing results.

FIGURE 6 illustrates the protocol in the presence of preexisting maternal vascular disease. The screening tests include an ultrasound evaluation for fetal growth and anatomy at 18–20 weeks and an ultrasound/amniotic fluid volume assessment/Doppler evaluation at 24–26 weeks of gestation. If the fetus is judged to be at risk based on these screening tests, patients are followed by intensive fetal surveillance; otherwise, only daily fetal kick counts are indicated. Follow-up ultrasound screening would be needed every 4–6 weeks. No pregnancies are allowed to continue beyond 40 weeks.

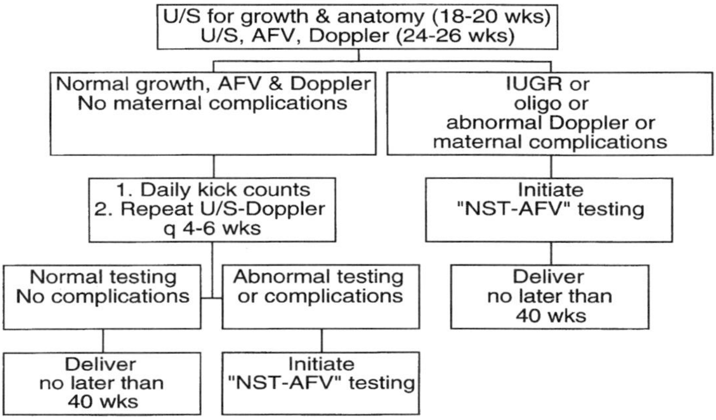

FIGURE 6. Antepartum fetal testing for preexisting maternal vascular disease (i.e., chronic hypertension, maternal renal or collagen disease, antiphospholipid syndrome, and so forth). Abbreviations as in FIGURE 1.

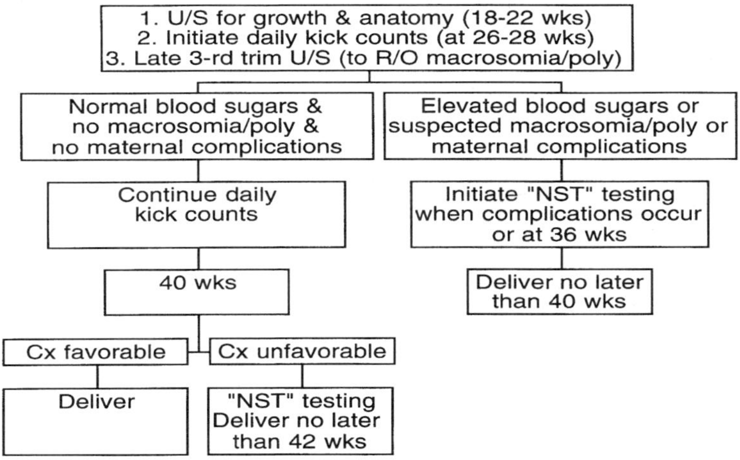

FIGURE 7. Antepartum fetal testing for gestational diabetes (diet-controlled). Abbreviations as in FIGURE 1.

FIGURE 7 illustrates the recommended protocol for diet-controlled diabetes. The presence of normal blood sugars during the antepartum period, absence of maternal complications, absence of fetal macrosomia, and absence of polyhydramnios indicate low fetal risk; and, therefore, daily kick counts are appropriate for surveillance. In the presence of elevated maternal sugars, suspected fetal macrosomia, polyhydramnios or any other maternal complications, NST testing is indicated for fetal surveillance. In the presence of one or more of these complications pregnancies should not be allowed to extend beyond 40 weeks.

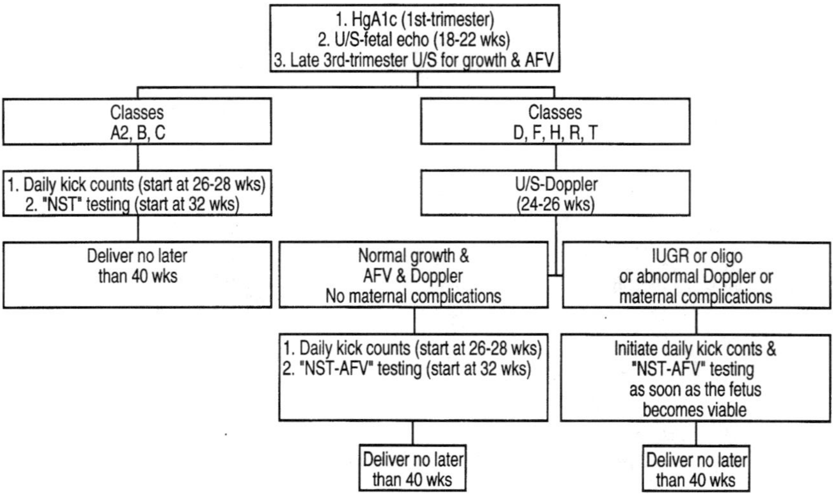

FIGURE 8. Antepartum fetal testing for insulin-dependent diabetes mellitus. Abbreviations as in FIGURE 1.

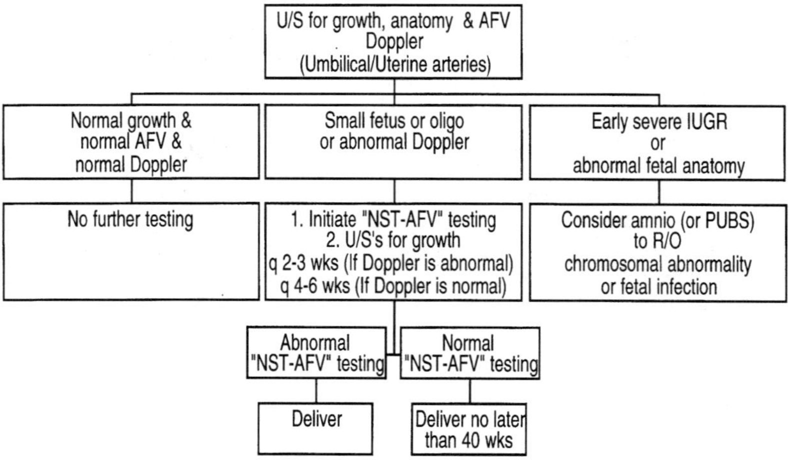

FIGURE 9. Antepartum fetal testing for suspected intrauterine growth restriction. Abbreviations as in FIGURE 1.

FIGURE 8 illustrates the recommended protocol for fetuses of insulin-dependent diabetics. Here, the screening tests are hemoglobin A1C (first trimester), an ultrasound with fetal echocardiography at 18–22 weeks, and a late third-trimester ultrasound to assess fetal growth and amniotic fluid volume. In classes A2, B, and C oligohydramnios is not expected, and these fetuses are followed with daily kick

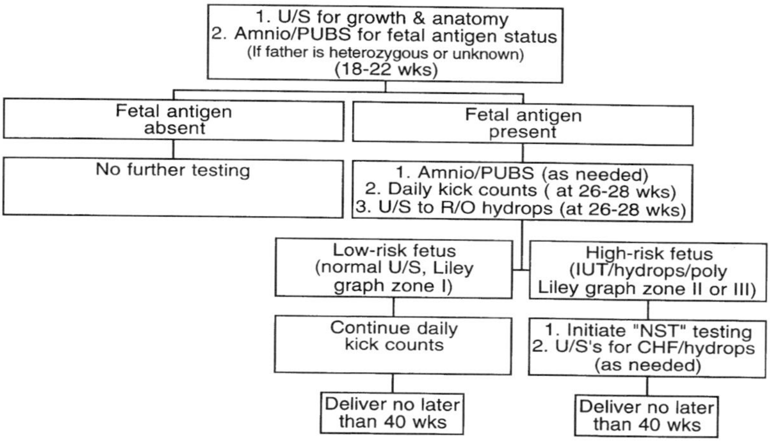

FIGURE 10. Antepartum fetal testing for maternal blood group immunization. Abbreviations as in FIGURE 1.

counts (starting at 26–28 weeks) and NSTs starting at 32 weeks. Classes D, F, H, R, and T are evaluated with an ultrasound/Doppler velocimetry at 24–26 weeks. The results of this ultrasound/Doppler velocimetry study will dictate the timing and frequency of biophysical surveillance in this group of fetuses. All fetuses of insulin-dependent diabetic mothers are delivered no later than 40 weeks of gestation.

FIGURE 9 shows the recommended protocol in cases of suspected IUGR. An ultrasound evaluation for fetal growth, amniotic fluid volume assessment, and Doppler velocimetry will differentiate between the fetuses who do not need further testing and those who should be followed by intensive testing using frequent growth and amniotic fluid volume assessment, as well as Doppler studies. In the presence of early severe IUGR or abnormal fetal anatomy, amniocentesis and/or cordocentesis to rule out fetal chromosomal abnormality or infection are the screening tests of choice.

FIGURE 10 illustrates the recommended protocol in cases of maternal blood group immunization. The determination of fetal blood antigen status (by amniocentesis or cordocentesis) is the main screening test. Fetuses are categorized as at no risk, low risk, or high risk. No testing is indicated for fetuses at no risk (with absent antigen). Low-risk fetuses (with positive antigen) are followed with daily kick counts, whereas high-risk fetuses are followed with frequent NSTs and ultrasounds. No fetus is delivered beyond 40 weeks gestation unless the fetus is negative for the antigen.

FIGURE 11 illustrates the recommended protocol of antepartum fetal testing for multiple gestations. The screening test is the ultrasonically determined placental chorionicity. The presence of dichorionic diamniotic placentation, normal fetal growth, and normal Doppler assessment is associated with very low-risk fetuses who do not need biophysical surveillance. On the other hand, the presence of monoamniotic placentation is an indication for frequent surveillance with non-stress tests, that is, daily testing. In the presence of monochorionic diamniotic placentation, the fetuses are at risk by definition and are followed with NST-amniotic fluid volume testing according to FIGURE 3.

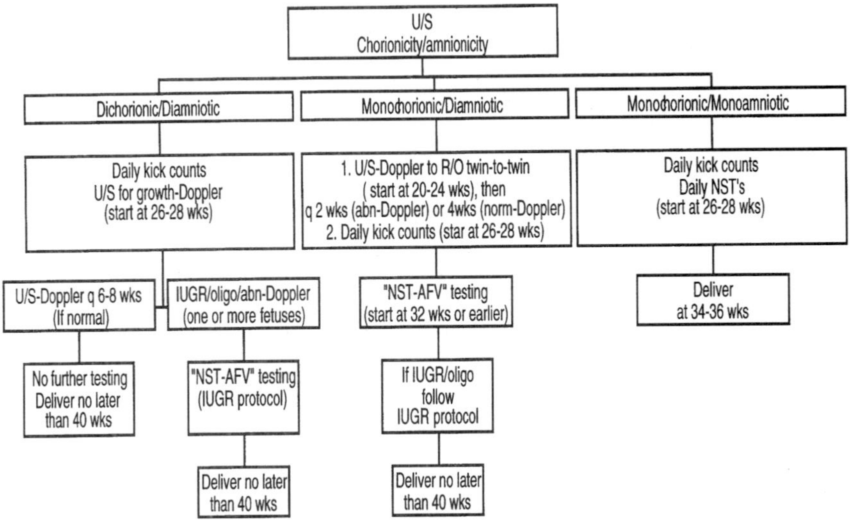

FIGURE 11. Antepartum fetal testing for multiple gestation. Abbreviations as in FIGURE 1.

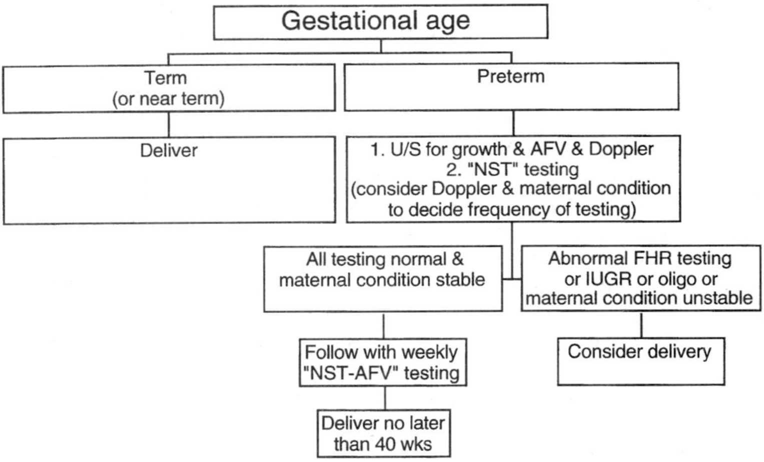

FIGURE 12. Antepartum fetal testing for preeclampsia. Abbreviations as in FIGURE 1.

FIGURE 12 illustrates the recommended protocol for fetal testing in preeclamptic mothers. In preeclampsia, the age of the fetus is the screening factor. At-term or near-term delivery is safer than fetal testing. In preterm gestations the results of ultrasound fetal growth, amniotic fluid volume assessment, NST, and Doppler veloci-

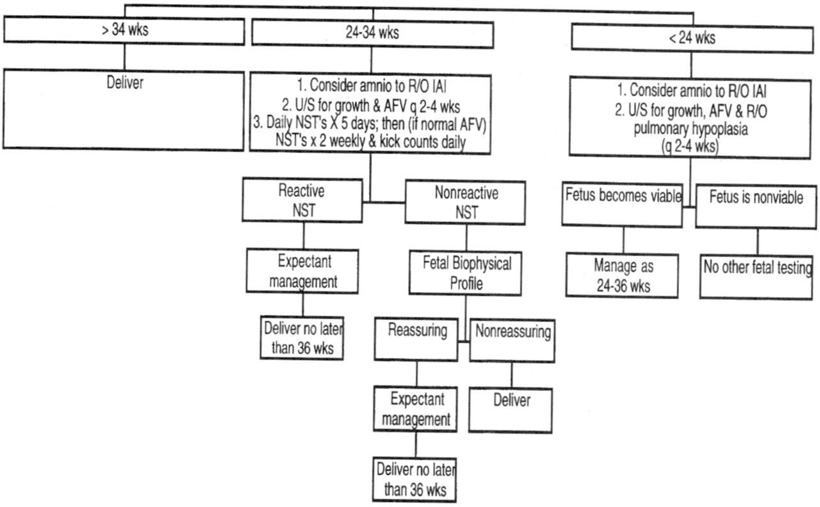

FIGURE 13. Antepartum fetal testing for premature rupture of the membranes. Abbreviations as in FIGURE 1.

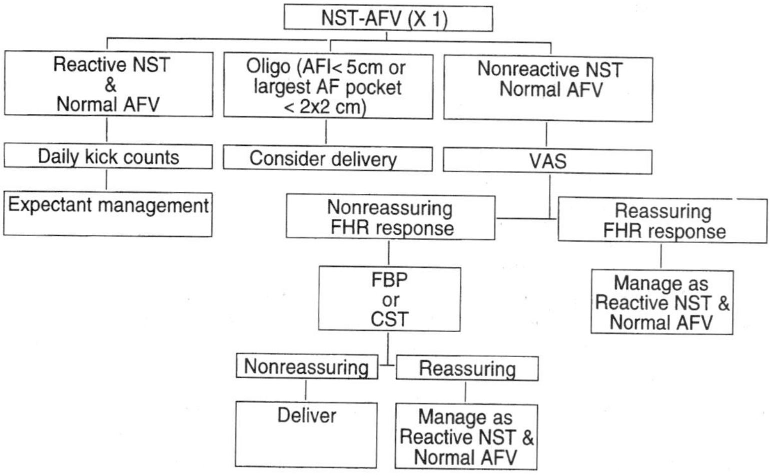

FIGURE 14. Antepartum fetal testing for cases of decreased fetal movement (or decreased kick-counts). Abbreviations as in FIGURE 1.

metry, as well as the maternal condition, will determine the timing and frequency of testing. No fetus should be delivered later than 40 weeks.

FIGURE 13 illustrates the recommended protocol of fetal testing in premature rupture of membranes. The most important screening criterion is the gestational age of the fetus. Delivery is recommended for gestational ages greater than 34 weeks. The screening test between 24 and 34 weeks is amniocentesis to rule out intraamniotic infection. In the absence of amniocentesis or if the amniocentesis is negative, then daily NST testing for 5 days followed by twice weekly NSTs with daily kick counts is appropriate. Because most fetuses with fetal distress or infection are delivered within the first 5 days after membrane rupture, the practice of reducing fetal testing after the first 5 days appears to be both safe and cost-effective. For gestations less than 24 weeks, the screening tests include amniocentesis (to rule out intraamniotic infection) and ultrasound to assess fetal growth, amniotic fluid volume, and presence or absence of lung hypoplasia. FIGURE 14 illustrates the recommended protocol for fetal biophysical surveillance in the presence of decreased fetal movement (or decreased kick counts).

COMMENTS

It is a well known fact that there is no ideal test for all high-risk fetuses. This should not be surprising because there are many different pathophysiological processes that can lead to fetal asphyxia, irreversible fetal damage, or death. The concept of indication-specific (or condition-specific) testing is supported by both clinical experience as well as recent literature. For instance, in postdates the use of Doppler is not beneficial,[7–12] whereas in IUGR[2,3] it helps in the early detection of at-risk fetuses. Another example is the strong predictive ability of oligohydramnios in post-dates, whereas in other high-risk conditions, for example diet-controlled gestational diabetes, normal fluid is the rule rather than the exception even in acidemic fetuses.[13]

Although there are no randomized controlled, trials to show the benefits of antepartum fetal testing, nonrandomized studies suggest that such testing has most likely accomplished its primary objective, which is to prevent fetal deaths.[14–17] Given the pressures of reducing health care costs and at the same time improving perinatal outcomes, the use of indication-specific antepartum fetal testing becomes a necessity. The purpose of the present article was to suggest fetal testing guidelines based on both clinical experience and existing literature. The goal was to have less antepartum fetal testing without compromising safety in order to improve cost-effectiveness. The concepts of indication and condition-specific testing are quite simple and call for the use of appropriate screening tests (or criteria) to differentiate between fetuses who are at risk and, therefore, in need for biophysical surveillance versus those who need little or no further testing. One of the three basic principles on the basis of which these protocols were constructed was the assumption that in some high-risk conditions fetal testing is not advisable beyond a certain gestational age because it may be neither safe nor cost-effective. For instance, postdates on a preexisting underlying high-risk condition such as maternal hypertension may increase the chances for a false negative fetal examination. The unique feature of the suggested protocols, therefore, is that they include guidelines for not only when to initiate but also when to terminate fetal surveillance.

The proposed indication-specific fetal testing will most likely reduce the total number of antepartum fetal tests by more than 50% as compared to current antepartum fetal testing protocols. Nowadays, most protocols call for twice weekly biophysical testing for high-risk conditions such as postdates, suspected IUGR, and insulin-dependent diabetes mellitus. The suggested indication-specific fetal testing calls for fetal surveillance only in at-risk fetuses. Accordingly, these at-risk fetuses are tested with biophysical surveillance only once a week supplemented by daily kick counts. This modification could possibly account for almost a 50% reduction in the total number of the currently performed fetal tests. Further reductions in the total number of fetal tests are achieved by not testing the fetuses who are judged to be at low risk.

Although some arguments could be made regarding the specifics of each proposed indication-specific (or condition-specific) testing scheme, we strongly believe that the concept of a two-tier approach of using screening tests (or criteria) to differentiate between low-risk fetuses who need little, if any, biophysical surveillance versus those who are at risk and therefore in need for intensive surveillance, is logical, safe, and cost-effective. We recognize that no protocol or set of guidelines will cover the needs of all fetuses. These guidelines, therefore, should be considered as general pathways that will cover the needs of most, but not all, fetuses.

Indication-specific antepartum fetal testing has been recommended in the past, but it has not achieved recognition by practicing physicians or the obstetrical literature.[1,15] Nevertheless, managed care and capitation are powerful forces necessitating wise and appropriate use of our health-care resources. Because there are no randomized, controlled trials for antepartum fetal testing, we have to use logic, clinical experience, and nonrandomized observational studies to make the best judgments about how to use fetal testing. In our opinion, the time has come for indication-specific antepartum fetal testing.

REFERENCES

1. Vintzileos, A.M. 1995. Forward in antepartum fetal surveillance. Clin. Obstet. Gynecol. **38:** 1–2.
2. Alfirevic, L. & J.P. Neilson. 1995. Doppler ultrasonography in high-risk pregnancies: systematic review with meta-analysis. Am. J. Obstet. Gynecol. **172:** 1371–1387.
3. Divon, M. 1995. Randomized controlled trials of umbilical artery Doppler velocimetry: How many are too many? Ultrasound Obstet. Gynecol. **6:** 377–379.
4. Vintzileos, A.M., W.A. Campbell, D.J. Nochimson, *et al.* 1986. Qualitative amniotic fluid volume versus amniocentesis in prediction infection in preterm premature rupture of the membranes. Obstet. Gynecol. **67:** 579–583.
5. Vintzileos, A.M., W.A. Campbell, D.J. Nochimson & P.J. Weinbaum. 1986. The use of the nonstress test in patients with premature rupture of the membranes. Am. J. Obstet. Gynecol. **155:** 149–153.
6. Vintzileos, A.M., W.A. Campbell, D.J. Nochimson & M.E. Connolly. 1985. The fetal biophysical profile in patients with premature rupture of the membranes—an early predictor of fetal infection. Am. J. Obstet. Gynecol. **152:** 510–516.
7. Stokes, H.J., R.V. Roberts & J.P. Newnham. 1991. Doppler flow velocity waveform analysis in postdate pregnancies. Aust. N.Z. J. Obstet. Gynecol. **31:** 27–30.
8. Guidetti, D.A., M.Y. Divon, R.L. Cavalieri, *et al.* 1987. Fetal umbilical artery flow velocimetry in postdate pregnancies. Am. J. Obstet. Gynecol. **157:** 1521–1523.
9. Ducey, J., E. Guzman, L. Saldana, *et al.* 1988. Uterine and umbilical Doppler velocimetry in posterm pregnancy. J. Reprod. Med. **33:** 259–261.
10. Bar-Hava, I., M.Y. Divon, M. Sardo & Y. Barnhard. 1995. Is oligohydramnios in post-term pregnancy associated with redistribution of fetal blood flow? Am. J. Obstet. Gynecol. **173:** 519–522.
11. Zimmermann, P., T. Albäck, *et al.* 1995. Doppler flow velocimetry of the umbilical artery, uteroplacental arteries and fetal middle cerebral artery in prolonged pregnancy. Ultrasound Obstet. Gynecol. **5:** 189–197.

12. WEINER, A., G. FARMAKIDES, H. SCHULMAN, *et al.* 1996. Central and peripheral haemodynamic changes in post-term fetuses: correlation with oligohydramnios and abnormal fetal heart rate pattern. Br. J. Obstet. Gynecol. **103:** 541–546. [Application of a technique which has been previously utilized in the study of pregnancies complicated by intrauterine growth restriction.]
13. SALVESEN, D.R., J. FREEMAN, J.M. BRUDENELL & K.H. NICOLAIDES. 1993. Prediction of fetal acidaemia in pregnancies complicated by maternal diabetes mellitus by biophysical profile scoring and fetal heart rate monitoring. Br. J. Obstet. Gynaecol. **100:** 227–233.
14. COOPER, R.L., R.L. GOLDENBERG, M.B. DUBARD, *et al.* 1994. Risk factors for fetal death in white, black and hispanic women. Obstet. Gynecol. **84:** 490–495.
15. NAGEOTTE, M.P., C.V. TOWERS, T. ASRAT, *et al.* 1994. The value of a negative antepartum test: contraction stress test and modified biophysical profile. Obstet. Gynecol. **84:** 231–234.
16. MILLER, D.A., Y.A. RABELLO & R.H. PAUL. 1996. The modified biophysical profile: antepartum testing in the 1990s. Am. J. Obstet. Gynecol. **174:** 812–817.
17. MANNING, F.A. 1995. Dynamic ultrasound-based fetal assessment: the fetal biophysical profile score. Clin. Obstet. Gynecol. **38:** 26–44.

Recent Advances in Respiratory Care of the Term Neonate

IAN GROSS[a]

Division of Perinatal Medicine, Department of Pediatrics, Yale University School of Medicine, New Haven, Connecticut 06520, USA

ABSTRACT: Persistent pulmonary hypertension is a major cause of morbidity and mortality in the term and near-term infant. Management of this condition, which is characterized by respiratory distress and cyanosis, has been greatly enhanced by inhaled nitric oxide (NO) therapy. The following treatment regime is suggested: Conventional ventilation should be used initially, and hyperventilation should be avoided. Surfactant should be administered early, preferably within 6 hours of diagnosis. If conventional ventilation fails, the next step is high-frequency ventilation or inhaled NO. Some infants who do not respond to inhaled NO when administered by conventional ventilation will respond to NO delivery via a high-frequency ventilator. If all of these therapies fail, extracorporeal membrane oxygenation (ECMO) should be considered. By the use of this approach, the mortality from PPH has been considerably reduced, and concerns today relate primarily to morbidity, particularly long-term neurologic outcome and chronic lung disease resulting from ventilation and barotrauma.

The most significant respiratory problem of the term neonate is persistent pulmonary hypertension of the newborn (PPH), and most of the recent advances in respiratory care relate to the management of this disease. PPH[1] often occurs in infants who are otherwise normal, and until recently this condition has been extremely refractory to therapy.

PATHOGENESIS OF PERSISTENT PULMONARY HYPERTENSION OF THE NEWBORN

In order to understand PPH, one must first consider the fetal circulation. During fetal life, oxygenation and gas exchange are functions of the placenta, and relatively little blood flows through the lungs. There is increased vascular tone in the pulmonary circulation with elevated pressures in the right side of the heart. As a result of this, blood entering the right atrium, particularly from the inferior vena cava, tends to be shunted from the right atrium to the left atrium through the foramen ovale. The

[a]Address for correspondence: Division of Perinatal Medicine, Department of Pediatrics, Yale University School of Medicine, 333 Cedar Street, New Haven, CT 06520. Phone: 203-688-2320; fax: 203-688-5426.

ian.gross@yale.edu

blood that enters the right ventricle and then the pulmonary artery may be shunted across the ductus arteriosus into the aorta. Much of the blood that originally entered the right atrium ultimately flows to the aorta, and the lungs are effectively bypassed.

After birth, vascular tone in the pulmonary circulation decreases, resulting in lower pressure in the right side of the heart. There is functional closure of the foramen ovale, and within hours the ductus arteriosus usually closes. The normal postnatal circulation is established, with blood entering the right atrium progressing to the right ventricle and pulmonary artery and reentering the heart via the pulmonary veins and the left atrium.

In some babies, for reasons that are not entirely clear, pulmonary vasoconstriction occurs again after birth, resulting in increased pressure in the right side of the heart and the shunting of blood from the right side to the left side across the foramen ovale and/or the ductus arteriosus. The decreased pulmonary blood flow causes hypoxemia and cyanosis.

Both short- and long-acting factors have been associated with increased pulmonary vascular resistance. Acute constriction can be caused by hypoxia and acidosis. Enhanced resistance of longer duration is thought to be due to increased thickness of the smooth muscle layer of the wall of small arterioles. The mechanism underlying this thickening is not entirely clear, but chronic low-grade intrauterine hypoxia has been implicated.

PPH is associated with asphyxia at birth, and for this reason it is also associated with post-mature delivery and meconium aspiration, another consequence of asphyxia. Pulmonary vasoconstriction also often complicates pulmonary hypoplasia, particularly that due to diaphragmatic hernia, and it is seen in babies with pneumonia and sepsis where vasoactive substances may play a role. The clinical criteria for the diagnosis of PPH are a PaO_2 of less than 70 torr in an FiO_2 of 1.0, absence of structural heart disease, and documentation of right-to-left shunting.

Because the lung fields in babies with PPH may be underperfused and clear on X-ray, it is important to differentiate this condition from cyanotic congenital heart disease. The only way this can be done with certainty is by means of an echocardiogram. This will exclude anatomic heart disease and reveal pulmonary hypertension and left-to-right shunting. It is also important to visualize the pulmonary veins, because anomalous pulmonary venous return can simulate many of the features of PPH.

MANAGEMENT OF PERSISTENT PULMONARY HYPERTENSION OF THE NEWBORN

The management of this condition is focused on mechanical ventilation, support of the circulation, and dilatation of the pulmonary arterioles. PPH is a transient condition, as the arterial spasm usually lasts 5–7 days; if the babies can be maintained for this time without producing significant injury to lung tissue, the chance of survival is enhanced.[2] Hyperventilation, which induces hypocarbic alkalosis, is effective in temporarily dilating the pulmonary arteries and improving oxygenation, but the long-term price that must be paid in terms of injury to the lungs has led many physicians to abandon this technique.[3] As will be discussed below, surfactant therapy and high-frequency ventilation have also been shown to enhance oxygenation in these infants.

It is important to maintain perfusion because there is often decreased blood pressure, in part due to decreased blood return to the left side of the heart. This is usually accomplished by a combination of intravenous fluids and pressors, such as dopamine and dobutamine.

Reversal of the constriction of the pulmonary arterioles is a critical component of management that only recently has yielded to therapy. In the past, alkalinization by hyperventilation or by infusion of bicarbonate was used, the latter technique being preferred. Attempts to dilate the pulmonary circulation with nonspecific vasodilators, such as tolazoline, were associated with limited success and considerable toxicity. With the advent of inhaled nitric oxide, it has finally become possible to effectively and selectively dilate the pulmonary arterioles in many of these infants.

Inhaled Nitric Oxide

Nitric oxide (NO) is produced in the endothelial cells of blood vessels and then diffuses into the adjacent vascular smooth muscle. It is capable of dilating both pulmonary and systemic arteries and is not a specific pulmonary vasodilator. When NO is administered by inhalation, however, it diffuses from the airways into the wall of the pulmonary vessels, dilating the arterioles. It then binds rapidly to hemoglobin in the vessel lumen and is inactivated. NO leaves the pulmonary circulation bound to hemoglobin and does not have significant effects on the systemic circulation. For this reason the effects of inhaled NO are limited to the pulmonary vasculature, and it acts as a *de facto* pulmonary vasodilator.

In addition to dilating constricted pulmonary arterioles, inhaled NO also has the effect of optimizing ventilation/perfusion matching. This is due to the fact that when NO is inhaled, it will most effectively dilate those blood vessels that are associated with the best ventilated alveoli. Thus, inhaled NO may be of benefit in a variety of pulmonary conditions and not only those associated with severe vasoconstriction.

Early reports had suggested that NO was toxic to the lungs, but recent animal and clinical studies have suggested that low levels of inhaled NO do not result in pulmonary toxicity. The reason for earlier concerns may relate to the fact that NO is often contaminated with NO_2, nitrogen dioxide, and this may have caused the toxicity. One of the side effects of inhaled NO is met-hemoglobinemia; and it has been shown in clinical trials that inhaled NO therapy can result in met-hemoglobin levels in the 2–5% range. Higher levels are usually seen with inhalation of high concentrations of NO (80 ppm) and tend to resolve rapidly when NO inhalation ceases. In this regard, it is worth noting that cigarette smoke contains between 600–1000 ppm of NO.

Another concern relates to platelet function. It has been shown that NO inhibits platelet aggregation and adhesion *in vitro*. Nevertheless, as will be discussed later, bleeding has not been a problem when NO has been used in term babies.

In 1997, two major multicenter randomized, controlled trials of NO were published. The first was that of Roberts *et al.*[4] Babies of more than 37 weeks' gestation or 2.5 kg in weight were eligible for entry into the study if they had a PaO_2 of less than 55 torr in 100% oxygen. Babies with pulmonary hypoplasia or cardiac disease were excluded and prior high-frequency ventilation was not permitted. Fifty-eight infants were assigned to placebo or NO therapy in this randomized, blinded trial. The initial dose of NO was 80 ppm, but this was weaned if there was a favorable response. It was determined that the baby had a successful immediate response if, 20 minutes after starting therapy, the PaO_2 was greater than 55 torr, there was no systemic hypotension, and the oxygenation index (OI) was less than 40. (The oxygenation index takes into account the baby's oxygenation and the amount of ventilator support that is required to accomplish it. The formula is: OI = mean airway pressure (MAP) $\times$ $FiO_2 \times 100 / PaO_2$.) Seven percent of the control infants and 53% of the NO-treated infants met this definition of "success." Therefore, just over half the babies had an immediate response to NO. It was not possible to determine which infants were most likely to respond to NO. In addition, the need for extracorporeal membrane oxygenation (ECMO) was reduced by about one-third in the babies who received NO.

A larger randomized, controlled study with 235 infants was published in 1997 by the NIH Neonatal Research Network.[5] Babies of over 34 weeks of gestation were eligible for entry into this trial if they had an OI of greater than 25 on two successive determinations. The infants could have received prior treatment with high-frequency ventilation. Diagnoses included PPH, meconium aspiration, pneumonia, and respiratory distress syndrome (RDS). Another 53 infants with diaphragmatic hernia were analyzed in a separate study. Babies who were assigned to NO treatment were started on a dose of 20 ppm, but this could be increased up to 80 ppm if oxygenation did not improve. The mode of ventilation before entry, high frequency or conventional, was continued. A good short-term response was again observed. The OI in the NO group decreased from 43 to 29 after treatment was started, and the PaO_2 went up by 58 torr. In addition, the percentage of babies who required ECMO was decreased by 30%.

Inhaled NO was not stopped in any infant because of toxicity, and there was no difference from controls in the incidence of intracranial, pulmonary, or gastrointestinal bleeds, nor was there any difference in the instance of stroke. Met-hemoglobinemia did not prove to be a problem in this study. There was, however, no change in the incidence of bronchopulmonary dysplasia or in the duration of ventilation or hospitalization.

Unfortunately the results in infants with diaphragmatic hernia were not encouraging. Essentially, there was no significant change in oxygenation after NO was started, and there was no decrease in the requirement for ECMO in these infants.[6]

The question of whether babies will respond more favorably to NO if they are also being managed with high-frequency ventilation is not resolved at present. The NIH study did not find a benefit in those infants who were on high-frequency ventilation. However, a multicenter study from Denver[7] with a crossover design did suggest that some infants who were in respiratory failure after receiving inhaled NO via a conventional ventilator responded favorably if they were switched to high-frequency ventilation.

We can conclude from the randomized trials with inhaled NO that about 55% of infants with PPH have an immediate increase in oxygenation, the need for ECMO is reduced by about a third, and in some babies NO may be more effective with high-frequency ventilation. It appears appropriate at this time to start with 20 ppm, but it may be necessary to increase the dose. NO does not appear to be a successful therapy for infants with diaphragmatic hernia.

Although term babies with respiratory disease respond positively to NO, its use in premature infants has been limited. This is partly due to concerns about the risk of intraventricular hemorrhage. There are reports of premature babies, particularly those with group B streptococcal sepsis, who have responded favorably to NO,[8] but large, randomized trials are needed so that the use of NO in the premature infant can be evaluated.

Surfactant Therapy

Surfactant has also proved to be a useful therapy in term infants with persistent pulmonary hypertension. The rationale for the use of surfactant is that surfactant is deficient in adults with adult respiratory distress syndrome (ARDS) and that surfactant administration improves gas exchange and lung mechanics in animal models of ARDS. In term infants with meconium aspiration, Findlay *et al.*[9] have shown that large doses of surfactant (150 mg of phospholipid per kg) started within 6 hours of birth resulted in improved oxygenation, particularly after the second and third dose. There was also decreased air leak, requirement for ECMO, days on oxygen, days on the ventilator, and days in the hospital. Lotze *et al.*[10] examined the effect of surfactant in babies with PPH, meconium aspiration, and sepsis. In this study, the standard dose of surfactant (100 mg per kg) was used, and therapy did not have to be started within 6 hours. They found that there was a significant reduction in the need for ECMO, but there was no difference in the incidence of air leak, pulmonary hemorrhage, days in oxygen, or days on the ventilator.

These studies indicate that surfactant therapy is beneficial in term infants with PPH. It is not clear that the higher dose used in the Findlay study is necessary, and standard doses of surfactant may be adequate. It is reasonable to administer surfactant to infants with meconium aspiration or PPH soon after intubation and ventilation. Up to 4 doses should be administered if the PO_2 is less than 60–70 torr in an FiO_2 of 1.0.

High-Frequency Ventilation

Although high-frequency ventilation is used empirically for patients with PPH by many centers, few studies have examined this treatment in a randomized, controlled fashion. Clark *et al.*[11] randomized infants of greater than 34 weeks' gestation, and in respiratory failure, to high-frequency or conventional ventilation. Those infants who failed conventional ventilation were then crossed over to high frequency, and similarly those who were failing high frequency were crossed over to conventional. The initial rate of response to high-frequency and conventional ventilation was similar. Whereas 38% of patients who failed conventional ventilation responded to rescue with high-frequency ventilation, however, only 10% of infants who failed high-frequency responded to conventional ventilation.

The results of this study have been borne out by clinical experience. Although it is currently not possible to predict which infants will respond to high-frequency ventilation, it is appropriate to try high-frequency ventilation in infants with PPH who fail conventional ventilation.

Liquid Ventilation

Liquid ventilation is another modality that offers some promise for the management of these children, although there is little published experience with liquid ventilation in term babies in pulmonary failure. In liquid ventilation, perfluorocarbons are instilled into the lungs. Perfluorocarbons are liquids with oxygen and carbon dioxide solubility far greater than that of blood, so that they can be saturated with oxygen and used as a vehicle for delivering oxygen to the alveoli. Perfluorocarbons also have low surface tension and can act as surfactants. They spread well and recruit collapsed alveoli, resulting in more uniform ventilation. This improves lung compliance and ventilation–perfusion matching. It has also been proposed that perfluorocarbons may wash out debris such as meconium and that they may be used to deliver drugs.

In total liquid ventilation,[12] the lungs are totally filled with fluid, and slow "breaths" are delivered by a liquid ventilator. The liquid is run in, allowed to stay in the lungs for a few seconds, and then run out again. An advantage of total liquid ventilation is that there is no alveolar air–liquid interface and therefore problems with surface tension do not exist. They can be administered under very low pressures and are good for delivery of drugs. The major disadvantage is that it is a complex procedure requiring special equipment.

Partial liquid ventilation is being studied more intensively due to its simplicity.[13] In this modality the lungs are filled with liquid to the functional residual capacity (FRC). Gas ventilation is then used with a standard ventilator, so that on inspiration the lungs are partly filled with the liquid and partly filled with air. On expiration the lungs will be filled only with the liquid. The advantage of partial liquid ventilation is that it is less complex and uses conventional equipment. The disadvantages are that an air–liquid interface remains, so that surface tension could still be a problem and higher inflationary pressures may be required. A number of studies have suggested that partial liquid ventilation may be valuable in premature infants with respiratory failure,[13] but there is currently little published information on partial liquid ventilation in term infants. Studies examining this therapy are currently under way.

Lung growth in the fetus is partly dependent on the internal distending pressure within the airways, which is generated by the lung liquid. An interesting experimental approach to the use of liquid ventilation in babies with diaphragmatic hernia involves placing the infant on ECMO and then using liquid ventilation to create a distending pressure in the lungs. It is hypothesized that this treatment will promote growth of the hypoplastic lungs.

Extracorporeal Membrane Oxygen

ECMO is the rescue treatment of last resort for infants with PPH. The use of ECMO is based on the assumption that the pulmonary vasospasm in this condition is transient, and if the infants can be supported for a period of about a week, the vasospasm will resolve, and the patients can be weaned from this form of life support. In this procedure, a catheter is usually placed into the right atrium via the jugular vein to withdraw blood from the heart. The blood is then anticoagulated and pumped through a membrane oxygenator that adds oxygen and removes carbon dioxide. The oxygenated blood is returned to the baby through the carotid artery. In an alternative method, known as veno-venous ECMO, the blood is both withdrawn and returned to the body by the venous system, obviating the need for ligation of the carotid artery.

ECMO is an expensive and labor-intensive therapy with a number of complications, including bleeding. However, for appropriate children, it can be life saving. In most centers, babies are considered to be candidates for ECMO if the OI is persistently greater than 40. (For example, if the mean airway pressure is 20, the FiO_2 is 1.0, and the PO_2 is 50, the baby will have an OI of 40.) ECMO is currently used in babies over 34 weeks' gestation, partly because of technical limitations in inserting catheters into smaller babies and partly because of the risk of intraventricular hemorrhage in premature infants.

Although many centers have established ECMO facilities during the past decade, this was done without careful evaluation of this therapy in randomized, controlled trials. The most comprehensive trial to date is the UK collaborative trial,[14] in which approximately 90 infants were assigned to ECMO and another 90 to conventional therapy. The survival rate to discharge was 71% in the ECMO group and 42% in the conventional ventilation group.

The use of ECMO in the United States peaked at about 1500 cases a year in 1992. Since then there has been a progressive decline, probably related to the availability of inhaled NO. Many centers are currently reporting that fewer babies with medical conditions are being treated with ECMO and that it is being primarily used for babies with surgical problems. This relates to the fact that medical disorders such as PPH tend to respond favorably to NO, whereas surgical conditions such as diaphragmatic hernia do not.

The neurodevelopmental outcome of infants treated with ECMO is reasonably encouraging. Glass *et al.*[15] have reported on the 5-year follow up of 103 infants treated with ECMO. About 17% had a major disability, and 49% reported some degree of academic problems at school. In general, the outcome for babies who are treated with ECMO and those with severe PPH, but who are not treated with ECMO, appears to be similar.

SUGGESTED APPROACH TO MANAGEMENT OF BABIES WITH PERSISTENT PULMONARY HYPERTENSION

Therapy should begin with conventional ventilation, and hyperventilation should be avoided. Surfactant should be administered early, preferably within 6 hours of diagnosis. If conventional ventilation is successful, it should be continued. If conventional ventilation fails, the next step is high-frequency ventilation, or inhaled NO. If NO therapy is unsuccessful with conventional ventilation, NO should be administered via a high-frequency ventilator. If all of these therapies fail, ECMO should be considered.

By the use of this approach, the mortality from PPH has been considerably reduced, and concerns today relate primarily to morbidity, particularly long-term neurologic outcome and chronic lung disease resulting from ventilation and barotrauma. The advent of inhaled NO has certainly had a major impact on the treatment of this disease, and the outlook is far more optimistic than it was 10 years ago.

REFERENCES

1. GROSS, I. 1994. Respiratory System. *In* Principles and Practice of Pediatrics. 2nd edit. F. Oski, C. DeAngelis, R. Feigin & J.B. Warshaw, Eds.: 365–379. J.B. Lippincott. Philadelphia.

2. Wung, J., L.S. James, E. Kilchevsky & E. James. 1985. Management of infants with severe respiratory failure and persistence of the fetal circulation without hyperventilation. Pediatrics **76:** 488–494.
3. Dworetz, A.R., F.R. Moya, B. Sabo, *et al.* 1989. Survival of infants with persistent pulmonary hypertension without extracorporeal membrane oxygenation. Pediatrics **84:** 1–6.
4. Roberts, J.D., J. Fineman, F.C. Morin, *et al.* 1997. Inhaled nitric oxide and persistent pulmonary hypertension of the newborn. N. Engl. J. Med. **336:** 605–610.
5. Neonatal Inhaled Nitric Oxide Study Group. 1997. Inhaled nitric oxide in full-term and nearly full-term infants with hypoxic respiratory failure. N. Engl. J. Med. **336:** 597–604.
6. The Neonatal Inhaled Nitric Oxide Study Group. 1997. Inhaled nitric oxide and hypoxic respiratory failure in infants with congenital diaphragmatic hernia. Pediatrics **99:** 838–845.
7. Kinsella, J.P., W.E. Truog, W.F. Walsh, *et al.* 1997. Randomized, multicenter trial of inhaled nitric oxide and high-frequency oscillatory ventilation in severe, persistent pulmonary hypertension of the newborn. J. Pediatr. **131:** 55–62.
8. Abman, S.H., J.P. Kinsella, M.S. Schaffer, *et al.* 1993. Inhaled nitric oxide in the management of a premature newborn with severe respiratory distress and pulmonary hypertension. Pediatrics **92:** 606–609.
9. Findlay, R.D., H.W. Taeusch & F.J. Walther. 1996. Surfactant replacement therapy for meconium aspiration syndrome. Pediatrics **97:** 48–52.
10. Lotze, A., B.R. Mitchell, D.I. Bulas, *et al.* 1998. Multicenter study of surfactant (beractant) use in the treatment of term infants with severe respiratory failure. J. Pediatr. **132:** 40–47.
11. Clark, R.H., B.A. Yoder & M.S. Sell. 1994. Prospective, randomized comparison of high-frequency oscillation and conventional ventilation in candidates for extracorporeal membrane oxygenation. J. Pediatr. **124:** 447–454.
12. Greenspan, J.S., M.R. Wolfson, S.D. Rubenstein & T.H. Schaffer. 1990. Liquid ventilation of human preterm neonates. J. Pediatr. **117:** 106–111.
13. Lowe, C.L., J.S. Greenspan, S.D. Rubenstein, *et al.* 1996. Partial liquid ventilation with perflubron in premature infants with severe respiratory distress syndrome. N. Engl. J. Med. **335:** 761–767.
14. UK Collaborative ECMO Trial Group. 1996. UK collaborative randomised trial of neonatal extracorporeal membrane oxygenation. Lancet **348:** 75–82.
15. Glass, P., A.E. Wagner, P.H. Papero, *et al.* 1995. Neurodevelopmental status at age five years of neonates treated with extracorporeal membrane oxygenation. J. Pediatr. **127:** 447–457.

Mechanisms of Perinatal Cerebral Injury in Fetus and Newborn

MARIA DELIVORIA-PAPADOPOULOS[a] AND OM PRAKASH MISHRA

Department of Pediatrics, MCP Hahnemann University, and St. Christopher's Hospital for Children, Philadelphia, Pennsylvania 19129, USA

ABSTRACT: Cerebral hypoxia in the fetus and newborn results in neonatal morbidity and mortality as well as long-term sequelae such as mental retardation, seizure disorders, and cerebral palsy. In the developing brain, determinants of susceptibility to hypoxia should include the lipid composition of the brain cell membrane, the rate of lipid peroxidation, the presence of antioxidant defenses, and the development and modulation of excitatory amino acid neurotransmitter receptors such as the *N*-methyl-D-aspartate (NMDA) receptor, the intracellular Ca^{2+}, and the intranuclear Ca^{2+}-dependent mechanisms. In addition to the developmental status of these cellular components, the response of these potential mechanisms to hypoxia determines the fate of the hypoxic brain cell in the developing brain. Using electron spin resonance spectroscopy of alpha-phenyl-*N*-tert-butyl-nitrone spin adducts, studies from our laboratory demonstrated that tissue hypoxia results in increased free radical generation in the cortex of fetal guinea pigs and newborn piglets. Pretreatment with $MgSO_4$ significantly decreased the hypoxia-induced increase in free radical generation in the term fetal brain. We also showed that brain tissue hypoxia modifies the NMDA receptor ion-channel recognition and modulatory sites. Furthermore, a higher increase in NMDA receptor agonist-dependent Ca^{2+} in synaptosomes was demonstrated. The increase in intracellular Ca^{2+} may activate several enzymatic pathways such as phospholipase A_2 and metabolism of archidonic acid by cyclooxygenase and lipoxygenase, conversion of xanthine dehydrogenase to xanthine oxidase by proteases, and activation of nitric oxide synthase. Using inhibitors of each of these enzymes such as cyclooxygenase (indomethacin), lipoxygenase (nordihydroguaiaretic acid), xanthine oxidase (allopurinol), and nitric oxide synthase (*N*-nitro-L-arginine), studies have shown that these enzyme reactions result in oxygen free radical generation, membrane peroxidation, and cell membrane dysfunction in the hypoxic brain. Specifically, generation of nitric oxide free radicals during hypoxia may lead to nitration and nitrosylation of specific membrane proteins and receptors, resulting in dysfunction of receptors and enzymes. We conclude that hypoxia-induced modification of the NMDA receptor leading to increased intracellular Ca^{2+} results in free radical generation and cell injury. We suggest that during hypoxia the increased intracellular Ca^{2+} may lead to increased intranuclear Ca^{2+} concentration and alter nuclear events including transcription of specific apoptotic genes and activation of endonucleases, resulting in programmed cell death.

[a]Address for correspondence: Maria Delivoria-Papadopoulos, M.D., Ann Preston Hall 2nd Floor, Department of Pediatrics, Medical College of Pennsylvania Hospital, 3300 Henry Avenue, Philadelphia, PA 19129, USA.

INTRODUCTION

Cerebral hypoxia in the fetus and newborn results in neonatal morbidity and mortality as well as long-term sequelae such as mental retardation, seizure disorders, and cerebral palsy.[37,43,44] Although the consequences of antepartum or perinatal hypoxia can be seen in babies, the specific cellular mechanisms of pathologic processes preceding the onset of cerebral dysfunction are not well understood. Several excellent reviews on subjects dealing with the mechanisms of hypoxic/ischemic brain damage were published recently.[13,16,24,27,30] This review primarily focuses on the generation of oxygen-free radical species during hypoxia in fetal and newborn animals, identification of free radical species, participation of various pathways and strategies in the inhibition of free radical generation during hypoxia by using specific enzyme inhibitors and antagonists of the *N*-methyl-D-aspartate (NMDA) receptor ion-channel complex.

In the developing brain, determinants of susceptibility to hypoxia-induced cell damage should include the lipid composition of the brain cell membrane; the rate of lipid peroxidation; the presence of enzymatic and nonenzymatic antioxidant defenses; development of free radical generating pathways; and development and modulation of the NMDA receptor, the intracellular and intranuclear Ca^{2+} influx mechanisms. In addition to the developmental stages of these cellular components, the response of these potential mechanisms to hypoxia determines the fate of the hypoxic cell in the developing fetus and newborn. Elucidation of basic cellular and molecular mechanisms in response to hypoxia in the developing brain will enable the development of novel strategies for preventing or attenuating the deleterious effects of hypoxia in the human newborn.

Free radicals are molecular species with unpaired electrons in the outer orbit with a strong tendency to initiate chain reactions that result in membrane peroxidation, protein oxidation, nucleic acid oxidation, and cell damage. Normally, more than 80% of the oxygen consumed by the cell is completely reduced by cytochrome oxidase to water without production of oxygen free radicals. The remaining 10–20% undergoes other oxidation reduction reactions in the cytoplasm and mitochondria that produce a superoxide anion radical. To protect cells from the deleterious effects of free radicals, a number of enzymatic and nonenzymatic defenses such as catalase, superoxide dismutase, glutathione peroxidase, ascorbic acid, and vitamin E are present in cells.

GENERATION OF OXYGEN-FREE RADICAL SPECIES DURING HYPOXIA IN THE FETUS

Studies from our laboratory provided evidence of increased levels of lipid peroxidation products in the cerebral cortex of fetal guinea pigs and newborn piglets following hypoxia, suggesting increased generation of oxygen-free radicals during hypoxia.[14,28,32] The hypoxia-induced increase in lipid peroxidation products was also associated with a decrease in cell membrane Na^+,K^+-ATPase activity.[31,38] Studies in newborn piglets showed that the hypoxia-induced increase in lipid peroxidation, which was associated with a decrease in Na^+,K^+-ATPase activity, was selective to synaptosomal membranes and was not seen in the myelin membranes.[38] Furthermore, the increase in membrane lipid peroxidation and the decrease in Na^+,K^+-ATPase activity during hypoxia were prevented by prior administration of alpha-tocopherol, suggesting the production of oxygen-free radicals during hypoxia.[42] These studies provided strong circumstantial evidence but did not directly demonstrate hypoxia-induced generation of free radicals. The direct demonstration of production of free radicals during hypoxia was documented by measuring the signal of spin adducts using electron spin resonance spectroscopy (ESR) which allows direct identification and characterization of free radicals.[28,29]

The effect of *in utero* hypoxia on free radical generation in the cerebral cortex of the guinea pig fetus was determined in fetuses obtained from six normoxic and six hypoxic pregnant Dunkin Hartley guinea pigs (60 days' gestation) purchased from Hilltop Research Animals, Scottdale, Pennsylvania. The study was approved by the Institutional Animal Care committee of the University of Pennsylvania. The mothers were exposed to either 21% or 7% oxygen for 60 minutes in a specially designed chamber fitted with a probe to monitor oxygen tension. After anesthesia (50 mg/kg), an incision was made in the lower abdomen, and fetuses were delivered and quickly decapitated. Within 4–10 seconds of decapitation, cortical tissue was placed in ice cold buffer containing alpha-phenyl-*N*-tert-butyl nitrone (PBN) for free radical measurements and in liquid nitrogen for biochemical analysis. PBN solution (100 mM) was prepared in deionized water and treated with activated charcoal until electron spin resonance spectroscopy signals from impurities were eliminated. The final concentration of PBN was determined using a molar extinction coefficient of 16,700 at 294 nm.

Free radical quantification and identification were performed using ESR spectroscopy according to the method of Sakamoto *et al.*[40] with toluene used as the organic solvent for extraction. For free radical quantification, cortical tissue was homogenized in a nitrogen-bubbled 2.5 ml, ice-cold, Krebs-Ringer's phosphate buffer solution (120 mM NaCl, 5 mM KCl, 1.3 mM $CaCl_2$, 1.3 mM $MgSO_4$, and 10 mM Na_2HPO_4) containing 100 mM PBN to trap oxygen-free radicals present in the tissue. The homogenate was mixed with 2 ml deoxygenated HPLC grade toluene and centrifuged at 7,000 *g* for 10 minutes at 0°C. 1.5 ml toluene phase was concentrated to 0.5 ml under nitrogen n and transferred to a 5-mm quartz capillary tube. The ESR measurements were performed at −20°C using a Varian E-4 spectrometer at the following settings: gain, 2×10^4; microwave power 20 mW, modulation amplitude 0.2 mT, time constant 3 seconds, scan range 10 mT, and scan time 8 minutes. Two scans were made and the signals were averaged. Spin adduct formation was calculated as follows: the peak to peak heights of the midfield doublet signals were added and regarded as the intensity of free radical generation. The signal intensity was divided by the dry weight of the tissue and expressed as signal height per gram of tissue. During hypoxia, there was a significant decrease in cerebral concentration of ATP from 3.24 μmol/g brain in the normoxic to 0.86 μmol/g brain in the hypoxic fetus, and phosphocreatine concentration decreased from 2.95 μmol/g brain in the normoxic to 0.56 μmol/g brain in the hypoxic fetus. The cerebral high energy phosphates data confirmed the cerebral tissue hypoxia.

Representative electron spin resonance spectra of the PBN adducts from the cortices of normoxic and hypoxic guinea pig fetuses are shown in FIGURE 1. Data from all animals on spin adduct formation as ESR signal intensity/g dry tissue weight was 33.8 ± 9.3 ($n = 13$) in normoxic fetuses as compared to 57.9 ± 9.26 in cortices of hypoxic fetuses. Thus, a 71% increase in spin adduct signal was observed in the hy-

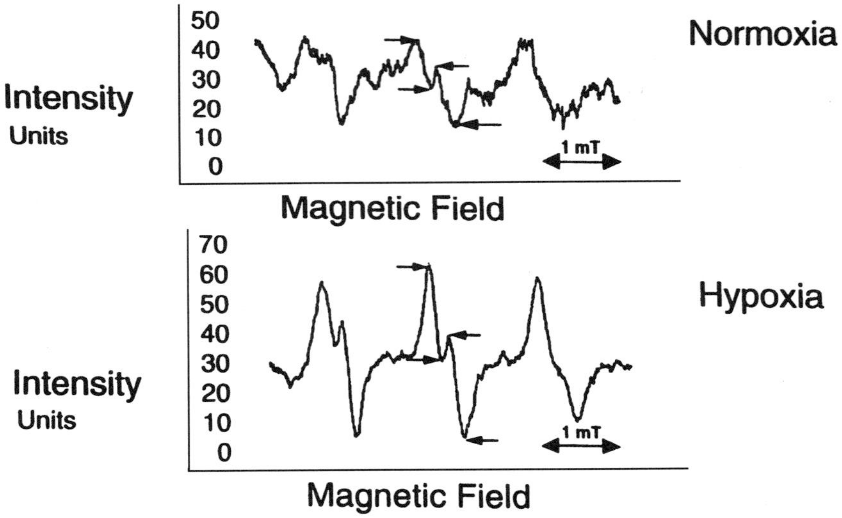

FIGURE 1. Electron spin resonance spectra of the PBN spin adducts from the fetal guinea pig brain cortices under normoxia (**A**) and hypoxia (**B**). Summation of the peak to peak amplitudes (as indicated by the *horizontal single arrows*) of the midfield doublet signals measures the free radical intensity. Note the increased free radical generation in the hypoxic fetal brain. The hyperfine splitting constants of the spectra are [α_N] of 13.9 G and [α_H] of 2.5 G.

poxic fetal cortices. The increase in free radical production during hypoxia was also associated with an increase in brain cell membrane lipid peroxidation products in the guinea pig fetus following hypoxia, as indicated by an increase in fluorescent compounds. The level of fluorescent compounds in the brain cell membranes of the hypoxic fetus increased from 0.639 ± 0.054 µg quinine sulfate/g brain in the normoxic fetus to 0.810 ± 0.102 µg quinine sulfate/g brain in the hypoxic fetus.

The ESR spectra from the cortical tissue were very similar to those of PBN-alkoxyl radical adducts. The hyperfine splitting constants [αN] for the PBN-alkoxyl radicals and cortical tissue specimen were almost identical, 14.1 G for the former and 13.9 G for the latter. The hyperfine splitting constants [αH] for the cortical tissue and PBN-alkoxyl radical adducts were 2.5 G and 4.2 G, respectively. Therefore the majority of spin adducts in the hypoxic fetal cortex appeared to be PBN-alkoxyl radicals.

FREE RADICAL GENERATION IN CEREBRAL CORTEX OF THE FETAL GUINEA PIG DURING GESTATION

Using the same strategy as just described, studies were conducted to examine free radical generation in the guinea pig fetal brain during maturation in preterm (40 days) and term (60 days) fetuses.[29] In addition, the effect of administration of Mg^{2+}, an *N*-methyl-D-aspartate (NMDA) receptor ion-channel blocker, prior to hypoxic exposure, on the hypoxia-induced free radical generation was also evaluated.[11] The Mg^{2+}-treated group received an initial bolus of $MgSO_4$ (600 mg/kg i.p.) 1 hour prior to hypoxia followed by a second dose (300 mg/kg i.p.). The results show that in a control group of term fetuses, cortical tissue from the hypoxic fetuses showed a significant increase (71% increase, $p < 0.01$) in phenyl-*N*-tert-butylnitrone (PBN) spin adducts. In the preterm group, cortical tissue from the hypoxic fetuses showed a 33% increase ($p < 0.001$) in PBN spin adducts. Baseline free radical generation during normoxia was 22.5% higher in preterm as compared to term (41.4 ± 3.5 units/g tissue vs 33.8 ± 9.3 units/g tissue, $p < 0.05$). In the Mg^{2+}-treated groups, spin adduct levels in cortical tissue from hypoxic fetuses did not significantly differ from those of the normoxic group (30.2 ± 9.9 units/g tissue, normoxic-Mg^{2+} vs 30.6 ± 8.1 units/tissue, hypoxic-Mg^{2+}). The studies indicate that the fetal brain may be more susceptible to hypoxia-induced free radical damage at term than at preterm and that Mg^{2+} administration significantly decreased the hypoxia-induced increase in oxygen-free radical generation in the term fetal guinea pig brain in comparison with the nontreated hypoxic group.

FREE RADICAL GENERATION IN CEREBRAL CORTEX OF NEWBORN PIGLETS

Studies from our laboratory demonstrated an increased peroxidation of brain cell membrane lipids during hypoxia in the newborn.[14,38,42] We examined the effect of hypoxia on the generation of free radicals, the identification of predominant free radical species, and the contribution of specific free radical-generation pathways such as cyclooxygenase,[2] xanthine oxidase,[1] and nitric oxide synthase.[34]

The production of free radicals during hypoxia was documented by measuring the signal of spin adducts with electron spin resonance spectroscopy. Newborn piglets of 3 to 5 days were assigned to either normoxia (PaO_2 80 to 120 mm Hg) or hypoxia (PaO_2 <20 mm Hg) for 1 hour. Cortical samples were obtained by biopsy from anesthetized, ventilated piglets. Cerebral tissue hypoxia was documented by a decrease in ATP and phosphocreatine. Cortex was homogenized in the presence of a spin trapping agent, *N*-tert-phenyl-butyl-nitrone. Lipids were extracted, and free radical formation was detected by acquiring the electron spin resonance spectra with a Varian-E-109 spectrometer. Signal height was measured and divided by the dry tissue weight. Whereas the hypoxic cortex showed a significantly higher ESR signal of 789 ± 82 mm/g tissue compared with a mean reference value of 265 ± 50 ($p < 0.001$), the normoxic cortex signal of 458 ± 84 mm/g tissue was not different from its corresponding mean reference value of 407 ± 55. The data provided direct evidence of increased free radical generation during hypoxia in the newborn model. On the basis of the characteristics of the spin adduct signal (hyperfine splitting constants; $\alpha N = 13.8$ G and $\alpha H = 2.2$ G), the free radical species present in the hypoxic tissue was identified to be an alkoxyl radical. Administration of allopurinol (20 mg/kg IV) reduced the hypoxia-induced increase in free radical generation by 59% in the cerebral cortex of newborn piglets. Studies investigating the role of nitric oxide synthase in free radical generation during hypoxia with a modified procedure for extraction and ESR analyses showed a significant decrease in free radical generation in the cerebral cortex of *N*-nitro-L-arginine-treated piglets.

These studies demonstrate increased free radical generation during hypoxia in the cerebral cortex of the fetus and the newborn, and intervening with the inhibitors of pathways of free radical generation reduced the hypoxia-induced production of free radical species. Alkoxyl radical appears to be the predominant free radical species identified during hypoxia, indicating that free radical-mediated lipid peroxidation is an ongoing event during cerebral hypoxia, a mechanism of hypoxic neuronal injury.

MECHANISMS OF FREE RADICAL GENERATION DURING HYPOXIA

There are a number of potential mechanisms of free radical generation under hypoxic conditions. During hypoxia, the increased accumulation of intracellular Ca^{2+} due to excessive activation of NMDA[45] and non-NMDA receptors is crucial in hypoxia-induced excitotoxicity. Increased intracellular Ca^{2+} can initiate a number of biochemical events that could lead to free radical generation and cell death such as: (1) activation of phospholipase A_2, leading to increased generation of oxygen-free radicals from cyclooxygenase and lipoxygenase pathways; (2) activation of nitric oxide synthase, leading to peroxynitrite formation and generation of free radicals; (3) activation of proteases, leading to conversion of xanthine dehydrogenase to xanthine oxidase and resulting in increased free radical generation; (4) activation of phospholipase C, leading to IP_3 formation and resulting in the release of Ca^{2+} from intracellular stores; and (5) free radical generation further triggering the release of additional excitatory amino acids neurotransmitters as well as influencing the activation of the NMDA receptor ion-channel activity through the redox site.

In addition to Ca^{+2} mediation, there are other potential mechanisms of free radical generation during hypoxia such as: (1) reduction of electron transport chain components including ubiquinone (a component that undergoes autooxidation to produce free radicals); (2) increased release of ferritin under the conditions of decreased cellular high energy compounds; and (3) increased degradation of ATP during hypoxia, increasing the substrate for the xanthine oxidase reaction and leading to increased free radical generation.

An increase in intracellular Ca^{2+} is considered to be a critical event in hypoxic-ischemic neuronal excitotoxicity. It appears that Ca^{2+}-dependent neuronal damage is an NMDA receptor-mediated excitotoxicity that is initiated as a result of hypoxia. During hypoxia, an increase in intracellular Ca^{2+} following the initial influx via the NMDA receptor ion channel may be a result of additional mechanisms, including the release of Ca^{2+} from intracellular stores such as endoplasmic reticulum and mitochondria. Studies suggest that mitochondria might be an important contributor of Ca^{2+}. The initial increase in intracellular Ca^{2+} leading to activation of phospholipases may increase the concentration of free fatty acids and inositol triphosphates. The increase in fatty acids is known to impair mitochondrial function. Because proton-motive force generated in mitochondria is necessary for Ca^{2+} uptake, a lack of such force impairs the Ca^{2+} buffering capacity of mitochondria during hypoxic conditions.

NITRIC OXIDE FREE RADICALS AND NEURONAL INJURY

The role of nitric oxide (NO) in neuronal injury, both *in vitro* and *in vivo*, has been controversial.[10,11] This controversy may be due to the use of nonspecific nitric oxide synthase (NOS) inhibitors. Three major isoforms of NOS have been identified: constitutive neuronal, constitutive endothelial, and inducible macrophage isoforms. Following ischemia, NO produced from neuronal NOS has toxic effects, but NO produced from endothelial NOS has protective effects in the brain.[23]

Hypoxic brain injury is associated with the formation of NO, a gaseous free radical.[4,9] Although under normal conditions NO physiologically mediates cerebral vasodilatation,[15] recent studies suggest that NO may react with superoxide anion to form peroxynitrite and cause neurotoxicity.[5,12,22] Furthermore, N^w-nitro-L-arginine (NNLA) administration in a middle cerebral artery occlusion model reduced the volume of cortical infarct in the mouse, indicating the role of NO in neurotoxicity.[33]

One effect of cerebral hypoxia is to cause an increase in extracellular glutamate and aspartate.[6,20] These excitatory amino acids can activate the *N*-methyl-D-aspartate (NMDA) receptor, which results in an increase in the level of intracellular calcium.[17,26] In the endothelium and neurons, calcium initiates the production of NO through the stimulation of NOS.[7,19] In addition, stimulation of non-NMDA glutamate receptors also generates NO.

Phospholipase A_2 activation, mediated via NMDA receptor stimulation, produces superoxide anion within the neuron.[25] Thus, cerebral hypoxia may increase the production of superoxide anion and NO, which together may react to form peroxynitrite.

Peroxynitrite has been shown to induce lipid preoxidation *in vitro* and is thought to be a mediator of direct cell damage.[25] Proxynitrite can diffuse for several micrometers before decomposing to produce two powerful cytotoxic oxidants, hydroxyl radical and nitrogen dioxide.[4,5] NOS inhibition appears to be neuroprotective, indicating the role of NO in ischemic neuronal damage.[8,22,35]

Nitric oxide (NO) is reported to cause neuronal damage through various mechanisms. We tested the hypothesis that NO synthase inhibition by N^w-nitro-L-arginine (NNLA) will result in decreased oxygen-derived free radical production, leading to the preservation of cell membrane structure and function during cerebral hypoxia.[34] Ten newborn piglets were pretreated with NNLA (40 mg/kg); five were subjected to hypoxia, whereas the other five were maintained with normoxia. An additional 10 piglets without NNLA treatment underwent the same conditions. Hypoxia was induced with a lowered FiO_2 and documented biochemically by decreased cerebral ATP and phosphocreatine levels. Free radicals were detected by using electron spin resonance spectroscopy with a spin trapping technique. Results demonstrated that free radicals, corresponding to alkoxyl radicals, were induced by hypoxia but were inhibited by pretreatment with NNLA before inducing hypoxia. NNLA also inhibited hypoxia-induced generation of conjugated dienes, products of lipid peroxidation. Na^+, K^+-ATPase activity, an index of cellular membrane function, decreased following hypoxia but was preserved by pretreatment with NNLA. This data demonstrated that during hypoxia NOS generates free radicals via peroxynitrite production, presumably causing lipid peroxidation and membrane dysfunction. These results suggested that NO is a potentially limiting factor in the peroxynitrite-mediated lipid peroxidation resulting in membrane injury.

The appearance of primary free radicals, such as superoxide anion or hydroxyl radical, may not indicate oxidative injury. The reactivity of superoxide radicals is limited,[3,41] but hydroxyl radicals are highly reactive to almost all molecules[21] so that they can target even noncritical molecules. Therefore, their concentration does not necessarily correlate with the degree of oxidative damage, particularly when assessing lipid peroxidation. Furthermore, these radicals damage cells in cooperation with other radical species or oxidants.[4,5] In contrast, the production of secondarily formed lipid free radicals provides strong evidence of peroxidative injury. This is particularly true for alkoxyl radicals, which are generated from lipid peroxide by either iron or copper ions and can abstract hydrogen atoms from polyunsaturated fatty acids, leading to further lipid peroxidation.[21] Our results suggested that NO has an *in vivo* role in the generation of alkoxyl radicals, leading to free radical-mediated lipid peroxidation.

The exact molecular mechanism of hypoxic membrane damage is not clear. An appealing hypothesis is that when peroxynitrite (formed by the reaction between superoxide anions and NO) is protonated, it decomposes rapidly to form nitrogen dioxide and hydroxyl radicals, both of which are strong oxidants and can initiate oxidative reactions.[4,5,36] It has been shown that peroxynitrite can cause lipid peroxidation *in vitro*.[36] Therefore, it appears that the hypoxia-induced high concentration of NO may result in an increased production of peroxynitrite, causing lipid peroxidation.

In summary, studies demonstrated that cerebral tissue hypoxia results in increased free radical generation that may lead to the oxidation of brain cell membrane lipids, membrane enzymes, receptor proteins, as well as the nuclear DNA precipitating the hypoxic neuronal injury in the fetus and newborn.

REFERENCES

1. Andersen, C.B., P.J. Marro, T. Ohnishi, A. Zhu & M. Delivoria-Papadopoulos. 1996. Effect of allipurinol on free radical formation during cerebral hypoxia in newborn piglets. Pediatr. Res. **39:** 43A.
2. Andersen, C.B., T. Ohnishi, J.E. McGowan, O.P. Mishra & M. Delivoria-Papadopoulos. 1995. Effect of indomethacin (INDO) on free radical formation during hypoxia. Pediatr. Res. **37:** 42A.
3. Baum, R.M. 1984. Superoxide theory of oxygen toxicity is center of heated debate. Chem. Eng. News **9:** 20–28.
4. Beckman, J.S. 1991. The double-edged role of nitric oxide in brain function and superoxide-mediated injury. J. Dev. Physiol. **15:** 53–59.
5. Beckman, J.S., T.W. Beckman, J. Chen, P.A. Marshall & B.A. Freeman. 1990. Apparent hydroxyl radical production by peroxynitrite: implications for endothelial injury from nitric oxide and superoxide. Proc. Natl. Acad. Sci. USA **87:** 1620–1624.
6. Benveniste, H., J. Drejer, A. Schousboe & N.H. Diemer. 1984. Elevation of the extracellular concentrations of glutamate and aspartate in rat hippcampus during transient cerebral ischemia monitored by intracerebral microdialysis. J. Neurochem. **43:** 1369–1374.
7. Bredt, D.S. & S.H. Snyder. 1989. Nitric oxide mediates glutamate-linked enhancement of cGMP levels in the cerebellum. Proc. Natl. Acad. Sci. USA **86:** 9030–9033.
8. Buisson, A., M. Plotkine & R.G. Boulu. 1992. The neuroprotective effect of a nitric oxide inhibitor in a rat model of focal cerebral ischaemia. Br. J. Pharmacol. **106:** 766–767.
9. Cazevielle, C., A. Muller, F. Meynier & C. Bonne. 1993. Superoxide and nitric oxide cooperation in hypoxia/reoxygenation-induced neuron injury. Free Radic. Biol. Med. **14:** 389–395.
10. Dawson, D.A. 1994. Nitric oxide and focal cerebral ischemia: multiplicity of actions and diverse outcome. Cerebrovasc. Brain Metab. **64:** 299–324.

11. DAWSON, T.M. & S.H. SNYDER. 1994. Gases as biological messengers: nitrix oxide and carbon monoxide in the brain. J. Neurosci. **14:** 5147–5159.
12. DAWSON, V.L., T.M. DAWSON, E.D. LONDON, D.S. BREDT & S.H. SNYDER. 1991. Nitric oxide mediates glutamate neurotoxicity in primary cortical cultures. Proc. Natl. Acad. Sci. USA **88:** 6368-6371.
13. DELIVORIA-PAPADOPOULOS, M. & O.P. MISHRA. 1998. Mechanisms of cerebral injury in perinatal asphyxia and strategies for prevention. J. Pediatr. **132:** S30–S34.
14. DIGIACOMO, J.E., C.R. PANE, S. GWIAZDOWSKI, O.P. MISHRA & M. DELIVORIA-PAPADOPOULOS. 1992. Effect of graded hypoxia on brain cell membrane injury in newborn piglets. Biol. Neonate. **61:** 25–32.
15. FARACI, F.M. 1991. Role of endothelium-derived relaxing factor in cerebral circulation: large arteries vs. microcirculation. Am J. Physiol. **261:** H1038–1042.
16. FERRER, I. 1996. Cell death in the normal developing brain, and following ionizing radiation, methylazoxy methanol acetate, and hypoxic-ischemia in the rat. Neuropathol. Appl. Neurobiol. **22:** 489–492.
17. FRANDSEN, A. & A. SCHOUSBOE. 1993. Excitatory amino acid-mediated cytotoxicity and calcium homeostasis in cultured neurons. J. Neurochem. **60:** 1202–1211.
18. FRITZ, K.I., F. GROENEDAAL, J.E. MCGOWAN, O.P. MISHRA & M. DELIVORIA-PAPADOPOULOS. 1996. Effect of cerebral hypoxia on NMDA receptor binding characteristics after treatment with 3-(2-carboxypiperizin-4-yl)propyl-1-phosphonic acid (CPP) in newborn piglets. Brain Res. **729:** 16–74.
19. GARTHWAITE, J. G. GARTHWAITE, R.M. PALMER & S. MONCADE. 1989. NMDA receptor activation induces nitric oxide syntesis from arginine in rat brain slices. Eur. J. Pharmacol. **172:** 413–416.
20. GLOBUS, M.Y.T., R. BUSTO, W.B. DIETRICH, E. MARTINEZ, I. VALDES & M.D. GINSBERG. 1988. Effect of ischemia on the *in vivo* release of striatal dopamine, glutamate, and y-aminobutryic acid studied by intracerebral microdialysis. J. Neurochem. **51:** 1455–1464.
21. HALLIWELL, B. 1992. Reactive oxygen species and the central nervous system. J. Neurochem. **59:** 1609–1623.
22. HAMADA, Y., T. HAYAKAWA, H. HATTORI & H. MIKAWA. 1994. Inhibitors of nitric oxide synthesis reduce hypoxic-ischemic brain damage in the neonatal rat. Pediatr. Res. **35:** 10–14.
23. HUANG, Z., P.L. HUANG, N. PANAHIAN, T. DALKARA, M.C. FISHMAN & M.A. MOSKOWITZ. 1994. Effects of cerebral ischemia in mice deficient in neuronal nitric oxide. Science **265:** 1883–1885.
24. JOHNSTON, M.V. 1995. Neurotransmitters and vulnerability of the developing brain. Brain Dev. **17:** 301–306.
25. LAFON, C.M., S. PIETRI, M. CULCASI & J. BOCKAERT. 1993. NMDA-dependent superoxide production and neurotoxicity. Nature **364:** 535–537.
26. LIPTON, S.A. & P.A. ROSENBERG. 1994. Excitatory amino acids as a final common pathway for neurological disorders. N. Engl. J. Med. **330:** 613–622.
27. LONGO, L.D. & S. PACKINTHAN. 1997. Hypoxia-ischemia and the developing brain: hypotheses regarding the pathophysiology of fetal-neonatal brain damage. Br. J. Obstet. Gynaecol. **104:** 653–662.
28. MAULIK, D., Y. NUMAGAMI, T. OHNISHI, O.P. MISHRA & M. DELIVORIA PAPADOPOULOS. 1998. Direct detection of oxygen free radical generation during in-utero hypoxia in the fetal guinea pig. Brain Res. **798:** 166–172.
29. MAULIK, D., S.A. ZANELLI, Y. NUMAGAMI, T. OHNISHI, O.P. MISHRA & M. DELIVORIA-PAPADOPOULOS. 1999. Oxygen free radical generation during in-utero hypoxia in the fetal guinea pig brain: the effects of maturity and of magnesium sulfate administration. Brain Res. **817:** 117–122.
30. MISHRA, O.P. & M. DELIVORIA-PAPADOPOULOS. 1999. Cellular mechanisms of hypoxic brain injury in the developing brain. Brain Res. Bull. **48:** 233–238.
31. MISHRA, O.P. & M. DELIVORIA-PAPADOPOULOS. 1988. Na^+, K^+-ATPase in developing fetal guinea pig brain and the effect of maternal hypoxia. Neurochem. Res. **17:** 1223–1228.
32. MISHRA, O.P. & M. DELIVORIA-PAPADOPOULOS. 1989. Lipid peroxidation in developing fetal guinea pig brain during normoxia and hypoxia. Dev. Brain Res. **45:** 129–135.

33. NOWICKI, J.P., D. DUVAL, H. POIGNET & B. SCATTON. 1991. Nitric oxide mediates neuronal death after focal cerebral ischemia in the mouse. Eur. J. Pharmacol. **204:** 339–340.
34. NUMAGAMI, Y., A.B. ZUBROW, O.P. MISHRA & M. DELIVORIA-PAPADOPOULOS. 1997. Lipid free radical generation and brain cell membrane alteration following nitric oxide synthase inhibition during cerebral hypoxia in the newborn piglet. J. Neurochem. **69:** 1542–1547.
35. QUAST, M.J., J. WEI & N.C. HUANG. 1995. Nitric oxide synthase inhibitor NG-nitro-L-arginine methyl ester decreases ischemic damage in reversible focal cerebral ischemia in hyperglycemic rats. Brain Res. **677:** 204–212.
36. RADI, R., J.S. BECKMAN, L.M. BUSH & B.A. FREEMAN. 1991. Peroxynitrite-induced membrane lipid peroxidation: the cytotoxic potential of superoxide and nitric oxide. Arch. Biochem. Biophys. **288:** 481–487.
37. RAICHLE, M.E. 1983. The pathophysiology of brain ischemia. Ann. Neurol. **13:** 2–10.
38. RAZDAN, B., P.J. MARRO, O. TAMMELA, R. GOEL, O.P. MISHRA & M. DELIVORIA-PAPADOPOULOS. 1994. Selective sensitivity of synaptosomal membrane function to cerebral cortical hypoxia in newborn piglet. Brain Res. **600:** 308–314.
39. ROSENKRANTZ, T.S., J. KUBIN, O.P. MISHRA, D. SMITH & M. DELIVORIA-PAPADOPOULOS. 1996. Brain cell membrane Na^+, K^+-ATPase activity following severe hypoxic injury in the newborn piglet. Brain Res. **730:** 52–57.
40. SAKAMOTO, A., S.T. OHNISHI, T. OHNISHI & R. OGAWA. 1991. Relationship between free radical production and lipid peroxidation during ischemia-reperfusion injury in the rat brain. Brain Res. **554:** 186–192.
41. SAWYER, D.T. & J.S. VALENTINE. 1981. How super is superoxide? Accounts Chem. Res. **14:** 393–400.
42. SHIN, S.M., B. RAZDAN, O.P. MISHRA, L. JOHNSON & M. DELIVORIA PAPADOPOULOS. 1994. Protective effect of α-tocopherol on brain cell membrane function during cerebral cortical hypoxia in newborn piglets. Brain Res. **553:** 45–50.
43. VANNUCCI, R.C. 1990. Experimental biology of cerebral hypoxia-ischemia: relation to perinatal brain damage. Pediatr. Res. **27:** 317–326.
44. VOLPE, J.J. 1995. Neurology of the Newborn, 3rd Ed. WB Saunders. Philadelphia.
45. ZANELLI, S.A., Y. NUMAGAMI, J.E. MCGOWAN, O.P. MISHRA & M. DELIVORIA-PAPADOPOULOS. 1999. NMDA receptor-mediated calcium influx in cerebral cortical synaptosomes of the hypoxic guinea pig fetus. Neurochem. Res. **24:** 437–446.

Angiogenic Factors in the Perinatal Period: Diversity in Biological Functions Reflected in Their Serum Concentrations Soon after Birth

ARIADNE MALAMITSI-PUCHNER,[a] JOHN TZIOTIS, EFTHIMIA PROTONOTARIOU, ANGELIKI SARANDAKOU, AND GEORGE CREATSAS

Second Department of Obstetrics and Gynecology, University of Athens, Athens 11528, Greece

ABSTRACT: These studies investigated whether serum levels of the angiogenic factors angiogenin, basic fibroblast growth factor (bFGF), and vascular endothelial growth factor (VEGF) change soon after birth due to the elimination of the placenta and to diminished angiogenic but increased adaptational demands in extrauterine life. Also investigated was whether serum levels correlate with sex, birth weight, or mode of delivery. Serum from healthy mothers and their healthy full-term infants at birth (umbilical cord, UC), day 1 (N1) and day 4 (N4) postpartum was analyzed by enzyme immunoassays. Angiogenin levels were higher in maternal serum and rose significantly from UC to N1 and N4, possibly because of the elimination of the placenta, which produces an angiogenin inhibitor. bFGF and VEGF maternal levels were lower than fetal and neonatal ones. Although neonatal bFGF levels did not differ from fetal levels, possibly reflecting diminished angiogenesis *ex utero*, VEGF levels increased in neonatal serum, possibly signifying adaptational demands. Neither factor depended on sex, mode of delivery, or birth weight. Thus, significant differences from normal reference values of the studied factors might reflect ill-defined situations of the placenta and fetus/newborn serving as early diagnostic markers.

Angiogenesis is the formation of new blood vessels from preexisting ones.[1] It is now known that the sprouting of new capillaries, taking place in angiogenesis, presupposes the secretion by various cells of soluble angiogenic factors. The latter, in general, have the ability to degrade the basement membrane of the capillary wall and to cause proliferation and migration of endothelial cells into the extracellular matrix after its proteolysis, as well as to form tubular structures—the new capillary sprout.[2] Angiogenesis predominantly occurs in fetal life and mainly in the third trimester,[3] as it is a prerequisite for rapid tissue growth and development.[4] The main source of angiogenic factors *in utero* derives from the placenta.[5] Nevertheless, this same organ also produces inhibitors of angiogenesis.[6,7]

The studies reported,[8,9] approved by the ethics committee of our teaching hospital, were based on the hypothesis that birth might signal a change in the serum con-

[a]Address for correspondence: A. Malamitsi-Puchner, M.D., 2nd Department of Obstetrics and Gynecology, University of Athens, Soultani 19, GR-100682 Athens, Greece. Phone: +30 1 3303110, +30 1 7286353; fax: +30 1 7233330.

centrations of the various angiogenic factors in the fetus/newborn for the following reasons: (a) the placenta is eliminated; (b) angiogenic demands are deminished in extrauterine life as compared to the large-scale angiogenesis occuring *in utero*[10]; (c) adaptation and stabilization in the independent extrauterine life is indispensable, and thus regulatory factors assuring the good function of various tissues and organs should be present. Some angiogenic factors were found to have such properties.[11]

The aim of these studies was to investigate serum levels of three main angiogenic factors in the perinatal period and to establish normal reference values. It is assumed that abnormal levels of these factors soon after birth might reflect ill-defined situations of the placenta and fetus/newborn, thus serving as early diagnostic markers.

METHODS

Subjects

Thirty healthy, appropriate for gestational age, full-term infants born from 30 healthy, nonsmoking mothers with uncomplicated single pregnancies were included in each study after obtaining informed concent from their parents. In the first study 13 were boys and 17 were girls, while in the second study 16 were boys and 14 girls. Mean (± SD) birth weight was 3376 ± 334 g (range 2800–4000) and 3265 ± 337 g (range 2530–3950), respectively. Mean gestational age was 39.5 ± 1.5 weeks and 38.8 ± 1.1 weeks, respectively. In the first study 17 infants were born by vaginal delivery (VD) and 13 by cesarean section (CS) because of a previous CS, whereas in the second study 20 were born by VD and 10 by CS. Apgar scores of all studied infants were ≥8 1 and 5 minutes after birth, and placentas were in all cases normal in appearance and weight.

Procedure

One milliliter of blood was drawn from a peripheral vein of all 30 infants in each study on day 1 and 4 of life. In 10 cases of each study blood was also drawn from the mother before delivery as well as from the umbilical cord at delivery. Blood was collected in pyrogen-free tubes, and serum was immediately separated by centrifugation after clotting and was kept frozen at –20°C until assayed. The analysis was performed by enzyme immunoassays, using commercially available kits (angiogenin human ELISA system RPN 2161, Amersham International plc, human basic fibroblast growth factor (bFGF) Quantikine™ HS, and human vascular endothelial growth factor (VEGF) Quantikine, R&D Systems Minneapolis, MN 55413). The minimum detectable concentrations and intra- and interassay coefficients were, respectively, for angiogenin, 0.6 μg/l, 2.8%, and 9.0%; for bFGF, 0.5 pg/ml, 7.2% and 8.1%; and for VEGF, 9.0 pg/ml, 4.8%, and 6.6%.

Data Analysis

Data on angiogenin serum concentrations showed a normal distribution (Kolmogorov-Smirnov test); therefore, parametric methods, *t*-test, and paired *t*-test were used, and Pearson's correlation coefficients were calculated. On the other hand, data on the other two angiogenic factors did not demonstrate normal distributions; there-

TABLE 1. Serum levels of the angiogenic factors angiogenin (μg/l, mean ± SD), bFGF (pg/ml, median; range), and VEGF (pg/ml, median; range) in the mothers, the umbilical cords, and the neonates on the first and fourth day of life

Serum source	Angiogenin	bFGF	VEGF
MS	226 ± 50	1.6 (0.5 – 4.8)	<9
UC	119 ± 34	6.9 (0.5 – 61.7)	127 (15 – 735)
N1	166 ± 45	10.4 (1.2 – 21.6)	366 (18 – 1346)
N4	241 ± 53	7.1 (0.5 – 53.6)	442 (19 – 1070)

NOTE: MS, mothers (n = 10); UC, umbilical cords (n = 10); N1, first day of life (n = 30); N4, fourth day of life (n = 30); bFGF, basic fibroblast growth factor; VEGF, vascular endothelial growth factor.

fore, nonparametric tests—Wilcoxon, Mann-Whitney U-test—were used, and Spearman's correlation coefficients were calculated.

RESULTS

Serum levels of all three angiogenic factors are presented in TABLE 1. In the first study, a statistically significant difference existed between maternal serum (MS) and umblilical cord serum (UC) ($p < 0.0002$) as well as between MS and neonatal day 1 (N1) serum ($p < 0.01$). Nevertheless, no difference existed between MS and neonatal day 4 serum (N4). On the other hand, UC showed a statistically highly significant difference from N1 ($p < 0.0002$) and N4 ($p < 0.0003$), as well as N1 from N4 ($p < 10^{-7}$). A statistically significant correlation was found between angiogenin serum concentrations in UC and N1 ($r = 0.84$, $n = 10$, $p < 0.002$) as well as between those in N1 and N4 ($r = 0.37$, $n = 30$, $p < 0.04$). No statistically significant difference was found in the UC, N1, and N4 samples between boys and girls as well as between infants born by VD and CS. Lastly, no serum concentration of angiogenin correlated with birth weight.

In the second study in all MS samples VEGF levels were below the lower limit of detection. bFGF and VEGF serum levels were statistically significantly lower in MS than in UC ($p = 0.02$ and 0.006, respectively), N1 ($p = 0.009$ and 0.006, respectively), and N4 ($p = 0.009$ and 0.006, respectively). Levels of bFGF in UC did not differ significantly from those in N1 and N4. In contrast, levels of VEGF in UC differed significantly from those in N1 ($p = 0.008$) and N4 ($p = 0.006$). Both factors did not change from N1 to N4. Furthermore, no statistically significant difference in the serum levels of bFGF and VEGF was found between boys and girls as well as between infants born by VD and CS. Also, no correlations existed between matched MS, UC, N1, and N4 serum samples of either bFGF or VEGF. Additionaly, serum samples of bFGF in MS, UC, N1, and N4 did not correlate with respective samples of VEGF. Finally, neither bFGF nor VEGF serum levels in UV, N1, and N4 correlated with birth weight.

DISCUSSION

The results of these studies indicate that serum levels of the three studied angiogenic factors are differently expressed in the perinatal period. Thus, angiogenin levels are higher in maternal serum than umbilical cord serum, as well as in neonatal day 1 serum, but they do not differ from neonatal day 4 serum levels, indicating a suppression of angiogenin in fetal life, probably through placental ribonuclease inhibitor (PRI).[7] As soon as the placenta is eliminated, angiogenin levels rise significantly even in N1 serum samples, not differing from MS levels in N4 samples. In contrast, bFGF and VEGF present lower levels in MS than in UC, because the placenta is the main source of angiogenic factors[5] and no placental inhibitor of the action of both factors has been documented. bFGF serum levels do not change significantly soon after birth, possibly because large-scale angiogenesis has slowed down at the end of a term pregnancy[5] and angiogenic demands in extrauterine life are considerably restricted[10] in comparison to intrauterine needs. On the other hand, N1 VEGF levels seem to increase in relation to UC levels. This finding could be attributed to the adaptation demands of extrauterine life for tissues expressing VEGF mRNA, such as epithelial cells of lung alveoli and cardiac myocytes,[12] as well as to the role of VEGF in these tissues in regulating microvascular permeability or maintaining the differentiated state of microvessels that otherwise might undergo involution, since VEGF is primarily considered a regulator of normal function.[13]

Perinatal stress, reflected in the mode of delivery, sex and birth weight do not influence serum levels of all angiogenic factors studied. In the case of angiogenin, this could be attributed to the existence of placental ribonuclease inhibitor (PRI), which inhibits all actions of angiogenin.[7] As for VEGF, which is known to be upregulated by hypoxia,[11] its increased serum levels in N1 samples could be partly due to a subclinical, delivery-induced hypoxia that is not evident from rough clinical scores, such as the Apgar score, but is known to accompany every delivery.

In conclusion, serum angiogenin levels increase soon after birth reaching maternal levels by day 4 of life. In contrast, bFGF and VEGF serum levels are significantly higher in the fetus and neonate than in the mother. Nevertheless, bFGF levels do not change significantly between fetal and early neonatal life, since large-scale angiogenesis has slowed down at term *in utero*, a finding that does not apply to VEGF, which, in addition to being angiogenic, is also a factor regulating normal function.

Thus, significant deviations in the serum levels of the above angiogenic factors from those determined in these studies might imply placental or neonatal abnormalities, allowing these factors to serve as diagnostic markers in pathological situations.

REFERENCES

1. Folkman, J. & M. Klagsbrun. 1987. Angiogenic factors. Science **235:** 442–447.
2. Gordon, J.D., J.L. Shifren, R.A. Foulk, *et al.* 1995. Angiogenesis in the human female reproductive tract. Obstet. Gynecol. Surv. **50:** 688–697.
3. Beck, L. Jr. & P.A. D'Amore. 1997. Vascular development: cellular and molecular regulation. FASEB J. **11:** 365–373.
4. Jackson, J.R., M.P. Seed, C.H. Kircher, *et al.* 1997. The codependence of angiogenesis and chronic inflammation. FASEB J. **11:** 457–465.

5. SHARKEY, A.M., D.S. CHARNOCK-JONES, C.A. BOOCOCK, *et al.* 1993. Expression of mRNA for vascular endothelial growth factor in human placenta. J. Reprod. Fertil. **99:** 609–615.
6. JACKSON, D., O.V. VOLPERT, N. BOUCK *et al.* 1994. Stimulation and inhibition of angiogenesis by placental proliferin and proliferin-related protein. Science **266:** 1581–1584.
7. SHAPIRO, R. & B.L. VALLEE. 1987. Human placental ribonuclease inhibitor abolishes both angiogenic and ribonucleolytic activities of angiogenin. Proc. Natl. Acad. Sci. USA **84:** 2238–2241.
8. MALAMITSI-PUCHNER, A., A. SARANDAKOU, G. GIANNAKI, *et al.* 1997. Changes of angiogenin serum concentrations in the perinatal period. Pediatr. Res. **41:** 909–911.
9. MALAMITSI-PUCHNER, A., J. TZIOTIS, E. PROTONOTARIOU, *et al.* 1999. Heparin-binding angiogenic factors (basic fibroblast growth factor and vascular endothelial growth factor) in early neonatal life. Pediatr. Res. **45:** 877–880.
10. SHALABY, F., J. ROSSANT, T.P. YAMAGUCHI, *et al.* 1995. Failure of blood-island formation and vasculogenesis in FLK-1-deficient mice. Nature **376**(6535)**:** 62–66.
11. FERRARA, N., K. HOUCK, L. JAKEMAN & D.W. LEUNG. 1992. Molecular and biological properties of the vascular endothelial growth factor family of proteins. Endocrinol. Rev. **13:** 18–32.
12. BERSE, B., L.F. BROWN, L. VAN DE WATER, *et al.* 1992. Vascular permeability factor (vascular endothelial growth factor) gene is expressed differentially in normal tissues, macrophages and tumors. Mol. Biol. Cell **3**(2): 211–220.
13. FERRARA, N. & B. KEYT. 1997. Vascular endothelial growth factor: basic biology and clinical implications. EXS **79:** 209–232.

Role of Leptin in Reproduction

CHRISTOS S. MANTZOROS[a]

Division of Endocrinology, Department of Internal Medicine, Beth Israel Deaconess Medical Center, Harvard Medical School, Boston, Massachusetts 02215, USA

ABSTRACT: Leptin is a 16-kDa adipocyte-secreted protein the serum levels of which reflect mainly the amount of energy stores but are also influenced by short-term energy imbalance as well as several cytokines and hormones. Leptin, by binding to specific receptors, alters the expression of several hypothalamic neuropeptides that regulate neuroendocrine function as well as energy intake and expenditure. More specifically, accumulating evidence suggests that this hormone may serve to signal to the brain information on the critical amount of fat stores that are necessary for LHRH secretion and activation of the hypothalamic-pituitary-gonadal axis. Rising leptin levels have been associated with initiation of puberty in animals and humans and normal leptin levels are needed for maintenance of menstrual cycles and normal reproductive function. Moreover, circadian and ultradian variations of leptin levels are associated with minute to minute variations of LH and estradiol in normal women. Falling leptin levels in response to starvation result in decreased estradiol levels and amenorrhea in subjects with anorexia nervosa or strenuously exercising athletes. In addition, leptin has a potentially important role during pregnancy and in the physiology of the neonate. Finally, recent evidence suggests that leptin may influence ovarian steroidogenesis directly, but the exact role of intra-ovarian leptin action in the physiology and pathophysiology of the human reproductive system needs to be further elucidated.

INTRODUCTION

The discovery of leptin 6 years ago has broadened significantly our understanding of body weight and energy balance regulation.[1] Over the last 6 years more than 1,400 papers have been published on leptin, leading to an ever advancing body of knowledge. Thus, although leptin was originally considered to be an "antiobesity hormone," the role of leptin is currently viewed as much broader and includes regulation of multiple hypothalamic-pituitary axes.[2] This paper focuses primarily on our current understanding of the role leptin plays in reproductive physiology and pathophysiology and is divided into three parts. The first part deals with the reproductive alterations associated with food deprivation and obesity, the second part with leptin biology and physiology, and the third part with the effect of leptin in reproductive function.

[a]Address for correspondence: C.S. Mantzoros, MD, DSc, Division of Endocrinology, RN 325, Beth Israel Deaconess Medical Center, 330 Brookline Avenue, Boston, MA 02215, USA. Phone: 617-667-2151; fax: 617-667-2927.

cmantzor@caregroup.harvard.edu

REPRODUCTIVE ALTERATIONS IN STATES OF FOOD DEPRIVATION AND OBESITY

Fertility and pregnancy require adequate nutrition and energy reserves. States of severe food deprivation–wasting (anorexia nervosa, insulin-dependent diabetes, ballet dancer's lifestyle, etc.) and obesity are associated with reproductive system abnormalities. In men, serum testosterone decreases as body mass increases, but free testosterone levels are decreased only in massively overweight individuals. By contrast, both estradiol and esterone concentrations rise in relation to weight gain, whereas severe food deprivation is associated with decreased estrogen levels and amenorrhea in women. Thus, it is evident that energy balance plays a significant role in reproductive function and fertility. This effect of nutrition and/or energy reserves on reproductive function has long been suspected to be mediated by metabolic signal(s) that link adipose stores with neuroendocrine function. The discovery of leptin 6 years ago and recent data suggesting that this hormone may influence reproduction provided the biochemical basis of the communication that exists between fat stores and the brain.

LEPTIN PHYSIOLOGY

Leptin mRNA, expressed in white adipose tissue,[3–5] stomach, placenta,[6] and mammary gland, encodes a 167 amino acid protein[1] that is a member of the long-chain helical cytokine family.[7–9] Leptin circulates in plasma in the free and bound form, and its levels display a significant circadian and ultradian variation. Serum leptin levels are closely associated with the amount of adipose stores[10–15] as well as short-term energy balance. The composition of the diet and hormonal factors regulate leptin levels too. Insulin levels increase,[16–30] whereas activation of the adrenergic system reduces leptin mRNA expression and circulating levels,[31–33] and the effect of glucocorticoids remains controversial.[34–39] Several cytokines, such as tumor necrosis factor α (TNFα) and interleukins 1 and 6, also alter serum leptin levels.[40–45] Finally, women have higher leptin levels than men[10,46–49] because of either their different body fat distribution or the inducing effects of estrogen/progesterone combined with the suppressive effect of androgens (Ref. 16 and references therein).

LEPTIN ACTION

Leptin acts by binding to specific leptin receptors in the brain and activating the JAK-STAT system (JAK-signal transducer and activator of transcription), which results in altered expression of many hypothalamic neuropeptides (Ref. 16 and references therein). Altered expression of neuropeptide Y (NPY), and possibly other neuropeptides, by leptin results in changes of energy homeostasis and activation of several neuroendocrine axes, including the hypothalamic-pituitary-gonadal axis. The fact that leptin receptors are also expressed in peripheral tissues, including ovaries, has been interpreted as a suggestion of a direct effect of leptin in the gonads, but the physiologic significance of gonadal leptin receptors has not yet been fully elucidated.

LEPTIN'S ROLE IN HUMAN PHYSIOLOGY AND PATHOPHYSIOLOGY

Leptin, like several other cytokines, displays extreme functional pleiotropy. In addition to regulating body weight and energy homeostasis, leptin stimulates a wide variety of biologic responses, including reproductive development and function. The actions of leptin related to the reproductive system will be reviewed herein.

Leptin in the Neonate

Leptin derived from both the placenta[6] and fetal adipose tissue[50,51] has been detected in neonatal cord blood.[33] Cord blood leptin levels are positively associated with body weight of the neonate and are lower in preterm and small-for-gestational-age but higher in large-for-gestational-age neonates.[33] Thus, it has been suggested that leptin may be signaling the amount of fat stores to the brain and influencing energy homeostasis. It has also been suggested that leptin may regulate growth[52] and promote hematopoiesis and lymphopoiesis in newborns.[53,54] but this view has recently been challenged on the basis of two arguments. It is known that ob/ob mice grow normally and that absence of leptin does not result in impairment of fetal growth in the two leptin-deficient children described to date.[55] However, the fact that subjects with leptin deficiency or impaired leptin action due to leptin receptor mutations have impaired linear growth in postnatal life suggests a role for leptin in growth. Thus, this issue remains to be solved conclusively when leptin or leptin antagonists become available for physiologic studies in humans. It was also recently shown that leptin is secreted in the milk and can pass from the gastrointestinal tract to the blood.[56] Whether, in addition to neonatal leptin, maternal leptin in milk may play a role in regulating neonatal food intake in humans, as in rodents, energy balance and/or growth[56] remains to be shown.

Leptin in Childhood–Puberty

Twenty-six years ago Frisch *et al.*[57] made the important observation that menarche occurs when a certain critical mass of body weight is reached. As a child approaches puberty, the percentage of body fat increases and appears to signal to the brain the onset of puberty and reproductive maturation. Similarly, the ceasing of menstruation that occurs in patients with anorexia nervosa, in ballet dancers, or in long distance runners who have extremely low body fat stores is also consistent with Frisch *et al.*'s "critical body weight" theory. Although the mechanism underlying this hypothesis had remained obscure for the last 26 years, the discovery of leptin 6 years ago provided a potential physiologic link between energy reserves and reproductive function. Thus, because leptin concentrations in rodents and children are directly proportional to their adiposity,[58] it has been proposed that leptin may serve to signal to the brain the critical amount of fat stores necessary for initiation of puberty and maintenance of menstrual cycles and reproductive ability. The foregoing hypothesis is in agreement with the hypogonadotropic hypogonadism of leptin-deficient ob/ob mice and the fact that leptin treatment corrects the reproductive system defects of these mice[59] independently of its effect on decreasing body weight. In addition, animal experiments have consistently shown that leptin administration to prepubertal mice and nonhuman primates accelerates puberty (Ref. 60 and references therein). In normal children, leptin levels rise before puberty as body fat mass increases, and they reach their peak at the onset of puberty, suggesting that leptin may trigger the initiation of puberty in humans too.[61] By contrast, subjects with inactivating mutations of the leptin receptor remain prepubertal and have hypogonadotrophic hypogonadism similar to that of the ob/ob mouse model of obesity.[62] Leptin, therefore, appears to provide a necessary signal to the brain regarding the amount of energy stores that would be necessary to successfully carry a pregnancy to term. However, whether leptin acts directly on the hypothalamic–pituitary–gonadal axis or whether leptin acts only as a permissive factor to allow reproductive pubertal maturation to proceed if and only when metabolic resources are adequate for pregnancy remains to be shown. Recent evidence demonstrates that leptin acts on hypothalamic cells to release LHRH, thereby regulating the release of gonadotropins.[63] The subsequent stimulation of gonadal steroid secretion leads to development of the reproductive tract and induction of puberty.[59,63] The exact mechanism by which leptin regulates LHRH secretion and the function of the hypothalamic–pituitry–gonadal axis as well as the potential indirect effects of leptin on the reproductive system are currently the subject of intensive research efforts.

Leptin in Normal Reproductive Function

As just mentioned, it appears that leptin plays a role in regulating reproductive function in cases of extreme energy deficiency or excess. Recent data also indicate that leptin is necessary for normal reproductive function in states of adequate energy reserves too. Leptin is secreted in a pulsatile manner, and its circulating levels display a distinct circadian rhythm in humans. Moreover, minute to minute variations in serum leptin levels are significantly related to minute to minute changes in ACTH and cortisol levels in normal men.[64] More importantly, minute to minute variations of serum leptin levels are also significantly associated with serum luteinizing hormore (LH) and estradiol levels in normal women,[65] indicating that leptin may contribute to physiologic levels and rhythmicity of reproductive hormones. Interestingly, leptin pulse amplitude is higher in women than in men, indicating that the strongest distinction between the sexes is not at the level of organization or oscillation frequency but rather in the amount of leptin released per unit time.[66] Animal experiments have shown that rats treated intracerebroventricularly with leptin antiserum have impaired LH pulsatility consistent with a direct role of leptin in regulating LHRH and LH pulsatile secretion. However, the pathophysiologic significance of these observations and the extent of the role leptin plays in normal reproductive function in humans remain to be fully clarified by future studies.

Leptin in Pregnancy

Serum leptin concentrations have been shown to increase in pregnant women and to correlate with serum levels of several hormones.[67] Leptin levels peak during the second and third trimester and return to normal within 24 hours of delivery.[67] These changes of circulating leptin levels coincide with the period during pregnancy in which energy metabolism shifts from an anabolic to a catabolic state and glucose demands decrease whereas lipolysis and use of fatty acids increase. Thus, it was previously suggested that leptin may be one of the factors that regulate maternal and fetal energy balance during gestation. These preliminary observations and the foregoing hypotheses need to be confirmed by future studies in order to advance our knowledge of the role leptin plays in pregnancy.

Leptin in Relation to the Reproductive Abnormalities in Response to Starvation

Because limited food availability is a state much more frequent than obesity worldwide, it has been suggested that leptin may have primarily evolved as an adaptive mechanism to starvation. Thus, one of leptin's main roles would be to conserve energy by decreasing thyroid hormone levels and to mobilize energy stores by increasing the secretion of glucocorticoids, while at the same time suppressing gonadal function during periods of starvation, that is, when the energy demands of pregnancy and lactation cannot be met.[68] This hypothesis was proved on the basis of animal physiology experiments 3 years ago[68] and recent "experiments of nature." More specifically, leptin administration to starving mice restores the neuroendocrine changes induced by falling leptin levels due to food deprivation, including the suppressed gonadal axis.[68] This effect is, at least in part, NPY mediated.[67] In addition, experiments of nature recently demonstrated that the foregoing observations are also part of human physiology. "Functional leptin deficiency" due to mutations of the leptin receptor gene results in abnormalities of the hypothalamic–pituitary–gonadal axis.[62] Furthermore, leptin deficiency associated with anorexia nervosa, a disease model of starvation, is also characterized by reproductive abnormalities (see below). Based on the foregoing observations, it can reasonably be claimed that leptin is the hormone that signals to the brain the state of starvation and thus results in teleologically appropriate changes of the reproductive system that would limit procreation under conditions of limited energy availability.

Leptin in Eating Disorders

Serum leptin levels in anorexia nervosa and nonspecific eating disorders[69] are low but similar to those of healthy subjects with comparable BMI.[70–72] However, patients with anorexia nervosa appear to have more efficient transport of leptin to the CSF at lower serum leptin concentrations[72] and have normalization of the CSF and serum leptin levels before the BMI returns to normal. These findings may explain the difficulty patients with anorexia nervosa have in gaining weight[73,74] and may provide the underlying mechanism for the neuroendocrine abnormalities seen in patients with anorexia nervosa[74,75] or strenuously exercising women. Amenorrhea in these women may indicate that fat content is sensed via leptin, and in low leptin states, that is, in women who do not have a certain amount of nutritional reserves, ovulation is inhibited.[57] In addition, it was recently shown that increasing serum luteinizing hormone levels in response to refeeding in women with anorexia nervosa track very closely their increase in serum leptin levels.[75] Thus, low leptin levels appear to cause amenorrhea in women with anorexia nervosa, and normalization of leptin levels should be a necessary factor for the resumption of menses in these patients.[74,75]

Leptin and Polycystic Ovarian Disease

Another syndrome in which the role of circulating leptin was recently investigated is the polycystic ovary syndrome (PCOS), a heterogeneous syndrome associated with insulin resistance.[76] In most studies, serum leptin levels in PCOS did not differ from those in normal women with similar adiposity.[77–81] In addition, leptin does not appear to be associated significantly with either hyperinsulinemia, hypernadrogenism, or higher LH levels in these women. However, because leptin receptors have been identified in the ovaries,[82] where leptin may have an inhibitory role in LH, insulin, and IGF-1–induced steroidogenesis,[83,84] recent data suggest that leptin action in the ovaries may be much more important than circulating leptin levels in predicting fertility (Mantzoros *et al.*, unpublished observations). Thus, the exact role of leptin in the pathogenesis of PCOS remains to be demonstrated by future studies.

LEPTIN VERSUS LEPTIN RESISTANCE AND REPRODUCTIVE ABNORMALITIES IN OBESITY

Numerous studies have revealed an association between nutritional status, adiposity, and reproductive function.[57] Not only extremely lean but also obese women have an increased incidence of oligomenorrhea or amenorrhea and infertility.[85] Similar to the role of leptin in regulating reproductive function in low energy availability states is its possible role in regulating reproductive function in obesity too. Interestingly, obese ob/ob mice are hypogonadal and infertile. Moreover, leptin administration to this mouse model of obesity results in maturation of the reproductive tract, as evidenced by increased gonadal hormones, as well as increased testicular weight and normalization of testicular histology in males and the timing of vaginal opening, and increased weights of uteri, ovaries, and oviduct in females.[57] However, it is now known that obesity in most humans is due probably to acquired leptin resistance and not to leptin deficiency as in the ob/ob mouse model of obesity. Although individuals with early onset obesity due to mutations of either the leptin or the leptin receptor gene have been identified,[55] the frequency of such mutations in the general population is probably very low.[86–88] It is of interest, however, that patients with impaired leptin action due to leptin receptor mutations present with dysfunction of their gonadal axis.[89,90] It is reasonable to expect that similar abnormalities of the reproductive system would be caused by the relative leptin deficiency that is common in most subjects with obesity. However, the exact role of leptin in reproductive abnormalities associated with obesity remains to be shown in future studies.

In summary, leptin appears to be the link between nutrition/energy reserves and reproductive function. Future studies are expected to further advance our knowledge in this area of human physiology and will hopefully broaden our therapeutic armamentarium, resulting in tangible benefits for our patients.

ACKNOWLEDGMENT

This study was supported by the Clinical Associate Physician Award (National Institutes of Health and Beth Israel Deaconess Medical Center), the Hershey Family and the Junior Investigator Award (Beth Israel Deaconess Medical Center and Harvard Medical School), and the Boston Obesity Nutrition Research Center Award.

REFERENCES

1. Zhang, Y., R. Proenca, M. Maffei *et al.* 1994. Positional cloning of the obese gene and its human homologue. Nature (Lond.) **372:** 425–432.
2. Flier, J.S. 1997. Leptin expression and action: new experimental paradigms. Proc. Natl. Acad. Sci. USA **94:** 4242–4245.
3. Gong, D.W., S. Bi, R.E. Pratley & B.D. Weintraub. 1996. Genomic structure and promoter analysis of the human obese gene. J. Biol. Chem. **271:** 3971–3974.
4. Lee, G.H., R. Proenca, J.M. Montez *et al.* 1997. Immunohistochemical localization of leptin and uncoupling protein in white and brown adipose tissue. Endocrinology **138:** 797–804.
5. Klein, S., S.W. Coppack, V. Mohamed-Ali & M. Landt. 1996. Adipose tissue leptin production and plasma leptin kinetics in humans. Diabetes **45:** 984–987.
6. Masuzaki, H., Y. Ogawa, N. Sagawa *et al.* 1997. Nonadipose tissue production of leptin: leptin as a novel placenta-derived hormone in humans. Nat. Med. **3:** 1029–1033.
7. Friedman, J.M. 1998. Leptin, leptin receptors and the control of body weight. Nutr. Rev. **56:** S38–46.
8. Zhang, F., M.B. Babinski, J.M. Beals *et al.* 1997. Crystal structure of the obese protein leptin E-100. Nature **387:** 206–209.
9. Madej, T., M.S. Boguski & S.H. Bryant. 1998. Threading analysis suggests that the obese gene product may be a helical cytokine. FEBS Lett. **373:** 13–18.
10. Lonnqvist, F., D. Arner, L. Nordfors & M. Schalling. 1995. Overexpression of the obese (ob) gene in adipose tissue of human obese subjects. Nature Med. **1:** 950–953.
11. Considine, R.V., M.K. Sinha, M.L. Heiman *et al.* 1996. Serum immunoreactive-leptin concentrations in normal-weight and obese humans. N. Engl. J. Med. **334:** 292–295.
12. Montague, C.T., J.B. Prons, L. Sanders *et al.* 1997. Depot- and sex-specific differences in human leptin mRNA expression. Diabetes **46:** 342–347.
13. Lonnqvist, F., L. Nordfors, M. Jansson *et al.* 1997. Leptin secretion from adipose tissue in women. Relationship to plasma levels and gene expression. J. Clin. Invest. **99:** 2398–2404.
14. Lonnqvist, F., A. Thorne, K. Nilsell *et al.* 1995. A pathogenic role of visceral fat b3-adrenoreceptors in obesity. J. Clin. Invest. **95:** 1109–1116.
15. Ronnemaa, T., S.-L. Karonene, A. Rissanen *et al.* 1997. Relation between plasma leptin levels and measures of body fat in identical twins discordant for obesity. Ann. Intern. Med. **126:** 26–31.
16. Tritos, N. & C.S. Mantzoros. 1997. Leptin: its role in obesity and beyond. Diabetologia **40:** 1371–1379.
17. Kolaczynski, J.W., R.V. Considine, J. Ohannesian *et al.* 1996. Responses of leptin to short-term fasting and refeeding in humans. Diabetes **45:** 1511–1515.
18. Kolaczynski, J.W., J.P. Ohannesian, R.V. Considine *et al.* 1996. Response of leptin to short-term and prolonged overfeeding in humans. J. Clin. Endocrinol. Metab. **81:** 4162–4165.
19. Caro, J.F., M.K. Sinha, J.W. Kolaczynski *et al.* 1996. Leptin: the tale of an obesity gene. Diabetes **45:** 1455–1462.
20. Jenkins, A.B., T.P. Markovic, A. Fleury & L.V. Campbell. 1997. Carbohydrate intake and short-term regulation of leptin in humans. Diabetologia **40:** 348–351.
21. Mantzoros C.S., AS. Prasad, F. Beck *et al.* 1998. Zinc regulates serum leptin concentrations in humans. J. Am. Coll. Nutr. **17:** 270–275.
22. Rentsch, J. &. M. Chiesi. 1996. Regulation of ob mRNA levels in cultured adipocytes. FEBS Lett. **379:** 55–59.
23. Wabitsch, M., P.B. Jensen, W.F. Blum *et al.* 1996. Insulin and cortisol promote leptin production in cultured human fat cells. Diabetes **45:** 1435–1438.
24. Kolaczyncki, J.W., M.R. Nyce, R.V. Considine *et al.* 1996. Acute and chronic effect of insulin on leptin production in humans. Diabetes **45:** 699–701.
25. Utriainen, T., R. Malmstrom, S. Makimattila & H. Yki-Jarvinen. 1996. Supraphysiological hyperinsulinemia increases plasma leptin concentrations after 4 h in normal subjects. Diabetes **45:** 1364–1366.

26. RYAN, A.S. & D. ELAHI. 1996. The effects of acute hyperglycemia and hyperinsulinemia on plasma leptin levels: its relationships with body fat, visceral adiposity, and age in women. J. Clin. Endocrinol. Metab. **81:** 4433–4438.
27. MALMSTROM, R., M.R. TASKINEN, S.L. KARONEN & H. YKI-JARVINEN. 1996. Insulin increases plasma leptin concentrations in normal subjects and patients with NIDDM. Diabetologia **39:** 993–996.
28. REMESAR, X., I. RAFECAS, J.A. FERNADEZ-LOPEZ & M. ALEMANY. 1997. Is leptin an insulin counter-regulatory hormone? FEBS Lett. **402:** 9–11.
29. HAFFNER, S.M., H. MIETTINEN, L. MYKKANEN *et al.* 1997. Leptin concentrations and insulin sensitivity in normoglycemic men. Int. J. Obes. Relat. Metab. Disord. **21:** 393–399.
30. MANTZOROS, C.S., A.D. LIOLIOS, N.A. TRITOS *et al.* 1998. Circulating insulin concentrations, smoking and alohol intake are important independent predictors of leptin in young healthy men. Obesity Res. **6:** 179–185.
31. DONAHOO, W.T., T.R. JENSEN, T.J. YOST & R.H. ECKEL 1997. Isoproterenol and somatostatin decrease plasma leptin in humans: a novel mechanism regulating leptin secretion. J. Clin. Endocrinol. Metab. **82:** 4139–4143.
32. MANTZOROS, C.S., D. QU, R.C. FREDERICH *et al.* 1006. Activation of beta(3) adrenergic receptors suppresses leptin expression and mediates a leptin-indepent inhibition of food intake in mice. Diabetes **45:** 909–914.
33. MANTZOROS, C.S., A, VARVARIGOU, V.G. KAKLAMANI *et al.* 1997. Effect of birth weight and maternal smoking on cord blood leptin concentrations of full-term and preterm newborns. J. Clin. Endocrinol. Metab. **82:** 2856–2861.
34. SLIEKER, L.J., K.W. SLOOP, P.L. SURFACE *et al.* 1995. Regulation of expression of ob mRNA and protein by glucocorticoids and cAMP. J. Biol. Chem. **271:** 5301–5304.
35. MIELL, J.P., P. ENGLARO & W.F. BLUM. 1996. Dexamethasone induces an acute and sustained rise in circulating leptin levels in normal human subjects. Horm. Metab. Res. **28:** 704–707.
36. LARSSON, H. & B. AHREN. 1996. Short term dexamethasone treatment increases plasma leptin independently of change in insulin sensitivity in healthy women. J. Clin. Endocrinol. Metab. **81:** 4428–4432.
37. PAPASPYROU-RAO, S., S.H. SCHNEIDER, R.N. PETERSEN & S.K. FRIED. 1997. Dexamethasone increases leptin expression in humans in vivo. J. Clin. Endocrinol. Metab. **82:** 1635–1637.
38. MASUZAKI, H., Y. OGAWA, K. HOSODA *et al.* 1997. Glucocorticoid regulation of leptin synthesis and secretion in humans: elevated plasma leptin levels in Cushing's syndrome. J. Clin. Endocrinol. Metab. **82:** 2542–2547.
39. CIZZA, G., A.J. LOTSIKAS, J. LICINIO *et al.* 1997. Plasma leptin levels do not change in patients with Cushing's disease shortly after correction of hypercortisolism. J. Clin. Endocrinol. Metab. **82:** 2747–2750.
40. BORNSTEIN, S.R., K. UHLMANN, A. HAIDAN *et al.* 1997. Evidence for a novel peripheral action of leptin as a metabolic signal to the adrenal gland. Leptin inhibits cortisol release directly. Diabetes **46:** 1235–1238.
41. MANTZOROS, C.S., S. MOSCHOS, I. AVRAMOPOULOS *et al.* 1997. Leptin concentrations in relation to BMI and the TNFa system in humans. J. Clin. Endocrinol. Metab. **82:** 3408–3413.
42. ZUMBACH, M.S., M.W.J. BOEHMA, P. WAHL *et al.* 1997. Tumor necrosis factor increases serum leptin levels in humans. J. Clin. Endocrinol. Metab. **82:** 4080–4082.
43. GRUNFELD, C., C. ZHAO J. FULLER *et al.* 1996. Endotoxin and cytokines induce expression of leptin, the ob gene product in hamsters. J. Clin. Invest. **97:** 2152–2157.
44. SARAF, P., R. FREDERICH, E. TURNER *et al.* 1997. Multiple cytokines and acute inflammation raise mouse leptin levels: potential role in inflammatory anorexia. J. Exp. Med. **185:** 171–175.
45. JANIK, J.E., B.D. CUTRI, R.V. CONSIDINE *et al.* 1997. Interleukin 1a increases serum leptin concentrations in humans. J. Clin. Endocrinol. Metab. **82:** 3084–3086.
46. SCHRAUWEN, P., W.D. VAN MARKEN LICHTENBELT, K.R. WESTERTERP & W.H.M. SARIS. 1997. Effect of diet composition on leptin concentration in lean subjects. Metabolism **46:** 420–424.

47. HICKEY, M.S., J.A. HOUMARD, R.V. CONSIDINE *et al.* 1997. Gender-dependent effects of exercise training on serum leptin levels in humans. Am. J. Physiol. **272:** E562–E566.
48. SAAD, M.F., S. DAMANI, R.L. GINGERICH *et al.* 1997. Sexual dimorphism in plasma leptin concentrations. J. Clin. Endocrinol. Metab. **82:** 579–584.
49. OSTLUND, R.E., JR., J.W. WANG, S. KLEIN & R. GINGERICH. 1996. Relation between plasma leptin concentration and body fat, gender, diet, age, and metabolic covariates. J. Clin. Endocrinol. Metab. **81:** 3909–3913.
50. SCHUBRING, C., W. KIESS, P. ENGLARO *et al.* 1996. Leptin concentrations in amniotic fluid, venous and arterial cord blood and maternal serum: high leptin synthesis in the fetus and inverse correlation with placental weight. Eur. J. Pediatr. **155:** 830–834.
51. SCHUBRING, C., W. KIESS, P. ENGLARO *et al.* 1997. Levels of leptin in maternal serum, amniotic fluid, and arterial and venous cord blood: relation to neonatal and placental weight. J. Clin. Endocrinol. Metab. **82:** 1480–1483.
52. CARRO, E., R. SENARIS, R.V. CONSIDINE *et al.* 1997. Regulation of *in vivo* growth hormone secretion by leptin. Endocrinology **138:** 2203–2206.
53. BENNETT, B.D., G.P. SOLAR, J.Q. YUAN *et al.* 1996. A role for leptin and its cognate receptor in hematopoiesis. Curr. Biol. **6:** 1170–1180.
54. MIKHAIL, A.A., E.X. BECK, A. SHAFER *et al.* 1997. Leptin stimulates fetal and adult erythroid and myeloid development. Blood **89:** 1507–1512.
55. MONTAGUE, C.T., S. FAROOQI, J.P. WHITEHEAD *et al.* 1997. Congenital leptin deficiency is associated with severe early-onset obesity. Nature **387:** 903–908.
56. CASABIELL, X., V. PINEIRO, M. TOME *et al.* 1997. Presence of leptin in colostrum and/or breast milk from lactating mothers: a potential role in the regulation of neonatal food intake. J. Clin. Endocrinol. Metab. **82:** 4270–4272.
57. FRISCH, R. & J.W. MCARTHER. 1974. Menstrual cycles: fatness as a determinant of minimum weight for height necessary for their maintenance or onset. Science **185:** 949–951.
58. HASSINK, S.G., D.V. SHESLOW, E. DE LANCEY *et al.* 1996. Serum leptin in children with obesity: relationship to gender and development. Pediatrics **98:** 201–203.
59. CHEHAB, F.F., M.E. LIM & R. LU. 1996. Correction of the sterility defect in homozygous obese female mice by treatment with the human recombinant leptin. Nat. Genet. **12:** 318–320.
60. ROGOL, A.D. 1998. Leptin and puberty. J. Clin. Endocrinol. Metab. **83:** 1089–1090.
61. MANTZOROS, C.S., J.S. FLIER & A.D. ROGOL. 1997. A longitudinal assessment of hormonal and physical alterations during normal puberty in boys. V: rising leptin levels may signal the onset of puberty. J. Clin. Endocrinol. Metab. **82:** 1066–1070.
62. CLEMENT, K., C. VAISSE, N. LAHLOU *et al.* 1998. A mutation in the human leptin receptor gene causes abesity and pituitary dysfunction. Nature **392:** 398–401.
63. YU, W.H., M. KIMURA, A. WALCZEWSKA *et al.* 1997. Role of leptin in hypothalamic-pituitary function. Proc. Natl. Acad. Sci. USA **94:** 1023–1028.
64. LICINIO, J., C. MANTZOROS, A.B. NEGRAO *et al.* 1997. Human leptin levels are pulsatile and inversely related to pituitary-adrenal function. Nat. Med. **3:** 575–579.
65. LICINIO, J., A.B. NEGRAO, C.S. MANTZOROS *et al.* 1998. Synchronicity of frequently sampled, 24 hour concentrations of circulating leptin, luteinizing hormone and estradiol in healthy women. Proc. Natl. Acad. Sci. **95:** 2541–2546.
66. LICINIO, J., A.B. NEGRAO, C.S. MANTZOROS *et al.* 1998. Sex differences in circulating human leptin pulse amplitude: clinical implications. J. Clin. Endocrinol. Metab. **83:** 4140–4147.
67. SIVAN, E., P.G. WHITTAKER, D. SINHA *et al.* 1998. Leptin in human pregnancy: the relationship with gestational hormones. Am. J. Obstet. Gynecol. **179:** 1128–1132.
68. AHIMA, R., D. PRABAKARAN, C.S. MANTZOROS *et al.* 1996. Role of leptin in the neuroendocrine response to fasting. Nature **382:** 250–252.
69. FERRON, F., R.V. CONSIDINE, R. PEINO *et al.* 1997. Serum leptin concentrations in patients with anorexia nervosa, bulimia nervosa and non-specific eating disorders correlate with the body mass index but are independent of the respective disease. Clin. Endocrinol. **46:** 289–293.
70. DEUSCHLE, M., W.F. BLUM, P. ENGLARO *et al.* 1996. Plasma leptin in depressed patients and healthy controls. Horm. Metab. Res. **28:** 714–717.

71. HEBERBRAND, J., W. BLUM, N. BARTH *et al.* 1997. Leptin levels in patients with anorexia nervosa are reduced in the acute stage and elevated upon short-term weight restoration. Mol. Psychiatry **2:** 330–334.
72. MANTZOROS, C.S., J.S. FLIER, M.D. LESEM *et al.* 1997. Cerebrospinal fluid in anorexia nervosa: correlation with nutritional status and potential role in resistance to weight gain. J. Clin. Endocrinol. Metab. **82:** 1845–1851.
73. MANTZOROS, C.S. 1997. Obesity, eating disorders and restrained eating. Is leptin the missing link ? Mol. Psychiatry **2:** 377–380.
74. AUDI, L., C.S. MANTZOROS, A. VIDAL-PUIG *et al.* 1998. Leptin in relation to the resumption of menses in anorexia nervosa. Mol. Psychiatry **3:** 544–547.
75. BALLAUFF, A., A. ZIEGLER, G. EMONS *et al.* 1999. Serum leptin and gonadotropin levels in patients with anorexia nervosa during weight gain. Mol. Psychiatry **4:** 71–75.
76. CONWAY, G.S. & H.S. JACOBS. 1997. Leptin: a hormone of reproduction. Hum. Reprod. **12:** 633–635.
77. MANTZOROS, C.S., A. DUNAIF & J.S. FLIER. 1997. Leptin concentrations in the polycystic ovary syndrome. J. Clin. Endocrinol. Metab. **82:** 1687–1691.
78. CHAPMAN, I.M., G.A. WITTERT & R.J. NORMAN. 1997. Circulating leptin concentrations in polycystic ovary syndrome; relation to anthropometric and metabolic parameters. Clin. Endocrinol. **46:** 175–181.
79. LAUGHLIN, G.A, A.J. MORALES & S.S.C. YEN. 1997. Serum leptin levels in women with polycystic ovary syndrome: the role of insulin resistance/hyperinsulinemia. J. Clin. Endocrinol. Metab. **82:** 1692–1696.
80. ROURU, J., L. ANTTILA, P. KOSKINEN *et al.* 1997. Serum leptin concentrations in women with polycystic ovary syndrome. J. Clin. Endocrinol. Metab. **82:** 1697–1700.
81. BRZECHFFA, P.R., A.J. JAKIMIUK, S.K. AGARWAL *et al.* 1996. Serum immunoreactive leptin concentrations in women with polycystic ovary syndrome. J. Clin. Endocrinol. Metab. **81:** 4166–4169.
82. KARLSSON, C., K. LINDELL, E. SVENSSON *et al.* 1997. Expression of functional leptin receptors in the human ovary. J. Clin. Endocrinol. Metab. **82:** 4144–4148.
83. SPICER, L.J. & C.C. FRANCISCO. 1997. The adipose obese gene product, leptin: evidence of a direct inhibitory role in ovarian function. Endocrinology **138:** 3374–3379.
84. HOGGARD, N., L. HUNTER, P. TRAYHURN *et al.* 1998. Leptin in reproduction. Proc. Nutr. Soc. **57:** 421–427.
85. ZACHOW, R.J. & D.A. MAGOFFIN. 1997. Direct intraovarian effects of leptin: impairment of the synergistic action of insulin-like growth factor 1 on follicle stimulating hormone dependent estradiol-17 beta production by rat ovarian granulosa cells. Endocrinology **138:** 847–850.
86. MAFFEI, M., M. STOFFEL & M. BARONE. 1996. Absence of mutations in the human OB gene in obese/diabetic individuals. Diabetes **45:** 679–682.
87. NIKI, T., H. MORI, Y. TAMORI *et al.* 1996. Human obese gene: molecular screening in Japanese and Asian Indian NIDDM patients associated with obesity. Diabetes **45:** 675–678.
88. CONSIDINE, R.V., E.L. CONSIDINE, C.J. WILLIAMS *et al.* 1995. Evidence against either a premature stop codon or the absence of obese gene mRNA in human obesity. J. Clin. Invest. **95:** 2986–2988.
89. CLEMENT, K., C. GARNER, J. HAGER *et al.* 1996. Indication for linkage of the human ob gene region with extreme obesity. Diabetes **45:** 687–690.
90. STROBEL, A., T. ISSAD, L. CAMOIN *et al.* 1998. A leptin missense mutation associated with hypogonadism and morbid obesity. Nat. Genet. **18:** 213–215.

The Potential Role of Intraovarian Factors on Ovarian Androgen Production

ATHANASSIOS CHRYSSIKOPOULOS[a]

Second Department of Obstetrics and Gynecology, University of Athens, "Areteion" Hospital, Athens, Greece

ABSTRACT: The circuit of gonadotropins (FSH, LH) and ovaries (theca and granulosa cells) in ovarian estrogen and androgen production is well established. Recent research has revealed an intraovarian network that may ultimately prove relevant to the understanding of ovarian hyperandrogenism. Most of these substances, such as growth factors and cytokines, do not have independent effects on basal androgen production, but exhibit their regulatory potential by modulating hCG- or LH-stimulated steroid production. Precise understanding of the regulatory role of intraovarian factors in ovarian androgen production would shed new light on the pathophysiology and therapy of hyperandrogenemic excess in women.

INTRODUCTION

Historically, the understanding of the ovarian function progressed from the very early perception of its role as a reproductive organ, a "female testis" (Galen, circa 200 A.D.), to its endocrine capacity as a gland capable of hormone—including androgen—production controlled mainly by pituitary principles.[1] The understanding of the endocrine system that regulates ovarian androgen production is one of the major goals of reproductive research.

THECA-INTERSTITIAL CELLS

In each growing follicle, two different cell populations proliferate and differentiate in hormone-producing cells. These cell populations are the theca-interstitial cells (TICs), the theca-lutein cells (TLCs), and the granulosa cells (GCs) contributing to estradiol (E_2) production. In contrast to the aboundance of information from literature refering to the GCs' function, little is known about the development and the secretory activity of the TICs.

"Thecogenesis," or the development of the TICs, constitutes a phenomenon including cell proliferation with increasing mitotic activity and cell differentiation with hormone production. In the initial stage, the newly recruited primordial follicle comprises one or two layers of cuboital GCs and the basal lamina surrounded by a

[a]Address for correspondence: Athanassios Chryssikopoulos, 2nd Department of Obstetrics & Gynecology, University of Athens, 76 Vas. Sophias Ave., GR-115 28 Athens, Greece.

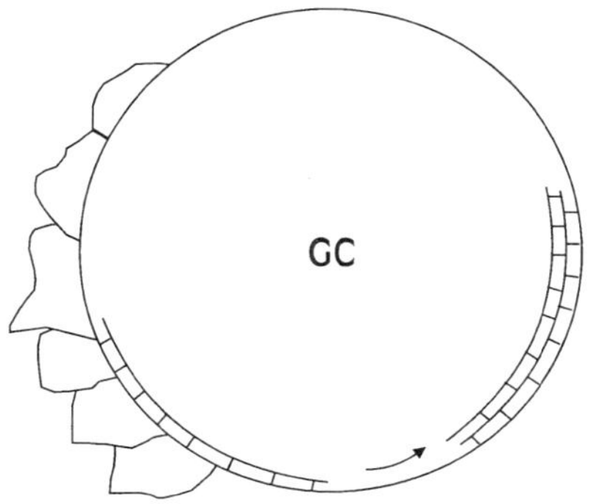

FIGURE 1. The primordial follicle encloses one or two layers of granulosa cells (GCs), and the basal lamina is surrounded from a few undifferentiated cells. The cells proliferate but do not undergo detectable differentiation.

few undifferentiated fibroblast-like cells. These cells proliferate but do not undergo detectable differentiation[2] (FIG. 1).

In the second developmental stage, GCs attain a critical mass of three or more layers, and the preantral follicle exerts autocrine/paracrine stimulation, converting the surrounding fibroblast-like cells into hormone-producing cells. This occurs with both the expression of LH receptors[3] and the production of two enzymes, P450scc[4] and 3β-hydroxysteroid dehydrogenase (3β-HSD).[5] In this stage the TICs secrete progesterone (P) (FIG. 2).

The third stage of development includes the formation of the antrum in the follicle[6] and the conversion from a P-producing TIC to an androstenedione (Δ^4-A)-producing TIC. These changes are achieved with the induction of the expression of the enzyme 17α-hydroxylase (P450c17) mRNA and protein[4,6] (FIG. 3). At the same time, the proliferating GCs begin to produce aromatic enzymes (P450arom) under the influence of FSH, thus giving the androgens produced a means of metabolizing in E_2 (FIG. 4).

The establishment of the GC–TIC interrelationship should secure the formation of a functional follicular unit. In the case of follicular atresia, TICs undergo hypertrophy and remain as clusters in the stroma.[2] Because of the integrity of their enzyme activity, especially of the P450c17 enzyme,[6] they continue their production of Δ^4-A under the influence of LH and insulin.[7]

In the fourth developmental stage the TIC of the dominant follicle, under the influence of the preovulatory LH surge, undergoes a conversion to TLC in the corpus luteum and a significant reduction of its P450c17 activity. Thus, TLCs produce mainly P.

The process of ovum maturation, the onset of ovulation, and the formation and function of the corpus luteum predispose a strict accordance in time of the parallel procedures of thecogenesis and folliculogenesis.

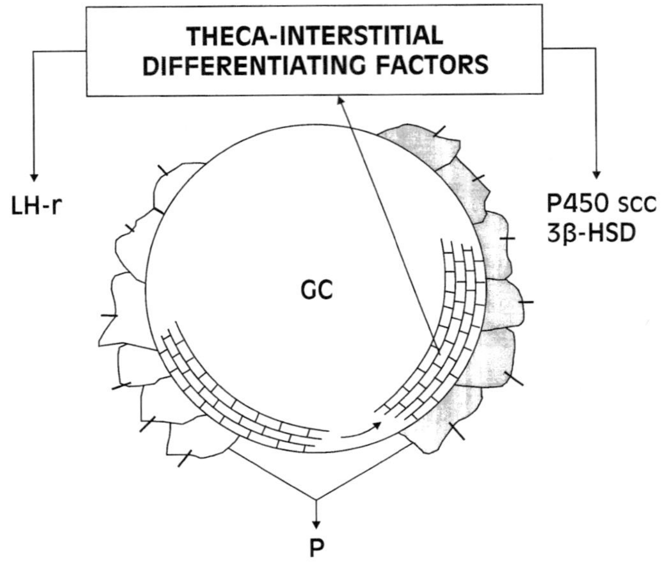

FIGURE 2. In the preantral follicle, the granulosa cells (GC) attain a critical mass of three or four layers and produce factor(s) that convert the surrounding undifferentiated cells into hormone-producing cells. This procedure occurs with both the expression of LH receptors (LH-r) and the production of two enzymes, P450scc and 3β-hydroxysteroid dehydrogenase (3β-HSD). The preantral follicle produces progesterone (P).

THE REGULATION OF ANDROGEN PRODUCTION

In the preantral follicle, the GCs do not possess aromatic enzymes. Thus, the produced androgens are not metabolized to E_2, and they accumulate. During this phase, several intraovarian substances—growth factors and cytokines—are recruited. These factors present autocrine/paracrine properties, and they suppress androgen production and avoid hyperandrogenemia (TABLE 1).

Fibroblast growth factor-β (FGF-β), a growth factor with mitogenic and cell-differentiating properties, is produced by bovine GCs.[8] This peptide has proven to exert modest inhibitory action on hCG-supported androsterone accumulation in the rat whole ovarian dispersates by inhibiting the P450c17 activity.[9] In human TIC, FGF-β reduced either forskolin- or dibutyryl cAMP–stimulated dehydroepiandrosterone production.[10]

Transforming growth factor-β (TGF-β), a member of a family with structural homology to inhibin, activin, and the Müllerian inhibitory substance, is also one of the possible intraovarian modulators of androgen biosynthesis. Its mRNA is expressed in rat TIC[11] and in human GC.[12]

Studies in rat TIC have shown that TGF-β displays a potent inhibitory action on ovarian androgen production[13,14] by inhibiting the P450c17 activity,[12,14] while the content of the enzyme is not decreased.[13]

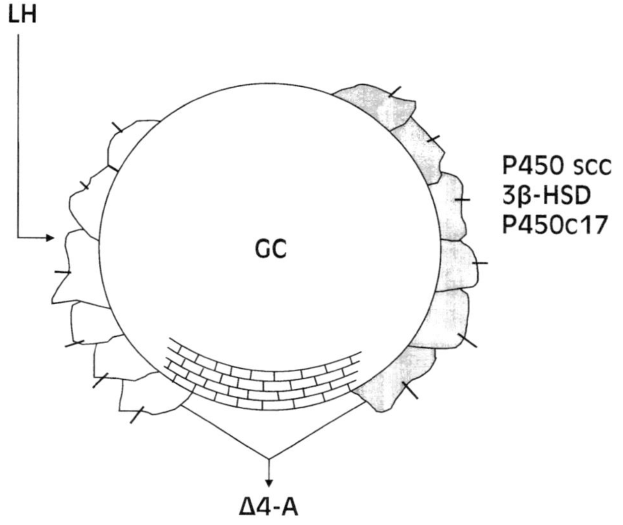

FIGURE 3. In the preantral follicle, progesterone is metabolized in Δ^4-androstenedione (Δ^4-A). This metabolic change is achieved through the production of the enzyme 17α-hydroxylase/17,20-lyase (P450c17).

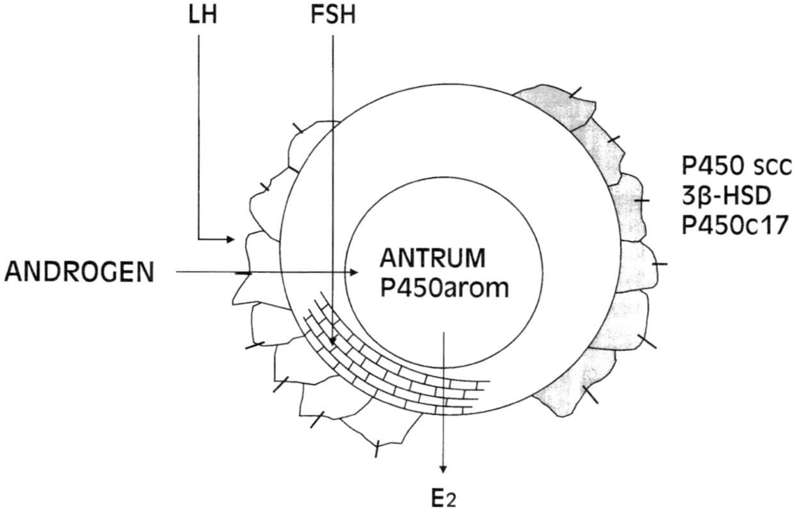

FIGURE 4. In the antral follicle the granulosa cells (GC), under the influence of FSH, begin to produce aromatic enzymes (P450arom) that metabolize the theca-interstitial cell–produced androgens, in estradiol (E_2). 3β-HSD: 3β-hydroxysteroid dehydrogenase.

TABLE 1. Factors inhibiting the LH-supported androgen production in the theca-interstitial cells (TIC) from preantral follicle

Cell origin	Factor/cytokine	LH-induced androgen production
GCs	FGF-β	↓
TIC, GCs	TGF-β (P450c17a↓)	↓
TIC, GCs	TGF-α	↓
GCs	Activin	↓
GCs, macrophages	IL-1β	↓
GCs, macrophages	TNF-α	↓

ABBREVIATIONS: GC: granulosa cell; FGF-β: fibroblast growth factor-β; TGF-α, -β: transforming growth factor-α, -β; IL-1β: interleukin-1β; TNF-α: tumor necrosis factor-α.

Transforming growth factor-α (TGF-α) gene experssion has been demonstrated in rat and human ovary.[15] In human growing follicles, TGF-α has been detected in both TIC and GC.[16] This growth factor modulates in autocrine/paracrine action the TIC androgen biosynthesis by inhibiting the LH-dependent androgen production in rat TIC *in vitro* through reduction of P450c17 enzyme activity.[17]

Activin, a homodimeric form of inhibin-β subunits synthesized by GCs during preantral and early antral follicle development, could suppress TIC androgen synthesis during this time.[18] *In vitro* studies of rat ovarian follicles showed that activin

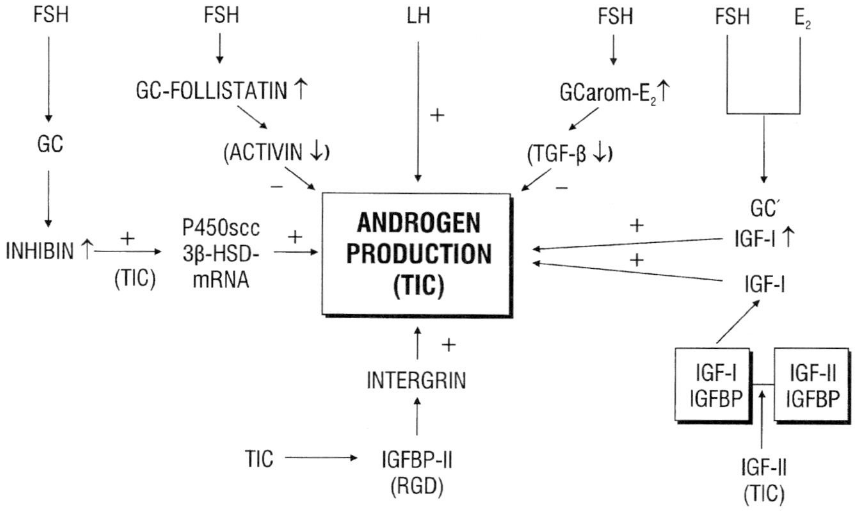

FIGURE 5. Factors that promote the LH-supported androgen production in the theca-interstitial cells (TIC) from the antral follicle. GC: granulosa cell; TGF-β: transforming growth factor-β; IGF-I, -II: insulin-like growth factor-I, -II; IGFBP-I, -II: IGF binding protein-I, -II; 3β-HSD: 3β-hydroxysteroid dehydrogenase; ↑,+: increase, stimulation; ↓,–: reduction, inhibition.

decreases LH-regulated androgen production.[19] Similarly, LH/IGF-I-treated human TICs display significant augmentation of androgen biosynthesis in response to inhibin[20] and inhibition of androgen production when exposed to activin.[21]

In parallel with the local action of growth factors, the cytokines, immunoregulatory molecules secreted by resident ovarian macrophages of somatic ovarian cells,[22] have been demonstrated to play a regulatory role during follicle development and ovulation.[23] Tumor necrosis factor-α (TNF-α) exerts potent inhibitory effects on LH-dependent androgen production by TICs,[24] probably through inhibition of the P450c17 enzyme activity. Interleukin-1 (IL-1) has also been demonstrated to inhibit LH/hCG-stimulated androgen biosynthesis in TIC cultures.[25] Previous studies with several experimental models have demonstrated that ovarian TICs are a site of IL-1β gene expression.[26] Moreover, recent findings have revealed the existence of a complete, highly compartmentalized, gonadotropin-dependent human intraovarian IL-1 system replete with ligands, a receptor, and a receptor antagonist.[27] Transcripts of IL-1β were found in macrophage-free follicular fluid, indicating that GCs may contribute to cytokine synthesis.[28] The steroidogenic pattern in the cultured TICs in the presence of IL-1 suggested inhibition of the P450c17 activity.[1] Gonadotropin-releasing hormone (GnRH) gene expression is detected in the rat ovary. Specific GnRH receptors have also been detected in the rat and human ovaries. Thus, GnRH could also act peripherally, modulating ovarian androgen production. In rat ovarian cell culture, GnRH and a potent GnRH agonist can inhibit basal and gonadotropin-supported androgen synthesis by reducing the P450c17 enzyme activity.[29]

In the preantral follicle, the reduction of the androgen production inhibits their accumulation, curtailing hyperandrogenemia, an essential factor of follicular atresia and reduced fertility. Although the precise identity of the inciting atretic signal remains controversial, an increased body of information indicates that sex steroids, mainly androgens, may play a role in the promotion of atresia. Treatment with antisera to either LH[30] or androstenedione[31] resulted in increased ovulation rates. On the contrary, the systematic application of dihydrotestosterone reduced the overall extent of atresia in pregnant mare serum gonadotropin-treated, immature rats.[32] Probably, the decrease in follicular estrogen concentrations, rather than the increase in follicular androgen content that correlates with the initiation of atresia, is significant.[33]

In the antral follicle, the presence of P450arom enzymes is responsible for the metabolism of androgens to E_2. Because the E_2 production increases during the follicle development to dominant follicle, androgens, being the precursor substances, must increase. In this phase of ovarian evolution, mechanisms that augment the increased production of androgens prevail (FIG. 5). Two of these mechanisms inactivate previous procedures that inhibit androgen production. The FSH-stimulated GCs produce follistatin,[19] which probably blocks the androgen-suppressing effect of activin, while simultaneously increasing E_2 production in growing follicles reduces the inhibitory effect of TGF-β in the LH-induced androgen production in TIC.[34] Both mechanisms indirectly promote the androgen production in the TIC.

The role of IGFs as intraovarian regulators is of interest. The IGF-I and IGF-II genes, as well as type I and II IGF receptors, are expressed in both in murine and human ovarian cells.[1] Although, IGF-I alone is without effect on androgen production, it amplifies the stimulatory effect of gonadotropins in TICs.[35] Growth hormone, FSH, and E_2 stimulate the expression of IGF-I by GC,[36] and it is possible that these hormones exert at least part of their effects on the ovary via the IGF system.

IGF-I enhances LH-dependent androgen production by enhancing the ability of LH to increase P450scc gene expression and enzyme activity such as P450c17 and protein content.[37,38]

Insulin-like growth factor-I concentrations further increase after the release of the growth factor from the IGF-binding proteins (IGFBPs) and its replacement by IGF-II produced in the TICs. It has been demonstrated that TICs express IGFBPs,[39] and their expression can be stimulatd by E_2 and IGF-I.[36,39] Because IGFBPs can regulate IGF-I activity, TIC-derived IGFBPs may play an important autocrine role in modulating any paracrine stimulatory effects of IGF-I on TIC androgen production.[36,39]

Simultaneously, FSH-stimulated inhibin production in GCs increases androgen synthesis in the TIC, augmenting P450scc enzyme activity and 3β-HSD mRNA expression.[36] Finally, IGFBP-2, derived from TICs, contains the RGD amino acid sequence that has been implicated as an integrin-binding site.[18]

In this follicle developmental stage, any dysfunction of the mechanisms that augment androgen production reduces the FSH-stimulated E_2 production in GCs resulting in follicular degeneration, whereas reduced P450arom production leads to hyperandrogenemia and follicular atresia.

Despite the fact that the dominant follicle produces increasing amounts of E_2 until ovulation, the E_2 production declines at mid-cycle. The reduction of E_2 synthesis in GCs and of androgen production in TICs are the result of the high E_2 concentrations via inhibition of the P450c17 enzymic activity.[40] Basal and hCG-stimulated androgen production in rat whole ovarian dispersates decreased significantly within 12 hours of *in vivo* estrogen administration in both intact and hypophysectomized animals.[41]

Estrogen may also act indirectly on ovarian androgen production through the catecholestrogens present in ovarian tissue. Catecholestrogens have been shown to inhibit both basal and LH-supported androgen production by porcine TIC cultures.[42] There is a significant report that high intrafollicular catecholestrogen concentrations are associated with high estrogen concentrations.[43]

In conclusion, in each growing follicle, intraovarian substances such as growth factors and cytokines, in time sequence, regulate via autocrine/paracrine procedures, the permanent LH action on the TICs with a subsequent fluctuation of androgen production. Any chronic and/or quantitative deviation leads to hyperandrogenemia as in the classic example of ovarian polycystic syndrome.

REFERENCES

1. Ruutiainen, K. & E.Y. Adashi. 1993. Intraovarian factors in hyperandrogenism. Semin. Reprod. Endocrinol. **11:** 324–328.
2. Erickson, G.F., D.A. Magoffin, C.A. Dyer & C. Hofeditz. 1985. The ovarian androgen producing cells: a review of structure/function relationships. Endocrinol. Rev. **6:** 371–399.
3. Yamoto, M., K. Shima & R. Nakano. 1992. Gonadotropin receptors in human ovarian follicles and corpora lutea throughout the menstrual cycle. Horm. Res. **37:** 5–11.
4. Suzuki, T., H. Sesano, M. Tamura, *et al.* 1993. Temporal and spatial localization of steroidogenic enzymes in premenopausal human ovaries: in situ hybridization and immunohistochemical study. Mol. Cell. Endocrinol. **97:** 135–143.

5. DUPONT, E., F. LABRIE, V. LUU-THE & G. PELLETIER. 1992. Immunocytochemical localization of 3β-hydroxysteroid dehydrogenase/Δ5-Δ4 isomerase in human ovary. J. Clin. Endocrinol. Metab. **74:** 994–998.
6. TAMURA, T., J. KITAWAKI, T. YAMAMOTO, *et al.* 1992. Immunohistochemical localization of 17α-hydroxylase/c 17-20 lyase and aromatase cytochrome P450 in the human ovary during the menstrual cycle. J. Endocrinol. **135:** 589–595.
7. BARBIERI, R.L., S. SMITH & K.J. RYAN. 1988. The role of hyperinsulinaemia in the pathogenesis of ovarian hyperandrogenism. Fertil. Steril. **50:** 197–212.
8. SUCHANEK, E., V. SIMUNIC, D. JURATIC & V. GRIZELJ. 1994. Follicular fluid contents of hyaluronic acid, follicle-stimulating hormone and steroids relate to the success of in vitro fertilization on human oocytes. Fertil. Steril. **62:** 347–352.
9. HURWITZ, A., E.R. HERNANDEZ & C.E. RESNICK. 1990. Basic fibroblast growth factor inhibits gonadotropin-supported ovarian androgen biosynthesis: mechanism(s) and site(s) of action. Endocrinology **126:** 3089–3095.
10. HULL, M.G.R., R.J. ARMATAGE & A. MCDERMOTT. 1994. Use of follicle-stimulating hormone alone to stimulate the ovaries for assisted conception after ovarian desensitization. Fertil. Steril. **62:** 997–1003.
11. MULHERON, G.W., D. DANIELPOUR & D.N. SCHOMBERG. 1991. Rat thecal/interstitial cells express transforming growth factor-β type 1 and 2, but only type 2 is regulated by gonadotropin in vitro. Endocrinology **129:** 368–374.
12. MULHERON, G.W., N.L. BOSSERT & J.A. LAPP. 1992. Human granulosa and cumulus cells express transforming growth factors-beta type 1 and 2 mRNA. J. Clin. Endocrinol. Metab. **130:** 1707–1715.
13. MAGOFFIN, D.A., B. CANCEDO & G.F. ERICKSON. 1989. Transforming growth factor-β promotes differentiation of ovarian thecal–interstitial cells but inhibits androgen production. Endocrinology **125:** 1251–1258.
14. HERNANDEZ, E.R., A. HURWITZ & D.W. PAYNE. 1990. Transforming growth factor-β1 inhibits ovarian androgen production: gene expression, cellular localization, mechanism(s) and site(s) of action. Endocrinology **127:** 2804–2811.
15. KUDLOW, J.E., M.S. KOBRIN & A.P. PUCHIO. 1987. Ovarian transforming growth factor-α gene expresion immunohistochemical localization to the theca-interstitial cells. Endocrinology **121:** 1577–1579.
16. DAYA, A., J. GUNBY & E.G. HUGHES, *et al.* 1995. Follicle-stimulating hormone versus human menopausal gonadotropin for in vitro fertilization cycles. Fertil. Steril. **64:** 347–354.
17. WEITSMANN, S.R. & D.A. MAGOFFIN. 1993. Transforming growth factor-α inhibits luteinizing hormone-stimulated androgen production by blocking 17α-hydroxylase/c 17-20 lyase activity in rat ovarian theca interstitial cells. Endocrinol. J. **1:** 109–115.
18. ZACHOW, R.J. & D.A. MAGGOFIN. 1997. Ovarian androgen biosynthesis: paracrine/autocrine regulation. *In* Androgen Excess Disorders in Women. R. Azziz, Ed.: 13–22. Lippincott-Raven. Philadelphia.
19. HSUEH, A.J.W., K.D. DAHL & J. VAUGHAN. 1987. Heterodimers and homodimers of inhibin subunits have different paracrine action in the modulation of luteinizing hormone-stimulated androgen biosynthesis. Proc. Natl. Acad. Sci. USA **84:** 5082–5086.
20. HILLIER, S.G., E.L. YONG & P.I. ILLINGWORT. 1991. Effect of recombinant inhibin on androgen synthesis in cultured human thecal cells. Mol. Cell. Endocrinol. **75:** R1–R6.
21. HILLIER, S.G., E.L. YONG & P.I. ILLINGWORT. 1991. Effect of recombinant activin on androgen synthesis in cultured human thecal cells. J. Clin. Endocrinol. Metab. **72:** 1206–1211.
22. ADASHI, E.Y. 1996. The ovarian follicular apparatus. *In* Reproductive Endocrinology, Surgery and Technology. E.Y. Adashi, J.A. Rock, Z. Rosenwaks, Eds.: 18–39. Lippincott-Raven. Philadelphia.
23. CHRYSSIKOPOULOS, A. 1997. The relationship between the endocrine and immune systems. Ann. N.Y. Acad. Sci. **816:** 83–93.
24. ANDREANI, C.L., D.W. PAYNE & J.N. PACKMAN. 1991. Cytokine mediated regulation of ovarian function. Tumor necrosis factor-α inhibits gonadotropin-supported ovarian androgen biosynthesis. J. Biol. Chem. **266:** 6761–6766.

25. HURWITZ, A., M. DUSHNIK, H. SOLOMON, *et al.* 1991. Cytokine mediated regulation of rat ovarian function: interleukin-1 inhibits gonadotropin-induced androgen biosynthesis. Endocrinology **129:** 1250–1256.
26. HURWITZ, A., E. RICCIARELLI, L. BOTERO, *et al.* 1991. Endocrine- and autocrine-mediated regulation of rat ovarian (theca–interstitial) interleukin-1β gene expression: gonadotropin-dependent preovulatory acquisition. Endocrinology **129:** 3427–3429.
27. HURWITZ, A., J. LOUKIDES, E. RICCIARELLI, *et al.* 1992. Human intraovarian interleukin-1 (IL-1) system: highly compartmentalized and hormonally dependent regulation of the gene encoding IL-1, its receptor and its receptor antagonist. J. Clin. Invest. **89:** 1746–1754.
28. KARAGOUNI, E.E., A. CHRYSSIKOPOULOS, T. MANTZAVINOS, *et al.* 1998. Interleukin-1β and interleukin-1α may affect the implantation rate of patients undergoing in vitro fertilization–embryo transfer. Fertil. Steril. **70:** 553–559.
29. MAGOFFIN, D.A., D.S. REYNOLDS & G.F. ERICKSON. 1981. Direct inhibitory effect of GnRH on androgen secretion by ovarian interstitial cells. Endocrinology **109:** 661–663.
30. TERRANOVA, P.F. & G.S. GREENWALD. 1981. Increased ovulation rate in the cyclic pig after a single injection of an antiserum to LH. J. Reprod. **61:** 37–42.
31. KARAMUZZI, R.J., W.G. DAVIDSON & P.F.A. VAN LOOK. 1977. Increasing ovulation rate in sheep by active immunization against an ovarian steroid androstenedione. Nature (London) **269:** 817–818.
32. KOHUT, J.K., J.F. JARRELL, L.Z. YOUNG & E.V. LAI. 1985. Does dihydrotestosterone induce atresia in the hypophysectomized immature female rats treated with pregnant mare's serum gonadotrophin? Am. J. Obstet. Gynecol. **151:** 250–255.
33. DHANASEKARAN, N. & N.R. MOUGDAL. 1989. Studies on follicular atresia: role of gonadotropins and gonadal steroids in regulating cathepsin-D activity in preovulatory follicles in the rat. Mol. Cell. Endocrinol. **63:** 133–142.
34. MAGOFFIN, D.A., D. HUBERT-LESLIE & R.J. ZACHOW. 1995. Estradiol-17β, insulin-like growth factor-I and luteinizing hormone inhibit secretion of transforming growth factor β by rat ovarian theca–interstitial cells. Biol. Reprod. **53:** 625–633.
35. HERNADEZ, E.R., C.E. RESNICK & J.E. SVOBODA. 1988. Somatomedin-C/insulin-like growth factor I as an enhancer of androgen biosynthesis by cultured rat ovarian cells. Endocrinology **122:** 1603–1612.
36. MAGOFFIN, D.A. & G.F. ERICKSON. 1994. Control systems of theca-interstitial cells. *In* Molecular Biology of the Female Reproductive System. J.K. Findlay, Ed.: 39–65. Academic Press. Orlando, FL.
37. MAGOFIN, D.A., K.W. KURTZ & G.F. ERICKSON. 1990. Insulin-like growth factor-I selectively stimulates cholesterol side chain cleavage expression in ovarian theca-interstitial cells. Mol. Endocrinol. **9:** 489–496.
38. MAGOFFIN, D.A. & S.R. WEITSMAN. 1997. Synergistic interactions between LH and insulin/IGFs. *In* The Ovary: Regulation, Dysfunction and Treatment. M. Filicori, Ed.: 79–85. Elsevier Science. Amsterdam.
39. ERICKSON, G.F., D. LI, S.R. WEITSMAN, S. SHIMASAKI, *et al.* 1995. Insulin-like growth factor-I (IGF-I) stimulate the IGF-binding protein system in the rat theca interstitial cells. Endocrine **3:** 525–531.
40. JOHNSON, J.C., H. MARTIN & C.H. TSAI-MORRIS. 1984. The in vitro and in vivo effect of estradiol upon the 17α-hydroxylase and C17,20-lyase activity in ovaries of immature hypophysectomized rats. Mol. Cell. Endocrinol. **35:** 199–204.
41. MAGOFFIN, D.A. & G.F. ERICKSON. 1981. Mechanism by which 17α estradiol inhibits ovarian androgen production in the rat. Endocrinology **108:** 962–969.
42. LEUNG, P.C.K. & D.T. ARMSTRONG. 1979. Estrogen treatment of immature rats inhibits ovarian androgen production in vitro. Endocrinology **104:** 1411–1417.
43. HAMMOND, J.M., R.M. JERSEY, M.A. WOLEGA & J. WEISZ. 1986. Catecholestrogen production by porcine ovarian cells. Endocrinology **118:** 2292–2299.

The Genetics of Obesity

Lessons for Polycystic Ovary Syndrome

RICHARD S. LEGRO[a]

Department of Obstetrics and Gynecology, Pennsylvania State University College of Medicine, Hershey, Pennsylvania 17033, USA

ABSTRACT: Both polycystic ovary syndrome (PCOS) and obesity are common disorders with a complex phenotype. Both are presumably heterogeneous in etiology. Understanding the genetics of obesity, which has a longer and richer history, may therefore illuminate the genetics of PCOS, where major projects are now underway. Obesity may be the penultimate condition in which the effects of heredity and environment will forever mingle. Most obesity mutations identified to date (with the exception of the *Agouti* mutation) are inherited in an autosomal recessive manner. Therefore, it is unlikely that such mutations, even when identified in a human population, could explain only a fraction of the cases that make up the high prevalence of both of these disorders. Although the mouse models of single gene defects causing obesity contain many similar aspects of the PCOS phenotype such as obesity and subfecundity, there is no mouse model that mimics all aspects of the syndrome, especially the circulating androgen excess. This elevation in circulating androgens may be the *sine qua non* of the syndrome as indicated by our findings in sisters of PCOS probands that hyperandrogenemia may be the distintinctive reproductive phenotype. Isolation of PCOS and obesity genes may allow the development of targeted interventions that will lead to effective and safe treatment of both obesity and PCOS.

INTRODUCTION

Obesity may be the most costly and most common health issue in the United States.[1] Up to one-third of adult women are affected, an estimated 35 million women. Polycystic ovary syndrome is also common and may be the most common endocrine disorder among women.[2] It is estimated to affect between 5 and 7% of the U.S. population.[3] Up to 50% of women affected with PCOS are thought to be obese.[4] Therefore, understanding the genetics of obesity, which has a longer and richer history, may illuminate the genetics of PCOS, where major projects are now just underway. The goal of this presentation is to review the genetics of obesity in both the mouse and human and to speculate on the utility of this effort in identifying PCOS genes.

[a]Address for correspondence: Richard S. Legro, Department of Obstetrics and Gynecology, PO Box 850, 500 University Drive, M.S. Hershey Medical Center, Hershey, PA 17033. Phone: 717-531-8478; fax: 717-531-6286.

rsl1@psu.edu

OBESITY: A NATIONAL EPIDEMIC

Evidence suggests that obesity is becoming more prevalent among U.S. adults.[5] The National Health and Nutrition Examination Surveys from 1960–1991 have found an ever greater prevalence of obesity. This reached 8% over the last decade. Mean body weight for all adult men and women increased 3.6 kg in this same period. Although obesity appears to increase with age, it peaks in middle age. Significant differences in the prevalence of obesity are based on ethnicity and gender. For instance, African American and Latino populations display a higher prevalence of obesity than does the non-Hispanic white population. Women also appear to have a higher prevalence of obesity than men, with prevalence estimates ranging from 33–49% for women versus 31–36% for men. The medical complications associated with obesity are protean and include an increased risk of type 2 diabetes, hypertension, cardiovascular disease, osteoarthritis, gout, sleep apnea, dysfunction uterine bleeding, and endometrial carcinoma.

The cost of obesity including medical care as well as dietary supplementation and weight loss programs is estimated to approach 100 billion dollars.[1] Unfortunately, there are no effective treatments that result in permanent weight loss, and it is estimated that 90–95% of patients who experience a weight decrease will relapse. There is a tendency to blame this high recidivism rate on character weakness rather than to acknowledge that this may reflect fundamental metabolic and potentially genetic differences in obese individuals.

There is no universal definition of obesity. Most commonly used definitions relate weight to height. The best correlation with body fat for such a ratio is with the body mass index (BMI), which is calculated as weight in kilograms divided by height in meters squared (kg/m^2). This is also known as Quetelet's Index. The 1985 National Institutes of Health Consensus Panel on Obesity defined obesity as a BMI greater than the 85% percentile.[6] This value is 27.3 kg/m^2. Approximately 40% of females of reproductive age are obese by this definition.

WHY IS OBESITY SO COMMON?

Obesity may be the penultimate condition in which the effects of heredity and environment will forever mingle. Are we an obese society because we expend our wealth on a constant flow of calorie-filled delights or are we genetically programmed to ever increase in girth? Studies suggest that the energy expenditure rate in obese persons is nearly identical to that in lean persons. This suggests that obese persons may be more efficient at storing energy. The ability to conserve rather than expend energy in fat would confer a survival advantage, especially in a hunter-gatherer society prone to periods of famine, war, and climactic upheaval. This has been referred to as the "thrifty gene" hypothesis.[7]

Studies in twins, adoptees, and nuclear family data suggest that 25–40% of body fat may be heritable. The risk of obesity is about two to three times higher if there is a family history of obesity. Segregation analyses do not show a consistent form of inheritance. Although multiple studies show a single major gene for high body mass that appears to segregate from parents to children, an equal number of studies suggest no segregating allele. At the present time the most important regions of the hu-

TABLE 1. Summary of mouse mutations causing obesity and their known human homologues

Gene	Mutation	Gene Product	Human Chromosome	Action
Lep	ob	Leptin	7q31.3	Central effect suppressing appetite and increasing energy expenditure
Lepr	db fa	Leptin receptor	1q32	Leptin signal precessing, transport, or clearance
Cpe	fat	Carboxypeptidase E	11p15	Prohormone processing (including neuropeptides)
Tub	tub	Phosphodiesterase	4q32 (?)	Hyopthalamic cellular apoptosis ?
Agouti	Ay	Agouti signaling protein	20q11.2	Blocking of melanocortin-4 receptor
UCP-2		Uncoupling Protein 2	11q13	Uncouples respiratory fuel oxidation; role in thermoregulation, energy balance, and body weight regulation
Nhlnh2		Basis helix-loop-helix transcription factor		Involved in neurogenesis in hypothalamus; disruption leads to hypothalamic-pituitary abnormalities and adult-onset obesity

man genome that show linkage are 1p, 3p, 6p, and 11q.[8] Support for a single gene causing obesity has come largely from mouse models.[9] These are discussed with reference to results of studies of homologous genes in humans.

MOUSE MODELS OF OBESITY

It is interesting that the first nongenetic mouse models were created in the early 1940s via iatrogenic hypothalamic brain lesions, which resulted in many of the characteristics of obesity found in mouse genetic models: hyperphagia, hyperinsulinemia, and a decreased metabolic rate. Six single gene obesity mutations have been described in mice. The affected protein and its mechanism of action as well as the location of its human homolog are found in TABLE 1. The *ob/ob* mouse was first described in 1950 at the Jackson Laboratory in Bar Harbor, Maine, USA. The *db/db* was described in the 1970s. These mice were identical in phenotype, that is, they were obese, infertile, and prone to diabetes at an early age, and both were the result of an autosomal recessive mutation. It was not until the cloning of the *ob* gene (both mouse and human), which coded for leptin, that a whole new chapter in the endocrinology and genetics of obesity was opened, a chapter that has just started to be written in the human.[10]

Leptin is a 167 amino acid peptide synthesized solely in adipose tissue. The name comes from the Greek for thin. It is thought to be a "satiety" hormone, sending a message to the brain from fat tissue about the adequacy of fat stores. Leptin concentrations in obese humans are increased in direct proportion to the fat mass. Per unit fat mass, obese persons produce exactly as much leptin as do lean people. Leptin deficiency appears to be a rare cause of obesity in humans. Leptin mutations have been described in infants and recently in adults. The two infants described were from a highly consanguineous Pakistani family.[11] Both children were severely obese, with very low serum levels of leptin. The patients had a frameshift mutation that resulted in a string of incorrect amino acids before terminating in a premature stop codon. The adults described were similar to their mouse homologs.[12] They displayed massive obesity, hyperphagia, lack of sexual development, and low levels of sex steroids. The mutation in the family was a C-T substitution, resulting in an Arg-Trp replacement, which impaired protein secretion from the fat cell. The phenotypes of these adults suggest that leptin is also important in reproductive function and perhaps vital to the initiation of puberty. Recently, a genome-wide scan and multipoint linkage analysis identified a locus on 2p21 that showed strong evidence of linkage with serum leptin levels (lod score 4.95).[13] The candidate gene in this region, which includes such genes as glucokinase regulatory protein (*GCKR*) and proopiomelancortin (*POMC*), has not been identified to date. There are also multiple family studies that show linkage with the chromosomal region where leptin is located including studies of Pima Indians, the Quebec Family Study, the Paris Cohort of Obese Sibling study, the University of Pennsylvania Family Obesity Study, and the San Antonio Family Diabetes Study.[8]

The leptin receptor is a member of the cytokine family of receptors and has several splice variants. Six, labeled *ra* through *rf*, have been described to date. They are located in a wide variety of tissues in addition to brain. The STAT docking site that is encoded by exon 18b is essential for activating the promoter regions of target genes. It is included only in the longest splice variant, *rf*, the one predominantly expressed in the hypothalamus. It is theorized that the shorter forms, many of which lack the transmembrane region of the receptor, may function as circulating carrier proteins for leptin. The intracellular region of the receptor utilizes transcription factors in the JAK/STAT family for signal transduction. Adding back leptin to the *Ob/Ob* mouse will correct the underlying abnormalities and restore a normal mouse phenotype. As expected with a receptor mutation, the addition of the hormone to the *db/db* mouse produces no modification of phenotype. The *db* mutation in mice produces a G-T substitution, resulting in a truncated and nonfunctional form of the long form. The *fa* mutation results in reduced intracytoplasmic transport and reduced function, whereas the fa^k results in stop codon. The leptin receptor has been cloned in the human.[14] A mutation in the human receptor gene has been identified.[15] Homozygous affected patients present with early onset morbid obesity and no pubertal development. In addition, their secretion of growth hormone and thyrotropin is reduced.

Tub and *fat* mutant mice are similar, but the *tub* mutants average a lower body weight. Anecdotally neither are hyperphagic. The homozygous *tub* mouse is hyperinsulinemic with postpubertal obesity and also has degeneration of retinal and cochlear ganglion cells. In fact, the mouse is blind. The *tub* gene codes for a protein, a phosphodiesterase, that may be involved in the establishment of hypothalamic neural circuits. The mutated gene may play a role in apoptosis in the affected neural cells, leading to blindness.

The fat gene results from mutation in *Cpe*, carboxypeptidase E. The *Cpe* mutation in its homozygous form results in elevated plasma proinsulin concentrations due to the lack of carboxypeptidase activity in the islet beta cell. Carboxypeptidase is required for excision of various residues remaining at the C-terminus of various peptide prohormone intermediates. These hormones include proinsulin, proopiomelanocortin (the precursor hormone to ACTH, melanocyte-stimulating hormone (MSH), and β-endorphin. The *fat* phenotype in mice tends to present later than does that from the aforementioned single gene mutations. Recently a mutation was identified in prohormone convertase (*PC-1*) in a 47-year-old women.[16] She weighed 89 kg at age 45 and had marked elevations of proinsulin with nondetectable insulin after glucose challenge. The woman was compound heterozygote with a Gly-Arg 483 that prevented secretion of the protein and a mutation in the donor splice site that led to the loss of exon 5 and a premature stop codon with no functional catalytic region. Three of the four children who inherited the first mutation were clinically unaffected as was the remaining child who inherited the latter mutation.

The *Agouti* mutation is a dominant one. This is unique among the mutations noted in mouse models as the previous mutations discussed were recessive. The *Agouti* gene regulates hair pigmentation, resulting in the agouti coat color (intermittent yellow and black pigment bands). The *Agouti* gene encodes agouti signaling protein (ASP), which blocks the action of MSH on hair follicle pigment-producing cells. This causes a switch from production of black hair pigment to yellow pigment. The human homolog of this protein was recently located to chromosome 16. The mechanism of insulin resistance is unknown, but it may be related to effects on intracellular calcium transport. Alternatively the hormone may exert an anorexiant effect by antagonizing the effect of α-MSH at melanocortin receptors. Recently, linkage was found in the Quebec family study between melanocortin receptor 3 (*MC3R*) and BMI 17 as well as with melanocortin receptor 5 (*MC5R*) and BMI.[18]

NEW CANDIDATES: UNCOUPLING PROTEINS AND TRANSCRIPTION FACTORS

A key gene involved in energy expenditure was recently identified that may play a role in human obesity.[19] Brown adipose tissue (BAT) in animals was found to be a discrete adipose tissue, whose function is to expend energy and generate heat. This heat production in BAT is stimulated by environmental cold or food intake. This activity is mediated by uncoupling of respiration from any fuel-consuming process, so that the only byproduct is heat. In brown adipocytes, this uncoupling of respiration is initiated by norepiephrine stimulation. The specific protein involved is uncoupling protein 1 (*UCP-1*) or thermogenin. This was thought to be a rather insignificant diversion of energy expenditure in humans, as BAT is found only in neonates or in humans living under extreme environmental conditions (either external such as arctic regions or internal such as a catecholamine-secreting tumor). A second uncoupling protein, *UCP-2*, was recently discovered that is expressed in a wide variety of tissues other than BAT, such as white adipose tissue, muscle, and kidney.[19] *UCP-2* is 59% identical to *UCP-1*. Because *UCP-2* is widely expressed, it may be more responsible for determining basal metabolic rate rather than responding to environmentally determined stimuli as is the case with UCP. Indeed, *UCP-2* mRNA levels are unaffected by cold exposure, but they are significantly increased by a high fat diet, suggesting differential regulation of the two proteins. Although *UCP-2* has been localized to human chromosome 11, no mutations in the human gene have been identified to date.

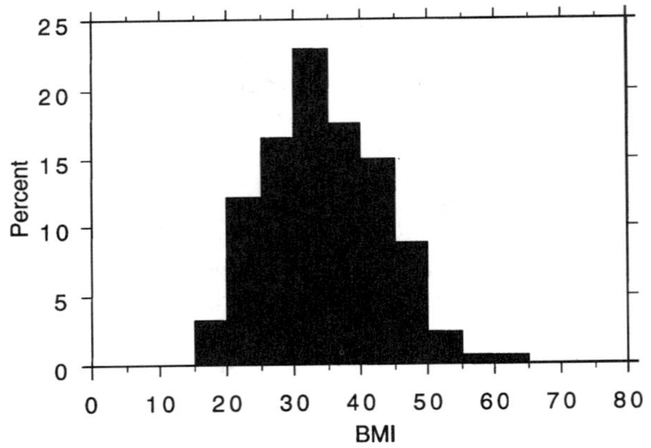

FIGURE 1. Histogram of distribution (%) of body mass index (BMI) among 280 consecutive women with polycystic ovary syndrome (PCOS) studied at Pennsylvania State University College of Medicine, Hershey, Pennsylvania.

Knockout mice for the transcription factor *Nhlh2* were recently generated to look at the effects of the absence of this basic helix-loop-helix transcription factor on the organism.[20] This gene is expressed in the ventromedial and lateral hypothalamus, Rathke's pouch, and the anterior lobe of the pituitary. Male mice were hypogonadal and infertile, as were female mice reared alone. Both males and females displayed progressive adult-onset obesity.

OBESITY IN POLYCYSTIC OVARY SYNDROME

Obesity and PCOS have often been linked, and obesity has been found to exacerbate the underlying insulin resistance in PCOS.[21] Obesity has also been linked to increased androgen production and hirsutism in women with PCOS.[22] Obesity in PCOS, as in the mouse models just described, has also been associated with increasing subfecundity above and beyond that of the PCOS diagnosis alone[22] and with resistance to ovulation induction treatments.[23] The exact prevalence of obesity among women with PCOS varies between countries and probably reflects both environmental and genetic factors. Even between western, industrialized countries, however, there can be vast differences in the prevalence of obesity. In Balen and Jacob's series of 1,741 consecutive women with PCOS, 38.4% had a BMI ≥ 26.[22] In our series of 280 women with PCOS characterized to date, 87.5% had a BMI ≥ 26, a nearly two-fold higher prevalence (FIG. 1). Some investigators have speculated that obesity may be the primary metabolic insult among women with PCOS[24]; however, this view is not held universally.

The mechanism of the increased prevalence of obesity in women with PCOS, just like the mechanism for insulin resistance, is not known currently. In our experience,

TABLE 2. Simple correlation between BMI and continuous variables that have been used to assign phenotypes in a cohort of 280 women with PCOS[a]

Variable	Count	F-value	R	P value
Total ovarian volume (R + L ovary)	118	1.68	0.12	0.20
Total testosterone level	275	2.50	0.10	0.11
Fasting glucose level	262	10.3	0.20	<0.01
Luteinizing hormone level	217	25.0	0.33	<0.0001
Fasting insulin level	212	83.4	0.53	<0.0001

[a]Strongest correlation with simple regression analysis between BMI is with fasting insulin and weakest is with ovarian volume.

obesity appears unrelated to circulating androgens (TABLE 2), but it does appear significantly to affect other stigmata of the PCOS phenotype including LH levels and markers of insulin action, fasting glucose and insulin. When we simply correlate BMI with this continuous stigmata of the phenotype, we find the strongest correlation with fasting insulin and the weakest with circulating androgen levels and ovarian size on transvaginal ultrasonography. Lower LH levels with increasing BMI in women with PCOS has been found by many investigators.[25,26] This elevation in circulating androgens may be the *sine qua non* of the syndrome, as indicated by our findings in sisters of PCOS probands that hyperandrogenemia is the distinctive reproductive phenotype.[27]

GENETICS OF PCOS: SUBPHENOTYPE OF OBESITY

Both PCOS and obesity are common disorders with a complex phenotype. Both are presumably heterogeneous in etiology. Most obesity mutations identified to date (with the exception of the *Agouti* mutation) are inherited in an autosomal recessive fashion. Therefore, it is unlikely that such mutations, even when identified in a human population, could explain only a fraction of the cases that make up the high prevalence of both of these disorders. Although mouse models of single gene defects causing obesity contain many similar aspects of the PCOS phenotype such as obesity and subfecundity,[28] there is no mouse model that mimics all aspects of the syndrome, especially the circulating androgen excess. Linkage studies among obese human families have consistently identified candidate gene regions of the genome, but specific genes and mutations have been less forthcoming. Although such studies among the families of women with PCOS are still in their infancy, several linkages have been reported.[29,30]

Although both disorders represent abnormalities of continuous variables, the definition of "abnormal" or "affected" phenotype for either disorder is investigator dependent. The cutoff point for determining obesity has often been debated, and quantitative linkage analyses that can use the full continuous information of BMI are intriguing. However, such analyses are currently not used routinely to examine the genetics of complex disorders and have not yet been applied to PCOS. Many different variables, potentially continuous such as circulating androgen levels, ovarian size and morphology, and menstrual interval have been used to define PCOS and could theoretically be used in a quantitative linkage analysis. We currently believe that hyperandrogenemia alone may be useful for assigning phenotypes to women of reproductive age in genetic analyses of PCOS families. Combinations of continuous variables such as hyperandrogenic chronic anovulation, based on circulating testosterone levels and severe oligomenorrhea, or anovulatory PCO based on ovarian morphology and oligomenorrhea may also identify smaller and more genetically homogeneous subphenotypes of obesity within PCOS families.[31,32] These studies are currently underway in our group and may add insight into the genetics of obesity.

SUMMARY

We are just beginning now to identify specific molecular mechanisms in humans that result in obesity. The mechanism of obesity in women with PCOS is unknown. The majority of known mutations causing obesity are the result of autosomal recessive mutations, and as such they are likely to account for a small fraction of this disorder of epidemic proportion. Subtle reduction in the function of these proteins through, as of yet, uncharacterized mutations may result in reduced function of some of these key proteins. Although the initial effect may be negligible, the cumulative effect of any mutation that shifts energy expenditure to the storage side may be the eventual and gradual development of obesity. These insights may allow development of targeted interventions that will allow more effective and safer treatment of both obesity and PCOS than we have established to date.

ACKNOWLEDGMENTS

This work was supported by Public Health Service grant K08 HDO118, The National Cooperative Program in Infertility Research (NCPIR) grant U54 HD 34449, and GCRC grant MO1 RR 10732 to Pennsylvania State University.

REFERENCES

1. ROSENBAUM, M., R.L. LEIBEL & J. HIRSCH. 1997. Obesity. N. Engl. J. Med. **337:** 396–407.
2. DUNAIF, A. 1997. Insulin resistance and the polycystic ovary syndrome: mechanism and implications for pathogenesis. Endocr. Rev. **18:** 774–800.
3. ALLEN, S.E., H.D. POTTER & R. AZZIZ.1997. Prevalence of hyperandrogenemia among nonhirsute oligo-ovulatory women. Fertil. Steril. **67:** 569–572.
4. FRANKS, S. 1995. Polycystic ovary syndrome. N. Engl. J. Med. **333:** 853–861.
5. KUCZMARSKI, R.J., M.D. CARROLL, K.M. FLEGAL & R.P. TROIANO. 1997. Varying body mass index cutoff points to describe overweight prevalence among U.S. adults: NHANES III (1988 to 1994). Obes. Res. **5:** 542–548.
6. BURTON, B.T., W.R. FOSTER, J. HIRSCH & T.B. VAN ITALLIE. 1985. Health implications of obesity: an NIH Consensus Development Conference. Int. J. Obesity **9:** 155–170.
7. WENDORF, M. & I.D. GOLDFINE. 1991. Archaeology of NIDDM. Excavation of the "thrifty" genotype. Diabetes **40:** 161–165.
8. BOUCHARD, C. 1997. Genetics of human obesity: recent results from linkage studies. J. Nutr. **127:** 1887S–18890S.
9. LEIBEL, R.L., W.K. CHUNG & S.C. CHUA, JR. 1997. The molecular genetics of rodent single gene obesities. J. Biol. Chem. **272:** 31937–31940.

10. ZHANG, Y., R. PROENCA, M. MAFFEI, M. BARONE, L. LEOPOLD & J.M. FRIEDMAN. 1994. Positional cloning of the mouse obese gene and its human homologue. Nature **372:** 425–432.
11. MONTAGUE, C.T., I.S. FAROOQI, J.P. WHITEHEAD *et al.* 1997. Congenital leptin deficiency is associated with severe early-onset obesity in humans. Nature **387:** 903–908.
12. STROBEL, A., T. ISSAD, L. CAMOIN, M. OZATA & A.D. STROSBERG. 1998. A leptin missense mutation associated with hypogonadism and morbid obesity. Nat. Genet. **18:** 213–215.
13. COMUZZIE, A.G., J.E. HIXSON, L. ALMASY *et al.* 1997. A major quantitative trait locus determining serum leptin levels and fat mass is located on human chromosome 2. Nat. Genet. **15:** 273–276.
14. LUOH, S.M., F. DI MARCO, N. LEVIN *et al.* 1997. Cloning and characterization of a human leptin receptor using a biologically active leptin immunoadhesin. J. Mol. Endocrinol. **18:** 77–85.
15. CLEMENT, K., C. VAISSE, N. LAHLOU *et al.* 1998. A mutation in the human leptin receptor gene causes obesity and pituitary dysfunction. Nature **392:** 398–401.
16. JACKSON, R.S., J.W. CREEMERS, S. OHAGI *et al.* 1997. Obesity and impaired prohormone processing associated with mutations in the human prohormone convertase 1 gene. Nat. Genet. **16:** 303–306.
17. LEMBERTAS, A.V., L. PERUSSE, Y.C. CHAGNON *et al.* 1997. Identification of an obesity quantitative trait locus on mouse chromosome 2 and evidence of linkage to body fat and insulin on the human homologous region 20q. J. Clin. Invest. **100:** 1240–1247.
18. CHAGNON, Y.C., W.J. CHEN, L. PERUSSE, M. CHAGNON, A. NADEAU & W.O. WILKISON. 1997. Linkage and association studies between the melanocortin receptors 4 and 5 genes and obesity-related phenotypes in the Quebec Family Study. Mol. Med. **3:** 663–673.
19. FLEURY, C., M. NEVEROVA, S. COLLINS *et al.* 1997. Uncoupling protein-2: a novel gene linked to obesity and hyperinsulinemia. Nat. Genet. **15:** 269–272.
20. GOOD, D.J., F.D. PORTER, K.A. MAHON, A.F. PARLOW, H. WESTPHAL & I.R. KIRSCH. 1997. Hypogonadism and obesity in mice with a targeted deletion of the Nhlh2 gene. Nat. Genet. **15:** 397–401.
21. DUNAIF, A., K.R. SEGAL, W. FUTTERWEIT & A. DOBRJANSKY. 1989. Profound peripheral insulin resistance, independent of obesity, in polycystic ovary syndrome. Diabetes **38:** 1165–1174.
22. BALEN, A.H., G.S. CONWAY, G. KALTSAS, K. TECHATRASAK, P.J. MANNING & C. WEST. 1995. Polycystic ovary syndrome: the spectrum of the disorder in 1741 patients. Hum. Reprod. **10:** 2107–2111.
23. LEGRO, R.S. 1998. Polycystic ovary syndrome: current and future treatment paradigms. Am. J. Obstet. Gynecol. **179** (6 Part 2, Suppl. S)**:** S101-S108.
24. OVESEN, P., J. MOLLER, H.J. INGERSLEV *et al.* 1993. Normal basal and insulin-stimulated fuel metabolism in lean women with the polycystic ovary syndrome. J. Clin. Endocrinol. Metab. **77:** 1636–1640.
25. TAYLOR. A.E., B. MCCOURT, K.A. MARTIN, E.J. ANDERSON, J.M. ADAMS & D.H. SCHOENFELD. 1997. Determinants of abnormal gonadotropin secretion in clinically defined women with polycystic ovary syndrome. J. Clin. Endocrinol. Metab. **82:** 2248–2256.
26. MORALES, A.J., G.A. LAUGHLIN, T. BUTZOW, H. MAHESHWARI, G. BAUMANN & S.S.C. YEN. 1996. Insulin, somatotropic, and luteinizing hormone axes in lean and obese women with polycystic ovary syndrome: common and distinct features. J. Clin. Endocrinol. Metab. **81:** 2854–2864.
27. LEGRO, R.S., D. DRISCOLL, J.F. STRAUSS, J. FOX & A. DUNAIF. 1998. Evidence for a genetic basis for hyperandrogenemia in the polycystic ovary syndrome. Proc. Natl. Acad. Sci. USA **95:** 14956–14960
28. BRAY, G.A.1992. Genetic, hypothalamic and endocrine features of clinical and experimental obesity. Prog. Brain Res. **93:** 333–340
29. WATERWORTH, D.M., S.T. BENNETT, N. GHARANI *et al.* 1997. Linkage and association of insulin gene VNTR regulatory polymorphism with polycystic ovary syndrome. Lancet **349:** 986–990.

30. Gharani, N., D.M. Waterworth, S. Batty *et al.* 1997. Association of the steroid synthesis gene CYP11a with polycystic ovary syndrome and hyperandrogenism. Hum. Mol. Genet. **6:** 397–402.
31. Franks, S., N. Gharani, D. Waterworth, S. Batty, D. White & R. Williamson. 1997. The genetic basis of polycystic ovary syndrome. Hum. Reprod. **12:** 2641–2648.
32. Legro, R.S., R. Spielman, M. Urbanek, D. Driscoll, J. F. Strauss, 3rd & A. Dunaif. 1998. Phenotype and genotype in polycystic ovary syndrome. Rec. Prog. Horm. Res. **53:** 217–256.

Insulin Sensitizers and Antiandrogens in the Treatment of Polycystic Ovary Syndrome

E. DIAMANTI-KANDARAKIS[a] AND E. ZAPANTI

1st Department of Internal Medicine, University of Athens Medical School, Athens, Greece

ABSTRACT: The heterogeneous origin of polycystic ovary syndrome (PCOS) has been demonstrated by several studies. Abnormalities in steroidogenesis and metabolism are present, but the exact link between these two pathologic features remains to be clarified. In clinical practice, more than one therapeutic approach for the treatment of this syndrome has been proposed over the last few decades. Because hyperandrogenism and hyperinsulinemia contribute to a different degree to the phenotype of PCOS, therapeutic efforts have focused on agents that could treat or modify the clinical manifestations of these disorders. Antiandrogens as a sole treatment or combined with oral contraceptives are considered the treatment of choice for the manifestations of hyperandrogenemia, but there is no agreement about their efficacy on the metabolic sequelae of PCOS (insulin resistance, hyperinsulinemia, dislipidemia). Furthermore, the improvement of insulin sensitivity by insulin sensitizers may be of therapeutic value directly and/or indirectly in the management of clinical manifestations of hyperinsulinemia and hyperandrogenemia.

INTRODUCTION

The polycystic ovary syndrome (PCOS) is a common endocrine disorder and also extremely heterogeneous. Because of the diversity of clinical and biochemical findings, there has been much debate about whether it represents a single disorder or associated pathologic conditions. Abnormalities in steroidogenesis and metabolism are both present to a different degree, but their causative relationship remains unresolved.[1]

Insulin resistance and compensatory hyperinsulinemia are characteristic metabolic disturbances of many women with PCOS and are probably central to the pathogenesis of the syndrome since they can induce hyperandrogenism and anovulation.[2] It has been demonstrated by *in vivo* and *in vitro* studies that hyperinsulinemia stimulates ovarian androgen production and decreases the synthesis of SHBG by the liver.[3] It has also been shown that chronic hyperandrogenemia and hyperinsulinemia affect the secretion of gonadotropins in favor of an increase in luteinizing hormone and contribute to the mechanism of anovulation.[4]

In addition, women with PCOS present other metabolic disorders like dyslipidemia (elevated levels of total and low-density lipoprotein cholesterol and triglyceride, with decreases in HDL) and may be exposed in increased risk for cardiovascular disease.[5,6]

[a]Address for correspondence: E. Diamanti-Kandarakis, Zefyrou 1a, 14578 Ekali, Greece.

Obesity, which is commonly associated with PCOS, can worsen both hyperandrogenism and anovulation. Studies of obese women with menstrual abnormalities have demonstrated the resumption of normal cycling and fertility after weight loss.[7,8]

Antiandrogens alone, or more often in combination with oral contraceptives, can correct the endocrine hallmark of the syndrome which is hyperandrogenism and are considered the most accepted type of therapy.[9,10] However there is not agreement to which degree antiandrogens can correct ovarian or adrenal dysfunction and also the long term consequences of the syndrome including the metabolic sequelae.

Because hyperinsulinemia may play a role in the pathogenesis of PCOS particularly in the obese women, therapeutic efforts have focused on the efficacy of insulin sensitizing agents in the management of women with PCOS. Recently, clinical studies have been done where old and new insulin-sensitizing agents have been tried as a sole treatment of metabolic as well as reproductive dysfunction.

METFORMIN

Metformin is a biguanide that has been extensively used in Europe and Canada for several years in the management of type II diabetes. It reduces plasma glucose concentrations by an average of 25% and can be used as a monotherapy or in combination with sulfonylureas.[11]

Mechanism of Action

The mode of action of metformin has not been explained by a single mechanism, and it's likely that the drug has effects on multiple metabolic pathways. These involve the suppression of glucose output and enhanced glucose uptake by tissues. Previous studies in experimental animals[12,13] have shown that the main effect of metformin is to decrease hepatic glucose output. Regarding the action of metformin on the liver, it seems that in the absence of insulin, high concentrations of the drug are required to suppress gluconeogenesis. In contrast, when insulin is present, the two agents acting together will suppress gluconeogenesis at low concentrations.[13]

The enhancing action of metformin on glucose uptake by tissues has been confirmed by *in vitro* and *in vivo* studies. It has been shown that metformin increases glucose uptake by fat and muscle, in the presence as well as in the absence of added insulin.[14,15] Studies with glucose clamp technique have demonstrated the ability of metformin to improve insulin-stimulated glucose disposal in diabetic insulin-resistant patients.[16,17] In addition, there is evidence that metformin reduces insulin requirements in insulin-treated NIDDM and IDDM patients. However, it remains to be clarified whether metformin potentiates the action of insulin or acts as a separate factor, yet one requiring the presence of insulin to exert effects on peripheral glucose uptake.[18]

It has been shown that metformin can improve tissue sensitivity to insulin in NIDDM patients by increasing insulin receptor binding, but this effect is uncertain under physiologic concentrations of insulin.[18] *In vitro* studies in animals have shown an increase by metformin in insulin receptor phosphorylation and tyrosine kinase activity in skeletal muscle, but a similar effect has not been demonstrated in adipose tissue.[14] Nevertheless, is not clear whether the amelioration of insulin sensitivity is a direct effect of metformin or a consequence of the improvement of the metabolic status of the animal (concept of glucose toxicity). Many investigators have shown that the increase by metformin of insulin-mediated glucose uptake is mainly exerted with enhanced nonoxidative glucose metabolism.[7,19] The increase in nonoxidative metabolism includes the formation of glycogen, the incorporation of glucose into triglyceride, and the conversion of glucose to lactate in the intestine. Despite the increase of lactate production in the intestine, changes in peripheral concentrations both in the basal and postprandial states are small. In addition, lactate is reutilized as a substrate for gluconeogenesis and therefore protects against hypoglycemia.[18,20]

Metformin Effects in PCOS

Several studies have demonstrated that the treatment with metformin has a favorable effect in women with PCOS. Velazquez *et al.* have shown that the administration of metformin in women with PCOS is associated with an improvement of insulin sensitivity, with a concurrent significant decrease in levels of androgens, and with a normalization of the LH/FSH ratio.[21]

There is evidence from both clinical and in vitro studies[24,25] that in PCOS there is an increase of the ovarian cytochrome P450c17a activity, stimulated by hyperinsulinemia and resulting in excessive ovarian androgen production. Nestler and coworkers[26] found that treatment with metformin in PCOS was associated with a reduction of ovarian cytochrome P450c17a activity and therefore with an amelioration of hyperandrogenism. Other studies have demonstrated an improvement of menstrual cyclicity and fertility under metformin therapy and also a small but significant reduction in body weight.[22] The later is in contrast to the findings reported by Diamanti-Kandarakis and coworkers, who found that metformin, when administered for six months in sixteen obese women with PCOS, caused a weight-independent increase in glucose utilization rate and a decrease in androgens levels.[23] There are studies, however, that do not support the beneficial effects of metformin in PCOS, and the associated weight loss is considered to be the main factor responsible for the amelioration of the manifestations of the syndrome.[27]

In conclusion, the biochemical and clinical benefits of metformin therapy in obese PCOS outweighed the results of negative trials. Future clinical studies should include lean women with PCOS in more extended randomized trials.

Adverse Effects

The major concern with biguanides has been the risk of lactic acidosis. The incidence of metformin-related lactic acidosis is about 1/20th that related to phenformin,[28] and the risk is estimated to be 0.08 per 1000 patient years).[18] Most cases of lactic acidosis have occurred in patients with renal failure or in patients in whom the drug is contraindicated (renal and hepatic disease, hypoxic conditions, severe infection, pregnancy).[18] Malabsorption syndromes have been reported, including decreased absorption of vitamin B12, but rarely caused clinical problems.[11]

THIAZOLIDINEDIONES

Troglitazone is the first oral thiazolidinedione approved for use in treating noninsulin-dependent diabetes melitus. It combines hypolipidemic and insulin-sensitizing properties.[29] Troglitazone reduces hyperglycemia in animal models of NIDDM without stimulating insulin secretion. It has multiple therapeutic effects on glucose metabolism, including actions on hepatic glucose metabolism and peripheral insulin action. It also reduces lipid levels and systemic blood pressure.[30] With regard to the hepatic effects of troglitazone, it has been shown that in rats the drug provokes a reduction of the hepatic glucose output by increasing hepatic sensitivity to the suppressive effects of insulin.[31]

In a study of type II diabetes in humans, a decrease in basal hepatic glucose output has been demonstrated, when measured by tritiated [^{3}H]-3 glucose turnover before and after the completion of treatment with 200 mg troglitazone twice daily for 6–12 weeks.[32] Several studies have assessed the peripheral insulin effects of troglitazone. Studies in animals have shown that troglitazone stimulates GLUT1 and GLUT4 gene expression and reduces tumor necrosis factor-α (TNF-α) and hepatic glucokinase expression through activation of specific nuclear receptors termed *peroxisome proliferator-activator receptors (PRARs).*[33,34] The effect of thiazolidinediones in expression of these and probably other genes contributes to the insulin-sensitizing and lipid-lowering properties of these compounds.[30]

In vivo, several studies using euglycemic clamp technique have been conducted in the type II diabetic population in order to evaluate the peripheral action of troglitazone. It seems that the insulin-mediated glucose tissue disposal is increased by troglitazone and is unaffected by ethnicity and the degree of obesity and hyperglycemia.[32,35] In general, troglitazone has beneficial effects in obese, as well as in lean diabetics, although obese patients or patients who have high fasting plasma insulin levels may derive the greatest benefit.[36]

Referring to the action of troglitazone on lipid levels, most studies have shown a favorable effect of troglitazone in triglyceride, free fatty acid, and LDL and HDL cholesterol levels. In the study of the multicenter European Troglitazone Study Group, 330 mildly obese NIDDM patients were treated with troglitazone for 12 weeks. The doses of troglitazone were 200, 400, 600, or 800 mg once daily, or 200 or 400 mg twice daily. Interestingly, all the doses of troglitazone were equally effective in lowering glycemia, whereas lipid profile was ameliorated at the highest troglitazone doses.[37]

Troglitazone Effect in PCOS

Most studies have shown that troglitazone exerts its metabolic effects, primarily by improving insulin sensitivity and without direct effects on insulin secretion. A double-blind study conducted by Dunaif *et al.*[38] has shown beneficial effects on metabolic profile and reproductive function in women with PCOS. The findings of Dunaif were also confirmed by a study by Ehrmann *et al.*[39]

Adverse Effects

Although troglitazone seems to be well tolerated, some minor adverse effects have been reported occurring in less than 10% of patients. They include somatic complaints, and they are rapidly reversible with drug discontinuation.[30] Troglitazone has been reported to cause mild anemia and neutropenia. These abnormalities have been observed mostly within the first 4–8 weeks of therapy and might be related to the dilutional effect of troglitazone.

Liver function abnormalities have also been noted, including increases in aspartate aminotransferase (AST), alanine aminotransferase (ALT), and lactate dehydrogenase (LDH). All of these abnormalities were reversible after the discontinuation of the drug.[30]

ANTIANDROGENS

Antiandrogens play an important role in the therapy of hyperandrogenic states such as polycystic ovary syndrome. Antiandrogens include compounds that inhibit androgen synthesis (ketoconazole), inhibit 5α reductase (finasteride), or interact with the androgen receptor (AR) preventing the biologic actions of androgens on their target tissue (cyproterone acetate, spironolactone, flutamide).

Ketoconazole

Ketoconazole is an imidazole derivative used for the treatment of fungal disease. It blocks adrenal and gonadal steroid synthesis by inhibiting $P450_{SCC}$ (cholesterol side chain cleavage enzyme), $P450_c17$(17α-hydroxylase and 17,20-lyase), 3β hydroxysteroid dehydrogenase, and $P450_c11$ (11 β-hydroxylase) enzymes.[40] Although treatment with ketoconazole may have beneficial effects on hirsutism, its use is not appropriate in benign conditions like PCOS. Long-term treatment with ketoconazole suppresses cortisol synthesis and can cause severe hepatotoxicity.

Finasteride

Finasteride is 5α-reductase inhibitor that is used for the treatment of benign prostatic hyperplasia. It inhibits androgen action by decreasing the production of 5α-DHT, the most potent ligand (for AR).[41] Finasteride has no effect on the levels of circulating testosterone and gonadotropins. In one controlled study, it was shown that 5 mg finasteride daily can be as effective as 100 mg spironolactone in reducing hair shaft diameter.[42]

No side effects have been noted in women treated with finasteride, but because it can cause ambiguous genitalia in male offspring of female rats, the drug should not be taken throughout the first trimester of pregnancy. [43]

Cyproterone Acetate

Cyproterone acetate (CPA) is one of the best known steroidal antiandrogens and derives from 17-hydroxyprogesterone. It is a potent progestin and also possesses antiandrogenic and mild glucocorticoid activity.[44] It has been extensively tried in Europe and has been found to be highly effective. It is probably the best established drug for treatment of hirsutism and is also effective against acne.[44,45]

Cyproterone acetate blocks androgen action by competitive binding to the AR. It binds to the receptor with about 21% of the affinity of testosterone.[46] Antiandrogenic effects of cyproterone acetate are exerted by blocking AR at the pilocebaceous unit, as well as by reducing serum testosterone levels and decreasing 5α-reductase activity.[47]

CPA, is almost never given alone in patients with PCOS in order to avoid menstrual bleeding. It is usually given in combination with an estrogen as a contraceptive preparation (2 mg in combination with 35 or 50 mg ethinylestradiol). Although this regimen decreases hair growth in many women, higher doses are usually used to treat hirsutism. Treatment with 50 mg cyproterone acetate daily for 10 days (with an oral contraceptive) suppresses serum gonadotropins and testosterone at least as much as a GnRH analogue.[43]

Satisfactory results have been obtained with other protocols using a wide range of doses of CPA (2–100 mg/day) in combination with ethinylestradiol (20–50 mg/day). These preparations were used continuously or in a cycle fashion. With the above therapeutic regimens, 4–9 months are usually required to improve hirsutism.[48,49]

Adverse Effects

The side effects of CPA are similar to those of medroxyprogesterone acetate and include weight gain, fluid retention, mood changes, headaches, breast tenderness, and decreased libido. Some of the side effects may be due to the glucocorticoid activity of the drug.[47] CPA in combination with estrogens has mild effects on lipid profile. Slight increases in total cholesterol, HDL cholesterol, the HDL/LDL ratio, and in triglycerides have been reported.[54]

Because of the potential hepatotoxicity of the drug, monitoring of serum transaminases every 3 to 6 months is recommended. The most common reaction is a transient mild elevation of liver enzymes, but drug-induced hepatitis, although rare, has also been reported.[47]

Spironolactone

Spironolactone (SP), an antihypertensive diuretic agent, used alone or as an adjunct, has been shown to be effective in more than 70% of hyperandrogenemic hirsute patients.[51] Spironolactone acts as an androgen receptor antagonist at the hair follicle, and also decreases androgen synthesis by inhibiting the microsomal cytochrome P-450 system.[52] Furthermore, SP has a direct inhibitory effect on 5α-reductase.

Therapy with SP results in a decrease in serum concentrations of total and free testosterone without significant alterations in the levels of LH, FSH, estradiol progesterone, DHEAS, and cortisol.[52] SP improves hirsutism, acne, and seborrhea. Beneficial effects of SP have been documented at doses as low as 50 mg/day. The dose might be increased gradually in those patients who do not respond to the starting dose of 50 mg daily. Normalization of menstrual cycles has also been reported, in women with PCOS, after three months of therapy with SP.[53] SP generally must be taken for 6 to 8 months before subjective or objective findings of improvement are significant.[54]

In a recent study, lean PCOS women were treated with SP alone for 3–4 months insulin resistance was partially reversed, although it remained lower than in controls and showed no further improvement after 1 year of treatment.[46]

Adverse Effects

Initially, SP administration may cause mild diuresis, weakness, and fatigue. Occasionally, use of SP may be associated with headaches, breast enlargement and tenderness (26%), weight gain, and dizziness (26%).[10] The most common side effect of SP is irregular uterine bleeding. For this reason the drug is often given cyclically (on days 4 through 21) or combined with oral contraceptives.[55]

SP may cause a slight rise in serum potassium levels and should not be used in women with renal insufficiency. Patients under this medication should be monitored for hyperkalemia at the start of the dosage regimen and once every 6 months thereafter during treatment.[56]

Flutamide

Flutamide is the best known nonsteroidal antiandrogen used for the treatment of prostate cancer. It has been found to be effective in the treatment of skin manifestations of hyperandrogenemia, acne, and hirsutism.[10,57,58] Flutamide has about 20% of the affinity of spironolactone for the AR but is used in higher doses (150–200 mg daily).[43] Flutamide itself is a weak antiandrogen, converted upon digestion to a potent antiandrogen, 2-hydroxyflutamide.[58,59] Both flutamide and hydroxyflutamide inhibit the binding of 5α–DHT to AR and reduce nuclear translocation of the AR.[58]

Several studies have been conducted to compare the efficacy of flutamide to that of other antiandrogens. One study has shown greater improvement in hirsutism scoring with flutamide than with spironolactone.[10] Other studies have found the two drugs equally effective.[60] It has been shown that treatment with flutamide corrected the signs of hyperandrogenism (hirsutism and particularly acne) in lean and obese PCOS.[61] Flutamide has also been shown to have beneficial effects in chronic anovulation. Six months of treatment with flutamide as monotherapy restored ovulatory cycles in all young women with PCOS with normalization of ovarian volume. This observation led the authors to the suggestion that flutamide inhibits androgen synthesis.[62] A decrease in circulating androgens in women with PCOS has been also demonstrated by other authors.[46,61]

Regarding the metabolic effects, flutamide has no significant (or minimally significant) effect on insulin resistance.[61] Interestingly it seems to have a beneficial effect on lipid profile in PCOS women with no alteration of insulin sensitivity.[63]

Adverse Effects

The most common side effect of flutamide is dry skin, which is noted in 70% of patients.[10] Increased appetite and weight gain have been reported. The major concern with flutamide is a potentially fatal drug-induced liver failure that occurs in less than 0.5% of patients under this medication.[64]

REFERENCES

1. DUNAIF, A. 1997. Insulin resistance and the polycystic ovary syndrome: mechanism and implications for pathogenesis. Endocrinol. Rev. **18**(6)**:** 774–800.
2. DUNAIF, A., G. GREEN & W. FUTTERWEIT. 1990. Suppression of hyperandrogenism does not improve peripheral or hepatic insulin resistance in the polycystic ovary syndrome. J. Clin. Endocrinol. Metab. **70:** 699–704.

3. BARBIERI, R.L. 1990. The role of adipose tissue and hyperinsulinemia in the development of hyperandrogenism in women. *In* Adipose Tissue and Reproduction. R. Frisch, Ed.: 42–57. Karger. Basel.
4. CONWAY, G.S., J.W. HONOUR & H.S. JACOBS. 1989. Heterogeneity of the polycystic ovary syndrome: clinical, endocrine and ultrasound features in 556 patients. Clin. Endocrinol. (Oxford) **30:** 459–470.
5. MATTSSON, L.A., G. GULLEBERG, L. HAMBERGER, *et al.* 1984. Lipid metabolism in women with polycystic ovary syndrome: possible implications for an increased risk of coronary heart disease. Fertil. Steril. **42:** 579–584.
6. WILD, R.A., B. GRUBB & A. HARTZ. 1990. Clinical signs of androgen excess risk factors for coronary artery disease. Fertil. Steril. **54:** 255–259.
7. BATES, G.W. & N.S. WHITWORTH. 1982. Effect of body weight reduction on plasma androgens in obese, infertile women. Fertil. Steril. **38:** 406–409.
8. PIJNEBORG, R., J. ANTHONY & D.A. DAVEY. 1991. Placental bed spiral arteries in the hypertensive disorders of pregnancy. Br. J. Obstet. Gynaecol. **98:** 648–655.
9. LOBO, R.A., U. GOEBELSMANN & R. HORTON. 1983. Evidence for the importance of peripheral tissue events in the development of hirsutism in polycystic ovary syndrome. J. Clin. Endocrinol. Metab. **57:** 393–397.
10. CUSAN, L., A. DUPONT, A. BELANGER, *et al.* Treatment of hirsutism with the pure antiandrogen flutamide. J. Am. Acad. Dermatol. **23:** 462–465.
11. GROOP, L.C. 1997. Drug treatment of non-insulin-dependent diabetes mellitus. *In* Textbook of Diabetes. J. Pickup & G. Williams, Eds.: 38.8. Blackwell Scientific. Oxford, England.
12. MEYER, F., M. IPAKTCHI & H. CLAUSER. 1967. Specific inhibition of gluconeogenesis by biguanides. Nature **213:** 203–204.
13. WOLLEN, N. & C.J. BAILEY. 1988. Inibition of hepatic gluconeogenesis by metformin: synergism with insulin. Biochem. Pharmacol. **37:** 4353–4358.
14. JACOBS, D.B., G.R. HAYES, J.A. TRUGLIA & D.H. LOCKWOOD. 1986. Effects of metformin on insulin receptor tyrosine Kinase activity in rat adipocytes. Diabetologia **29:** 798–801.
15. MATTHAEI, S., A. HAMMAN, H.H. KLEIN, *et al.* 1991. Association of metformin effects to increase insulin stimulated glucose transport with potentiation of insulin induced translocation of glucose transporters from intracellular pool to plasma membrane in rat adipocytes. Diabetes **40:** 850–857.
16. REAVEN, G.M., P. JOHNSTON, C.B. HOLLENBECK, *et al.* 1992. Combined metformin–sulfanylurea treatment of patients with non-insulin dependent diabetes in fair to poor glycemic control. J. Clin. Endocrinol. Metab. **74:** 1020–1026.
17. DE FRONZO, R.A., N. BARZILAI & D. SIMONSON. 1991. Mechanism of metformin action in obese and lean non-insulin-dependent diabetic subjects. J. Clin. Endocrinol. Metab. **73:** 1294–1301.
18. BAILEY, C.J. 1993. Minireview: metformin an update. Gen. Pharmacol. **24(6):** 1299–1309.
19. JOHNSON, A.B., J.M. WEBSTER, C.F. SUM, *et al.* 1993. The impact of metformin on hepatic glucose production and skeletal muscle glycogen synthase activity in overweight type II diabetic patients. Metabolism **42:** 1217–1221.
20. STUMVOLL, M., N. NURJHAN, G. PERIELLO, *et al.* 1995. Metabolic effects of metformin in non insulin dependent diabetes mellitus. N. Engl. J. Med. **333:** 550–554.
21. VELAZQUEZ, E.M., S. MENDOZA, T. HAMER, *et al.* 1994. Metformin therapy in polycystic ovary syndrome reduces hyperinsulinemia, insulin resistance, hyperandrogenemia, and systolic blood pressure, while facilitating normal menses and pregnancy. Metabolism **43**(5)**:** 647–654.
22. VELAZQUEZ, E., A. ACOSTA & S.G. MENDOZA. 1997. Menstrual cyclicity after Metformin therapy in polycystic ovary syndrome. Obstet. Gynecol. **90**(3)**:** 392–395.
23. DIAMANTI, E., C. KOULI, T. TSIANATELLI & A. BERGIELLE. 1998. Therapeutic effects of metformin on insulin resistance and hyperandrogenism in polycystic ovary syndrome. Eur. J. Endocrinol. **138**(3)**:** 269–274.
24. GILLING-SMITH, C., D.S. WILLIS, R.W. BEARD & S. FRANKS. 1994. Hypersecretion of androstenedione by isolated thecal cells from polycystic ovaries. J. Clin. Endocrinol. Metab. **79:** 1158–1165.

25. CAREY, A.H., D. WATERWORTH, K. PATEL, *et al.* 1994. Polycystic ovaries and premature male pattern baldness are associated with one allele of the steroid metabolism gene CYP17. Hum. Mol. Genet. **3:** 1873–1876.
26. NESTLER, J.E., J.N. CLORE & W.G. BLACKARD. 1992. Effects of insulin on steroidogenesis in vivo. *In* Polycystic Ovary Syndrome. A. Dunaif, G.R. Givens, F.P. Haseltine & G.R. Merriam, Eds.: 265–268. Blackewell Scientific. Oxford, England.
27. EHRMANN, D., M. COVAGHAM, J. IMPERIAL, *et al.* 1997. Effects of metformin on insulin secretion, insulin action, and ovarian steroidogenesis in women with P.C.Os. J. Endocrinol. Metab. **82:** 524–530.
28. SIRTORI, C.R. & C. PASIK. 1994. Reevaluation of a biguanide metformin: mechanism of action and tolerability. Pharmacol. Res. **30:** 187.
29. YOSHIOKA, T., Y. AIZAWA, T. FUJITA, *et al.* 1991. Studies on hindered phenols and analogues. V. Synthesis, identification and antidiabetic activity of the glucuronide of CS-045. Chem. Pharm. Bull. **39:** 2124–2125.
30. HENRY, R. 1997. Thiazolidinedions: in current therapies for diabetes. Endocrinol. Metab. Clin. N. Am. **26**(3)**:** 553–573.
31. LEE, M.K. & J.M. OLEFSKY. 1995. Acute effects of troglitazone on in vivo insulin action in normal rats. Metabolism **44:** 1166–1169.
32. SUTER, S.L, J.J. NOLAN, P. WALLACE, *et al.* 1992. Metabolic effects of new oral hypoglycemic agent CS-045 in NIDDM subjects. Diabetes Care **15:** 193–203.
33. BAHR, M., M. SPELLEKEN, M. BOCK, *et al.* 1996. Acute and chronic effects of troglitazone (CS-045) on isolated rat ventricular cardiomyocytes. Diabetologia **39:** 766–774.
34. DE VOS, P., A-M. LEFEBVRE, S.G. MILLER, *et al.* 1996. Thiazolidinediones repress ob gene expression in rodents via activation of peroxisome proliferator-activated receptor α. J. Clin. Invest. **98:** 1004–1009.
35. MIMURA, K., F. UMEDA, S. HIRAMATSU *et al.* 1994. Effects of a new oral hypoglycaemic agent (CS-045) on metabolic abnormalities and insulin resistance in type 2 diabetes. Diabet. Med. **11:** 685–691.
36. CHEN, C. 1998. Troglitazone: an antidiabetic agent. Am. J. Health Syst. Pharm. **55**(9)**:** 905–925.
37. KUMAR, S., A.J.M. BOULTON, H. BECK-NIELSEN, *et al.* 1996. Troglitazone, an insulin action enhancer, improves metabolic control in NIDDM patients. Diabetologia **39:** 701–709.
38. DUNAIF, A., D. SCOTT, D. FINEGOOD, *et al.* 1996. The insulin-sensitizing agent troglitazone improves metabolic and reproductive abnormalities in the polycystic ovary syndrome . J. Clin. Endocrinol. Metab. **81:** 3299–3306.
39. EHRMANN, D.A., D.J. SCHNEIDER, B.E. SOBEL, *et al.* 1997. Troglitazone improves defects in insulin action, insulin secretion, ovarian steroidogenesis and fibrinolysis in women with P.C.Os J. Clin. Endocrinol. Metab. **82:** 2108–2011.
40. VENTUROLI, S., *et al.* 1990. Ketoconazole therapy for women with acne and/or hirsutism. J. Clin. Endocrinol. Metab. **71:** 335–337.
41. GROUP, TM-FS. 1991. One year experience in the treatment of benign prostatic hyperplasia with finasteride. J. Androl. **12:** 372.
42. WONG, I.L., R.S. MORRIS, L. CHANG, *et al.* 1995. A prospective randomised trial comparing finasteride to spironolactone in the treatment of hirsutism J. Clin. Endocrinol. Metab. **80:** 233–238.
43. RITTMASTER, R.S. 1995. Medical treatment of androgen-dependent hirsutism: clinical review. J. Clin. Endrinol. Metab. **80**(9)**:** 2559–2563.
44. BELISLE, S. & E.J. LOVE. 1986. Clinical efficacy and safety of cyproterone acetate in severe hirsutism: results in a multicentered Canadian study. Fertil. Steril. **46:** 1015–1020.
45. HAMMERSTEIN, J., J. MECKIES, I. LEO-ROSSBERG, *et al.* 1975. Use of cyproterone acetate (CPA) in the treatment of acne, hirsutism. and virilism. J. Steroid Biochem. **6:** 827–836.
46. MOGHETTI, P., F. TOSI, R. CASTELLO, *et al.* 1996. The insulin resistance in women with hyperandrogenism is partially reversed by antiadrogen treatment: evidence that androgens impair insulin action in women. J. Clin. Endocrinol. Metab. **81:** 952–960.

47. HUMPEL, M., H. WENDT, P.E. SCHULZE, *et al.* 1977. Bioavelability and pharmacokinetics of cyproterone acetate after oral administration of 2.0 mg cyproterone acetate in combination with 50 μg ethinyloestradiol to 6 young women. Contraception **15:** 579–582.
48. EDEN, J.A. 1991. The polycystic ovary syndrome presenting as resistant acne successfully treated with cyproterone acetate. Med. J Aust. **155:** 677–681.
49. GREENWOOD, R., L. BRUMMITT, B. BURKE & W.J. CUNLIFFE. 1983. Acne: double-blind clinical and laboratory trial of tetracycline, oestrogen-cyproterone acetate, and combined treatment. Br. Med. J. **291:** 1231.
50. STIVEL, M.S., R. KAULI, H. KAUFMAN & Z. LARON. 1982. Adrenocortical function in children with precocious sexual development during treatment with cyproterone acetate. Clin. Endocrinol. **16:** 163–166.
51. PITTAWAY, D.E. 1985. Evaluation and treatment of unresponsive hirsutism. Sex Med. Today **3:** 14–18.
52. CUMMING, D.C., J.C. YANG, R.W. REBAR, *et al.* 1982. Treatment of hirsutism with spironolactone. JAMA **247**(9)**:** 1295–1298.
53. MILEWICZ, A., D. SILBER & M.A. KIRSCHNER. 1983. Therapeutic effects of spironolactone in polycystic ovary syndrome. Obstet. Gynecol. **61**(4)**:** 42–432.
54. ADASHI, E.Y. & Z. ROSENWAKS. 1987. Hirsutism and virilization. *In* Gynecology: Principles and Practice. Z. Rosenwaks, F. Benjamin & M.L. Stone, Eds.: 611–646. Macmillan. New York.
55. HELFER, E.L., J.L. MILLER & L.I. ROSE. 1988. Side-effects of spironolactone therapy in the hirsute woman. J. Clin. Endocrinol. Metab. **66**(1)**:** 208–211.
56. STULBERG, D.L. & B.S. CARUTHERS. 1990. Hirsutism—a practical approach to improving physical and mental well-being. Postgrad. Med. **87:** 8.
57. BRODGEN, R. & P. CHRISP. 1991. Flutamide. Drugs Aging **1:** 104–107.
58. SCHULTZ, M., A. SCHMOLDT, F. DONN & H. BECKER. 1988. The pharmacokinetics of flutamide and its major metabolites after a single oral dose and during chronic treatment. Eur. J. Pharmacol. **34:** 633–635.
59. DIAMANTI, E., N. KAKLAS, J. SPINA, *et al.* 1992. Intraovarian regulators and P.C.Os. The effect of an androgen receptor blocker on gonadotropin release and androgen levels in P.C.Os. Satellite symposium of the 9th International Congress of Endocrinology, Abstr. No 79.
60. ERENUS, M., O. GURBUZ, F. DURMUSOGLU, *et al.* 1994. Comparison of the efficacy of spironolactone versus flutamide in the treatment of hirsutism. Fertil. Steril. **61:** 613–616.
61. DIAMANTI-KANDARAKIS, E., A. MITRAKOU, M.M.I. HENNES, *et al.* 1995. Insulin sensitivity and antiandrogenic therapy in women with polycystic ovary syndrome. Metabolism **44:** 525–531.
62. DEL LEO, V., D. LANZETTA, A. D'ANTONA, *et al.* 1998. Hormonal effects of flutamide in young women with polycystic ovary syndrome. J. Clin. Endocrinol. Metab. **83:** 99–102.
63. DIAMANTI-KANDARAKIS, E., A. MITRAKOU, S. RAPTIS, *et al.* 1998. The effect of a pure antiandrogen receptor blocker, flutamide, on the lipid profile in the polycystic ovary syndrome. J. Clin. Endocrinol. Metab. **83**(8)**:** 2699–2705.
64. WYSOWSKI, D.K. & J.L. FOURCROY. 1994. Safety of flutamide? Fertil. Steril. **62:** 1089–1090.

Optimizing Estrogen Replacement in Adolescents with Turner Syndrome

R.L. ROSENFIELD,[a] N. PEROVIC, AND N. DEVINE

The University of Chicago, Department of Pediatrics, 5825 S. Maryland (M/C 5053), Chicago, Illinois 60637-1470, USA

Because estrogen has a biphasic effect on growth, determining the estrogen replacement regimen that is optimal for use with growth hormone (GH) therapy has become a practical issue in the management of Turner syndrome. Designing optimal sex hormone replacement treatment involves considering the timing and route of estrogen administration as well as the form and dose of estrogen. Contraceptive doses of estrogen are known to inhibit growth.[1] We carried out a pilot study which suggests that optimal estrogen replacement should consist of a small dose of estradiol administered systemically.

We organized a multicenter study of Turner syndrome patients who had been on GH therapy for 0.5 year or more.[2] Beginning at 12–15 years of age in 9 patients, we added depot estradiol (Depo-Estradiol, estradiol cypionate) in monthly intramuscular doses of 0.2, 0.4, 0.6, and, in a subgroup of $n = 7$, 0.8 mg at successive 6-month intervals. We compared them to a matched group of 37 patients with Turner syndrome who were started on standard estrogen treatment and received a similar course of GH therapy (Genentech National Cooperative Growth Study database). To estimate standard estrogen dosage, we determined that 5 of 11 girls who took conjugated estrogen (Premarin) received 0.3 mg or more daily.

The tempo of pubertal feminization seemed normal on depot estradiol therapy. All patients advanced at least one Tanner breast stage, and only two of the nine patients menstruated during the 2-year study period.

On a combination of depot estradiol and GH treatment, height increased 2.6 cm more in 2.0 years than it did with standard estrogen therapy plus GH treatment ($p < 0.001$).[2] This difference in growth is equivalent to the gain obtained with 1 year of GH therapy.[3] With depot estradiol, bone age advanced in proportion to chronologic age, so that this difference in height indicates a gain in adult height potential. Most of the gains occurred during the first year of depot estradiol therapy, at a depot estradiol dose of 0.2–0.4 mg monthly. This is equivalent to 140–280 μg per month of estradiol itself, which is less than half the dose of ethinyl estradiol, the more potent estradiol derivative that is the active estrogen in "low-dose" oral contraceptive pills.

We conclude that the predicted height of Turner syndrome patients on GH therapy is apparently improved by very low doses of systemic estradiol (E_2) rather than customary doses of estrogen to induce puberty.

[a]Phone: 773-702-6432; fax: 773-702-0443.
robros@peds.bsd.uchicago.edu

REFERENCES

1. ROSS, J., F. CASSORLA, M. SKERDA, I. VALK, D. LORIAUX & G.J. CUTLER. 1983. A preliminary study of the effect of estrogen dose on growth in Turner's syndrome. N. Engl. J. Med. **309:** 1104–1106.
2. ROSENFIELD, R.L., N. PEROVIC, N. DEVINE, N. MAURAS, T. MOSHANG, A.W. ROOT & J.P. SY. 1998. Optimizing estrogen replacement treatment in Turner syndrome. Pediatr. **102:** 486–488.
3. ROSENFELD, R.G., J. FRANE, K.M. ATTIE *et al.* 1992. Six-year results of a randomized prospective trial of human growth hormone and oxandrolone in Turner syndrome. J. Pediatr. **121:** 49–55.

Contraception in Women at High Risk or with Established Cardiovascular Disease

CHRISTOS PITSAVOS,[a] CHRISTODOULOS STEFANADIS, AND PAVLOS TOUTOUZAS

Cardiology Department, Hippokration Hospital, University of Athens, Greece

ABSTRACT: Oral contraceptives are one of the most effective and widely used reversible contraceptive methods. Over 90 million women worldwide, including over 44 million in developing countries, are now using oral contraceptives. Despite their advantages, there is concern about the links between combined oral contraceptives and the risk of cardiovascular disease. The risk attributable to oral contraceptive use in women <35 years of age is small, even if they smoke, but there are substantially increased risks in older women who both smoke and use oral contraceptives. Differences between oral contraceptive types in the relative risk of venous thromboembolism contribute little to the total cardiovascular mortality associated with oral contraceptive use, even though the total number of cardiovascular events is increased. It is important to consider the user's age and smoking status when determining oral contraceptive-attributable risks. Hormonal oral contraceptives have changed and now contain lower doses of estrogen and progestagen.

INTRODUCTION

Combined oral contraceptives containing ethinyl estradiol and a progestin have emerged worldwide as one of the most popular forms of family planning. Clearly, prescribers consider the benefits of this extraordinarily reliable method to outweigh the risks, a confidence that withstands periodic "pill scares" over breast cancer or venous thrombosis.[1] With increasing experience, we have learned that hormonal methods are safer than initially thought, particularly with the lower dose formulations currently prescribed. Furthermore, the pill offers many noncontraceptive health benefits; and although progestins, in contraceptive doses, have a slight adverse impact on the lipoprotein profile, there has been no parallel increase in clinical cardiovascular disease.[2]

Oral contraceptives are among the most effective and widely used reversible contraceptive methods. Thromboembolic disease associated with the use of oral contraceptives has been widely reported. In recent years, attempts to understand the pathogenesis of oral contraceptive–induced thromboembolic disease have found a correlation between larger estrogen doses and increased risk for a thrombotic event. Because the newer triphasic oral contraceptives provide effective contraception with a method of administration that mimics normal hormonal fluctuations during the

[a]Address for correspondence: Christos Pitsavos, M.D., 86 Pellis Str., 15234 Chalandri, Athens, Greece. Phone: 6008114; fax: 7784590.

menstrual cycle, some prescribers may infer that these products are associated with a decreased incidence of adverse effects over alternative oral contraceptives.[3]

CARDIOVASCULAR DISEASE

Over 90 million women worldwide, including over 44 million in developing countries, are now using oral contraceptives. Despite their advantages, there is concern about the links between combined oral contraceptives and the risk of cardiovascular disease. Although most contraceptive users are healthy with a low background incidence of major disease, the very large number of women using oral contraceptives throughout the world means that even modest elevations in risk have the potential to affect a large number of women. Possible biological mechanisms for the effects of combined oral contraceptives on cardiovascular disease include the interplay between lipoprotein metabolism; humoral regulators such as insulin, coagulation, and fibrinolysis; the products of the endothelium of blood vessels; and the renin–angiotensin–aldosterone system. These factors may predict, for individual women, an increased risk of cardiovascular effects with use of different hormonal contraceptives. Whether the various compositions of combined oral contraceptives have different risk profiles for cardiovascular disease should be assessed carefully.[4]

Mortality rates for cardiovascular diseases are very low in women of reproductive age. Myocardial infarction mortality rates rise from <0.4 per 100,000 woman-years at age 15–24 years to the range 2 to 7 per 100,000 woman-years at age 35–44 years. Stroke mortality rates similarly rise steeply with age and are between 3 and 5 times higher than those for myocardial infarction. The increased risk of stroke and myocardial infarction dominate the patterns of mortality in oral contraceptives users and smokers. The additional risks attributable to smoking are greater than the additional risks attributable to oral contraceptives use. The risk attributable to oral contraceptives use in women <35 years of age is small, even if they smoke, but there are substantially increased risks in older women who both smoke and use oral contraceptives. The additional mortality attributable to oral contraceptive use can be reduced by screening users, as this results in lower relative risks of ischemic stroke and myocardial infarction. Differences between oral contraceptive types regarding the relative risk of venous thromboembolism contribute little to the total cardiovascular mortality associated with oral contraceptive use, even though the total number of cardiovascular events is increased. A potential reduction in the risk of myocardial infarction with desogestrel- and gestodene- compared with levonorgestrel-containing oral contraceptives would have little difference on overall mortality rates in women in their 20s and 30s, but it may result in a net reduction in oral contraceptive-attributable mortality in women aged 40–44 years who smoke. An overall quantification of the risks for different types of oral contraceptive users is necessary for an informed choice of contraceptive method, and any assessment of the balance of cardiovascular risks is complex. It is important to consider the user's age and smoking status when determining oral contraceptive–attributable risks.[5]

The attitudes of gynecologists from 11 European centers provided guidance in contraception to women at high risk of developing cardiovascular disease and women with cardiovascular disease. In women with venous thrombosis, deep venous thrombosis, coagulation disorders, and stroke, it is preferable to prescribe methods other than combined oral contraceptives. A history of myocardial infarction was considered a relative contraindication and some experts suggested that, in some cases, the use of third-generation combined oral contraceptives may be possible. Combined oral contraceptives were not recommended in women with severe cardiovascular disease and in those over 35 years of age with light or moderate cardiovascular disease, heavy smokers (over 20 cigarettes per day), or those presenting with severe hyperlipidemia. The pill is not considered appropriate for women with clinically established cardiovascular diseases or in cases where more than two coronary risk factors exist. Combined oral contraceptive may safely be given to women with elevated blood pressure as long as it is lower than 160/100 mmHg, in cases of light and moderate cardiovascular disease as long as the patient is less than 35 years of age, in women who are not heavy smokers, in the presence of a mild or moderate degree of hyperlipidemia, and in uncomplicated diabetes mellitus provided that there are no additional risk factors. In these cases, third-generation combined oral contraceptives are preferred. The cooperation of the cardiologist is desirable in order to classify cardiovascular disease and for the patient's follow-up.[6]

Based on combined data from Africa, Asia, Europe, and Latin America collected in the World Health Organization Collaborative Study, odds ratios for cardiovascular disease combined, strokes, venous thromboembolism, and acute myocardial infarction were calculated. Among 3697 cardiovascular disease cases (59% stroke, 31% venous thromboembolism, and 10% acute myocardial infarction), 53, 37, and 13 women, respectively, were current users of oral and injectable progestogen-only and combined injectable contraceptives. Overall, the adjusted odds ratios for all cardiovascular disease combined compared with nonusers of any type of steroid hormone contraceptive associated with current use of oral and injectable progestogen-only contraceptives and combined injectable contraceptives, respectively, were 1.14 (95% CI: 0.79–1.63), 1.02 (0.68–1.54), and 0.95 (0.49–1.86). No significant changes in odds ratios were apparent for strokes, venous thromboembolism, or acute myocardial infarction in association with any of these types of contraception. However, a small, nonsignificant increase in odds ratios for venous thromboembolism was apparent in association with oral and injectable progestogen-only contraceptives. Although limited by the small number of cases and control subjects using the types of contraceptives under investigation, these data suggest that there is little or no increased risk of stroke, venous thromboembolism, or acute myocardial infarction associated with the use of oral or injectable progestogen-only or combined injectable contraceptives. However, further investigation into a possible adverse effect on stroke risk of progestogen-only contraceptives used by women with a history of high blood pressure are indicated.[7]

Primary care physicians, especially obstetrician/gynecologists, have a pivotal role to play in the reduction of cardiovascular disease. Behavior modification is the key to integrating prevention into the regular annual visit.[8]

HYPERTENSION

Premenopausal women have a lower incidence of hypertension than do postmenopausal women. Nevertheless, premenopausal women can be hypertensive, and this is an important factor in selecting a contraceptive method. Among women with a history of hypertension, odds ratios for stroke, as compared with that for nonusers of any type of steroid hormone contraceptive with no history of hypertension, rose from 7.2 (6.1–8.5) among nonusers of any type of steroid hormone contraceptive to 12.4 (4.1–37.6) among current users of all oral progestogens.[7] Women who were current users of oral contraceptives and had a history of hypertension (detected before the current period of oral contraceptive use, but not during pregnancy) had a substantially increased risk (10-fold to 15-fold) of hemorrhagic stroke compared with women who did not use oral contraceptives and had no history of hypertension.[9] A possible mechanism for the oral contraceptive-induced increase in blood pressure might be an exaggerated response of renin substrate to pharmacologic estrogen, resulting in elevated plasma renin levels. However, oral contraceptive-induced hypertension cannot be explained by this mechanism alone because similar elevations in renin substrate have been noted in normotensive and hypertensive oral contraceptive users.[10,11]

Ambulatory blood pressure levels in mild (stage 1) hypertensive women using oral contraceptives were compared with respective values in nonusers of oral contraceptives with similar office blood pressure. No significant differences in ambulatory diastolic blood pressure between the two groups were found. Hypertensive oral contraceptive users with the same office blood pressure as that in hypertensive noncontraceptive users have a significantly higher ambulatory systolic blood pressure. Alternative methods of contraception should be considered for hypertensive women in place of oral contraceptives.[12]

DIABETES MELLITUS

Diabetes mellitus is a serious chronic illness. It affects approximately 16 million people in the United States, half of whom are undiagnosed. The prevalence of non-insulin-dependent diabetes is higher in women than in men, and more women die each year from diabetes than from breast cancer. Its complications, retinopathy, nephropathy, neuropathy, and cardiovascular disease, exact a heavy toll on the individual with diabetes, as well as on society. Because of its significant morbidity and mortality in women, diabetes deserves a place in the concerns designated "women's health issues." It deserves more research attention and especially more public awareness, because many of its devastating complications can be prevented by improved detection and control.[13] If the disease is well controlled, oral contraceptives containing the lowest possible dose of ethinyl estradiol together with a third-generation progestin would be suitable, but only if the woman does not smoke.[14] Close monitoring of insulin requirements and glucose levels is mandatory.

THROMBOEMBOLISM

The effect on the risk of venous thromboembolism, ischemic and hemorrhagic stroke, and myocardial infarction differs and is strongly influenced by smoking and the presence of other cardiovascular risk factors, such as hypertension and diabetes mellitus. The incidence of each disease rises with age, and there are differences in risk among different hormonal contraceptive preparations.[5] Venous thromboembolism mortality rates rise less steeply with age and are approximately one-tenth the myocardial infarction mortality rates at age 35–44 years. The adverse effect of oral contraceptives on the risk of venous thromboembolism is the most important contributor to the total number of cardiovascular cases attributable to oral contraceptive use.[5]

Current users of low-estrogen dose combined oral contraceptives containing desogestrel or gestodene appear to be at higher risk of venous thromboembolism than users of combined oral contraceptives containing levonorgestrel. The possibility that these unexpected results on a secondary study objective are due to chance, bias, or residual confounding cannot be excluded entirely; and the results need to be confirmed by independent studies. They are at variance with the apparently more favorable metabolic effects of the newer progestagens.[15]

A multinational hospital-based case-control study of the risk of venous thromboembolic disease associated with combined oral contraceptives done in 1989–1993 prompted a separate inquiry comparing the risk of venous thromboembolism associated with low-estrogen (<35 μg ethinylestradiol) oral contraceptives containing levonorgestrel with risks in low-estrogen preparations containing the third-generation progestagens desogestrel or gestodene. This analysis of data from nine countries involved 769 cases and 1979 age-matched hospital controls and, in one center, 246 community controls matched by age and general practice.[15]

COAGULATION

The cumulative thrombotic risk of factor V (FV) Leiden and oral contraceptives (OC) leads to a recommendation that screening for the mutation be performed. Assuming that a family history of thrombosis increases the patient's likelihood of bearing factor V Leiden, a selective rather than universal screening would be performed. Factor V Leiden carriers, both heterozygotes and homozygotes, do not suffer from thromboembolism earlier than patients without the mutation. Family history is an unreliable criterion to detect factor V Leiden carriers. Screening for factor V Leiden can be worthwhile even if the advantages of oral contraception are assessed as higher than the thrombotic risk. Affected women who were aware of their additional risk could contribute to the prevention of thrombosis in risk situations.[16]

Venous thrombosis represents a manifestation of disordered hemostatic balance. The classical presentation is of pain and swelling of the lower limb, although clinical history and examination are notoriously misleading in reaching a diagnosis. A number of acquired predispositions have been associated with a tendency toward thrombosis, for example, immobilization, surgery, malignancy, and certain types of oral contraception, but in at least half of the instances no predisposition can be identified. A variety of genetic risk factors have also been identified. Mutations within the genes for antithrombin, protein C, and protein S are associated with a venous thromboembolic phenotype. The commonest thrombophilic predisposition, however, is a variant of coagulation factor V, factor V Leiden, which results from a single amino acid substitution rendering the factor V molecule resistant to activated protein C. Factor V Leiden is present in approximately 5% of individuals of European origin and is found in up to 40% of those with confirmed venous thrombosis. Increasingly, it is recognized that venous thrombosis should be considered a polygenic disorder, with interactions between the various single gene defects that predispose an individual to thrombosis, as well as normal genetic variation between persons in the levels of both procoagulant and anticoagulant proteins, all determining which individuals will express the phenotype of venous thrombosis.[17]

Sickle cell disease is an incurable, debilitating disease affecting the Afro-Caribbean population. The combined oral contraceptive pill, an effective and popular method of contraception, is often denied to women with sickle cell disease for fear that the disease process may have a synergistic effect on the coagulation changes associated with contraceptive steroids. Therapeutic concentrations of estradiol and progesterone did not appear to influence red cell deformability in women with sickle cell disease or normal AA hemoglobin.[18]

STROKE

The rate of stroke in young women has been falling for some years. The relative risk associated with oral contraceptive use also is falling. This is probably due to a combination of younger age at use of oral contraceptives, lower steroid dose of preparations, and more systematic screening of potential users, particularly with respect to blood pressure. The risk associated with oral contraceptive use is greater for occlusive stroke but increases with age in hemorrhagic stroke. Risk of occlusive stroke increases with increasing doses of estrogen. The evidence for risk related to type or dose of progestogen is less consistent, but there is no support for an increase in risk associated with use of desogestrel or gestodene.[19]

The risk of hemorrhagic stroke associated with use of oral contraceptives is less well established than that for ischemic stroke. WHO reported a collaborative, case-control study, in which the association between risk of hemorrhagic stroke and use of combined OCs in 1068 cases, aged 20–44 years, and 2910 age-matched controls has been assessed. We also assessed risks for all strokes combined (hemorrhagic, ischemic, and unclassified) based on 2198 cases and 6086 controls. Overall, current use of combined oral contraceptives was associated with slightly increased risk of hemorrhagic stroke; the increase was significant in the developing countries (odds ratio 1.76 [95% CI 1.34–2.30]) but not in Europe (1.38 [0.84–2.25]). Use of oral contraceptives in women younger than 35 years did not affect risk of hemorrhagic stroke in either group of countries, whereas in women aged older than 35 years, odds ratios were greater than 2. Odds ratios among current oral contraceptive users who were also current cigarette smokers were greater than 3. In both groups of countries, past use of oral contraceptives, dose of estrogen, and dose and type of progestagen had no effect on risk; and risks were similar for subarachnoid and intracerebral hemorrhage. The odds ratios for any type of stroke associated with current use of low-dose (<50 μg estrogen) and higher dose oral contraceptives were 1.41 (0.90–2.20) and 2.71 (1.70–4.32), respectively, in Europe and 1.86 (1.49–2.33) and 1.92 (1.48–2.50) in the developing countries. From these data, we estimated that about 13% and 8% of all strokes in women aged 20–44 in Europe and the developing countries, respectively, are attributable to the use of oral contraceptives. The risk of hemorrhagic stroke attributable to oral contraceptive use is not increased in younger women and is only slightly increased in older women. The estimated excess risk of all stroke types associated with use of low-estrogen and higher estrogen dose oral contraceptives in Europe was about two and eight, respectively, per 100,000 woman-years of oral contraceptive use. However, findings need to be considered within the context of other risks and benefits associated with oral contraceptive use, as well as those associated with the use of other forms of contraception.[9]

Hormonal oral contraceptives have changed and now contain lower doses of estrogen and progestagen. In an international study the risk of oral contraceptive–associated first stroke in women from Europe and other countries throughout the world has been assessed. The diagnosis of ischemic stroke was almost exclusively based on computed tomography, magnetic resonance imaging, or cerebral angiography carried out within 3 weeks of the clinical event. All cases and controls were interviewed while in hospital with the same questionnaire, which included information on medical and personal history, details of lifetime contraceptive use, and blood-pressure measurements before the most recent episode of oral contraceptives use. The incidence of ischemic stroke is low in women of reproductive age and any risk attributable to oral contraceptive use is small. The risk can be further reduced if users are younger than 35 years, do not smoke, do not have a history of hypertension, and have blood pressure measured before the start of oral contraceptive use. In such women oral contraceptive preparations with low estrogen doses may be associated with even lower risk.[20]

MYOCARDIAL INFARCTION

Estrogens and progestins for contraception or hormonal replacement therapy are widely used by practitioners. These steroids have substantial effects on lipids and lipoproteins that appear to be primarily related to chemical structure of the compound, dosage, and a patient's hormonal status. Although the mechanisms by which alterations in lipid and lipoproteins affect atherogenesis are not fully understood, epidemiologic studies clearly associate alterations with risk of coronary heart disease. Attention to these alterations by progestins and estrogens, as well as further research on how these steroids may exert other cardiovascular effects, is important because atherosclerotic heart disease is a major cause of morbidity and mortality for women as they age.[21]

Use of oral contraception is associated with increased risk of ischemic stroke and increased risk of myocardial infarction (only in heavy smokers), but no increased risk of angina. These increased risks need to be considered within the context of the very low absolute risks of cardiovascular disease in a population of 17 family planning clinics in England and Scotland. The population consisted of 17,032 women aged between 25 and 39 years at entry to the study. Five thousand eight hundred eighty women need to take oral contraception for one year to cause one extra stroke, and 1060 women who are heavy smokers need to take it for one year to cause one extra myocardial infarction.[22]

The association between oral contraceptive use and acute myocardial infarction (AMI) was established in studies from northern Europe and the United States, which took place during the 1960s and 1970s. In a hospital-based case-control study, the association between a first AMI and current oral contraceptive use in women from Africa, Asia, Europe, and Latin America (21 centers) was examined. The overall odds ratio for acute myocardial infarction was 5.01 (95% CI 2.54–9.90) in Europe and 4.78 (2.52–9.07) in the non-European (developing) countries; however, these risk estimates reflect the frequent coexistence of other risk factors among oral contraceptive users who have acute myocardial infarction. Very few acute myocardial infarctions were identified among women who had no cardiovascular risk factors and who reported that their blood pressure had been checked before oral contraceptive use; odds ratios associated with oral contraceptive use in such women were not increased in either Europe or the developing countries. Among oral contraceptive users who smoked 10 or more cigarettes per day, the odds ratios in Europe and in the developing countries were over 20. Similarly, among oral contraceptive users with a history of hypertension (during pregnancy or at any other time), odds ratios were at least 10 in both groups of countries. No consistent association between odds ratios for acute myocardial infarction and age of oral contraceptive users or estrogen dose was apparent in either group of countries. No significant increase in odds ratios was apparent with increasing duration of oral contraceptive use among current users, and odds ratios were not significantly increased in women who had stopped using oral contraceptives, even after long exposure. The study had insufficient power to examine whether progestagen dose or type had any effect on acute myocardial infarction risk. Current use of combined oral contraceptives is associated with an increased risk of acute myocardial infarction among women with known cardiovascular risk factors and among those who have not been effectively screened, particularly for blood pressure. Acute myocardial infarction is extremely rare in younger (<35 years), non-smoking women who use oral contraceptives, and the estimated excess risk of acute myocardial infarction in such women in the European centres is about 3 per 10(6) woman-years. The risk is likely to be even lower if blood pressure is screened before, and presumably during, oral contraceptive use. Only among older women who smoke is the degree of excess risk associated with oral contraceptives substantial (about 400 per 10(6) woman-years).[23]

MITRAL VALVE PROLAPSE

Mitral valve prolapse is defined as a displacement of the mitral leaflets in a posterior and superior direction relative to their normal position in systole. The main risk is that of bacterial endocarditis in patients with structural abnormality of the mitral valve, which can lead to chordal rupture, increased mitral insuficiency, and congestive heart failure. Whereas most women do not have symptoms, one study found that patients with mitral valve prolapse who experienced cerebrovascular insufficiency while taking oral contraceptives showed a reduction in platelet survival time.[24] In general, oral contraceptives can be safely used by women with mitral valve prolapse as long as they are without symptoms other than anxiety. At present, oral contraceptive use among patients with mitral valve prolapse is limited to those with an echocardiographically confirmed diagnosis but no mitral regurgitation. Specifically, oral contraceptives should not be used by patients who smoke or by women who have symptoms. In women who have experienced thrombotic complications, it may be advisable to perform coagulation screening. If abnormalities are discovered in blood clotting factors, other methods of contraception should be considered.[10]

PATHOPHYSIOLOGICAL CONSIDERATIONS

The possible pathophysiologic mechanisms for the association of oral contraceptives with vascular disease, including effects on coagulation, circulating lipoproteins, and glucose metabolism is reviewed. The new, low-dose estrogen oral contraceptives appear to affect coagulation minimally, and anticoagulant as well as procoagulant effects have been documented. Such concomitant factors as cigarette smoking, obesity, a family history of thrombosis, lack of physical activity, and blood type influence coagulation more strongly. Myocardial infarction and stroke are strongly correlated with the levels and pattern of circulating lipoproteins. The estrogen components of oral contraceptives have a favorable effect on lipids, whereas the effect of progestins, particularly potent androgenic progestins, is unfavorable and could be significant. Oral contraceptives containing high-dose androgenic progestins can produce abnormal glucose tolerance resulting in increased cardiovascular risk. Low-dose oral contraceptives are associated with early, transient breakthrough bleeding. However, educating patients in the management of breakthrough bleeding can help reduce the number of women who must be switched to higher dose oral contraceptives. Epidemiologic evidence confirms the safety of low-dose oral contraceptives. By selecting patients carefully, the risk of vascular disease from oral contraception can be reduced to very low levels.[25]

The mechanism of the vascular complications related to oral contraception is still unclear. Three mechanisms are discussed: (a) the possibility of accelerated atherosclerosis, suggested by the presence of a number of risk factors, a hypothesis that is not confirmed by pathological findings; (b) the possibility of a coagulation disease leading to thrombosis; and (c) the arguments in favor of an immunological mechanism. This hypothesis is supported by the strong correlation between vascular complications and presence of antibodies against the synthetic hormones contained in the drug. It is also consistent with the aspect of the lesions that might be induced by circulating immune complexes and antibodies. It is proposed that women at risk should be detected by systematic determination of antiethinylestradiol antibodies.[26]

MENOPAUSE

Despite the obvious predominance of coronary heart disease in middle-aged men, cardiovascular disease including coronary heart disease and cerebrovascular accidents is currently the major cause of death in women (54% cardiovascular mortality, 46% coronary mortality; 28% of all deaths). Before menopause, coronary heart disease is infrequent, which suggests that female hormones and metabolism offer protection. Without hormone replacement therapy after menopause, women may develop coronary atherosclerosis. Aging is among the nonmodifiable risk factors for coronary heart disease in women, whereas genetic predisposition and environmental factors remain controversial. The modifiable risk factors are mostly common to both sexes and include heavy cigarette smoking (especially in women under oral contraception) dyslipidemia, high blood pressure, and diabetes; some factors are peculiar to women. The delayed onset of coronary heart disease in women, roughly 10 years later than in men, and greater female longevity (81 years vs. 74 in men on average) points to the potential benefit of post-menopause hormone replacement therapy together with reduction of other modifiable risk factors. After menopause, the protective HDL cholesterol decreases, whereas high LDL cholesterol, high triglycerides, and high blood pressure are major risk factors for coronary heart disease as well as for cerebrovascular accident. The role of hormone replacement therapy in the prevention of cardiovascular disease in women is still controversial despite the results of meta-analyses that suggest a 25% to 44% reduction in coronary heart disease following estrogen therapy alone or in combination with progestogen, depending on the hormonal regime. Menopause, now considered as the marker for the end of natural protection against coronary heart disease, should be followed by early and prolonged combined hormone replacement therapy in order to reduce the low compliance with long-term hormone replacement therapy.[27]

The aorta is a potential target for an estrogen effect, because estrogen receptors have been demonstrated in aortic tissue of several species. The aorta of postmenopausal women with documented coronary artery disease is characterized by impaired elasticity compared to postmenopausal women without coronary artery disease. Intravenous 17β-estradiol produced an improvement of the elastic properties of the aorta in menopausal women both with and without coronary artery disease. Furthermore, 17β-estradiol led to reduced wave reflection in the arterial periphery indicating peripheral vasodilation.[28]

CONTRACEPTIVE SELECTION

The most frequent major adverse effect of hormonal contraception is an increased risk of cardiovascular disease. The side effects of oral contraceptives can be minimized by appropriate oral contraceptive selection. Side effects or perceived side effects that manifest themselves physically (e.g., weight gain, breakthrough bleeding, nausea, headache, breast tenderness, mood swings, acne, and hirsutism) are the most common causes of premature discontinuation of oral contraception. The relative androgenicity of the progestin component of combination oral contraceptives has become an important differential in selecting oral contraceptive formulations. Several studies have indicated that preparations with less androgenic potential can minimize some of the "physical" side effects and adverse metabolic effects traditionally associated with oral contraception. Acne and hirsutism, common preexisting conditions that are clearly related to the androgenicity of the progestin component, can be eliminated or improved by use of oral contraceptives with low androgenic activity. Many women perceive that oral contraceptives cause weight gain; although weight gain is to some extent androgen related, most studies comparing low-androgenic oral contraceptives with medium- or high-androgenic preparations have found little or no change in weight regardless of formulation. Breakthrough bleeding, which usually subsides within a few months, is related to the dose, potency, and ratio of the estrogen and progestin in the oral contraceptive formulation. Low-estrogen-dose oral contraceptives (≤35 μg ethinyl estradiol) containing fewer androgenic progestins are associated with bleeding patterns that are as acceptable as older low-estrogen-dose formulations. The same analysis found that smoking cigarettes promotes breakthrough bleeding in women who use oral contraceptives. There is no convincing evidence that the use of one progestin or another is less likely to cause or exacerbate headache; however, changing preparations sometimes reduces the incidence. Women with persistent headaches during the pill-free interval may benefit from a longer cycle of oral contraceptive treatment. Nausea and breast tenderness are primarily estrogen-related effects; if a women experiences persistent nausea, switching to an oral contraceptive formulation containing 20 μg ethinyl estradiol may be appropriate as long as the patient is cautioned that breakthrough bleeding is more likely. Mood changes are a common, highly subjective complaint whose relationship to oral contraceptives use is hard to assess. Concerns about the potentially deleterious effects of combination oral contraceptives on lipid/lipoprotein and carbohydrate metabolism have been substantially diminished by new epidemiologic findings relative to cardiovascular disease as well as by the development of low-androgenic progestins. Formulations containing these progestins lower LDL cholesterol and increase HDL cholesterol; they do not affect carbohydrate metabolism as much as older, more androgenic formulations.[29]

Injectable contraceptions appeal to women who value the efficacy, convenience, and safety provided by this reversible birth control option. Since FDA approval for contraceptive use in 1992, depot medroxyprogesterone acetate—already used by millions of women worldwide—has been used by several million women in the United States. Although women using this 3-month progestin-only injectable often experience irregular bleeding and spotting (initially), long-term depot medroxyprogesterone acetate use typically results in amenorrhea. Many users, including adolescents, choose depot medroxyprogesterone acetate because of its convenience—nearly 100% contraceptive effectiveness is achieved with four injections per year. Because depot medroxyprogesterone acetate does not contain estrogen, it represents an appropriate contraceptive choice for postpartum or lactating women, as well as those whose medical status precludes use of contraceptive doses of estrogen. Some examples include: women over age 35 who smoke, those with increased thromboembolism risk, women with cardiovascular or liver disease, and women with complex migraines. Although fertility resumes, on the average, 10 months after the last injection, suppression of ovulation occasionally persists for as long as 22 months. Consequently, depot medroxyprogesterone acetate is not an appropriate choice for women who may wish to conceive within the next two years. Because the use of depot medroxyprogesterone acetate lowers ovarian estradiol production, reversible loss of bone mineral density may occur. Studies currently in progress may clarify its long-term impact, if any, on bone mineral density. Therapeutic uses of depot medroxyprogesterone acetate include treatment of dysmenorrhea, menorrhagia (including that associated with fibroid uterine tumors), endometriosis, endometrial hyperplasia, ovulatory pain, pain associated with ovarian adhesive disease, premenstrual dysphoria, and perimenopausal symptoms.[30,31]

CONCLUSIONS

Women with hypertension, angina pectoris, or mitral valve prolapse require special considerations when selecting an appropriate method of contraception. All three effective, reversible options (oral contraceptives, intrauterine devices, or progestin implants) carry some degree of added risk for these patient populations. However, pregnancy itself presents certain risks and, in the event of contraceptive failure, certain women with these disorders are at increased risk of developing serious cardiovascular sequelae that affect both mother and fetus. These negative effects can carry far into the neonatal period.[10]

Concerns regarding thrombotic complications of oral contraceptives use have lessened considerably during the past 20 years. This remarkable change may reflect both decreased estrogen content of modern preparations and the use of case-control study design to assess relative risk. The thrombotic risks associated with current formulations of oral contraceptives are minimal and probably are negligible for myocardial infarction and stroke. The incidence of pill-associated thromboembolic disease is much lower than thought in the past and may be significantly lower than the thrombotic risk associated with pregnancy. Smoking remains a major risk factor for thrombotic complications in both women and men and should be actively discouraged in women who take oral contraceptives.[27] Although contraceptive choices are sometimes difficult in high-risk individuals with medical illness, it must be remembered that the risk of pregnancy is often much greater than the risks associated with contraceptive use.[28]

ACKNOWLEDGMENTS

The contribution of John Dernellis, M.D., to this work is gratefully acknowledged by the authors.

REFERENCES

1. Crook, D., N. Hampton & I. Godsland. 1997. Oral contraceptives and heart disease. *In* Women and Heart Disease. D.G. Julian & N.K. Wenger, Eds.: 265–277. Martin Dunitz, Ltd. London.
2. Plourd, D.M. 1996. Contraceptive options for perimenopausal women. Medscape Womens Health **1**(9)**:** 2.
3. Miwa, L.J., A.L. Edmunds, M.S. Shaefer & S.C. Raynor. 1989. Idiopathic thromboembolism associated with triphasic oral contraceptives. DICP **23**(10)**:** 773–775.
4. World Health Organization. 1998. Cardiovascular disease and steroid hormone contraception. Report of a WHO Scientific Group. World Health Organ Tech. Rep. Ser. **877:** i–vii; 1–89.
5. Farley, T.M., J. Collins & J.J. Schlesselman. 1998. Hormonal contraception and risk of cardiovascular disease. An international perspective. Contraception **57**(3)**:** 211–230.
6. Creatsas, G., C. Pitsavos, J.J. Amy, *et al.* 1996. A multicenter European survey of the attitudes to contraception in women at high risk or with established cardiovascular disease. Eur. J. Contracept. Reprod. Health Care **1**(3)**:** 267–273.
7. World Health Organization. 1998. Cardiovascular disease and use of oral and injectable progestogen-only contraceptives and combined injectable contraceptives. Results of an international, multicenter, case-control study. World Health Organization Collaborative Study of Cardiovascular Disease and Steroid Hormone Contraception. Contraception **57**(5)**:** 315–324.
8. Wild, R.A., E.L. Taylor & A. Knehans. 1994. The gynecologist and cardiovascular disease: a window of opportunity for prevention. J. Soc. Gynecol. Investig. **1**(2): 107–117.
9. World Health Organization. 1996. Haemorrhagic stroke, overall stroke risk, and combined oral contraceptives: results of an international, multicentre, case-control study. WHO Collaborative Study of Cardiovascular Disease and Steroid Hormone Contraception. Lancet **348**(9026)**:** 505–510.

10. SULLIVAN, J.M. & R.A. LOBO. 1993. Considerations for contraception in women with cardiovascular disorders. Am. J. Obstet. Gynecol. **168:** 2006–2011.
11. 1993. The fifth report of the Joint National Committee on Detection, Evaluation, and Treatment of High Blood Pressure. Arch. Intern. Med. **153:** 154–183.
12. NARKIEWICZ, K., G.R. GRANIERO, D. D'ESTE, *et al.* 1995. Ambulatory blood pressure in mild hypertensive women taking oral contraceptives. A case-control study. Am. J. Hypertens. **8**(3)**:** 249–253.
13. WISHNER, K.L. 1996. Diabetes mellitus: its impact on women. Int. J. Fertil. Menopausal Stud. **41**(2)**:** 177–186.
14. SKOUBY, S.O., L. MOLSTED-PEDERSEN & K. PETERSEN. 1993. Contraception for women with diabetes. Clin. Obstet. Gynecol. **168:** 2012–2020.
15. WORLD HEALTH ORGANIZATION. 1995. Effect of different progestagens in low oestrogen oral contraceptives on venous thromboembolic disease. World Health Organization Collaborative Study of Cardiovascular Disease and Steroid Hormone Contraception. Lancet **346**(8990)**:** 1582–1588.
16. SCHAMBECK, C.M., S. SCHWENDER, I. HAUBITZ, *et al.* 1997. Selective screening for the factor V Leiden mutation: is it advisable prior to the prescription of oral contraceptives? Thromb. Haemost. **78**(6)**:** 1480–1483.
17. APPLEBY, R.D. & R.J. OLDS. 1997. The inherited basis of venous thrombosis. Pathology **29**(4)**:** 341–347.
18. YOONG, W.C., S.M. TUCK & A. YARDUMIAN. 1998. The effect of ovarian steroids on sickle cell deformability. Clin. Lab. Haematol. **20**(3)**:** 151–154.
19. THOROGOOD, M. 1998. Stroke and steroid hormonal contraception. Contraception **57**(3)**:** 157–167.
20. WORLD HEALTH ORGANIZATION. 1996. Ischaemic stroke and combined oral contraceptives: results of an international, multicentre, case-control study. WHO Collaborative Study of Cardiovascular Disease and Steroid Hormone Contraception. Lancet **348**(9026)**:** 498–505.
21. BURKMAN, R.T. 1988. Lipid and lipoprotein changes in relation to oral contraception and hormonal replacement therapy. Fertil. Steril. **49**(5)**:** 39S–50S.
22. MANT, J., R. PAINTER & M. VESSEY. 1998. Risk of myocardial infarction, angina and stroke in users of oral contraceptives: an updated analysis of a cohort study. Br. J. Obstet. Gynaecol. **105**(8)**:** 890–896.
23. WORLD HEALTH ORGANIZATION. 1997. Acute myocardial infarction and combined oral contraceptives: results of an international multicentre case-control study. WHO Collaborative Study of Cardiovascular Disease and Steroid Hormone Contraception. Lancet **349**(9060)**:** 1202–1209.
24. ELAM, M.B., M. VIAR, T.E. RATTS & C.M. CHESNEY. 1986. Mitral valve prolapse in women with oral contraceptive-related cerebrovascular insufficiency. Arch. Intern. Med. **146:** 73–77.
25. STUBBLEFIELD, P.G. 1989. Cardiovascular effects of oral contraceptives: a review. Int. J. Fertil. **34:** 40–49.
26. BEAUMONT, V. & J.L. BEAUMONT. 1989. Vascular risk of oral contraceptive agents: realities and mechanisms. II. Mechanisms of vascular accidents: their prevention. Presse Med. **18**(25)**:** 1249–1253.
27. BROCHIER, M.L. & P. ARWIDSON. 1998. Coronary heart disease risk factors in women. Eur. Heart J. **19:** A45–52.
28. STEFANADIS, C., E. TSIAMIS, J. DERNELLIS & P. TOUTOUZAS. 1999. Effect of estrogen on aortic function in postmenopausal women. Am. J. Physiol. **276:** H658–662.
29. DARNEY, P.D. 1997. OC practice guidelines: minimizing side effects. Int. J. Fertil. Womens Med. **1:** 158–169.
30. KAUNITZ, A.M. 1998. Injectable depot medroxyprogesterone acetate contraception: an update for U.S. clinicians. Int. J. Fertil. Womens Med. **43**(2)**:** 73–83.
31. COMP, P.C. & A.Z. HOWARD. 1993. Contraceptive choices in women with coagulation disorders. Am. J. Obstet. Gynecol. **168:** 1990–1993.

Oral Contraceptives' Effects on the Vascular Component

Thrombophilic Parameters

IRENE KONTOPOULOU

1st Regional Transfusion and Haemophilia Center, Hippocration Hospital, 115 27 Athens, Greece

INTRODUCTION

Following the introduction of oral contraceptives (OCs) into clinical practice in 1960, the first published suggestion of their association with an increased risk of cardiovascular disease was a case report of a 40-year-old woman who developed pulmonary embolism after taking Enovid.[1] Subsequently, a series of case control studies evaluated the risk of venous thromboembolism associated with OCs.[2–6] Relative risk estimates varied between 2 and 11 and tended to be higher when only idiopathic cases were included.[7]

From the beginning of 1990, it became obvious that the association between OC use and venous thromboembolism requires further evaluation, as apart from estrogen,[8,9] the type of progestogen seemed to play a role in the development of venous thromboembolism.[10–12] For that, an extended collaborative study was undertaken by the World Health Organization (WHO).[13]

The WHO collaborative study, in a separate inquiry,[14] compared the risk of venous thromboembolism associated with low-estrogen (<35 μg ethinyloestradiol) OCs containing levonorgestrel and low-estrogen preparations containing the third-generation progestogens desogestrel or gestodene. This study revealed that whereas users of low estrogen-combined OCs containing levonorgestrel had 3.5 times the risk of venous thromboembolism than nonusers, OCs containing third-generation progestogens (desogestrel or gestrogence) were associated with significantly higher risks (9.1 compared with nonusers). These findings resulted in renewed interest in the biologic mechanisms underlying venous thrombosis during oral contraceptive use. Parallel to the epidemiologic studies on the influence of the different types of OCs on the risk of developing deep vein thrombosis and pulmonary embolism, a very large number of studies have investigated the effect of various OCs on hemostasis.[15–21]

HEMOSTATIC SYSTEM AND ORAL ANTICOAGULANTS

The natural balance between coagulation, anticoagulation, and fibrinolysis may be disturbed by many different environmental factors, such as oral contraceptive use, or by hereditary defects in procoagulation, anticoagulation, or fibrinolysis. As it is known, the procoagulant factors are the platelets and the coagulation factors (fibrinogen, FII, FV, FVII, FVIII, FIX, FX, FXI, FXII, and FXIII). The coagulation factors circulate in blood in an inactive form and, with the appropriate stimulus, are converted by enzymatic processes to the active state. These stimuli may result from tissue damage (extrinsic pathway) or within the blood itself (intrinsic pathway).

The main anticoagulant factors are the natural anticoagulants, antithrombin III (ATIII), protein C (PrC), and protein S (PrS). Antithrombin III inactivates FIIa and FXa as well as FIXa, FXIa, and FXIIa. Protein C and protein S inactivate FVa and FVIIIa through activated protein C (APC). An inherited deficiency of ATIII, PrC, and PrS with a reduction of natural anticoagulants to less than 60% causes thrombophilia. This defect is very rare. Fibrinolysis, on the other hand, is a proteolytic process that causes the breakdown of fibrin and the lysis of thrombus. The main factor in the fibrinolytic system is plasminogen which, through the action of activators (tPA) and inhibitors (PAI), is activated to plasmin.

Recently, Dahlback[22] reported that a lower sensitivity of activated factor V to the anticoagulant action of APC is the most common thrombophilic factor. In most cases the defect is inherited as a result of a single point mutation[23] to factor V gene (G⇒A at nucleotide 1691), and the mutant factor is known as FV Leiden. The FV Leiden is extremely rare among non-Caucasians, whereas its prevalence among Caucasians is between 2.0 and 7.0% with the higher prevalence among the North European populations.[24] Another recently described genetic variant associated with an increased risk of venous thrombosis is that of the prothrombin factor mutation (PT 20210A). The variant is located in the 3′-untranslated region of the gene at position 20210, where one nucleotide is changed (a G to A transition). This variant is associated with elevated levels of prothrombin in plasma, which is related to an increased risk of thrombosis.[25] The PT 20210 A prothrombin variant is a common abnormality, with a prevalence of carriership between 1.0 and 4.0%. It is believed to be more common in southern than in northern Europe and it has a low prevalance among Africans and Asians,[26] similar to that reported for FV Leiden.

Many studies document that OCs may stimulate procoagulation, inhibit anticoagulation, and stimulate fibrinolysis.[15–21] Most studies on the hemostatic and fibrinolytic effects of OCs have been conducted in healthy volunteers.

Although many controversies exist among the different studies, most have found increased aggregation of platelets;[16–18] however, other investigators found no evidence of *in vivo* platelet activation, as no changes in circulating platelet aggregates, release of beta thromboglobulin from alpha granules, or any modification of the mega thrombocyte percentage were detected.[17] Most also found increased levels of fibrinogen[15–17] and vitamin K-dependent procoagulant factors II, VII, IX, X, and factors VIII, XI, and XII, whereas levels of anticoagulant factors antithrombin III as well as PrS were decreased in most studies; however, findings are not consistent in all of them. On the contrary, the level of protein C is reportedly increased during the use of OCs.[27] On the other hand, an increase in fibrinolytic activity due to elevated levels of tPA was considered an efficient mechanism to shift the hemostatic balance to a more physiologic state.[17]

The study of fibrinopeptide A (FPA), which is a molecular marker of the split of fibrinogen by thrombin, showed slight but significant blood clotting activation after only 1 month of treatment, but it did not further increase after three cycles and it showed a tendency to decrease after six cycles. The changes in FPA observed during treatment with monophasic and triphasic formulation were similar.[17]

Contrary to the foregoing studies, which were conducted in healthy women, a recent study by the Leiden Thrombophilia study group assessed the effects of OCs on hemostatic variables in patients with venous thrombosis (thrombosis while on OCs) and in healthy control subjects on OCs.[28] They found the following: (1) There was mainly an increase in factors VII, XII, as well as PrC and a decrease in ATIII, APC sensitivity ratio, and PrS, (2) Less marked effects that were nonsignificant or only significant in either patients or controls were an increase in factor VIII, fibrinogen, and prothrombin and a decrease in the APTT and free PrS. In the former thrombosis patients, several of these effects of OCs were more pronounced than in healthy women, specifically factor VII, ATIII, APC sensitivity ratio, and PrC. Apparently some women become "high hemostatic responders" when exposed to oral contraceptives, and they may be most vulnerable to thrombogenic effects.

HEREDITARY THROMBOPHILIA AND ORAL CONTRACEPTIVES

In the last decade, our knowledge of thrombophilia, and mainly hereditary thrombophilia, has been developed extensively. Resistance to activated PrC due to FV Leiden mutation, PrC and PrS deficiency, and recently prothrombin polymorphism have been added to antithrombin III (ATIII) deficiency. The risk of thrombosis among women with hereditary ATIII deficiency taking OCs proved to be high for venous thromboembolism.[29] During an observation period of 36.3 years, the incidence of thrombosis per patient years was 27.3% for those on OCs compared to 3.4% for patients not on OCs. On the contrary, for patients with PrC or PrS deficiency, the incidence of thrombosis among OC users was 12% and 6.5%, whereas that among non-OC users was 6.9% and 8.6%, respectively. Therefore, OC should be strictly avoided in women with known ATIII deficiency, and ATIII measurements should be mandatory in women related to ATIII-deficient patients before starting OCs.

Patients with PrC deficiency had no significant increase in thrombosis, but an increased risk cannot be excluded. On the contrary, patients with PrS deficiency have no evidence of an excess thrombotic risk with OC intake.[29]

As referred to already, since 1994, a new hereditary abnormality in familial thrombophilia has been described. The poor anticoagulant response or resistance to APC (APC-R) of the FVa[22] is responsible for venous thrombosis.[30] In the majority of cases, APC-R is explained by a single point mutation in the factor V gene, which makes factor V insensitive to inactivation by APC.[23]

Acquired APC-R, in addition to the hereditary APC-R, does exist.[30–34] Henkens *et al.*[31] demonstrated that APC sensitivity in the absence of FV Leiden is influenced by the gender of the person and by the use of OCs (FIG. 1). The observed difference in the APC ratio between men and women was in agreement with the findings of other investigators.[34]

More than 18% of women using OCs had an APC ratio below normal, a prevalence much higher than that of 5–7% in the general population. This suggests an acquired APC-R in these women. Both the difference in APC sensitivity between men and women not using OCs and oral contraceptive users suggested a hormonal influence on PrC sensitivity. It has been demonstrated before that OCs influence the plasma levels of several clotting factors and natural inhibitors.[16,17, 21,27]

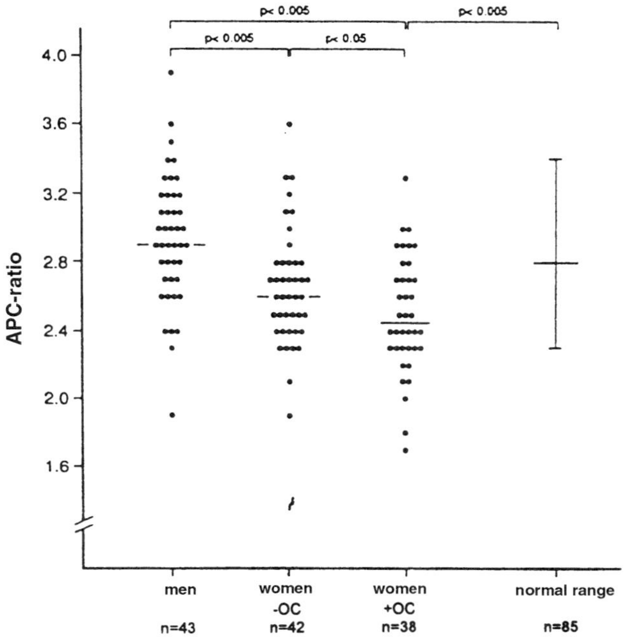

FIGURE 1. Difference in APC ratio between men and women.

These changes in plasma coagulation and anticoagulant factors theoretically support the concept of a hypercoagulable state due to OCs. The APC-R suggests an additional factor contributing to this concept.

Cumming *et al.*[33] proved that a significant reduction in the mean APC sensitivity ratio (APC-SR) was also observed at all stages of pregnancy (FIG. 2). The study was performed in 20 healthy women. APC-R was found in 8 of 19 women at 14–20 weeks of gestration, in 11 of 20 women at 28 weeks, and in 13 of 17 women at 36 weeks. At 8 weeks postpartum, the APC ratio was normal again. The development of resistance to APC may contribute to the increase risk of thrombosis during pregnancy.

In addition to the foregoing observations on APC-R, a research group from Maastricht[34] transformed an old *in vitro* test for thrombin formation into a very sensitive APC-R test not through APTT but through the endogenous thrombin product (ETP) and proved that[35]: (1) Third generation OCs induce resistance to the blood's natural anticoagulation system (APC-R) of almost the same magnitude as the resistance induced by FV Leiden. (2) Second-generation contraceptives show only part of this effect in the users of second-generation pills and can be clearly demarcated in both in women not on OCs and those on third-generation pills. (3) In women heterozygous for the FV Leiden mutation who take OCs, APC-R is as high as that among those who are homozygous for the mutation. These results agree with epidemiologic data.

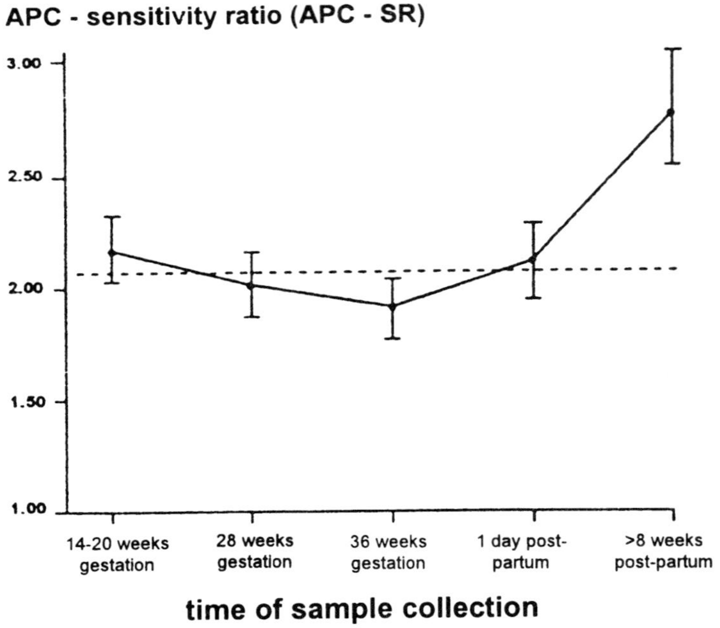

FIGURE 2. APC sensitivity ratio at all stages of pregnancy. (From Ref. 33.)

Until now, the increased risk for venous thrombosis during OC therapy has always been linked to the effects of estrogen on the coagulation system. The study of Rosing *et al.*[34] provides a strong indication of the biologic effect of the progestagen component on hemostasis and shows that with respect to the risk of venous thrombosis, the role of progesterone cannot be ignored (FIG. 3).

From the same study comes the observation that the effect of OCs on the APC response takes place within a few days after starting OC therapy and that the APC-SR drops during pill-free periods (FIG. 4). That information about the underlying mechanism is valuable. Unfortunately, the data do not yet allow further conclusions regarding changes in the hemostatic system to be linked to the impaired APC response and to the increased thrombotic risk of OC users. It has to be stressed, however, that the major difference between ETP-based and APTT-based methods is that initiation of coagulation in the case of the ETP occurs via the extrinsic pathway of coagulation, which means through tissue factor/factor VIIa, whereas in APTT-based systems, coagulation is initiated via the intrinsic coagulation pathway. This indicates that the basis of the impaired APC response in women using OCs may have to be sought in the activity and/or regulation of the extrinsic pathway of coagulation.

The recent discovery of the transition from guanine to adenine at position 20210 of the prothrombin gene[25] has widened the spectrum of inherited thrombophilia. Next to the mutation in the factor V gene,[23] the prothrombin gene mutation is the most common genetic determinant of deep vein thrombosis of the lower extremi-

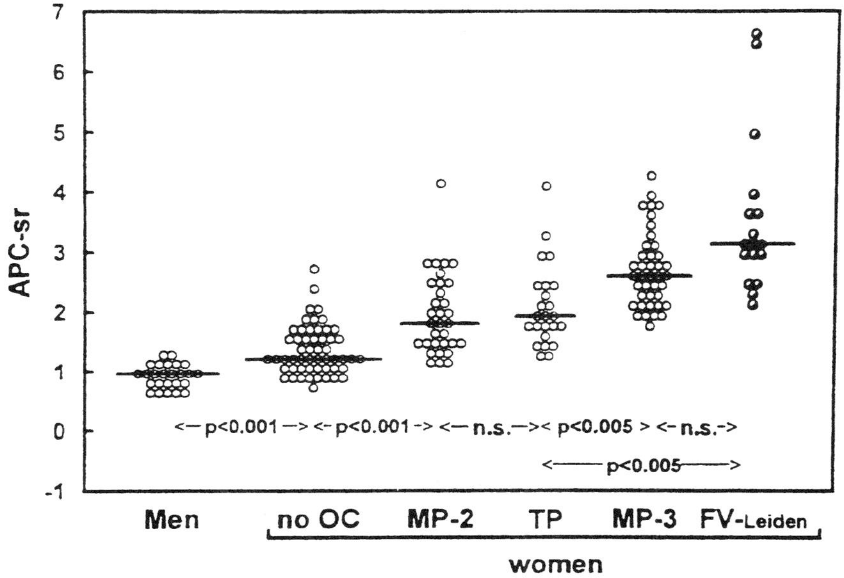

FIGURE 3. APC-sr/EPI of men, women using and not using OCs, and heterozygous females for LV Leiden. MP, second generation monophasic OC; TP, triphasic OC; and MP3, third generation monophasic OC. (From Ref. 34.)

ties.[37] Mutations in the prothrombin gene and factor V gene are also associated with cerebral vein thrombosis.[38–40] The use of OCs is also strongly and independently associated with the disorder. In a recent study,[41] the prevalence of the PT 20210A gene was higher in patients with cerebral vein thrombosis (20%) than in healthy controls (3%; OR 10.2; 95% CI 2.3–31.0) and it was similar to that in patients with deep vein thrombosis (18%). Similar results were obtained for the mutation in the factor V gene.

The use of OCs was more frequent among women with cerebral vein thrombosis (96%) than among controls (32%; OR 22; 95%; CI 5.9–84.2) and among those with deep vein thrombosis (61%; OR 4.4; 95% CI 1.1–17.8). For women who were taking OCs and who also have the prothrombin gene mutation (seven patients with cerebral vein thrombosis but only one control), the OR for cerebral vein thrombosis rose to 149.3 (95% CI 31.0–711.0). Because both the prothrombin gene mutation and the use of OCs cause hypercoagulability, their combination probably enhances the individual effects on coagulation. In particular, both increase plasma levels of prothrombin, the zymogen responsible for thrombin formation in the coagulation system.

Two questions are raised. The first is whether screening for the most common thrombophilic factors, the FV Leiden and prothrombin gene mutation, in young women before they are prescribed OCs would be useful.[42,43] The other question is whether withholding OCs from carriers of the mutations would be worthwhile.[35] Vandenbroucke and Rosendaal[35] suggested that indiscriminate screening would not be cost effective, even though the risk of deep vein thrombosis in oral contraceptive

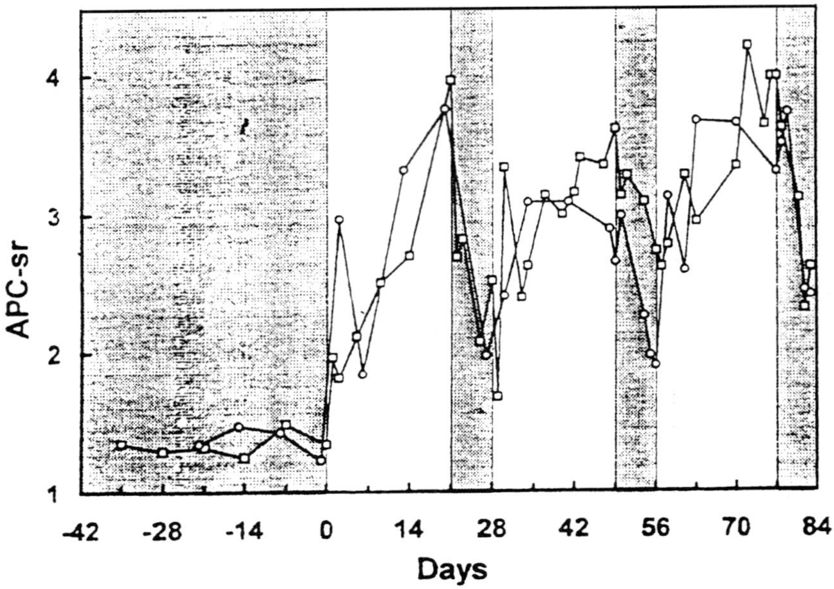

FIGURE 4. Effects of OCs on APC-sr in two women who started OC on day 0 and third generation monophasic. OC-free periods are indicated by *shaded bars*. (From Ref. 34.)

users who are carriers of the FV Leiden or FII mutation is greater than the risk in those without mutation. With respect to the second question, withholding the most effective mode of contraception might lead to more pregnancies, which would also increase the risk of venous thromboembolism. Therefore, it is recommended[35,42,43] that carriers of the prothrombin gene mutation or FV Leiden who have had an episode of thrombosis discontinue taking OCs. For asymptomatic carriers who are usually identified in family studies, counseling on alternative methods of contraception should be considered. In addition, the presence of other risk factors for thrombosis must be taken into account in these patients.

As it has already been stressed, known carriers of ATIII deficiency must strictly avoid OCs, and ATIII measurement must be mandatory for women relatives of ATIII-deficient persons before starting OCs.

In conclusion, it is obvious that we need even safer OCs, but until recently this was not possible, as the development of safe pills was "coagulation guesswork" due to the fact that the effect of OCs on hemostatic variables is not constant. Now, with the help of sensitive new tests like the APC-ratio, it is possible to discriminate the thrombogenic potential of the different pills during the process of developing new contraceptives. In the near future we can anticipate the production of safer oral contraceptives.

REFERENCES

1. JORDAN, W.M. 1961. Pulmonary embolism. Lancet **ii:** 1146–1147.

2. Vessey, M.P. & R. Doll. 1969. Investigation of relation between use of oral contraceptives and thromboembolic disease: a further report. Br. M.J. **ii:** 651–657.
3. Sartwell, P.E., A.T. Masi, F.D.G. Arthes *et al.* 1969. Thromboembolism and oral contraceptives: an epidemiologic case control study. Am. J. Epidemiol. **90:** 365–380.
4. Vessey, M.P., R. Doll, A.E. Fairburn & G. Glober. 1970. Prospective thromboembolism and use of oral contraceptives. Br. Med. J. **iii:** 123–126.
5. Maquire, M., J. Tonosia, P.E. Sartwell *et al.* 1979. Increased risk of thrombosis due to oral contraceptives: a further report. Am. J. Epidemiol. **110:** 188–195
6. Vessey, M.P., D. Mant, A. Smith & D. Yeates. 1986. Oral contraceptive and venous thromboembolism: findings in a large prospective study. Br. Med. J. **292:** 526.
7. Helmrich, S.P., L. Rosemberg, D.W. Kaufman *et al.* 1987. Venous thromboembolism in relation to oral contraceptive use. Obstet. Gynecol. **69:** 91–95.
8. Stalley, P.D., J.A. Tonascia, M.S. Tockman *et al.* 1975. Thrombosis with low estrogen oral contraceptives Am. J. Epidemiol. **102:** 197.
9. Inman, W.H.W., M.P. Vessey, B. Westerholm & A. Engelnud. 1970. Thromboembolic disease and the steroidal content of oral contraceptives: a report to the Committee on Safety of Drugs. Br. Med. J. **ii:** 203–209.
10. Gestmann, B.B., J.M. Piper, J.P. Freiman *et al.* 1990. Oral contraceptive oestrogen and progestin potencies and the incidence of deep venous thromboembolism. Am. J. Epidemiol. **4:** 931–936.
11. Jick, H., S. Jick, V. Gurewick, M. Mayers & C. Vasilakis. 1995. Risk of idiopathic caridiovascular death and nonfatal venous thromboembolism in women using oral contraceptives with differing progestagen components. Lancet **346:** 1589–1593.
12. Spitzer, W., M. Lewis, L. Heinemann *et al.* on behalf of Transnational Research Group on Oral Contraceptives and the Health of Young Women. 1996. Third generation oral contraceptives and risk of venous thromboembolic disorders: an international case-control study. Br. Med. J. **312:** 83–88.
13. World Health Organization. Collaborative Study of Cardiovascular Disease and Steroid Hormone Contraception. 1995. Venous thromboembolic disease and combined oral contraceptives: result of international multicentre case-control study. Lancet **346:** 1575–1581.
14. World Health Organization. Collaborative Study of Cardiovascular Disease and Steroid Hormone Contraception. 1995. Effect of different progestagens in low oestrogen oral contraceptives on venous thromboembolic disease. Lancet **346:** 1582–1588.
15. Poller, L. 1978. Oral contraceptives, blood clotting and thrombosis. Br. Med. Bull. **34:** 151–156.
16. Bonnar, J. 1987. Coagulation effects of oral contraception. Am. J. Obstet. Gynecol. **157:** 1042–1048.
17. Bruni, V., R. Abbate, S. Pinto *et al.* 1987. Effects of gestodene on haemostasis. Gynecological Endocrinology. : 523–532. Parthenon Publishing. Carnforth, U.K.
18. Cohen, H., I.J. Mackie, K. Walshe *et al.* 1988. A comparison of the effects of two thriphasic oral contraceptives on haemostasis. Br. J. Haematol. **69:** 259–263.
19. Abbate, R., S. Pinto, C. Rostagno *et al.* 1990. Effects of long-term gestodene-containing oral contraceptive administration on haemostasis. Am. J. Obstet. Gynecol. **163:** 424–430.
20. Fotherby, K. 1994. Are changes in haemotological factors and cardiovascular risk during oral contraceptives use dose related? Fertil. Control Rev. 3: 11–15.
21. Creatsas, G., I. Kontopoulou-Griva, E. Deligeorgiou *et al.* 1997. Effects of two combined monophasic and thriphasic ethinylestradiol gestrodene oral contraceptives on natural inhibitors and other hemostatic variables. Eur. J. Contracept. Reprod. Health Care **2:** 1–8.
22. Dahlback, B., M. Carlsson & P.J. Svensson. 1993. Familiar thrombophilia due to a previously unrecognised mechanism characterized by poor anticoagulant response to activated protein C: prediction of a cofactor to activated protein C. Proc. Natl. Acad. Sci. USA **90:** 1004–1008.
23. Bertina, R.M., B.P.C. Koeleman, T. Koster *et al.* 1994. Mutation in blood coagulation factor V associated with resistance to activated protein C. Nature **369:** 64–67.
24. Rees, D.C., M. Cox & J.B. Clegg. 1995. World distribution of factor V Leiden. Lancet **346:** 1133–1134.

25. POORT, R.S., F.R. ROSENDAAL, P.H. REITSMA & R.M. BERTINA. 1996. A common genetic varation in the 3'-untranslated region of the prothrombin gene is associated with elevated plasma prothrombin levels and an increase in venous thrombosis. Blood **88:** 3699.
26. ROSENDAAL, F.R., C.J.M. DOGGEN, A. ZIVELIN *et al.* 1998. Geographic distibution of the 20210 G to A prothrombin variant. Thromb. Haemostasis **79:** 706–708.
27. MALM, J., M. LAURELL & B. DAHLBACK. 1998. Changes in the plasma levels of vitamin K–dependent protein C and S and of C4b–binding protein during pregnancy and oral contraception. Br. J. Haematol. **68:** 437–443.
28. BLOEMENKAMP, K., F. ROSENDAAL, F. HELMERSHOST *et al.* 1998. Hemostastic effects of oral contraceptives in women who developed deep-vein thrombosis while using oral contraceptives. Thromb. Haemostasis **80:** 382–387.
29. PABINGER, I. & B. SCHNEIDER and the GTH Study Group on Natural Inhibitors. 1994. Thrombotic risk of women with hereditary antithrombin III, -protein C- and protein S-deficiency taking oral contraceptive medication. Thromb. Haemostasis **71:** 548–552.
30. SVENSSON, P.J. & B. DAHLBACK. 1994. Resistance to activated protein C as a basis for venous thrombosis. N. Engl. J. Med. **330:** 517–522.
31. HENKENS, C., V. BOM, A. SEINEN & J. VAN DER MEER. 1995. Sensitivity to activated protein C. Influence on oral contraceptives and sex. Thromb. Haemostasis **73:** 402–404.
32. OLIVIERI, O., S. FRISO, F. MANZATO & A. GUELLA. 1995. Resistance to activated protein C in healthy women taking oral contraceptives. Br. J. Haematol. **91:** 465–470.
33. CUMMING, A.M., R.C. TAIT, S. FILDES *et al.* 1995. Development of resistance to activated protein C during pregnancy. Br. J. Haematol. **90:** 725–727.
34. ROSING, J., G. TANS, G. NICOLAES *et al.* 1997. Oral contraceptives and venous thrombosis: different sensitivities to activated protein C in women using second- and third-generation oral contraceptives. Br. J. Haematol. **97:** 233–238.
35. VANDENBROUCKE, J. & F. ROSENDAAL. 1997. End of the line for "third-generation-pill" controversy? Lancet **349:** 1113–1114.
36. HELMERHOST, F.M., K.W.M. BLOEMENKAMP, E. BRIET *et al.* 1996. Factor V Leiden mutation and contraception. Gynecol. Endocrinol. **10:** 85–87.
37. SOUTO, J.C., I. COLL, D. LIOBE *et al.* 1998. The prothrombin 20210 A allele is the most prevalent genetic risk factor for venous thromboembolism in Spanish population. Thromb. Haemostasis **80:** 366–369.
38. MARTINELLI, I., G. LANDI, G. MERATI *et al.* 1996. Factor V gene mutation is a risk factor for cerebral venous thrombosis. Thromb. Haemostasis **75:** 393–394.
39. MARTINELLI, I., F.R. ROSENDAAL, J.P. VANDENBROUCKE & P.M. MANNUCCI. 1996. Oral contraceptives are a risk factor for cerebral vein thrombosis. Thromb. Haemostasis **76:** 477–478.
40. DE BRUIJN, S.F.T.M., J. STAM, M.M.W. KOOPMAN & J.P. VANDENBROUCKE for the Cerebral Venous Sinus Thrombosis Study Group. 1998. Case control study of risk of cerebral sinus thrombosis in oral contraceptive users who are carriers of hereditary prothrombotic conditions. Br. Med. J. **316:** 589–592.
41. MARTINELLI, I., E. SACCHI, G. LANDI *et al.* 1998. High risk of cerebral-vein thrombosis in carriers of a prothrombin-gene mutation and in users of oral contraceptives. N. Engl. J. Med. **338:** 1793–1797.
42. VANDERBROUCKE, J.P., F.J.M. VAN DEN MEER, F.M. HELMERHORST & F.R. ROSENDAAL. 1996. Factor V Leiden: should we screen oral contraceptive users and pregnant women? Br. J. Med. **313:** 1127–1130.
43. ROSENDAAL, F.R. 1995. Oral contraceptives and screening for factor V Leiden. Thromb. Haemostasis **75:** 524–533.

Dysmenorrhea

E. DELIGEOROGLOU[a]

2nd Department of Obstetrics and Gynecology, Division of Pediatric–Adolescent Gynecology and Reconstructive Surgery, University of Athens "Aretaieion" Hospital, Athens, Greece

ABSTRACT: Dysmenorrhea presents as painful periods that start two to three years after menarche. The pain usually begins when the bleeding starts and lasts for 48–32 hours. The cause of menstrual cramps and associated symptoms in primary dysmenorrhea is related to prostaglandin production. In secondary dysmenorrhea, there is documented pelvic pathology that causes the painful menstrual cramps, and treatment is cause related. Available treatments for primary dysmenorrhea—NSAIDS, oral combined contraceptives, β-blockers, psychotherapeutic methods, and crevical dilatation—are discussed.

INTRODUCTION

The Greek term "dysmenorrhea," translated literally, means "difficult menstrual flow." It is a common menstrual disorder during adolescence. In this period of life dysmenorrhea presents as painful periods, which usually start two to three years after menarche, with the onset of ovulation. It is one of the most common causes of recurrent absence from work, school, or other activities in a woman's life. It can reduce the quality of life and general well-being.[1]

In most cases no organic disease is present, so dysmenorrhea is characterized as primary. Menstrual pain due to pelvic pathology, such as endometriosis, pelvic inflammatory disease, or congenital anomalies of the Müllerian system, is classified as secondary dysmenorrhea.

The pathogenesis of pain in dysmenorrhea is believed to be primarily related to over-contractility of the myometrium, which causes ischemia of the uterus. Prostaglandin synthetase inhibitors and oral contraceptives have been shown to be effective in relieving menstrual pain. The treatment of secondary dysmenorrhea is cause related.

PRIMARY DYSMENORRHEA

Incidence

The incidence of dysmenorrhea varies a great deal, depending on the type of patient and the method used to evaluate the pain.[2] According to several studies, it can vary from 8 to 60%[3–5] or more. The term dysmenorrhea is reserved for those individuals whose pain is severe enough to limit normal activity or to require medical

[a]Address for correspondence: Efthimios Deligeoroglou M.D., 48, Marathonos Street, 152 35 Vrilissia, Athens, Greece. Phone: +301 7286353, +301-7286282; fax: +301 7233330.
geocre @ aretaieio.uoa.gr

TABLE 1. Scoring system for assessment of dysmenorrhea

	Grade	Working ability	Systemic symptoms	Analgesics
Grade 0	Menstruation is not painful, and daily activity is unaffected.	Unaffected	None	Not required
Grade 1	Menstruation is painful but seldom inhibits normal activity; analgesics are seldom required; mild pain.	Rarely affected	None	Rarely required
Grade 2	Daily activity affected; analgesics required and give sufficient relief so that absence from work or school is unusual; moderate pain.	Moderately affected	Few	Required
Grade 3	Activity clearly inhibited; poor effect of analgesics; vegetative symptoms (e.g., headache, fatigue, nausea, vomiting and diarrhea); severe pain.	Clearly inhibited	Apparent	Poor effect

treatment. The scoring system used for dysmenorrhea is shown in TABLE 1, as reported by Andersch and Milsom in "An Epidemiologic Study of Young Women with Dysmenorrhea."[6]

Disturbances of menstrual bleeding and dysmenorrhea are a major medical problem not only for women but also for their families and for health services.[7] In a study of about 1000 women in Mexico City, students with a mean age of 18 years (12–24), the prevalence of dysmenorrhea was 52.1% for the group <15 years of age, 63.8% for women between 15 and 19 years of age, and 52.3% for the 20- to 24-year-old group.[8]

Etiologic Theories

Several theories regarding the cause of primary dysmenorrhea have been presented over the years. Both purely physiological and purely psychological causes have been proposed. Theories on the cause of dysmenorrhea were proposed as early as the fifth century B.C.

Obstruction Theory

Hippocrates believed that cervical obstruction and stagnation of menstrual blood were responsible for painful menstruation. Nulliparus women experience more intense dysmenorrhea than parous women.[9,10] The frequency decreases with increasing parity.

Myometrial Activity

Recent studies have demonstrated that primary dysmenorrhea is associated with increased myometrial activity.[11] Investigators have reported that high intrauterine pressure during contraction causes pain. Further studies have revealed that increased intrauterine pressure is associated with decreased blood flow, and resulting uterine ischemia may be the primary cause of dysmenorrhea.

Neuromuscular Factors

Many authors have suggested neuromuscular activity as the cause of dysmenorhea. Altered neuromuscular activity in the uterus after pregnancy may explain the decreased menstrual pain after delivery.

Hormonal Influence

Primary dysmenorrhea does not emerge until the onset of ovulatory cycles (6–12 months after menarche), so in the first cycles after menarche adolescents do not experience pain.[1] Women with anovulatory cycles also do not experience menstrual pain.

Prostaglandins

There is evidence that metabolites of arachidonic acid are implicated in the pathophysiology of primary dysmenorrhea:

a. The high levels of PGF_{2a} and PGE_2 found in the menstrual fluid and endometrium of dysmenorrheic adolescents is now the most accepted theory to explain the etiology of this syndrome.[12–15] PGF_{2a} and PGE_2 cause vasoconstriction and myometrial contraction, which lead to ischemia and pain. They may also cause an "over-sensitivity" of the target neurons in physical and chemical stimulations.[16]

b. An elevated PGF_{2a}/PGE_2 ratio occurs in patients with primary dysmenorrhea.[17]

c. Intrauterine administration of PGF_{2a} induces uterine contractility and dysmenorrhea-like pain.[18,19]

d. Endometrial release of LTC_4, LTD_4, and LTE_4 is higher in women with dysmenorrhea.

e. Administration of anti-PG agents results in a marked improvement of pain in nearly 80% of dysmenorrheic women.

Vasopressin

The role of vasopressin has been the subject of intensive study: (a) Plasma concentrations of vasopressin during menstruation are higher in dysmenorrheic women, and (b) the administration of vasopressin stimulates uterine activity and causes symptoms of primary dysmenorrhea, but results suggest that this effect does not involve a mechanism of increased PGF synthesis.[20] These results suggest a direct effect of vasopressin on myometrium or an alternative mechanism for vasopressin to stimulate uterine contractility.

Psychological Factors

The literature regarding the etiology of primary dysmenorrhea has traditionally emphasized the role of psychological factors. The most recent data show that premenstrual symptoms were associated with other emotional distress factors in adolescents, whereas dysmenorrhea was not.[21] It has been widely claimed that exercise is beneficial for dysmenorrhea.[22]

Clinical Presentation

Primary dysmenorrhea presents as a lower midline, dull abdominal ache or cramping, generally occurring with ovulatory menstruation. The pain tends to be spasmodic and cyclic, often beginning approximately two days before the onset of menses, and is quite severe (sometimes feels like labor) the first day of menstruation.

Primary dysmenorrhea is differentiated from the more commonly reported cramps of a great number of women during menstruation the need for treatment, usually because the woman is unable to perform normal activities. FIGURE 1 shows the

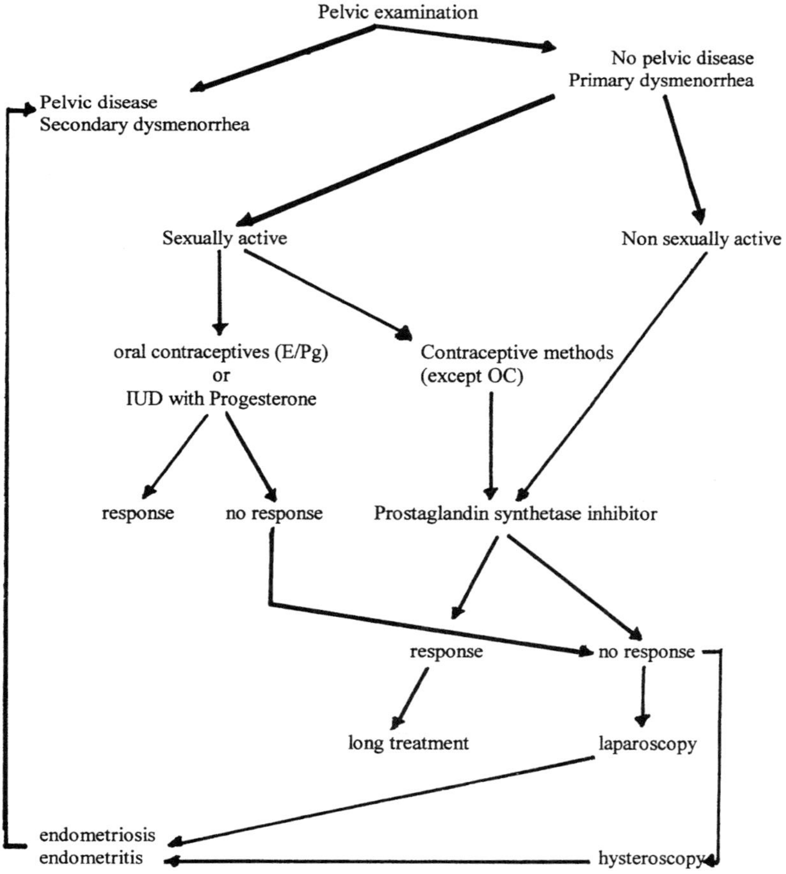

FIGURE 1. Evaluation and treatment of dysmenorrhea.

evaluation and the treatment of dysmenorrhea.[24] Often noticed are nausea, vomiting, diarrhoea, headache, and vertigo. Other symptoms that have been associated with dysmenorrhea are nervousness, depression, irritability, and insomnia.[8] Lack of sleep, stress, and caffeine consumption may increase the intensity of pain.[16]

Evaluation

For the evaluation of dysmenorrhea, a thorough history should be obtained, and a complete physical evaluation should be carried out. This includes a pelvic examination or rectal examination in the young adolescent. Pelvic examination with negative findings strongly supports the diagnosis of primary dysmenorrhea and must be differentiated from all other causes of secondary dysmenorrhea.

Management

The two principal pharmacotherapeutic agents employed in the treatment of primary dysmenorrhea are oral contraceptives and the nonsteroidal anti-inflammatory drugs.

Oral Contraceptives

Oral contraceptives reduce menstrual fluid levels to below normal (a) through reduction in menstrual fluid volume secondary to suppression of endometrial tissue growth and (b) through suppression of ovulation, giving rise to an anovulatory endocrine milieu when prostaglandin levels are low.[25] If there is not good relief of the dysmenorrhea, prostaglandin synthetase inhibitor can be added.[26]

Prostaglandin Synthetase Inhibitor

In young women who do not wish to use oral contraceptives as a method of birth control, the drug of choice for treating primary dysmenorrhea is a prostaglandin synthetase inhibitor.[26,27] Nonsteroidal anti-inflammatory drugs should be given as soon as pain begins after the onset of menstrual flow and should be continued throughout the first 48 or 72 hours of menstrual flow. Prostaglandin synthetase inhibitor relieves primary dysmenorrhea through suppression of menstrual fluid prostaglandins.[28] These drugs also have direct analgesic properties, and the rationale for giving them for the first 48 hours or 3 days is based on the observation that prostaglandin release is maximal during the first 48 hours of the menstrual flow. Studies have shown that ibuprofen appears to have the most favorable risk/benefit ratio.[29,30]

Other Therapeutic Suggestions

Spasmolytics,[31] calcium channel blockers, nonspecific analgesics, cervical dilatation, curettage, presacral neurectomy, transcutaneous electrical nerve stimulation (TENS),[32] accupuncture,[33] progestogens, LH-RH analogues, and magnesium may all be tried.[34,35] Further research to develop lipoxygenase inhibitors and leukotriene antagonists, in combination with cyclooxygenase inhibitors, may be used to treat all dysmenorrheic cases. Additionally, psychiatric help to modulate the reactive component of pain may be helpful.

TABLE 3. The most important causes of secondary dysmenorrhea

- Endometriosis
- Adenomyosis
- Pelvic inflammation
- Uterine fibroids — endometrial polyps
- Malformations of the Mullerian ducts
- Uterine retroversion in fixed position
- Small ovarian cysts
- IUD
- Stenosis of the cervical channel
- Pelvic varicocele

SECONDARY DYSMENORRHEA

Secondary dysmenorrhea, by definition, is due to an organic pelvic lesion. This type of dysmenorrhea usually occurs a few years after menarche, the pain may start 1 or 2 days before menses. Common causes of secondary dysmenorrhea are endometriosis, pelvic inflammatory disease (PID), and the use of intrauterine device (IUD).[36]

The pelvic examination may reveal tenderness, adnexal mass, or uterine myomas. Endometriosis may present a similar clinical picture but the pain usually increases for two to three days before menses and is most severe on the days with heaviest menstrual flow. Dyspareunia, infertility, heavy menstrual blood loss, or dysmenorrhea suggest organic disease.

Investigations that can be helpful for the work-up of secondary dysmenorrhea include cultures from the cervix and vagina, pelvic ultrasonography, or vaginal ultrasound, hysterosalpingography, hysteroscopy, and other adequate laboratory tests. Finally, the single most useful diagnostic procedure is laparoscopy. TABLE 2 shows the most important causes of secondary dysmenorrhea.

Management

If pelvic disease is discovered, the appropriate therapy should be directed toward it to alleviate the dysmenorrhea.

REFERENCES

1. ZONDERVAN, K.T., P.L. YUDKIN, M.P. VESSEY, *et al.* 1998. The prevalence of chronic pelvic pain in women in the U.K.: a systematic review. Br. J. Obst. Gyn. **105**(1)**:** 93–9.
2. SPEROFF, L. 1984. Diagnostica e terapia ostetrico-ginecologica attuale. Piccin Editore Padova.
3. AVANT, R.F. 1988. Dysmenorrhea. Prim. Care **15**(3)**:** 549–559.
4. NG, T.P., N.C. TAN & G.K. WANSAICHEONG. 1992. A prevalence study of dysmenorrhea in female residents aged 15–54 years in Clementi Town, Singapore. Ann. Acad. Med. Singapore **21**(3)**:** 323–327.
5. CREATSAS, G., N. ELEFTHERIOU, D. LOUTRADIS, *et al.* 1988. Menstrual disorders during adolescence. Proceedings of the 4th Pan-Hellenic Congress of Obstetrics and Gynecology. September 21–24. Thessaloniki, Greece.

6. NDERSCH, B. & I. MILSOM. 1982. An epidemiologic study of young women with dysmenorrhea. Am. J. Obstet. Gynecol. **144:** 655–660.
7. COLL-CAPDEVILA, C. 1997. Dysfunctional uterine bleeding and dysmenorrhea. Eur. J. Reprod. Health Care **2**(4)**:** 229–237.
8. PEDRON-NUWVO, N., L.N. GONZALEZ-UNZAGA, R. DE CELIS CARRILLO, *et al.* 1998. Incidence of dysmenorrhea and associated symptoms in women aged 12–24 years. Ginecol. Obstet. Mex. **66:** 492–494.
9. FORLEO, R., C. SBIROLI & U. DI TONDO. 1982. Mestruazione. Fisiopatologia della riproduzione femminile. Vol. **9:** 321–323. Edizione Gelmini. Milano.
10. HUFFMAN, J.W., C.J. DEWHURST & V.J. CAPRARO. 1981. The Gynecology of Childhood and Adolescence. W.B. Sauders. Philadelphia. pp. 469–484.
11. PICKLES, V.R. 1957. A plain muscle stimulant in the menstrum. Nature **180:** 1198–1199.
12. COLL-CAPDEVILA, C. 1997. Dysfunctional uterine bleeding and Dysmenorrhea. Eur. J. Reprod. Health Care **2**(4)**:** 229–237.
13. POIZAT, R. 1985. Prostaglandines: Physiologie de la Reproduction Humaine. Volume **9:** 119–134. Paris.
14. LUDWIG, H. 1996. Dysmenorrhoe. Ther. Umsch. **53**(6): 431–441.
15. YEN, S.S.C. 1986. The human menstrual cycle. *In* Reproductive Endocrinology. 2nd edit. S.S.C. Yen & R.B. Jaffe, Eds.: 126–151. W.B. Saunders. Philadelphia.
16. STOLL, S.L. 1992. Dismenorrea. Secrets in Ostetricia e Ginecologia. Volume **4:** 17–24. Edizione Italiana, Intramed Communications. Milan.
17. PICKLES, V.R. 1967. Prostaglandins in the human endometrium. Int. J. Fertil. **12:** 335–338.
18. WIQVIST, N., B. LINDHLOM, M. WIKLANS & L. WIHELMSSON. 1983. Prostaglandins and uterine contractility. Acta Gynecol. Scand. (Suppl.) **113:** 23–29.
19. BYDGEMAN, M., J. BREMME, S. GILLESPIE, *et al.* 1979. Effects of the prostaglandins on the uterus. Acta Obstet. Gynecol. Scand. (Suppl.) **87:** 33–38.
20. EKSTROEM, P., M. AKERLUD, M. FORLING, *et al.* 1992. Stimulation of vasopressin release in women with primary dysmenorrhea and after oral contraceptive treatment—effect on uterine contractility. Br. J. Obstet. Gynec. **99**(8)**:** 680–684.
21. FREEMAN, E.W., K. RICKELS & S.J. SONDHEIMER. 1993. Premenstrual symptoms and dysmenorrhea in relation to emotional distress factors in adolscents. J. Psychosom. Obstet. Gynaecol. **14:** 41–50.
22. GOLOMB, L.M., A.A. SOLIDUM & M.P. WARREN. 1998. Primary dysmenorrhea and physical activity. Med. Sci. Sports Exer. **30**(6)**:** 906–909.
23. GORLERO, F. 1990. La Dysmenorrhea. Parke & Davis. Lainate (Milano).
24. LITT, I.F. 1983. Menstrual problems during adolescence. Pediatr. Rev. **4:** 203.
25. CREATSAS, G., E. DELIGEOROGOU, *et al.* 1990. Prostaglandins: PGF_{2a}, PGE_2, 6-keto-PGF_{1a} and TXB_2 serum levels in dysmenorrheic adolescents before, during and after treatment with oral contraceptives. Eur. J. Obstet. Gynecol. Reprod. Biol. **36:** 292–298.
26. ALVIN, P.E. & I.F. LITT. 1982. Current status of the etiology and management of dysmenorrhea in adolescence. Pediatrics **70:** 516–521.
27. CHAN, W.Y. 1983. Prostaglandins and non-steroidal anti-inflammatory drugs in dysmenorrhea. Annu. Rev. Pharmacol. Toxicol. **23:** 131–149.
28. CREATSAS, G., N. GOUMALATSOS, N. ELEFTHERIOU, *et al.,* Eds. 1988. Dysfunctional uterine Bleeding during Adolescence. Proceedings of the IVth European Congress on Pediatric and Adolescent Gynecology. September 29–October 3. Rhodes, Greece.
29. ZHANG, W.Y. & A. LI WAN PO. 1998. Efficacy of minor analgesics in primary dysmenorrhea: a systematic review. Br. J. Obstet. Gynaecol. **105**(7)**:** 780–789.
30. PEDRON NUEVO, N., M. GONZALEZ UNZAGA & R. MEDINA SANTILLAN. 1998. Preventive treatment of primary dysmenorrhea with ibuprofen. Ginecol. Obstet. Mex. **66:** 248–252.
31. HERNANDEZ BUENO, J.A., J. DE LA JARA DIAZ, F. SEDENO CRUZ & F. LLORENS TORRES. 1998. Analgesic–antispasmodic effect and safety of lysine clonixinate and L-hyoscinbutylbromide in the treatment of dysmenorrhea. Ginecol. Obstet. Mex. **66:** 35–39.

32. KAPLAN, B., D. RABINERSON, S. LURIE, *et al.* 1997. Clinical evaluation of a new model of a transcutaneus electrical nerve stimulation device for the management of primary dysmenorrhea. Gynecol. Obstet. Invest. **44**(4)**:** 255–259.
33. TSENOV, D. 1996. The effect of acupunture in dysmenorrhea. Akush. Ginecol. Soffiia **35**(3)**:** 24–25.
34. DAWOOD, M.Y. 1986. Current concepts in the etiology and treatment of primary dysmenorrhea. Acta Obstet. Gynecol. Scand. (Suppl.) **138:** 7–10.
35. PICCIONE, E., G. NOCCIOLI, L. CASSADEI & F. SESTI. 1988. Attuali aspetti di terapia medica della dismenorrea. Giorn. It. Ost. Gyn. **4:** 277–281.
36. PESCETTO, G., D. PECORARI, L. DE CECCO & N. RAGNI. 1992. Manuale di Ginecologia ed Ostetricia. Edizione SEU. Roma. pp. 231–232.

Combined Oral Contraceptive Treatment of Adolescent Girls with Polycystic Ovary Syndrome

Lipid Profile

GEORGE CREATSAS,[a] CAROLINA KOLIOPOULOS, AND GEORGE MASTORAKOS

Athens University, 2nd Department of Obstetrics and Gynecology, Athens 11528, Greece

ABSTRACT: The clinical signs and neuroendocrine features of adolescents with polycystic ovary syndrome (PCOS) resemble those found in adult women with PCOS. These adolescent patients are candidates for long-term treatment by one of the different therapeutic approaches that have been proposed. It is therefore essential that the treatment does not induce unfavorable metabolic effects. We investigated and compared the effects of cyproterone acetate (CA) and desogestrel (D), as part of combined oral contraceptives (COC), on lipid metabolism and hirsutism in adolescents with PCOS. Twenty-four girls with clinical signs of PCOS were recruited. They were all hyperandrogenemic and euthyroid and had normal prolactin plasma levels. Nonclassic congenital adrenal hyperplasia was ruled out by the ACTH stimulation test. Blood samples were obtained for sex hormone binding globulin (SHBG), total cholesterol (TC), LDL cholesterol, HDL cholesterol, triglycerides (TGs), apolipoproteins A-I, A-II, B, and lipoprotein (a) (Lp(a)) measurements. After the initial examination, therapy was initiated in a randomly selected order (12 and 12 patients were treated daily by 2 mg CA and 0.150 mg D, respectively, plus 0.035 and 0.030 mg ethinylestradiol, respectively). The degree of hirsutism and the lipid profile were reevaluated every 3 months after initiation of therapy for 1 year. Our data show that after 12 months of treatment with the D or CA COC, the Ferriman-Gallway hirsutism score decreased and TC and LDL-C increased. TGs and HDL-C were raised significantly in the CA COC group, whereas apolipoprotein A1 increased during D COC treatment. The atheromatic indices did not change. These data suggest that treatment of adolescent girls with PCOS is comparably effective with the two contraceptive formulations and that the desogestrel COC could be considered in the treatment of adolescent PCOS patients because it does not have side effects on lipid metabolism.

INTRODUCTION

Polycystic ovary syndrome (PCOS) is among the most common disorders of premenopausal women, affecting 5–10% of this population. It is characterized by hyperandrogenism, chronic anovulation, and insulin resistance, which results in hirsutism, irregular menses, infertility as well as a higher risk of diabetes mellitus

[a]Address for correspondence: Prof. George Creatsas, 76, Vas. Sophias Av., Athens 11528 Greece. Fax: 3-01-723333.
geocre@aretaieio.uoa.gr

and cardiovascular disease. The etiology of this syndrome has been under investigation for many decades. It is now suspected that more than one genetic defect may cause the reproductive abnormalities as well as the insulin resistance that characterize this syndrome. It was recently shown that among 37 candidate genes, the strongest evidence for linkage and association with PCOS was with the follistatin gene.[1]

Only a few studies closely examined PCOS during adolescence and pointed to the pubertal onset of the syndrome. Girls affected by PCOS may fail to establish a regular menstrual cycle immediately after menarche, or they may have a regular cycle at first followed by menstrual irregularity and often weight gain. They may also develop signs of hyperandrogenism associated with augmented luteinizing hormone (LH) pulsatility, an increased LH/FSH ratio as well as selective elevation of ovarian androgens compatible with enhanced 17α-hydroxylase activity (testosterone, Δ_4-androstenedione).[2] These patients demonstrate increased ovarian volume due to increased ovarian stroma and multiple small follicles that are histologically atretic and are located peripherally along with a thickened sclerotic ovarian cortex.[3,4] Hyperinsulinemia reflecting insulin resistance and reduced IGFBP-1 and SHBG levels were also reported in these pubertal patients.[5] The finding that these neuroendocrine features in hyperandrogenic girls resemble those found in adult women with PCOS suggests the peripubertal onset of this syndrome. Furthermore, an association between premature adrenarche and PCOS was suggested recently. In certain girls with premature adrenarche, hyperandrogenism may be the first sign of PCOS and/or insulin resistance. The link between these disorders could be serine phosphorylation of P450c17 and/or the insulin receptor. The phosphorylation of the 17,20-lyase activity of P450c17 is held responsible for the hyperandrogenism of adrenarche and/or PCOS,[6] whereas that of the insulin receptor decreases its protein tyrosine kinase activity, causing a postbinding defect in insulin action, thereby inducing insulin resistance.[7]

Different therapeutic approaches have been proposed in the treatment of PCOS. Most of them, such as combinations of estrogens and progestogens in oral contraceptives (COC), aim at decreasing androgens. More specifically, the antiandrogenic progestogen, cyproterone acetate (CA), in COC is commonly used to treat the PCOS-related hirsutism.[8] As a progestogen, it inhibits LH and androgen production and increases the hepatic clearance of testosterone. As an antiandrogen, it exerts its effect by competing with androgens at their receptor sites. On the other hand, the ethinyl estradiol (EE) increases the levels of SHBG, resulting in lower free androgen levels, thus ensuring cyclicity and preventing pregnancy. The new oral contraceptives containing progestogens, such as desogestrel (D), with very low androgenic activity may prove to be effective in the treatment of hirsutism by decreasing SHBG levels and suppressing ovarian androgen production by reducing gonadotropins.

Dyslipidemia characterized by increased total cholesterol (TC), LDL-C, and triglycerides (TG) as well as decreased HDL-C is frequently found in women with PCOS, independently of the excess weight that is often found in these patients.[9–13] The foregoing abnormal lipid profile associated with the hyperinsulinemia and hypertension often observed in women with PCOS suggests that PCOS may be a risk factor for cardiovascular disease (CVD). Furthermore, differences in the lipid profile between cases and controls are more significant in women less than 40 years of age. This is probably interpreted by the age-associated rise in LDL-C.[14] Thus, the thera-

TABLE 1. Clinical characteristics of adolescents with polycystic ovary syndrome receiving either ethinyl estradiol (EE) plus desogestrel or EE plus cyproterone acetate[a]

Characteristics	Desogestrel + EE (n = 12)	Cyproterone acetate + EE (n = 12)
Age (y)	17.3 ± 1.7	17.5 ± 1.2
Hirsutism score	16.2 ± 6.2	16.8 ± 4.7
Waist/hip	0.76 ± 0.07	0.75 ± 0.05
Body mass index (BMI)	24.9 ± 4.7	23.4 ± 3.8
Testosterone (ng/ml)	1.06 ± 0.3	0.9 ± 0.3
Free testosterone (pg/ml)	3.2 ± 0.9	2.9 ± 0.6
Δ_4-Androstenedione (ng/ml)	3.9 ± 0.9	3.6 ± 1
SHBG (nmol/L)	70 ± 51	67 ± 40

[a]Values are represented as mean ±SD.

peutic use of COC in women with PCOS and their influence on the lipid profile are an important issue. The estrogens and progestogens of COC exert different action on blood lipids. Estrogens stimulate hepatic synthesis of HDL and TG and inhibit enzyme lipoprotein lipase. Conversely, progestogens may lower HDL by increasing this enzymic activity.[15] The metabolic effects of the new COC in healthy women using them for contraception are minimal to negligible. According to recent data, the use of COC containing D has the lowest metabolic impact on lipid metabolism compared to other low dose COC.[15–17] It has even been suggested that further studies of these new products could prove to have beneficial effects on lipid metabolism and cardiovascular disease.[18]

COMBINED ORAL CONTRACEPTIVE TREATMENT OF ADOLESCENT GIRLS WITH PCOS

To investigate the effect of COC on the PCOS lipid profile, we treated PCOS adolescent girls with contraceptive formulations containing (1) EE and CA, and (2) EE and D, and compared their effects on hirsutism and lipids (C. Koliopoulos *et al.*, paper under preparation).

Twenty-four 14- to 19-year-old girls with clinical signs of PCOS were recruited for this study. All patients were seen in the Gynecology Clinic of Areteion-University Hospital because of oligomenorrhea or secondary amenorrhea and/or hirsutism. They were all hyperandrogenemic, in good health, and euthyroid and had normal plasma prolactin levels. The ACTH stimulation test ruled out congenital adrenal hyperplasia caused by 21-hydroxylase deficiency. No subject had used any hormonal medication, including COC, for at least 3 months before the study. The body mass index (BMI), waist-to-hip (W/H) ratio, and Tanner stage were calculated for each patient. The degree of hirsutism was evaluated according to Ferriman-Gallway criteria.[19] The patients and their parents were informed and gave their consent.

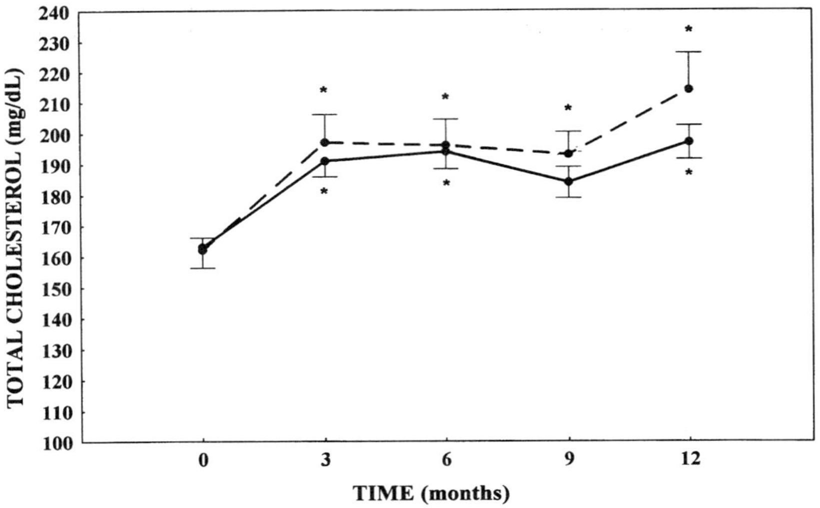

FIGURE 1. Serum total cholesterol values in the two groups of PCOS adolescent girls treated, respectively, with a D COC (*continuous line*) and a CA COC (*discontinuous line*). *Asterisk* indicates statistically significant difference ($p \leq 0.05$) from the baseline value of each group. Statistical analysis was performed by ANOVA repeated measures. Values are given as mean ± SE.

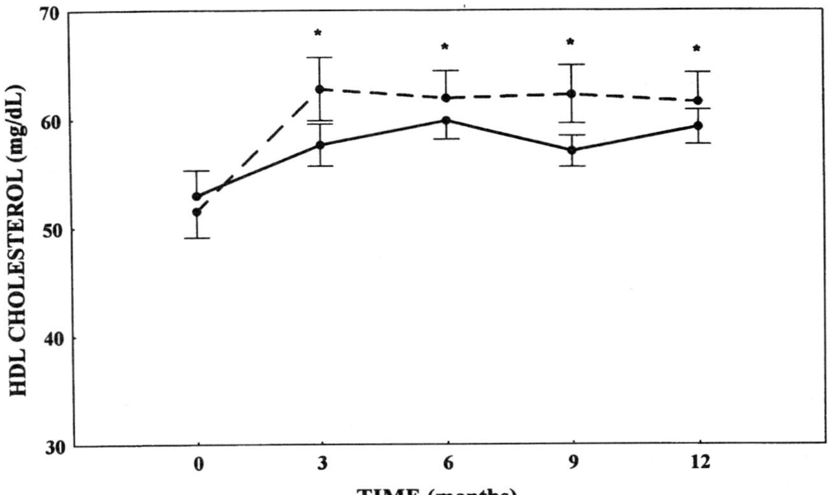

FIGURE 2. Serum HDL values in the two groups of PCOS adolescent girls treated, respectively, with a D COC (*continuous line*) and a CA COC (*discontinuous line*). *Asterisk* indicates statistically significant difference ($p \leq 0.05$) from the baseline value of each group. Statistical analysis was performed by ANOVA repeated measures. Values are given as mean ± SE.

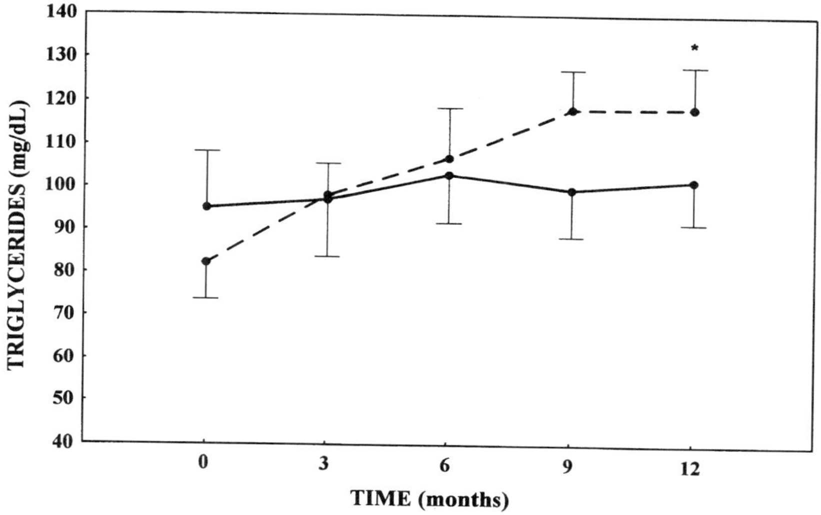

FIGURE 3. Serum triglyceride values in the two groups of PCOS adolescent girls treated, respectively, with a D COC (*continuous line*) and a CA COC (*discontinuous line*). *Asterisk* indicates statistically significant difference ($p \leq 0.05$) from the baseline value of each group. Statistical analysis was performed by ANOVA repeated measures. Values are given as mean ± SE.

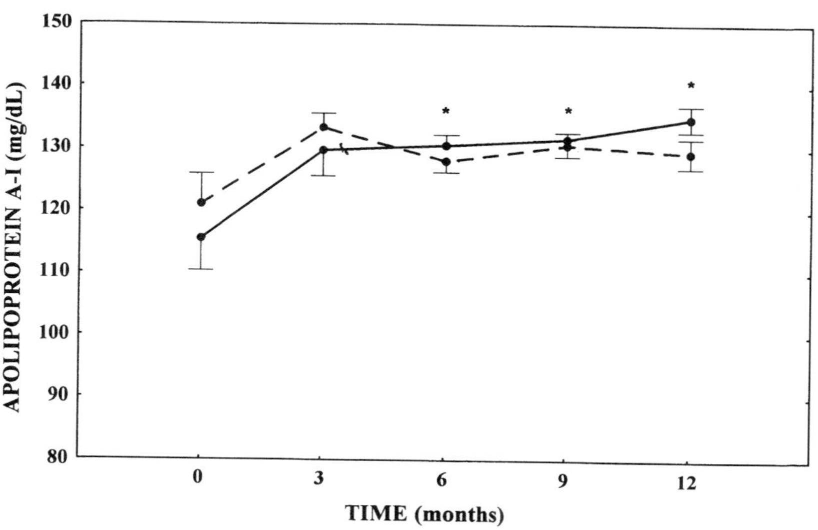

FIGURE 4. Serum apolipoprotein A-I values in the two groups of PCOS adolescent girls treated, respectively, with a D COC (*continuous line*) and a CA COC (*discontinuous line*). *Asterisk* indicates statistically significant difference ($p \leq 0.05$) from the baseline value of each group. Statistical analysis was performed by ANOVA repeated measures. Values are given as mean ± SE.

Blood samples were obtained for TC, LDL-C, HDL-C, TG, apolipopreins (A-I, A-II, B, Lp[a]), and SHBG on days 3–7 for cycling patients or on a random day for amenorrheic patients. Abdominal ultrasonography to assess the morphology and volume of the uterus and ovaries was also performed with a 5-mHz transducer on the same day of blood sampling.

After the initial examination, patients were randomly assigned to one of the following treatment groups: (A) 2 mg CA plus 0.035 mg EE (12 patients) or (B) 0.15 mg D plus 0.03 mg EE (12 patients). Treatment was given daily for 21 days followed by a 7-day rest for a period of 1 year. The initial clinical and endocrine characteristics did not differ between treatment groups (TABLE 1). Hirsutism and lipid profile were reevaluated every 3 months after initiation of therapy for 1 year.

Both drugs were well tolerated by PCOS adolescent patients, ensuring cyclicity. A significant decline in the Ferriman-Gallway hirsutism score was observed from the sixth month of therapy. Hirsutism score continued to decline until the twelfth month of treatment (p >0.001), but the difference between the ninth and twelfth months was not statistically significant.

LIPID PROFILE OF PCOS ADOLESCENT GIRLS BEFORE AND AFTER TREATMENT

During treatment, BMI and W/H remained unchanged in both groups of adolescent (r = 0.569 and 0.544, respectively). They were also positively correlated with W/H ratio (r = 0.688 and 0.681). Serum LDL-C and and TG levels demonstrated a positive correlation with W/H ratio (r = 0.490 and 0.592, respectively), whereas HDL-C levels were negatively correlated with BMI, W/H ratio, and Ferriman-Gallway score (r = –0.543, –0.635, and –0.419, respectively). Furthermore, TG, TC/HDL-C, and LDL/HDL-C ratios were negatively correlated with SHBG (r = –0.476, –0.529, and –0.479), whereas HDL-C was positively correlated (r = 0.607) with SH-BG. A weak positive correlation was observed between Lp(a) and either BMI or the W/H ratio (r = 0.382 and 0.358, respectively). No correlation was observed between androgens (testosterone, free testosterone, Δ_4-androstenedione, and S-DHEA) and lipids.

During treatment with both D and CA COC formulations, serum TC increased, reaching the highest level at 12 months of therapy (s = 0.005 and p >0.00, respectively) (FIG. 1.). A significant rise in LDL-C serum levels was demonstrated after 12 months of treatment with both COC formulations ($p = 0.029$ and $p = 0.001$, respectively). After a year of therapy, HDL-C serum levels were elevated by both COC formulations, but the rise was significant only with the CA formulation ($p = 0.03$) (FIG. 2). Atheromatic indexes were not affected by any treatment modality, whereas serum TG levels were raised significantly at the twelfth month of therapy with the CA COC ($p = 0.037$) (FIG. 3). In the case of apolipoproteins, only A-I demonstrated a significant rise from the sixth month of treatment, with the D COC reaching the highest level at the twelfth month ($p = 0.001$) (FIG. 4).

CONCLUSIONS

Both COC formulations are effective in ensuring normal menstrual cycles and reducing hirsutism in adolescent PCOS patients. The significant positive correlation of W/H ratio with lipid profile is in accord with other data indicating an association of central obesity with myocardial infarction, angina pectoris, and stroke.[10,20]

In our study the documented rise of TG and HDL-C by the CA COC indicates weak opposition of CA to the action of estrogens. Most studies of lipid metabolism of adult women on CA COC found this rise of TG and HDL-C.[21,22] In our cases we documented a rise of LDL-C also. The increase of A-I apolipoprotein, the major apolipoprotein of HDL-C, in adolescent patients on D COC, which was not paralleled by a significant increase in HDL-C, should be further investigated. This could possibly indicate that the two COC formulations regulate differently the various HDL-C subfractions, suggesting an increase in HDL_2 (containing only apolipoprotein A-I) and HDL_3 (containing both apolipoproteins A-I and A-II) by the D and CA COC, respectively. A definite conclusion could be withdrawn by measuring these subfractions in a larger number of patients.

Women with PCOS often have an increased prevalence of risk factors for CVD such as insulin resistance, hyperinsulinemia, obesity, impaired glucose tolerance, NIDDM, hyertension, dyslipidemia, and atherosclerotic cardiovascular disease. These abnormalities appear to be further enhanced by coexisting abdominal obesity and occur with increased frequency with advancing age. It is therefore most appropriate to practice preventive medicine from adolescence. Obese teenage patients should be encouraged to lose weight, because this would improve the clinical signs and metabolic aspects of the syndrome. Furthermore, psychologic support should be available. Until now the use of various agents in the form of COC has been very effective in controlling unwanted hair, but direct comparison studies of their effect on lipid metabolism especially in adolescent PCOS patients have not been performed. From our study we conclude that the COC containing the less androgenic progestogen, desogestrel, does not have unfavorable effects on lipid metabolism while limiting hyperandrogenism, and it is therefore suitable for long-term treatment of young patients with PCOS.

ACKNOWLEDGMENTS

We acknowledge the invaluable help of Analytiki Laboratories in the measurement of androgens and lipids.

REFERENCES

1. URBANEK, M. *et al.* 1999. Thirty-seven candidate genes for polycystic ovary syndrome: strongest evidence for linkage is with follistatin. Proc. Natl. Acad. Sci. USA **96:** 8573–8578.
2. APTER, D. *et al.* 1994. Accelerated 24-hour LH pulsatile activity in adolescent girls with ovarian hyperandrogenism: relevance to the developmental phase of polycystic ovarian syndrome. J. Clin. Endocrinol. Metab. **79:** 119–125.

3. HERTER, L.D. *et al.* 1996. Relevance of the determination of ovarian volume in adolescent girls with menstrual disorders. J. Clin. Ultrastruct. **24:** 243–248.
4. VERTOUROLI, S. *et al.* 1995. Longitudinal change of sonographic ovarian aspects and endocrine parameters in irregular cycles of adolescence. Pediatr. Res. **38:** 974–980.
5. APTER, D. *et al.* 1995. Metabolic features of polycystic ovary syndrome are found in adolescent girls with hyperandrogenism. J. Clin. Endocrinol. Metab. **80:** 2966–2973.
6. ZHANG, L.H. *et al.* 1995. Serine phosphorylation of human P450c17 increases 17,20-lyase activity: implications for adrenarche and the polycystic ovary syndrome. Proc. Natl. Acad. Sci. **92:** 10619–10623.
7. DUNAIF, A. *et al.* 1995. Excessive insulin receptor serine phosphorylation in cultured fibroblasts and in skeletal muscle. A potential mechanism for insulin resistance in the polycystic ovary syndrome. J. Clin. Invest. **96:** 801–810.
8. CREATSAS, G. 1993. Treatment of polycystic ovarian disease during adolescence with ethinyl estradiol ? cyproterone acetate versus a D-Tr-6 LHRH analog. Int. J. Gynaecol. Obstet. **42:** 147–153.
9. ROBINSON, S. *et al.* 1996. Dyslipidaemia is associated with insulin resistance in women with polycystic ovaries. Clin. Endocrinol. Oxf. **44:** 277–284.
10. NORMAN, R.J. *et al.* 1995. Metabolic approaches to the subclassification of the polycystic ovary syndrome. Fertil. Steril. **63:** 329–335.
11. WILD, RA.1995. Obesity, lipids, cardiovascular disease and androgen excess. Am. J. Med. **98:** 275–325.
12. HOLTE, *et al.* 1994. Serum lipoprotein lipid profile in women with the polycystic ovary syndrome: relation to anthropometric, endocrine and metabolic variables. Clin. Endocrinol. Oxf. **41:** 463–471.
13. CONWAY, G.S. *et al.* 1992. Risk factors for coronary artery disease in lean and obese women with the polycystic ovary syndrome. Clin. Endocrinol. Oxf. **37:** 119–125.
14. TALBOTT, E. *et al.* 1998. Adverse lipid and coronary heart disease risk profiles in young women with polycystic ovary syndrome: results of a case control study. J. Clin. Epidemiol. **51:** 415–422.
15. GODSLAND, I.F. *et al.* 1990. The effects of different formulations of oral contraceptive agents on lipid and carbohydrate metabolism. N. Engl. J. Med. **323:** 1375–1381.
16. CROOK, D. *et al.* 1998. Safety evaluation of modern oral contraceptives. Effects on lipoprotein and carbohydrate metabolism. Contraception **57:** 189–201.
17. LOBO, R.A. *et al.* 1996. Plasma lipids and desogestrel and ethinyl estradiol: a metaanalysis. Fertil. Steril. **65:** 1100-1109.
18. SPEROFF, L. *et al.* 1994. Clinical Gynecologic Endocrinology and Infertility. Williams & Wilkins. Baltimore, MD.
19. FERRIMAN, D. *et al.* 1961. Clinical assessment of body hair growth in women. J. Clin. Endocrinol. Metab. **21:**1440–1447.
20. PASQUALI, R. 1994. Body fat distribution has weight-independent effects on clinical, hormonal and metabolic features in women with the polycystic ovary syndrome. Metabolism **43:** 706–713.
21. FALSSETTI, L. *et al.* 1995. Effects of long term administration of an oral contraceptive containing ethinylestradiol and cyproterone acetate on lipid metabolism in women with polycystic ovary syndrome. Acta Obstet. Gynecol. Scand. **74:** 56–60.
22. PORCILE, A. *et al.* 1991. Longterm treatment of hirsuitism: desogestrel compared with cyproterone acetate in oral contraceptives. Fertil. Steril. **55:** 877–881.

Laparoscopic Approach to Ovarian Cysts in Women over 40 Years of Age

G. SCARSELLI,[a] G.L. BRACCO, L. PICIOCCHI, AND M.E. COCCIA

Department of Obstetrics and Gynecology, University of Florence, 50134 Firenze, Italy

For many years, the traditional treatment of ovarian cysts has been laparotomy. This approach is characterized, however, by elevated morbidity given that the majority of these cysts are very often benign. The main problem regarding the laparoscopic approach to the ovarian cyst is the risk of treating an ovarian cancer. As a consequence, there can be a worsening of prognosis, due to spillage at the time of laparoscopic surgery.

According to the literature, the incidence of ovarian carcinoma among patients who have undergone operative laparoscopy for adnexal masses varies from 0.1% to 4.2%.[1–8] Canis *et al.*[6] reported 19 cases of ovarian tumors out of 819 adnexal masses in 757 patients. The 19 ovarian tumors (2.32%) were classified as ($n = 7$) ovarian carcinomas and low malignant potential tumors ($n = 12$). If we consider the incidence of these tumors in relation to age, 1.8% were found in women under 50 and 7.6% were found in women over 50 years of age.

In a retrospective study, Maiman *et al.*[2] reported a total of 42 cases of malignancy after laparoscopic treatment of ovarian masses. However, only 12% of the physicians interviewed had used tumor markers, and only 40% had requested an intraoperative frozen section. Moreover, four of the most accepted benign characteristics of cysts, that is, diameter less than 8 cm, cystic neoplasm, unilaterality, and uniloculariety, were present in 31% of the cases.

Some retrospective studies[9–13] on the problem of spillage have reported that surgical rupture of the capsule in stage I epithelial ovarian cancer has an adverse influence on survival prognosis. However, other retrospective studies have reported that surgical rupture of a malignant cyst is not a negative prognostic factor, at multivariate analysis. In fact, some authors affirm that prognosis is not influenced at all if the patient is immediately treated.[14–16]

We would like to stress that the majority of ovarian cysts (87%) are benign[17] and are therefore eligible for endoscopic treatment. Following strict guidelines (echographic criteria of benignity: unilaterality, uniloculariety, absence of septa > 3 mm and intracystic vegetation, and pure borders; CA 125 levels < 35 IU/ml; benign laparoscopic appearance of cyst and the peritoneal cavity) and using cautious management, laparoscopic treatment of ovarian cysts can be reliable and safe.

On the other hand, Canis *et al.*[6] reported on two malignant tumors that had been macroscopically suspicious and were treated as benign masses. The false negative diagnoses (1.5%) were due to inadequate sampling. Thus, Canis suggested that the

[a]Address for correspondence: Department of Obstetrics and Gynecology, University of Florence, Viale Morgagni 85, 50134 Firenze, Italy. Phone: +39 055 4220168; fax: +39 055 434330. scarselli@endosphere.it

complete cyst, and not only a fragment or small bioptic sample, be submitted for intraoperative histologic examination. Chapron *et al.*[18] treated 26 patients with suspected signs of ovarian malignancy using laparoscopic adnexectomy with an endoscopic bag. The results of the intraoperative histological examination for all these patients were benign. The definitive histological results confirmed the frozen section findings. Using the same strategy, we have been able to avoid laparotomy, especially in postmenopausal patients, who, at ultrasound, present with complex adnexal masses. Laparotomy should not be considered a complication when managing suspicious adnexal masses. Immediate vertical laparotomy remains the gold standard for macroscopically suspicious masses. Although this approach is acceptable in postmenopausal patients,[6] laparoscopic adnexectomy of suspicious masses at ultrasound is not acceptable in young patients. The false positive rate of diagnosis of malignancy at ultrasound is still very high.

One pressing question must be asked: Can we distinguish a benign tumor from a malignant one? Appropriate patient selection for laparoscopic ovarian surgery requires information on the characteristics of the cyst. This can be obtained by ultrasound examination. One of the most important advances in gynecological ultrasound diagnosis has been the introduction of transvaginal sonography, which gives a good image of the pelvic organs given the closeness of the ultrasound transducer to the genital organs.

The protocol at our departement for the diagnosis and management of ovarian persistent cysts is based on a multimodal approach using clinical examination, case history, transabdominal and transvaginal ultrasonography, transvaginal color Doppler, and serum values of CA125 and other markers (CA19.9, CA15.3, CA72.4, CEA, αFP, βhCG).

The echographic criteria for distinguishing benign cysts are the following: unilateral mass, unilocular cyst, absence of both septa > 3 mm and intracystic vegetations, and pure borders.[19,20] However, using Sassone's score, which considers 9 as the cutoff point used to distinguish malignant from nonmalignant cysts,[21] several complex benign cysts, such as dermoid cysts, could be considered malignant.

If the above-mentioned criteria are respected, such as those evaluated by a transvaginal probe, and the dosage of CA125 employed is < 35 IU/ml,[8] the probability of finding a benign formation is very high. Some authors have noted that by using these specific ultrasonographic criteria, the negative predictive value has been 96%[19]; in post-menopausal women, the same values range from 95% to 100%.[22,23] When an ovarian mass is sonographically defined as a unilocular and nonechogenic cyst, the negative predictive value reported has been between 90% and 95%.[19,24] Other authors have reported 100% specificity by using a combination of the clinical examination, CA125 dosage < 35 IU/ml, and transvaginal ultrasound.[25,26]

In a prospective study that included 1769 asymptomatic postmenopausal patients, Conway[27] found ovarian cysts in 116 patients at ultrasound. The prevalence was 6.6%. Out of the 116 patients, 27 (23.28%) had simple cysts that disappeared spontaneously, 60 (50.48%) had persistent cysts, and 20 (17.24%) were lost to follow-up study. Eighteen out of the 60 women (26.09%) with persistent simple ovarian cysts underwent surgery. No malignant ovarian aspects were identified. Simple ovarian cysts are more common in postmenopausal women than had been previously believed. However, given that such cysts are unlikely to be or become malignant, conservative treatment can be followed. In fact, Kroon *et al.*[28] reported that 12 out of 32 (37.5%) cysts had spontaneously disappeared in a group of postmenopausal women with small, simple anechoic ovarian cysts.

Recently, the use of transvaginal color Doppler (TV-CDS) has allowed us to increase our knowledge on the state of neovascularization of the ovarian cyst wall.[29,30] It has become clear that this technique is a valuable tool for differentiating benign from malignant ovarian tumors.[30–33]

A low pulsatility index (PI) or resistance index (RI) indicates a low impedance to blood flow in the distal vasculature, as seen in neoplasias; a high PI or RI (associated with absent intratumoral neovascularization with color Doppler) is said to exclude ovarian cancer. According to the literature, the percentage of true positives varies from 80% to 100%, with a false positivity of 0%–20%. Fleischer[33] compared transvaginal color-Doppler ultrasonography with histologic findings in 126 ovarian masses. He reported a sensitivity level of 92%, a specificity level of 86%, a PPV of 86%, and a NPV of 98%. Furthermore, in 3 out of the 126 cases, the CD was highly suggestive of ovarian cancer, although the morphologic findings had not been suspicious. The mean and SD of the PI values in the benign group (1.4 ± 0.6) showed a statistically significant difference when compared to the malignant groups (0.6 ± 0.4) ($p = 0.04$). However, there was overlap in the range of PI values of the benign (0.8 to 2.0) and malignant groups (0.3 to 1.2).

According to Zanetta,[34] color Doppler is more accurate than conventional ultrasound and CA125 in discriminating malignancies from benign tumors. The best uses of this technique seem to be the gathering of ulterior preoperative information concerning masses with uncertain sonographic characteristics, and that of allowing better timing and tailoring of surgery.

CA125 is an antigen, identified by OC125 monoclonal antibody, found in cells cultured from patients with serous papillary ovarian carcinoma. Eighty percent of patients with known epithelial ovarian cancer respond positively to CA125 assay. It is correlated with tumor volume, but the percentage can be high in benign epithelial cysts such as endometrioma, adenomyosis, myoma, and PID. In the presence of certain factors such as a pelvic mass, however, a serum level of CA125 > 50 IU/ml and postmenopausal age, the probability of a malignant neoplasia is from 80 to 90%.

Furthermore, during laparoscopy we can obtain information by observing both the cyst and the peritoneal cavity. An aspiration of the peritoneal fluid sample, a careful examination of the cystic ovary, and a complete inspection of the pelvic peritoneum, the contralateral ovary, and the omentum can be performed using laparoscopy. Endoscopic bags can be used to remove the cyst or the whole ovary without spillage. Thus, intraoperative histological examination can be performed. In this way, it is possible to reduce the risk of treating an ovarian cancer during laparoscopy.[1,3,35]

Canis *et al.*[6] compared the accuracy of laparoscopic diagnosis with that of histodiagnosis in 819 adnexal masses. They found that all the malignant tumors that had been considered cancerous or suspicious at laparoscopy were confirmed histologically (sensitivity 100%). The positive predictive value was 41.3%, and the negative predictive value was 100%.

During laparoscopy, we can also study the ovarian cyst by laparoscopic ultrasound imaging (LUI). LUI is performed by using a high-frequency, multiple focus transducer (7.5 MHz): sector, convex, or linear. The possibility of having real-time multiplane imaging of the organs increases the accuracy of diagnosis.

The transducer (UST-5521, Aloka, Japan) is a 7.5-MHz linear array designed for easy insertion through a 10-mm trocar; it is applicable to SSD 620 (Aloka, Japan) ultrasound equipment and can be used to perform intraoperative ultrasound examinations.

The closeness of the LUI probe to the ovary, the use of a high-frequency transducer with high resolution, and the possibility of using color Doppler are among the advantages of this technique. It is even possible to identify very small papillary formations on the internal wall of the cysts. Identification of these formations is not possible when using conventional abdominal ultrasonography: it is difficult even when using transvaginal ultrasonography.

After using this imaging approach, our preliminary evaluation of LUI is that this type of ultrasonography can be a reliable diagnostic tool during gynecological operative endoscopy. It can also be helpful in intraoperative decision-making.[36]

An ovarian cyst may be sometimes histopathologically diagnosed as being a carcinoma of low malignant potential or a borderline ovarian tumor. Unilateral salpingo-oophorectomy, or, in some cases, cystectomy, is a valid alternative treatment in young women with localized (stage IA) disease.[37] These borderline tumors present a high survival rate (93%) at five years. A study of 254 cases was carried out by Mangioni *et al.*,[38] and they reported that not one of these patients had died because of the malignancy. Conservative surgery is a valid alternative in those patients still at reproductive age. Pelvic and para-aortic lymphadenectomy are indicated in stage III subjects with peritoneal spread: laparoscopic follow-up is suggested. However, even if no specific sonographic aspect exists for the identification of borderline tumors, ultrasonography is the best way to detect their recurrence. Conservative treatment of borderline ovarian tumors includes a laparoscopic procedure. Even if there appears to be a high risk of intraoperative rupture, the rate of recurrence is similar to that of laparotomic treatment.[39] Available data indicate that fertility, pregnancy outcome, and survival in such patients remain excellent.[40]

In 1993, the Italian Society of Endoscopy and Laser Therapy in Gynecology (S.I.E.L.G.) decided to perform a multicenter prospective study. The aim of the study was to verify whether laparoscopic treatment of ovarian cysts could be reliable and safe even in women over 40, when cautious management and strict guidelines were used. Forty-seven Italian Centers of Gynecological Endoscopy participated (from June 1994 until December 1995). The safety of laparoscopic treatment in women over 40 with ovarian persistent cysts was evaluated. Four hundred and six patients over 40 years of age (37.2% in postmenopause) took part in the study. All patients were divided into two groups according to the ultrasonographic characteristics of the cysts (benign or suspect). A comparison was made between 289 patients with benign ultrasonographic findings (group A) and 117 patients of the same age with ultrasonographic criteria that included septa, vegetation, solid components, or complex masses (group B).

The average age of group A subjects was 51.4 ± 8. Age ranged from 40 to 78 years. Histological diagnosis of the 289 ultrasonically identified benign cysts confirmed that they were all nonmalignant. In the 117 patients with suspicious ultrasonographic criteria (group B), four cases of malignancy were found: two were cases of serous cystoadenocarcinoma, one was a moderately differentiated Leydig cell tumor, and one was a low-malignant-potential tumor.

Statistical elaboration was carried out using the χ^2 method. Considering the prevalence of carcinoma in relation to the ultrasonographic findings, there was a significant statistical difference between the two groups ($p = 0.009$). Moreover, in the patients with no benign ultrasonographic criteria, there were no significant statistical differences between those in premenopause and those in postmenopause ($p = 0.612$).

At our department we treated a series of 276 ovarian cysts using laparoscopy. Sixty-eight patients were over 40 years of age. In 15 of the 68 cases (22%), the serum levels of the tumoral ovarian markers were abnormal. The ovarian markers were abnormal in endometriotic cysts and in dermoid cysts, as well as in paraovarian and in simple serous cysts. The diameters of all the cysts were 43 ± 13 mm (range 5–80). The duration of surgery was 59 ± 26 min (range: 15–120 min.). In two cases where severe adhesion was present, two laparoscopic (0.7%) procedures were converted into laparotomies. The duration of hospital stay was 2.6 ± 1.3 days. No relapses were noted at follow-up in the ultrasonographic controls. In this series we performed excision of the cyst in 45% of the cases and an adnexectomy in 55% of the cases. We did not find any case of malignancy.

In conclusion, operative laparoscopy represents a valid alternative for the treatment of benign adnexal masses, even in women over 40. The majority of cysts in this age group of women are benign. Patient selection for laparoscopic surgery is very important. Patient selection should be based on transvaginal ultrasound, color Doppler, dosage of CA125, clinical examination, and case history. This multimodal approach is fundamental for avoiding treatment of malignant masses. If the benign ultrasonographic criteria, (unilateral mass, unilocular cysts, absence of septa >3 mm and intracystic vegetations, defined borders) are respected and the serum level of CA125 is <35 IU/ml, the probability of the presence of a benign cyst is very high. Furthermore, during laparoscopy, we can obtain information from the cyst itself and from the peritoneal cavity. Endoscopic bags can be used to remove the cyst or the whole ovary without any spillage. Thus, intraoperative histological examination can be carried out. In this way, it is possible to reduce the risk of treating an ovarian cancer at laparoscopy.

Laparoscopic treatment of ovarian masses can be considered useful and safe, even in post-menopausal patients. However, the following criteria must be met: benign sonographic aspects, CA125 <35 IU/ml, and benign laparoscopic features. On the other hand, if vegetation, septa, and/or solid or complex cysts are present, there is no diagnostic possibility of eliminating the risk of finding and treating ovarian malignant masses. Ultrasonography is perhaps the most important tool available for distinguishing benign from malignant adnexal masses.

REFERENCES

1. PARKER, W. & J. BEREK. 1990. Management of selected cystic adnexal masses in postmenopausal women by operative laparoscopy: a pilot study. Am. J. Obstet. Gynecol. **163:** 1574–1579.
2. MAIMAN, M., V. SELTZER & J. BOYCE. 1991. Laparoscopic excision of ovarian neoplasms subsequently found to be malignant. Obstet. Gynecol. **77:** 563–565.

3. MANN, W.J. & H. REICH. 1992. Laparoscopic adnexectomy in postmenopausal women. J. Repr. Med. **37:** 254–256.
4. NEZHAT, F., C. NEZHAT, C.E. WELANDER, *et al.* 1992. Four ovarian cancers diagnosed during laparoscopic management of 1011 women with adnexal mass. Am. J. Obstet. Gynecol. **167:** 790–796.
5. METTLER, R., G. CAESAR, S. NEUNZLING & K. SEMM. 1993. Value of endoscopic ovarian surgery: critical analysis of 626 pelviscopically operated ovarian cysts at the Kiel University Gynecologyc Clinic 1990–1991. Geburtshilfe Frauenheilk. **53:** 253–257.
6. CANIS, M., G. MAGE, J.L. POULY, *et al.* 1994. Laparoscopic diagnosis of adnexal masses: a 12-year experience with long term follow-up. Obstet. Gynecol. **83:** 702–712.
7. SHALEV, E., S. ELIYAHU, D. PELEG, *et al.* 1994. Laparoscopic management of adnexal cystic masses in postmenopausal women. Obstet. Gynecol. **83:** 594–596.
8. GUGLIELMINA, J.N., G. PENNEHOUAT, B. DEVAL, *et al.* 1997. Treatment of ovarian cysts by laparoscopy. Contracept. Fertil. Sex. **25:** 218–229.
9. PUROLA, E. & U. NIEMINEN. 1968. Does rupture of cystic carcinoma during operation influence the prognosis? Ann. Chir. Gynaecol. Fenn. **57:** 615–617.
10. WEBB, M.J., D.G. DECKER, E. MUSSEY & T.J. WILLIAMS. 1973. Factors influencing survival in Stage I ovarian cancer. Am. J. Obstet. Gynecol. **116:** 222–228.
11. EINHORN, N., B. NILSSON & S. KERSTIN. 1985. Factors influencing survival in carcinoma of the ovary. Cancer **55:** 2019–2025.
12. FINN, C.B., B.M. LUESLEY, E.J. BUXTON, *et al.* 1992. Is Stage I epithelial ovarian cancer overtreated both surgically and systemically? Results of a five-year cancer registry review. Br. J. Obstet. Gynecol. **99:** 54–58.
13. SAINZ DE LA CUESTA, R., B.A. GOFF, A.F. FULLER, *et al.* 1994. Prognostic significance of intraoperative rupture of malignant ovarian neoplasm. Gynecol. Oncol. **52:** 111.
14. DEMBO, A.J., M. DAVY, A.E. STENWIG, *et al.* 1990. Prognostic factors in patients with stage I epithelial ovarian cancer. Obstet. Gynecol. **75:** 263–272.
15. SIGURDSSON, K., P. ALM & B. GULLBERG. 1983. Prognostic factor in malignant epithelial ovarian tumours. Gynecol. Oncol. **15:** 370–380.
16. SEVELDA, P., N. VAVRA, M. SCHEMPER & H. SALZER. 1990. Prognostic factors for survival in Stage I epithelial ovarian carcinoma. Cancer **65:** 2349–2352.
17. CREASMAN, W.T. & J.T. SOPER. 1986. The undiagnosed adnexal mass after the menopause. Clin. Obstet. Gynecol. **29:** 446–450.
18. CHAPRON, C., J.B. DUBUISSON, O. KADOCH, *et al.* 1998. Laparoscopic management of organic cysts: is there a place for frozen section diagnosis? Hum. Reprod. **13:** 324–329.
19. HERRMANN, U.J., G.W. LOCHER & A. GOLDHIRSCH. 1987. Sonographic patterns of malignancy: prediction of malignancy. Obstet. Gynecol. **69:** 777–781.
20. GRANDBERG, S., A. NOSTROM & A. WIKLAND. 1990. Tumors in the pelvis as imaged by vaginal sonography. Gynecol. Oncol. **37:** 224–229.
21. SASSONE, A.M., I.E. TIMOR-TRITSCH, A. ARTNER, *et al.* 1991. Transvaginal sonographic characterization of ovarian disease: evaluation of a new scoring system to predict ovarian malignancy. Obstet. Gynecol. **78:** 70–76.
22. RULIN, M.C. & A.L. PRESTON. 1987. Adnexal masses in postmenopausal women. Obstet. Gynecol. **70:** 578–583.
23. GOLDSTEIN, S.R., B. SUBRAMANYAM, J.R. SNYDER, *et al.* 1989. The postmenopausal cystic adnexal mass: the potential role of ultrasound in conservative management. Obstet. Gynecol. **73:** 8–10.
24. MEIRE, H.B., P. FARRANT & T. GUTHA. 1978. Distinction of benign from malignant ovarian cysts by ultrasound. Br. J. Obstet. Gynecol. **85:** 893–897.
25. FINKLER, N.J., B. BENACERERRAF, P.T. LAVIN, *et al.* 1988. Comparison of serum CA 125, clinical impression and ultrasound in the preoperation evaluation of ovarian masses. Obstet. Gynecol. **72:** 659–664.
26. JACOBS, I., I. STABILE, J. BRIDGES, *et al.* 1988. Multimodal approach to screening for ovarian cancer. Lancet **1:** 268–273.
27. CONWAY, C., I. ZALUD, M. DILENA, *et al.* 1998. Simple cyst in the postmenopausal patient: detection and management. J. Ultrasound Med. **17:** 369–372.
28. KROON, E. & E. ANDOLF. 1995. Diagnosis and follow-up of simple ovarian cysts detected by ultrasound in postmenopausal women. Obstet. Gynecol. **85:** 211–214.

29. LEIBMAN, A.J., B. KRUSE & M.B. MCSWEENEY. 1988. Transvaginal sonography: comparison with transabdominal sonography in the diagnosis of pelvic masses. Am. J. Roentgenol. **151:** 89–92.
30. BOURNE, T., S. CAMPBELL, C. STEER, *et al.* 1989. Transvaginal colour flow imaging: a possible new screening technique for ovarian cancer. Br. Med. J. **299:** 1367–1370.
31. KURJAK, A., I. ZALUD & Z. ALFIREVIC. 1991. Evaluation of adnexal masses with transvaginal color ultrasound. J. Ultrasound Med. **10:** 295–297.
32. FLEISCHER, A.C., W.H. RODGERS & B.K. RAO, *et al.* 1991. Assessment of ovarian tumor vascularity with transvaginal color Doppler sonography. J. Ultrasound Med. **10:** 563–568.
33. FLEISCHER, A.C., J.A. CULLINAN, C.V. PEERY, *et al.* 1996. Early detection of ovarian carcinoma with transvaginal color Doppler ultrasonography. Am. J. Obstet. Gynecol. **174:** 101–106.
34. ZANETTA, G., P. VERGANI & A. LISSONI. 1994. Color Doppler ultrasound in the preoperative assessment of adnexal masses. Acta Obstet. Gynecol. Scand. **73:** 637–641.
35. LEVINE, R.L. 1990. Pelviscopic surgery in women over forty. J. Reprod. Med. **35:** 597–600.
36. COCCIA, M.E., G.L. BRACCO & G. SCARSELLI. 1994. Laparoscopic sonography and multimodal diagnostic approach in case of endoscopic treatment of ovarian cyst. *In* Growth and Differentiation in Reproductive Organs. A.R. Genazzani, F. Petraglia, A.D. Genazzani & G. D'Ambrogio, Eds.: 173–175. CIC Edizioni Internazionali. Roma.
37. LIM TAN, S.K., H.E. CJIGAS & R.E. SCULLY. 1988. Ovarian cystectomy for serous borderline tumors: a follow-up study of 35 cases. Obstet. Gynecol. **72:** 755–778.
38. MANGIONI, C. & U.A. BIANCHI. 1996. Tumori maligni dell'ovaio. *In* La Clinica Ostetrica e Ginecologica. II Edizone. G.B. Candiani, V. Danesino & A. Gastaldi, Eds.: 1723–1725. Masson. Milano, Italy.
39. DARAI, E., J. TEBOUL, F. WALKER, *et al.* 1996. Epithelial ovarian carcinoma of low malignant potential. Eur. J. Obstet. Gynecol. Reprod. Biol. **66:** 141–145.
40. GOTLIEB, W.H., S. FLIKKER, B. DAVIDSON, *et al.* 1998. Borderline tumors of the ovary: fertility treatment, conservative management, and pregnancy outcome. Cancer **82:** 141–146.

Management of Hydrosalpinx: Reconstructive Surgery or IVF?

JOHN N. BONTIS AND KONSTANTINOS D. DINAS

Second Department of Obstetrics and Gynecology, Aristotelian University of Thessaloniki, Hippokration Hospital, 546 42 Thessaloniki, Greece

ABSTRACT: Tubal disease remains the most important factor in female infertility. Many investigators reported that patients with hydrosalpinx had a decreased clinical pregnancy rate and an increased miscarriage rate, resulting in a decreased ongoing pregnancy rate when compared to that of patients with other types of tubal disease. Different studies showed a deleterious effect of the presence of hydrosalpinx on the outcome of *in vitro* fertilization–embryo transfer, because toxic agents flowing from the hydrosalpinx to the uterus impair the implantation rate. Operative laparoscopy is effective in the treatment of hydrosalpinges (Stage I or II). Fertility outcome is related to tubal damage. Patients with Stage III and IV disease should be managed from the beginning with *in vitro* fertilization. Excision of hydrosalpinx(-ges) improves the pregnancy potential after *in vitro* fertilization. We believe that assisted reproductive technology and reproductive surgery can be complementary. The development of laparoscopic surgery and *in vitro* fertilization improved the pregnancy rate in patients with tubal factor infertility.

INTRODUCTION

Tubal factor infertility resulting from various forms of tuboperitoneal damage remains an extremely common cause of female infertility, accounting for more than 35% of all cases of female infertility. Endosalpingeal destruction, proximal or distal oviduct occlusion, and peritubal or periovarian adhesions disrupt not only the anatomic integrity but also the functional capacity of the tubes, thus inducing indirectly the commonest causes of female infertility.

Conventional surgery, which was introduced in the 1960s in the management of diseases of the inner genital tract and particularly of hydrosalpinx, was later improved with the introduction of microsurgical techniques, which included, besides greater magnification, greater accuracy and less trauma. With the application of the basic principles of microsurgery, the surgeon confines notably the possibility of new adhesion formation in the pelvic organs.

Laparoscopic surgery, introduced in the late 1970s, with its improved optics and use of video equipment and the laser beam, is currently considered absolutely indicated in the management of tubal diseases.

The opportunity to overcome the lack of tubal function by *in vitro* fertilization (IVF) and embryo transfer in the 1980s raises a question about the treatment strategy in cases of tubal factor infertility. In most centers the tubal factor still remains the main indication for IVF.

TABLE 1. Causes of hydrosalpinx

Causes	Patients (*n*)
Abortion	60
PID	55
Endometriosis	43
Previous operations	32
Tuberculosis	5
Unknown	24
Total	**219**

The main causes of hydrosalpinx are pelvic inflammatory disease, ectopic pregnancy, endometriosis, previous abdominal operations, and a history of peritonitis and tuberculosis. In our study of 219 women with hydrosalpinx, 60 reported at least one termination of pregnancy, 55 had pelvic inflammatory disease, 43 had endometriosis, 32 had previous operations, and 5 had secondary location of tubal tuberculosis[1] (TABLE 1). The presence of hydrosalpinx can easily be diagnosed with the use of hysterosalpingography, vaginal ultrasound scan and mainly laparoscopy and salpingoscopy.

RESULTS OF THE SURGICAL MANAGEMENT OF HYDROSALPINX

The surgical management of tubal diseases in infertile women offers remarkable help to couples. The rate of pregnancy after salpingoplasty depends on the degree of destruction of the epithelium of the hydrosalpinx. Recently, certain criteria have been established to guide the surgical management of hydrosalpinx. As a result, the surgical management of hydrosalpinx larger than 3 cm, with a thick wall, multilocullar, with extended adhesions and completely destroyed mucosa has produced disappointing results.

According to the previous criteria, most investigators suggest four stages for the classification of hydrosalpinx, Stages I, II, III, and IV. Currently, almost every center proposes IVF to women with hydrosalpinges of Stage III and IV. The possibility of successful intrauterine pregnancy in Stages I and II varies from 30–80%; on the other hand, this rate in Stages III and IV is under 10%.

In our unit 258 patients with complete obstruction of the distal part of the tube were surgically managed by microsurgery and laparoscopic surgery.[1] The pregnancy rate resulting from the former or latter technique did not show a statistically significant difference. In total, the rate of intrauterine pregnancies was 17.4%, whereas that of ectopic pregnancy was 10% (TABLE 2, FIG. 1). These results are similar to those of other investigators such as Marana and Quagliarello[2] with 27% intrauterine pregnancies and 8% ectopic pregnancies, Audibert and Viala[3] with 28.6% and 11.9% respectively, Winston and Margara[4] with 32% and 9%, respectively, and Singhal *et al.*[5] with 27% and 9%, respectively.

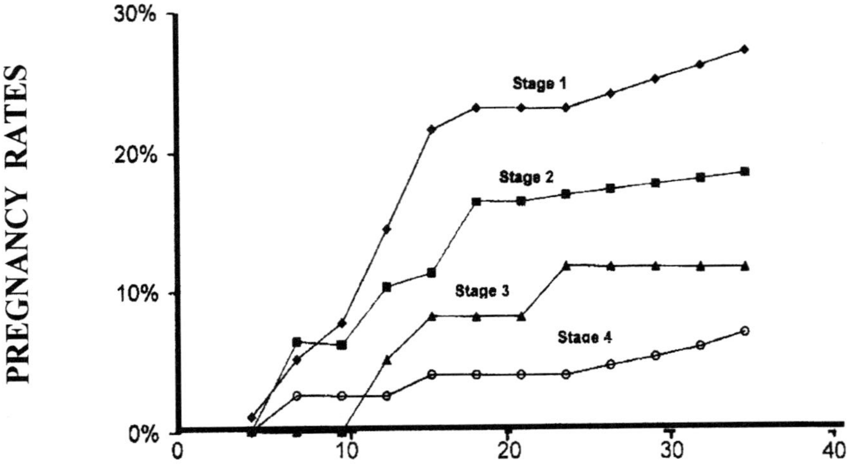

FIGURE 1. Salpingostomy. Pregnancy rates according to the hydrosalpinx stage.

TABLE 2. Conception rates after microsurgical and laparoscopic salpingostomy

Stage	Method	Patients (*n*)	Pregnancies	Intrauterine	Ectopic
Stage I	Microsurgery	75	30 (40.0%)	20 (26.6%)	10 (13.3%)
	Lap. surgery	23	5 (21.7%)	4 (17.4%)	1 (4.3%0)
Stage II	Microsurgery	62	16 (25.8%)	11 (17.7%)	5 (8%)
	Lap. surgery	14	2 (14.3%0	2 (14.3%)	0
Stage III	Microsurgery	38	9 (23.7%)	4 (10.5%)	5 (13.2%)
	Lap. surgery	2	0	—	—
Stage IV	Microsurgery	44	5 (11.4%)	3 (6.8%)	2 (4.5%0
	Lap. surgery	—	—	—	—
Total	Microsurgery	219	60 (27.4%)	38 (17.4%)	22 (10.0%)
	Lap. surgery	39	7 (17.9%)	6 (15.4%)	1 (2.6%)

The success of pregnancy depends on the pathoanatomic condition of the tube, particularly on the degree of epithelial destruction, the flattened folds, the absence of cilia on the ciliated cells, and the deficiency of secretory cells particularly in the ampulla. We have confirmed these findings in our study, obtaining microbiopsies before salpingostomy, which we studied by scanning and transmission electron microscopy[1] (FIGS. 2, 3, 4, and 5).

Distention of the distal tube is a result of high hydrostatic pressure following obstruction after infection, mainly pelvic inflammatory disease, usually caused by chlamydia. It should be emphasized that a large percentage of the women in our study reported previous termination of pregnancy and other operations.

The recent development of endoscopic surgery makes it the obligatory approach to the management of tubal diseases and an absolute indication in the management of hydrosalpinx(-ges). The advantages of this method are a shorter hospital stay, less

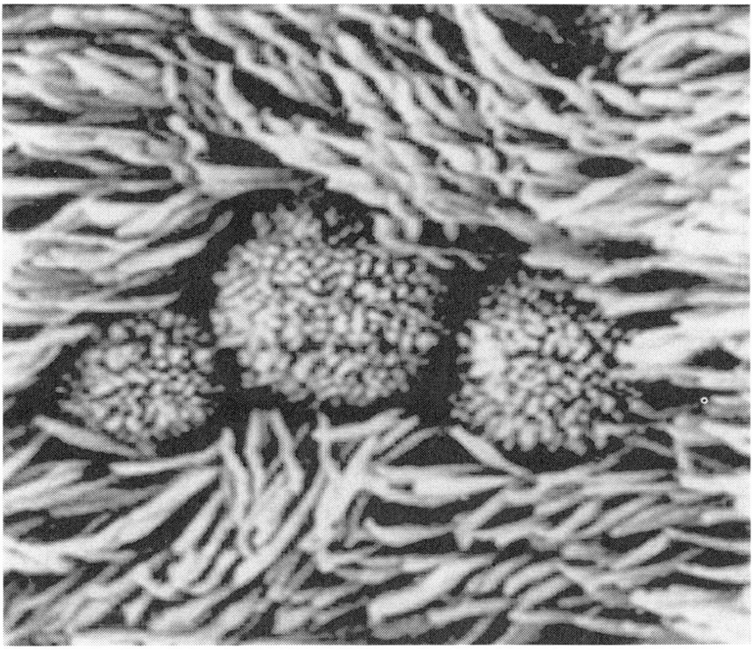

FIGURE 2. Normal tubal epithelium from the ampulla by scanning electron microscope. Ciliated and secretory cells are discerned. Magnification 5000×.

abdominal pain, and fewer possibilities for the formation of new adhesions, while the pregnancy rates are similar to those of microsurgery, according to the literature.

HYDROSALPINX AND *IN VITRO* FERTILIZATION

IVF/ET was developed to overcome mechanical obstruction attributable to tubal disease, particularly in cases of hydrosalpinx(ges). The pregnancy rate is significantly decreased when the distal end of the tube is significantly obstructed, which does not occur with other tubal diseases of varying etiology.

Sims *et al.*[6] reported a reduced rate of clinical pregnancy and an increased rate of miscarriage in women with hydrosalpinges compared with those of other types of tubal factor-related infertility. Strandell *et al.*[7] found that women with unilateral or bilateral hydrosalpinges had a significantly lower pregnancy rate than did women with tubal disease but without obstruction of its distal end. The pregnancy rate was 13% in women with hydrosalpinges compared with 26% in women with mild tubal damage. The investigators concluded that salpingectomy or salpingostomy could possibly increase the pregnancy rate.

Andersen *et al.*[8] reported a marked reduction in implantation rate when hydrosalpinges were visible on transvaginal ultrasound, and they noted pregnancy rates of

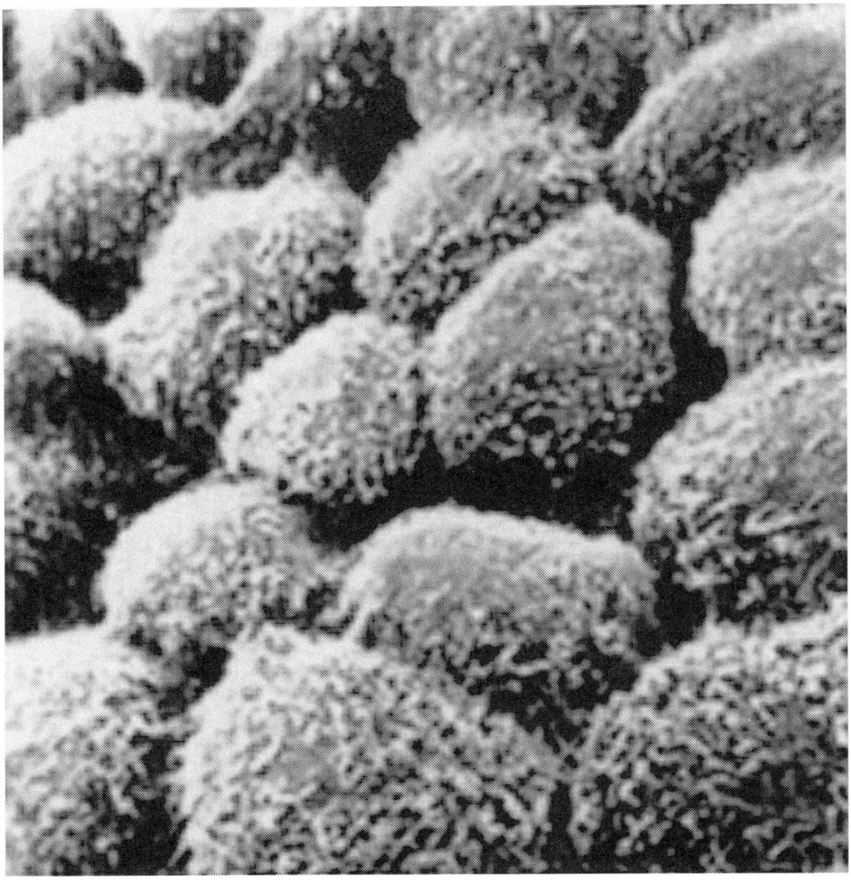

FIGURE 3. Total absence of ciliated and secretory cells in hydrosalpinx Stage IV.

22% with IVF in cases of hydrosalpinx compared with 36% in cases of tubal disease of other origin. The rate of miscarriage was 70% in hydrosalpinges compared with 36% in the other group. Vandrome *et al.*[9] confirmed the findings of the previous authors, with a pregnancy rate 10% in the group with hydrosalpinges and 23% in the other group.

Vejtorp *et al.*[10] in 1995, in a multicentral study in Denmark, studied 104 women with hydrosalpinges and 125 with other pathologic conditions and demonstrated a decreased pregnancy rate in the group with hydrosalpinges (6% and 23%, respectively). They also observed that delay in the application of IVF in women with hydrosalpinges decreased the possibility of conception.

Fleming *et al.*,[11] in a retrospective study of 79 women with hydrosalpinges of inflammatory etiology, demonstrated that the success of IVF was significantly affect-

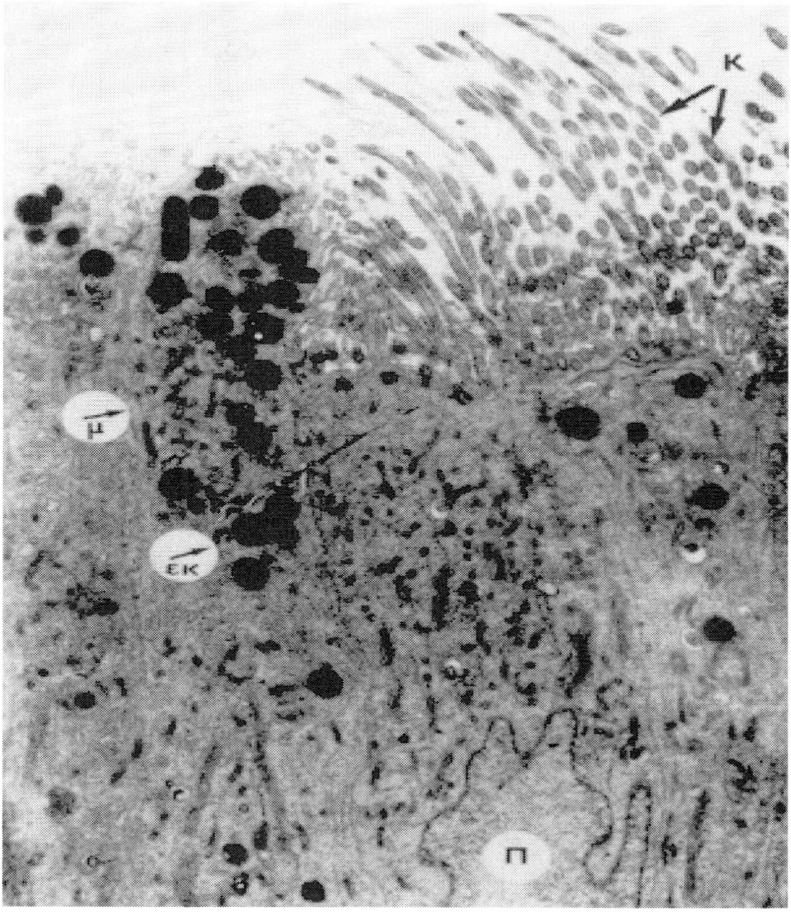

FIGURE 4. Normal tubal epithelium by electron transmission microscope. Magnification 6000×. EK, secretory cells; μ, mitochondria; Π, nucleus of ciliated cell.

ed. The authors suggested salpingectomy or salpingostomy to improve the results of IVF. In a recent study of 846 women with tubal disease by Katz *et al.*,[12] the pregnancy rate was 17% in the group with hydrosalpinx(ges) compared with 37% in the group with other tubal pathology. This study, which included 1,766 cycles, is considered the biggest retrospective study to prove that implantation and pregnancy are reduced in patients with hydrosalpinx(ges). Freeman *et al.*[13] agreed with the aforementioned results of other investigators, finding pregnancy rates of 15% in hydrosalpinx and 29% in diseases of other etiology. These authors suggest that hydrosalpinx affects not only the implantation rate but also the quality of ovum. Hy-

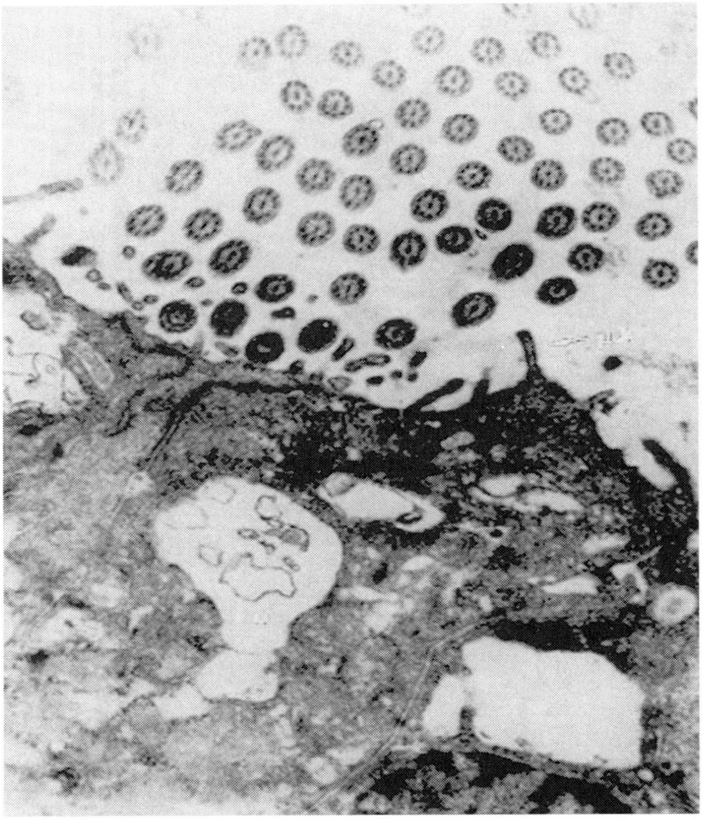

FIGURE 5. Abnormal epithelium of hydrosalpinx Stage III. Magnification 6000×. Absence of cilia and destruction of cytoplasm with the presence of vacuoles are discerned.

drosalpinx(ges) was found to affect the implantation rate of the fertilized ovum even in nonstimulated cycles.[14]

Hydrosalpinx(ges) predisposes to ectopic pregnancy in cases of IVF as well. Moreover, the first human pregnancy achieved by Edwards and Steptoe in 1977 was a tubal ectopic pregnancy. Zouves *et al.*[15] reported an ectopic pregnancy rate of 12% in 891 cycles in women with tubal obstruction; for that reason, they suggested ligating the uterine part of the tube with resection, clipping, or coagulation with CO_2 laser or diathermy.

Sharara *et al.*[16] studied 63 patients with hydrosalpinges and 60 without and found those with positive antibody titers against chlamydia. Providing antibiotics to patients with both hydrosalpinx and positive titers before IVF did not affect the results. In conclusion, IVF in patients with hydrosalpinges results in a lower pregnancy rate (10%), an increased possibility of ectopic pregnancy, a higher rate of inflammation after aspiration of tubal fluid during ultrasound, and, finally, an increased rate of miscarriage.

FACTORS AFFECTING IMPLANTATION IN HYDROSALPINX

Various factors affect the implantation rate of the fertilized ovum after IVF. A very important and yet unclarified factor is the environment of the uterine cavity and the mechanism by which the fluid contained in the hydrosalpinx disturbs the receptivity of the endometrium.

The proposed mechanisms by which hydrosalpinx decreases the success of implantation are: (1) reflux of hydrosalpinx' fluid into the uterine cavity,[17] (2) irreversible endometrial damage simultaneously with the acute phase tubal damage,[7] (3) release of intrauterine cytokines, prostaglandins, leukotrienes, and other inflammation compounds directly to the endometrium or via the circulatory or lymphatic system,[18,19] (4) alteration in integrin expression,[20] (5) delayed hypersensitivity response secondary to increased production of a 57-kDa heat-shock protein, leading to miscarriage,[21] and (6i) chronic endometritis caused mainly by *Chlamydia trachomatis*; 41% of endometrial biopsies obtained from asymptomatic women at risk for chlamydial infection were positive for *C. trachomatis*.[22] It is believed that the fluid contained in the hydrosalpinx is transferred directly into the endometrial cavity, affecting with its toxicity the endometrium and the embryo. The fluid contained in abnormal tubes probably contains microorganisms, debris, lymphocytes, and other toxic substances, whereas reflux of the fluid into the uterus has destructive results in the endometrium and the fertilized ovum. Hill *et al.*[23] reported in 1986 that hydrosalpinx may enlarge during ovarian stimulation protocols for IVF, thereby increasing tubal secretion. Aboulghar *et al.*[24] observed decreased ovarian response in ovarian stimulation with gonadotropins, whereas drainage of the hydrosalpinx before IVF insured a better ovarian response to stimulation.

Hydrosalpinx can be the result of chlamydial infection. By measuring IgG antibodies, it is possible to detect previous infection caused by chlamydia more in women with tubal damage than in women with infertility of other etiology. Rowland *et al.*[25] observed that previous infection from chlamydia reduces the success rate of IVF to 50%. It was also observed that women with previous chlamydial infection have high abortion rates after IVF. Licciardi *et al.*[26] found a 20% abortion rate among 145 women who had IVF treatment. Of those women 70% had IgG antibodies against chlamydia, whereas only 23% had a successful pregnancy after IVF/ET.

Shenk *et al.*[27] suggest a direct relation between toxicity of the contents of the hydrosalpinx and the embryo. These investigators observed degenerated embryos in 68%.

Recently a connection between endometrial receptivity and release of integrins and abnormal production of the latter was observed in patients with reduced endometrial receptivity. Lessey *et al.*[20] measured β-integrin with immunohistochemical methods from endometrial biopsies in women with hydrosalpinges. They observed notably low levels of $\alpha v\beta 3$-integrin in those with hydrosalpinges than in those without. They also demonstrated that in women whose tubes were surgically managed, integrins returned to normal.

SURGICAL MANAGEMENT OF HYDROSALPINX BEFORE *IN VITRO* FERTILIZATION

Hydrosalpinx(-ges) constitutes the main disturbance of the environment of the endometrial cavity, obstructing implantation of the embryo. It is generally accepted that salpingostomy, salpingectomy, or ligation of the uterine part of the tubes returns the rate of conception after IVF to normal.

One of the first studies to prove that surgical management of the tubes improves the pregnancy rate was that by Vandromme *et al.*[9] in 1995. They compared three groups of women with (1) hydrosalpinx, (2) salpingectomy, and (3) normal tubes. The pregnancy rate was 10%, 22%, and 31%, respectively. Kassabji *et al.*[28] compared 118 patients with hydrosalpinges and 157 patients who underwent salpingectomy and found that the pregnancy rate after IVF was 18% and 31%, respectively. Levy *et al.*[29] in a retrospective study compared three different operations in patients with hydrosalpinx. In the group with no surgical treatment the pregnancy rate was 8.5%, in the group with salpingostomy it was 17%, in the group with salpingectomy it was 28%, and in the group with tubal ligation it was 26%.

The first prospective study to show that excision of hydrosalpinx improves the pregnancy rate was performed by Shelton *et al.*[30] The pregnancy rate after salpingectomy rose to 25%. Murray *et al.*[31] reported a pregnancy rate of 8.5% in 26 women with hydrosalpinges and 38.6% in 97 women without hydrosalpinges.

In our study, which is still in progress, among 80 patients with hydrosalpinges of Stage III and IV the clinical pregnancy rate was 10%, whereas among 17 patients with severe pelvic inflammatory disease and hydrosalpinx (frozen pelvis) it was 8%. In 26 patients with hydrosalpinges who had at least one unsuccessful IVF attempt and underwent salpingectomy, the pregnancy rate was 18%. In 45 women with Stage I and II hydrosalpinx who underwent salpingostomy with laparoscopic surgery, the pregnancy rate was 17%, whereas 22 patients with hydrosalpinx who underwent resection of the final part of the tubal isthmus with CO_2 laser, the pregnancy rate was 15%.

It is not clear if salpingectomy harms the blood and nerve supply of the ovary, which are important parameters of follicle production, hormone production, and the number and quality of the ova. Other disadvantages of salpingectomy are the appearance of functional ovarian cysts and the preclusion of surgical management of the tube (salpingostomy) after recurrent failed IVF attempts. Verhulst *et al.*[32] suggested that bilateral salpingectomy does not compromise ovarian stimulation in IVF/ET. The aforementioned investigators found no statistically significant difference in the stimulation period, preovulatory levels of estradiol, and the number of oocytes retrieved between the two groups. When a woman decides to undergo salpingectomy, regardless of the method employed, it is very important that resection be made as close as possible to the tube to minimize damage to the ovarian blood supply. It is particularly emphasized that the surgeon must maintain the blood supply of the anastomotic vessels between the tube and the ovary.

Some authors suggest puncture of the hydrosalpinx and aspiration of fluid before the collection of ova, achieving relatively good results. The danger of subsequent infection is obvious, whereas an increased miscarriage rate, caused by reaccumulation of hydrosalpinx fluid after drainage, is hypothesized.[31] Andersen *et al.*[8] observed a high abortion rate (70%) among women with hydrosalpinx after IVF, whereas this rate among women without hydrosalpinx was 36%.

Salpingoscopy constitutes an important diagnostic tool for estimating the tubal epithelial condition and allows a precise definition of the abnormal status of the epithelium.[33] Defining the type of hydrosalpinx according to the criteria approved by the International Federation of Gynecologists helps the surgeon to determine and to suggest either the reconstructive surgical management of hydrosalpinx or IVF. Puttemans and Brosens,[34] after a debate in 1996, finally agreed that salpingectomy should not be performed before serious tubal abnormality is precisely diagnosed and, especially, an abnormality of its epithelium or some specific chronic tubal infection. These authors suggest obligatory salpingoscopy before surgical procedures to precisely estimate the tubal epithelial condition. If there is no severe damage, treatment should be salpingostomy.

Our own strategy towards patients with hydrosalpinges includes, first, an estimation of other infertility factors as well, such as age, ovarian function, and the male factor. Then, laparoscopy and salpingoscopy are performed. If Stage I or II hydrosalpinx is diagnosed, salpingostomy is performed at the same time and a period of 16–18 months is usually allowed for a pregnancy to occur without further intervention. On the other hand, if Stage III or IV hydrosalpinx is diagnosed, salpingectomy or tubal resection as near to the uterus as possible with CO_2 laser or diathermy is performed and then IVF is applied. Unfortunately there are no published studies in which the tubes are assessed with salpingoscopy before salpingectomy and the following results of IVF. Prospective randomized studies are needed to show improvement in IVF results after salpingectomy or other surgical methods in patients with hydrosalpinx.

CONCLUSION

Hydrosalpinx in infertile patients leads to low implantation and clinical pregnancy rates, on the one hand, and high abortion and ectopic pregnancy rates, on the other. The precise mechanism by which serious pathologic changes, particularly of tubal epithelium and of fluid in the hydrosalpinx, affect the implantation and development of the embryo is not clearly understood. Embryotoxic action of the fluid in the hydrosalpinx is considered by most to be responsible for the disappointing conception results.

Surgical management of hydrosalpinx (salpingostomy) in Stages I and II is suggested, whereas in severe hydrosalpinx, salpingectomy and then IVF are proposed.

More intimate knowledge of the pathophysiology of the tubes and the mechanism of gamete transfer into the uterine cavity is needed as well as prospective studies comparing the pregnancy outcome after various surgical techniques and IVF in patients with obstruction of the distal end of the tube.

REFERENCES

1. Bontis, J., B.V. Tarlatzis, G. Grimbizis *et al.* 1996. Microsurgical and laparoscopic management of tubal infertility: report of 763 cases. Middle East Fertil. Soc. J. **1:** 17–29.
2. Marana, R. & J. Quagliarello. 1988. Distal tubal occlusion: microsurgery versus *in vitro* fertilization. A review. Int. J. Fertil. **33:** 107–115.

3. AUDIBERT, F. & J.L. VIALA. 1991. Therapeutic strategies in tubal infertility with distal pathology. Hum. Reprod. **6:** 1439–1442.
4. WINSTON, R.M.L. & R.A. MARGARA. 1991. Microsurgical salpingostomy is not an obsolete procedure. Br. J. Obstet. Gynecol. **98:** 637–642.
5. SINGHAL, W., T.C. LI & I.D. COOKE. 1991. An analysis of factors influencing the outcome of 232 consecutive tubal microsurgery cases. Br. J. Obstet. Gynecol. **98:** 628–636.
6. SIMS, J.A., D. JONES, L. BUTLER & S.J. MUASHER. 1993. Effect of hydrosalpinx on outcome in in-vitro fertilization (IVF). Presented at the 49th annual meeting of the American Fertility Society 1993. American Fertility Society, program supplement: S95.
7. STRANDELL, A., U. WALDENSTROM, L. NILSSON & L. HAMBERGER. 1994. Hydrosalpinx reduces in-vitro fertilization/embryo transfer pregnancy rates. Hum. Reprod. **9:** 861–863.
8. ANDERSEN, A., Z. YUE, F. MENG & K. PETERSEN. 1994. Low implantation rate after in-vitro fertilization in patients with hydrosalpinges diagnosed by ultrasonography. Hum. Reprod. **9:** 1935–1938.
9. VANDROMME, J., E. CHASSE, B. LEJEUNE *et al.* 1995. Hydrosalpinges in in-vitro fertilization: an unfavorable prognostic feature. Hum. Reprod. **10:** 576–579.
10. VEJTORP, M., K. PETERSEN, A.N. ANDERSEN *et al.* 1995. Fertilization in vitro in the presence of hydrosalpinx and in advanced age. Ugeskr. Laeger. **157:** 4131–4134.
11. FLEMING, C. & M.J.R. HULL. 1996. Impaired implantation after in-vitro fertilization treatment associated with hydrosalpinx. Br. J. Obstet. Gynecol. **103:** 268–272.
12. KATZ, E., M.A. AKMAN, M.D. DAMEWOOD & J.E. GARCIA. 1996. Deleterious effect of the presence of hydrosalpinx on implantation and pregnancy rates with in vitro fertilization. Fertil. Steril. **66:** 122–125.
13. FREEMAN, M.R., C.M. WHITWORTH & G.A. HILL. 1996. Hydrosalpinx reduces in vitro fertilization – embryo transfer rates and in vitro blastocyst development. Presented at the 52nd annual meeting of the American Fertility Society 1996. American Fertility Society, program supplement: s211.
14. AKMAN, M.A., J.E. GARCIA, M.D. DAMEWOOD *et al.* 1996. Hydrosalpinx affects the implantation of previously cryopreserved embryos. Hum. Reprod. **1:** 1013–1014.
15. ZOURVES, C., M. ERENUS & V. GOMEL. 1991. Tubal ectopic pregnancy after in vitro fertilization and embryo transfer: a role for proximal occlusion or salpingectomy after failed distal tubal surgery. Fertil. Steril. **56:** 691–695.
16. SHARARA, F.I., R.T. SCOTT, JR., E.L. MARUT & J.T. QUEENAN, JR. 1996. In-vitro fertilization outcome in women with hydrosalpinx. Hum. Reprod. **11:** 526–530.
17. MANSOUR, R.T., M.A. ABOULGAR, G.I. SEROUR & R. RIAD. 1991. Fluid accumulation of the uterine cavity before embryo transfer: a possible hindrance for implantation. J. In Vitro Fert. Embryo Transf. **8:** 157–159.
18. RIFO, J.A., J. JEREMIAS, W.J. LEDGER & S.S. WITKIN. 1989. Interferon gamma in the pathogenesis of pelvic inflammatory disease. Am. J. Obstet. Gynecol. **160:** 26–31.
19. BEN-RAFAEL, Z. & R. ORVIETO. 1992. Cytocines-involvement in reproduction. Fertil. Steril. **58:** 1093–1099.
20. LESSEY, B.A., A.J. CASTELBAUM, M. RIBEN *et al.* 1994. Effect of hydrosalpinges on markers of uterine receptivity and success in IVF. Presented at the 50th annual meeting of the American Fertility Society 1994. American Fertility Society, program supplement: S45.
21. WITKIN, S.S., K.M. SULTAN, G.S. NEAL *et al.* 1994. Unsuspected *Chlamydia trachomatis* infection and *in vitro* fertilization outcome. Am. J. Obstet. Gynecol. **171:** 1208–1214.
22. JONES, R.B., J.B. MAMMEL, M.K. SHEPARD *et al.* 1986. Recovery of *Chlamydia trachomatis* from the endometrium of women at risk for chlamydial infection. Am. J. Obstet. Gynecol. **155:** 35–39.
23. HILL, G.A., C.M. HERBERT, A.S. FLEISCHER *et al.* 1986. Enlargement of hydrosalpinges during ovarian stimulation protocols for in-vitro fertilization and embryo replacement. Fertil. Steril. **45:** 883–885.
24. ABOULGHAR, M.A., R.T. MANSOUR, G.I. SEROUR *et al.* 1990. Transvaginal ultrasonic needle guided aspiration of pelvic inflammatory cystic masses before ovulation induction for *in vitro* fertilization. Fertil. Steril. **53:** 311–314.

25. ROWLAND, G.F., T. FORSEY, T.R. MOSS *et al.* 1985. Failure of *in vitro* fertilization and embryo replacement following replacement with *Chlamydia trachomatis*. J. In Vitro Fertil. Embryo Transfer **2:** 151–155.
26. LICCIARDI, F., J.A. GRIFO, Z. ROSENWAKS & S. WITKIN. 1992. Relation between antibodies to *Chlamydia trachomatis* and spontaneous abortion following *in vitro* fertilization. J. Assist. Reprod. Genet. **9:** 207–209.
27. SCHENK, L.M., J.W. RAMEY, S.A. TAYLOR *et al.* 1996. Embryotoxicity of hydrosalpinx fluid. Presented at the 43rd annual meeting of the Society of Gynecologic Investigators 1996. J. Soc. Gynecol. Invest. :88A.
28. KASSABJI, M., J. SIMS, L. BUTLER & S. MUASHER. 1994. Reduced pregnancy rates with unilateral or bilateral hydrosalpinx after *in vitro* fertilization. Eur. J. Obstet. Gynecol. Reprod. Biol. **56:** 129–132.
29. LEVY, M.J., D. MURRAY & A. SAGOSKIN. 1996. The adverse effect of hydrosalpinges on IVF success rates are reversed equally well by salpingectomy, proximal tubal occlusion and neosalpingostomy. Presented at the meeting of the American Society of Reproductive Medicine 1996. American Society for Reproductive Medicine, program supplement :S64.
30. SHELTON, K.E., L. BUTLER, J.P. TONER *et al.* 1996. Salpingectomy improves the pregnancy rate in *in-vitro* fertilization with hydrosalpinx. Hum. Reprod. **11:** 523–525.
31. MURRAY, D., A. SAGOSKIN, E. WIDRA & M. LEVY. 1998. The adverse effect of hydrosalpinges on *in vitro* fertilization pregnancy rates and the benefit of surgical correction. Fertil. Steril. **69:** 41–45.
32. VERHULST, G., N. VANDERSTEEN, A. VAN STEIRTEGHEM & P. DEVROEY. 1994. Bilateral salpingectomy does not compromise ovarian stimulation in an *in-vitro* fertilization/ embryo transfer programme. Hum. Reprod. **9:** 624–628.
33. VASQUEZ, G., W. BOECKS & I. BROSENS. 1995. Prospective study of tubal mucosal lesions and fertility in hydrosalpinges. Hum. Reprod. **10:** 1075–1078.
34. PUTTEMANS, P.J. & I.A. BROSENS. 1996. Preventive salpingectomy of hydrosalpinx prior to IVF. Salpingectomy improves *in-vitro* fertilization outcome in patients with a hydrosalpinx: blind victimization of the fallopian tube? Hum. Reprod. **11:** 2079–2081.

Adhesions: Laparoscopic Surgery versus Laparotomy

S. MILINGOS, G. KALLIPOLITIS, D. LOUTRADIS, A. LIAPI, K. MAVROMMATIS, P. DRAKAKIS,[a] J. TOURIKIS, G. CREATSAS, AND S. MICHALAS

Infertility Department, 1st Gynecologic and Obstetrics Clinic of the University of Athens, "Alexandra" Maternity Hospital, Athens, Greece

ABSTRACT: This study was undertaken to assess the effectiveness in pregnancy rates of microsurgery and operative laparoscopy in adhesiolysis. Adhesions were found to be the sole infertility factor in 15% of our patients. One hundred and ninety infertile patients with periadnexal adhesions as the only cause of their infertility were treated by microsurgery (86) or operative laparoscopy (104) and were followed up for 24 months. Our results indicate that advanced laparoscopic surgery in general is as effective as microsurgery in healthy infertile patients with adhesions but offers some advantages in comparison to laparotomy. Factors that adversely affect the postoperative success rates are the age of the women, the duration of infertility, and the severity of the adhesions.

INTRODUCTION

The association between peritoneal adhesions and infertility has long been established. Adhesiolysis has been shown to significantly improve pregnancy rates among infertile women with adhesions.[1,2] Intraabdominal adhesions are usually the consequences of surgical or gynecological operations, pelvic inflammatory disease, or endometriosis.[3–5] Periadnexal adhesions can impair fertility mainly by the disruption of the ovarian–fibrial relationship, thus interfering with the ovum pick-up mechanism and gamete transportation.[4–7] Some authors also suggested that the infertility may be related to a constricting effect of the adhesions on the development of the follicles or the ovarian blood supply.[8,9] There is no widely accepted terminology and classification for adhesions.

The American Fertility Society has recommended a system for describing adnexal adhesions in which a numerical value is assigned to each adnexa, and the prognosis of adhesiolysis is estimated.[10]

For many years, the only way to approach the problem of adhesions was laparotomy. Microsurgery, being delicate surgery itself, minimized the factors that contribute to the formation of postoperative adhesions and has almost doubled the term pregnancy rates in comparison to the gross dissection of adhesions.[11,12] Operative laparoscopy, which by its nature adheres to microsurgical principles, has also been used in adhesiolysis; and many reports have described its efficacy.[2,13–16]

To minimize the postoperative adhesion formation and reformation in both these surgical techniques, different tools and adjuvants have been used, and their efficacy has

[a]Address for correspondence: Dr. Peter Drakakis, Byzantiou 55, Papagou 156 69, Athens, Greece. Phone: 30-93-2433002; fax: 30-1-6546546.

been reported.[2,15–21] This study has several purposes. The first is to evaluate pregnancy rates after microsurgical and laparoscopic adhesiolysis. The second is to compare postoperative adhesion reformation after both of these operational techniques. The third is to analyze the prognostic factors for pregnancy outcome after adhesiolysis.

MATERIALS AND METHODS

Incidence of Pelvic Adhesions

To determine the incidence of pelvic adhesions, their cause, and concomitant infertility factors, we reviewed the clinical and operative records of 733 infertility patients who underwent a complete investigation in the Infertility Department of Alexandra Maternity Hospital, (Athens, Greece) during the last 5 years.

Microsurgical versus Laparoscopic Adhesiolysis

Adhesiolysis and restoration of the tubo-ovarian relationship was carried out in 190 patients suffering from infertility who presented in the Infertility Department of Alexandra Maternity Hospital during the last 10 years. In 86 of these patients, adhesiolysis was achieved by microsurgery, and in the remaining 104 laparoscopy was performed. The selection of the surgical modality was based only on the availability of operational facilities.

For the purposes of this study, the included patients' infertility was exclusively due to pelvic adhesions. The severity of adhesions was staged at laparotomy or laparoscopy and was adjusted to the American Fertility Society classification system of 1988.[10] On the basis of this staging, the patients were divided into three groups. The first group included patients with minimal or mild adhesions (score ≤10); the second group, those with moderate adhesions (score 11–20); and the third, those with severe adhesions (score >21). Cases involving extremely dense and extended adhesions, the so-called frozen pelvis, were excluded from the study. Operative laparoscopy was performed under video control, using a standard three- or four-puncture technique, depending on the extent and localization of the adhesions and the requirements of the operation.

Instrumentation included 5-mm scissors, atraumatic grasping foceps and holders, fine bipolar forceps, and microtip monopolar electrocoagulators. For irrigation we used Ringer's lactate solution. For adhesiolysis we followed a step-by-step approach: First, after a thorough inspection of the peritoneal cavity, we identified the intraabdominal structures. Once the anatomic landmarks were identified, the bowel adhesions were severed, followed by adhesiolysis of the ovaries and then by adhesiolysis of the fallopian tubes. This approach allows the progressive exposure of the pelvic organs and facilitates the operation. For the women in the laparotomy group, a Pfannestiel incision was performed, and microsurgery was used. For adhesiolysis we followed the same operative approach as that used in laparoscopy. Postoperatively, all patients received preventive antibiotic therapy and had an uneventful course. All women attempted to become pregnant after the operation and were followed up from the time of surgery to their last menstrual period if pregnancy occurred or at least for 24 months if not pregnant.

TABLE 1. Incidence of periadnexal adhesions in 733 infertile patients who underwent laparoscopy

Adhesion status	Patients (n)
Without adhesions	462 (63%)[a]
With adhesions	271 (37%)
Minimal	101 (37.2)
Mild	59 (21.7%)
Moderate	50 (18.5%)
Severe	61 (22.6%)
Adhesions plus tubal occlusion	47 (17.3%)
Adhesions plus endometriosis	45 (16.6%)
Adhesions plus other infertility factors	138 (51%)
Adhesions as the sole infertility factor	41 (15%)

[a]Values are number of patients with percentages in parentheses.

Factors Affecting Pregnancy Rate after Adhesiolysis

In 104 women who underwent laparoscopic adhesiolysis, we evaluated the effect of age, duration of infertility, and severity and cause of adhesions on pregnancy outcome.

Postoperative Adhesion Formation

Adhesion reformation was evaluated laparoscopically 3 to 6 months after the initial operation in 11 and 10 women who underwent microsurgical and laparoscopic adhesiolysis, respectively. For the statistical evaluation of postoperative pregnancy rates and for the factors that affected these rates, life table analysis was used. The patients' characteristics, the severity of the adhesions, the estimated operative time, blood loss and recovery time were compared in both groups with Student's t-test or the χ^2 test.

RESULTS

Incidence of Pelvic Adhesions

In 271 (37%) of the 733 patients, laparoscopy revealed the occurrence of different kind of adhesions. In 37%, 22%, 18.5%, and 22.5% of the cases, these adhesions were classified as minimal, mild, moderate, and severe, respectively (see TABLE 4), according to the American Fertility Society classification system.[10] In 26% the location of the adhesions was unilateral and in 74% bilateral. In 66.1% of the patients, the adhesions were the only laparoscopic finding, in 17.3% there was unilateral or bilateral tubal occlusions and in the remaining 16.6% endometriosis (TABLE 1). Reviewing the medical records of the 271 infertile patients with adhesions and comparing them with the laparoscopic findings, we did not find any apparent etiological factors in 32% of them. From the remaining 68% of the patients, the most probable etiological factors were previous gynecological operations (in 25%) and endometri-

TABLE 2. Possible etiologic factors related to adhesion formation in 271 infertile women

Etiologic factor	Patients (n)
Pelvic inflammatory disease related to pregnancy	19 (7%)[a]
Pelvic inflammatory disease not related to pregnancy	38 (14%)
Previous abdominal operations (appendectomy etc.)	16 (6%)
Previous abdominal operations (ectopic pregnancies, cyctectomy, myomectomy, etc.)	68 (25%)
Endometriosis	43 (16%)
Non apparent etiologic factors	87 (32%)

[a]Values are number of patients with percentages in parentheses.

TABLE 3. Patient characteristics

Variable	Laparotomy (n = 86)	Laparoscopy (n = 104)	Probability value
Age (years)	30.7 ± 4.0 (23–39)[a]	31.5 ± 4.5 (22–39)	$p > 0.1$[c]
Duration of infertility (years)	3.5 ± 2.3 (1–9)	3.6 ± 2.3 (1–11)	$p > 0.1$[c]
Primary infertility	56 (65%)[b]	62 (60%)	$p > 0.1$[d]
Secondary infertility	30 (35%)	42 (40%)	$p > 0.1$[d]
Length of follow-up (momths)	24	24	

[a]Values are means ±SD with ranges in parentheses.
[b]Values are number of patients with percentages in parentheses.
[c]Student's t-test.
[d]χ^2-test.

osis (in 16%). Pelvic inflammatory disease not related to pregnancy (14%) or related to pregnancy (7%) and previous abdominal operations (6%) were less common etiological factors (TABLE 2).

Microsurgical versus Laparoscopic Adhesiolysis

The general characteristics of patients who were operated either by laparotomy (86) or laparoscopy (104) are shown in TABLE 3. The women in both groups were comparable with respect to age, duration of infertility, gravidity, medical history, and length of follow-up. The total score of adhesions and the ovarian and tubal adhesions' score, according to the American Fertility Society classification system, were also comparable between the two groups (TABLE 4). Blood loss during the operation, the length of hospitalization and recovery time were significantly higher in the laparotomy than in the laparoscopy group ($p < 0.05$). On the contrary, there was no significant difference between the two groups in operational time ($p > 0.1$) (TABLE 5). As it has been mentioned, all women after the operation attempted to become pregnant. As a result, 34.9% from those that underwent microsurgery and 39.4% from those that underwent operative laparoscopy became pregnant during the two-year postoperative follow-up period (FIG. 1). All pregnancies were intrauterine except two in the laparoscopy group and one in the laparotomy group, which were ectopic.

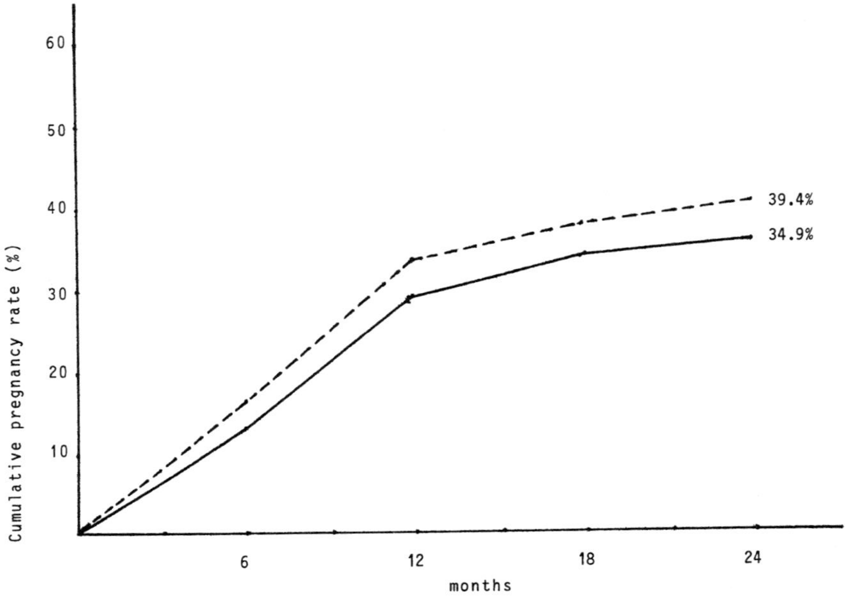

FIGURE 1. Cumulative probability of conception among women with periadnaxal adhesions who were treated by laparotomy (*solid line*) and laparoscopy (*broken line*).

TABLE 4. Characteristics of the adhesions in the patients included in the study

Variable	Laparotomy ($n = 86$)	Laparoscopy ($n = 104$)	Probability value
AFS total score	21.9 ± 12.0 (6–48)[a]	25.3 ± 14.6 (4–56)	$p > 0.1$[c]
AFS tubal score	14.6 ± 9.3	16.6 ± 9.3 (0–32)	$p > 0.1$[c]
AFS ovarian score	7.3 ± 6.8 (0–32)	8.7 ± 8.5 (0–28)	$p > 0.1$[c]
Stage mild	20 (23%)[b]	22 (21%)	$p > 0.1$[d]
Stage moderate	37 (43%)	32 (31%)	$p > 0.1$[d]
Stage severe	29 (34%)	50 (48%)	$p > 0.1$[d]

[a]Values are means ±SD with ranges in parentheses.
[b]Values are number of patients with percentages in parentheses.
[c]Student's *t*-test.
[d]χ^2-test.

The ectopic pregnancies were not included in the above-mentioned pregnancy percentages. These differences were not statistically significant ($p > 0.1$).

The estimated cumulative intrauterine pregnancy rates at 6, 12, 18, and 24 months were 12.8%, 29%, 33.6%, and 34.9%, respectively, for the laparotomy and 16.3%, 33.6%, 37.6%, 39.4%, respectively, for the laparoscopy group, as is shown in FIGURE 1 (NS; $p > 0.1$). As is also shown in this figure, most of the pregnancies in both groups took place during the first postoperative year (83% and 86% for the laparot-

TABLE 5. Surgical characteristics in our cases

Variable	Laparotomy ($n = 86$)	Laparoscopy ($n = 104$)	Probability value[c]
Estimated blood loss (cc)[a]	120.7 ± 45.4 (65–220)[b]	58 ± 18	$p < 0.001$
Operating time	2.1 ± 0.5 (1.2–3.2)	1.8 ± 0.6 (1–3)	$p > 0.1$
Hospitalization (days)	4.6 ± 1.0 (3–8)	1.5 ± 0.6 (1–3)	$p < 0.001$
Recovery time (days)	23.7 ± 4.1 (20–35)	6.2 ± 1.4 (5–10)	$p < 0.01$

[a]Blood loss was estimated by irrigation versus suction volumes and sponge counts.
[b]Values are means ±SD with ranges in parentheses.
[c]Student's *t*-test.

omy and laparoscopy group, respectively). According to the American Fertility Society classification of adhesions, 23% of the patients in the laparotomy group were staged as having mild disease, 43% as having moderate, and 34% as having severe disease. For the laparoscopy group, 21%, 31%, and 48% of the patients had a mild, moderate, and severe degree of adhesions, respectively. The distribution of patients for the different stages of adhesions was not statistically different between the two groups (TABLE 4). The cumulative intrauterine pregnancy rates for the two years of follow-up for the patients with mild, moderate, and severe disease were 60%, 35%, and 17.2%, respectively, for the laparotomy group and 54.5%, 43.7%, and 30%, respectively, for the laparoscopy group (NS; $p > 0.1$) (FIGS. 2, 3, and 4). The distribu-

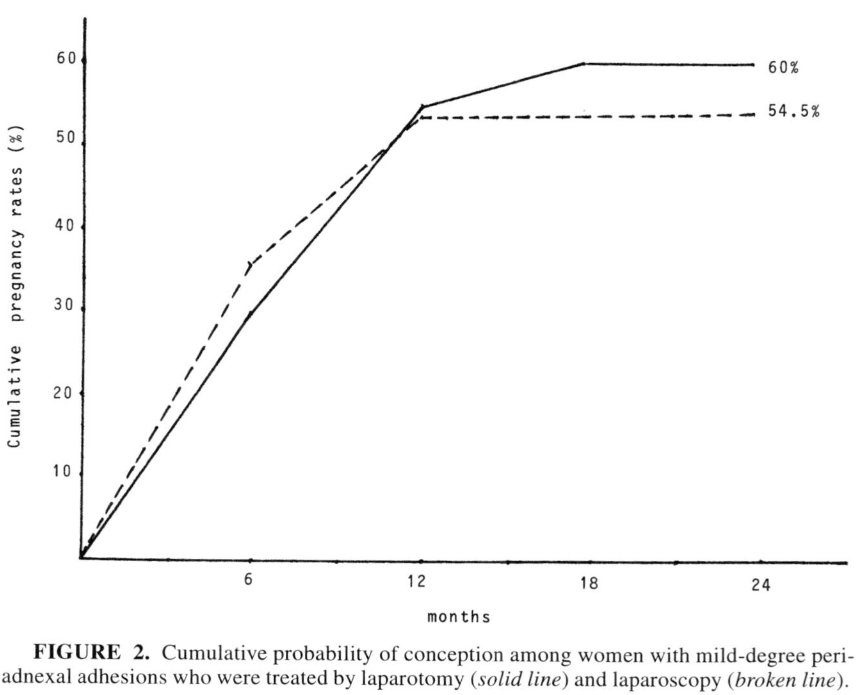

FIGURE 2. Cumulative probability of conception among women with mild-degree periadnexal adhesions who were treated by laparotomy (*solid line*) and laparoscopy (*broken line*).

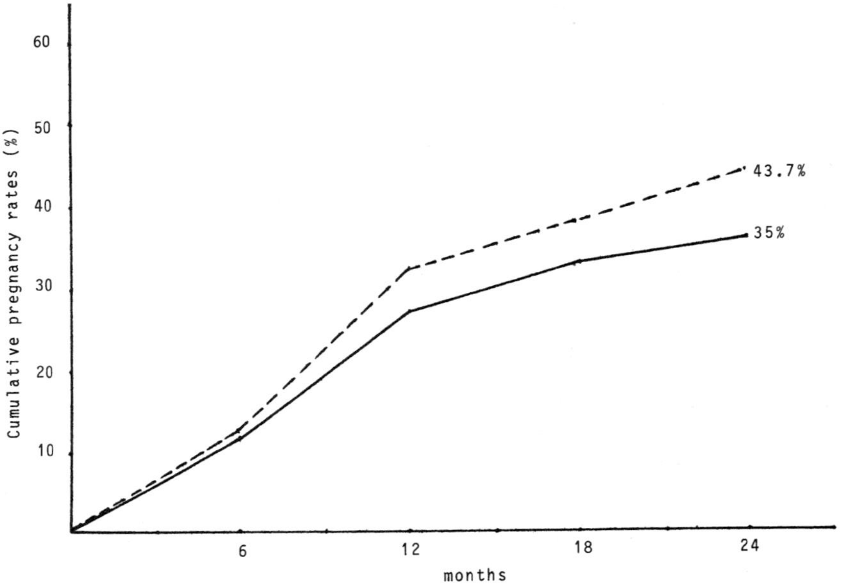

FIGURE 3. Cumulative probability of conception among women with moderate-degree periadnexal adhesions who were treated by laparotomy (*solid line*) and laparoscopy (*broken line*).

tion of the achieved pregnancies was rather the same in all stages of both groups of patients.

Factors Affecting Pregnancy Rate after Laparoscopic Adhesiolysis

From the evaluation of the laparoscopic findings and the other associated infertility factors, we regarded adhesions as the only or main etiological factor of infertility in 15% of the cases and as an additional factor in the remaining 85% (TABLE 1). Life table calculations were performed on several variables in order to evaluate their effect on the probability of conception. Thus, we analyzed the influence of age, duration of infertility, parity, and severity and etiology of adhesions on the success rate of laparoscopic adhesiolysis.

Age: The age of the operated women varied from 22 to 39 years. From TABLE 6, it can be concluded that age has a significant influence on the outcome of surgery and that women aged over 35 years are less likely to conceive than those below age 30.

Duration of infertility: The duration of preoperative infertility varied from 1 to 11 years. The pregnancy rate in women with duration of infertility more than 4 years was 30.8% in 24 months post-operatively in comparison to 43.7% when the duration of infertility was less than 4 years (TABLE 6) ($p < 0.05$).

Severity of adhesions: Lower conception rates were found with increasing severity of pelvic adhesions. The likelihood of women with mild, moderate, and severe

TABLE 6. Factors influencing the outcome of laparoscopic adhesiolysis in the patients of our study (n = 104)[a,b]

Variable	Women n (%)	Intrauterine pregnancy n (%)
Duration of infertility (years)		
1-4	78 (75%)	33 (42%)[c]
>4	26 (25%)	8 (31%)[c]
Age		
22-30	38 (36.5%)	18 (47%)[d]
31-35	46 (44%)	18 (39%)
36-39	20 (19.5%)	5 (25%)[d]
Severity of adhesions		
Mild	22 (21%)	12 (54.5%)[d]
Moderate	32 (31%)	14 (44%)
Severe	50 (48%)	15 (30%)[d]
Parity		
Primary infertility	62 (59.5%)	25 (40%)[e]
Secondary infertility	42 (40.5%)	16 (38%)[e]

[a]All values are number of patients with percentages in parentheses.
[b]Probability values were determined by the χ^2-test.
[c]$p < 0.05$.
[d]$p < 0.01$.
[e]$p < 0.1$.

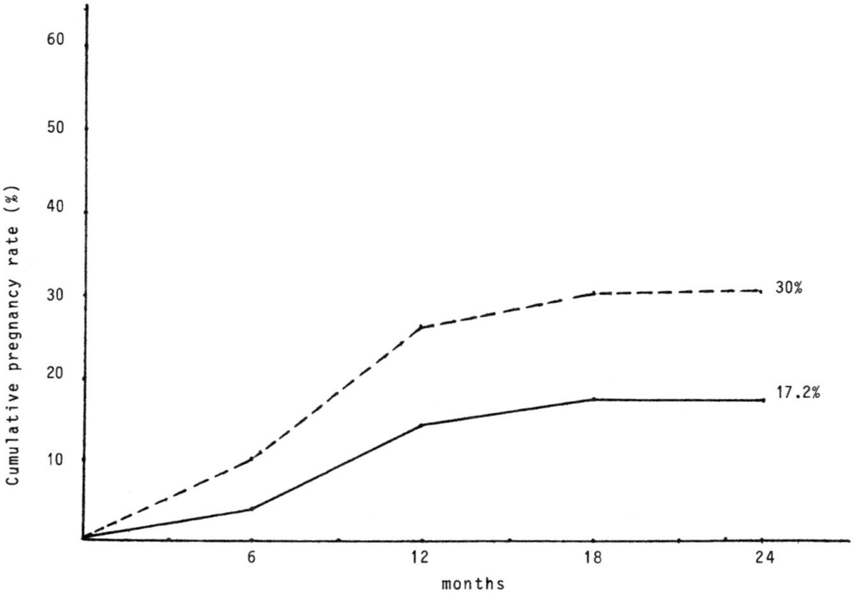

FIGURE 4. Cumulative probability of conception among women with severe-degree peri-adnexal adhesions who were treated by laparotomy (*solid line*) and laparoscopy (*broken line*).

TABLE 7. Adhesion scores at the time of infertility surgery and at second look laparoscopy in patients operated on by laparoscopy (n = 10) and laparotomy (n = 11)[a]

Operation	Total adhesion score at infertility surgery	Adhesion score at second-look laparoscopy
Laparotomy (n=11)	27.3 ± 9.3 (16–40)[c]	16.1 ± 8.8 (6–30)[c]
Laparoscopy (n=10)	26.8 ± 9.8 (12–40)[d]	9.2 ± 4.4 (0–17)[d]
Laparoscopy versus laparotomy	$p > 0.1$	$p < 0.05$

[a]All values are means ±SD with ranges in parentheses.
[b]Probability values were determined by theStudent's t-test
[c]$p < 0.01$.
[d]$p < 0.001$.

adhesions to conceive in the two postoperative years was 54.5%, 43.7%, and 30%, respectively (TABLE 6). As far as the location of adhesions is concerned, both peritubal and periovarian adhesions influence the post-operative success rate adversely, but the effect is worse in periovarian than in peritubal adhesions.

Postoperative Adhesion Formation

In TABLE 7, the adhesion scores in 11 and 10 patients who underwent microsurgical and laparoscopical adhesiolysis, respectively, are shown before and after the operation. The second-look laparoscopy was performed 3 to 6 months after the initial operation. As is shown in the table, a significant reduction of adhesion scores was found in both groups ($p = 0.01$ and $p = 0.001$). The reduction of adhesion reformation was significantly higher in laparoscopy than in laparotomy ($p = 0.05$).

DISCUSSION

Incidence of Pelvic Adhesions

Gynecologic surgeons have been addressing the problem of pelvic adhesions and its association with infertility for a long time. Many studies have demonstrated that the main reasons for pelvic adhesion formation are surgical or gynecological operations, inflammatory disease, or endometriosis.[3–5,22] Although the diagnosis of the adhesions is not difficult via laparoscopy, establishing their cause is not easy. This is due to the fact that the morphological appearance of the adhesions is rarely related to the cause. A causal association with the adhesions was found in only 68% of our cases. In the rest of the cases, the cause of adhesions was regarded as unknown. In some of these cases, silent infections, mainly from chlamydiae, could be responsible.[5,23] Periadnexal adhesions were found to be the sole abnormality and cause of infertility in 15% of our patients. More frequently, they coexisted with tubal occlusion (17.3%), endometriosis (16.6%), or other infertility factors (51%). Murphy reported that adhesions were the only infertility factor in only 5% of their patients.[24] Others reported infertility secondary to pelvic adhesions in 15–30% of the cases observed.[4,22] This coexistence of adhesions with other infertility factors appears to limit the success of infertility surgery or other treatment.[22,25,26]

Microsurgical versus Laparoscopic Adhesiolysis

Our results indicate that laparoscopic surgery is as effective as microsurgery in treating infertility due to adhesions. The comparison between the patients of each groups was feasible because, as is shown in TABLES 3 and 4, the relevant patients' parameters and the characteristics of the adhesions were comparable. In order to evaluate the effectiveness of the used surgical technique for adhesiolysis on conception rates, we included in our study only those patients for whom adhesions were the sole identified cause of infertility. The 1988 American Fertility Society classification system for adhesions[10] was used because it is the most widely employed. Simple and life table estimated cumulative intrauterine pregnancy rates were comparable for the laparoscopy and the laparotomy group (39.4% versus 34.9%). Although both operational techniques have been used for a large number of patients, and many studies have reported their efficacy on adhesiolysis and restoration of infertility, the clinical results from endoscopic surgery cannot be compared easily with those obtained by microsurgery. This is due to differences in patients' population, nature, and classification of the existing adhesions, presence of other infertility factors, experience of the surgeons, and absence of control groups and proper randomization. The reported pregnancy rates in the literature range from 29 to 81% after laparoscopy and from 41 to 75% after laparotomy.[13–17,22,27,28] Only a few studies in the literature have used proper randomization to compare fertility outcome between patients undergoing adhesiolysis by laparotomy and by laparoscopy. They have all shown nonsignificant differences between the two techniques.[14,15,17] A significantly increased pregnancy rate was found for the first year of the follow-up compared to the second. This trend of increased early postoperative pregnancy rates after laparoscopic or laparotomic adhesiolysis is also reported by others.[1,22] Although the achieved pregnancy rates in the laparotomy group (34.9%) did not differ significantly from those in the laparoscopy group (39.4%), we observed a greater difference concerning the effect of the surgical technique on patients with severe adhesions. Thus, in patients with severe adhesions treated laparoscopically, the pregnancy rate was 30.0% in comparison to 17.2% for patients treated by laparotomy. Though this difference does not reach the conventionally accepted level of statistical significance ($0.05 < p < 0.1$), there is an indication that women with severe adhesions are more likely to have increased pregnancy rates after laparoscopic adhesiolysis than after laparotomy. This may be due to reduced postoperative adhesion formation using laparoscopy in comparison to laparotomy.[2,12,29–33]

As shown in TABLE 3, the laparoscopic treatment of adhesions provides some noteworthy advantages to the patients compared to laparotomy. First, hospitalization time and recovery time to normal activity were significantly shorter after laparoscopic adhesiolysis. Second, diagnosis and treatment of the disease can be achieved by the same operative procedure. Third, the postoperative pain and the cosmetic results favor laparoscopy.

Factors Affecting Pregnancy Rate after Laparoscopic Adhesiolysis

Our results indicate that advanced laparoscopic surgery is effective for treating periadnexal adhesions. The statistical analysis of our data can also be used to determine the influence of the extent of the adhesions on pregnancy rates and the impact of several factors, namely the age of the patient, duration of infertility, parity, and cause of adhesions on the operational outcome. Our findings indicate that patients with thicker, more vascular, and more extensive adhesions have a much poorer prognosis after surgery. Thus, the intrauterine pregnancy rates were found to decrease gradually in relation to the severity of adhesions. The pregnancy rates achieved in patients with mild adhesions (54.5%) were statistically higher than those in patients with severe disease (30%) ($p < 0.05$). Although, as has already been mentioned, it is difficult to compare the different reports on adhesiolysis, our findings are comparable to those of many authors reporting the adverse effect of the severity of adhesions on pregnancy rates after adhesiolysis.[1,17,22,34]

Among the other studied variables, only the duration of infertility (>4 years) and the age of the patients (>35 years) were significantly associated with decreased pregnancy rates. Similar results on the association of these two factors with pregnancy rates have been reported in other studies for patients after adhesiolysis and surgical treatment of endometriosis.[22,25,35]

The likelihood of conception was not influenced in our patients by parity or the various causes of adhesions. These findings have also been reported by others.[22] Our data provide evidence that the major factors that influence the successful outcome of laparoscopic adhesiolysis are the severity and the extent of adhesions and the combined effect of age and duration of infertility.

Postoperative Adhesion Formation

The major determinant of the success of infertility surgery is the postoperative adhesion formation at and beyond the surface of the wound. In our material, although the number of cases is limited, the reduction in the mean adhesion scores was significantly greater postoperatively in both groups. The reduction was significantly greater in the laparoscopy than in the laparotomy group of patients. Adhesion reformation, though, occurred in all women of both groups except in two in the laparoscopy group, who were found free of postoperative adhesion reformation by second-look laparoscopy.

To address further the problem of postoperative adhesion reformation after laparoscopy and laparotomy, we summarize the data of the few experimental and clinical studies that compared the two techniques. From three experimental animal studies, which have compared postoperative adhesion formation following operative laparoscopy versus laparotomy, a significant advantage for laparoscopic surgery over laparotomy was demonstrated.[36–38] The most convincing clinical study comparing operative laparoscopy versus laparotomy in postoperative adhesion formation was conducted by Lundorff *et al.*[29] They prospectively randomized the surgical treatment of patients with ectopic pregnancy to either operative laparoscopy or laparotomy and found at second-look laparoscopy that the patients who have been treated by laparotomy developed significantly more adhesions than those treated by laparoscopy.

Many other clinical studies have shown that operative laparoscopy results in comparable or significantly greater reduction in adhesion reformation and lower *de novo* adhesion formation than laparotomy.[2,12,30–33] However, it is important to emphasize that laparoscopic surgery is not adhesion free. The operative laparoscopy study group reported adhesion reformation in 97% of women who underwent laparoscopic adhesiolysis by various techniques, and in 12% *de novo* adhesion formation occurred. Nevertheless, these authors reported that the score of postoperative adhesions was significantly lower than that of preoperative ones.[30,31] Other studies have also reported that 30% to 45% of laparoscopically resected adhesions had been reformed.[30]

CONCLUSIONS

Clinical experience and our results indicate that advanced laparoscopic surgery in general is as effective as microsurgery in treating infertility patients with adhesions, but laparoscopic surgery offers some advantages compared to laparotomy. The adhesiolysis can be performed during the initial diagnostic laparoscopy. The hospital stay and recovery time of the patient is brief. It avoids the inherent complications and drawbacks of laparotomy. It is associated with minimal discomfort to the patient. In addition, patients with severe adhesions treated laparoscopically have a higher likelihood of conceiving than patients treated by laparotomy. The postoperative adhesion reformation is lower after laparoscopic versus laparotomic adhesiolysis. Factors that adversely affect postoperative success, as far as fertility is concerned, are the age of the woman, duration of infertility, and the severity of the disease. It must, however, be emphasized that laparoscopic adhesiolysis can be a complex and difficult operation and that it needs much skill and experience. Therefore, each surgeon must determine the best surgical approach according to his or her own experience, in order to act in the patients' best interest.

REFERENCES

1. Tulandi, T., J.A. Collins & E. Burrows. 1990. Treatment-dependent and treatment-independent pregnancy among women with periadnexal adhesions. Am. J. Obstet. Gynecol. **162:** 354–357.
2. Evantash, E.G. 1997. Laparoscopy in the management of pelvic adhesions. *In* Update in Laparoscopy E.G. Evantash, Ed. Infertil. Reprod. Med. Clin. N. Am. **8**(3)**:** 383–397.
3. Levinson, C.J. & K. Swolin. 1980. Postoperative adhesions: etiology, prevention and therapy. Clin. Obstet. Gynecol. **23:** 1213–1218.
4. Drollette, C.M. & S.Z.A. Badawy. 1992. Pathophysiology of pelvic adhesions. Modern trends in preventing infertility. J. Reprod. Med. **37:** 107–122.
5. Grainger, D.A. 1994. Incidence and causes of pelvic adhesions. *In* Adhesions. R.E. Leach, Ed. Infertil. Reprod. Med. Clin. N. Am. **5**(3)**:** 391–404.
6. Corfman, R.S. & O. Badram. 1994. Effect of pelvic adhesions on pelvic pain and fertility. *In* Adhesions. R.E. Leach, Ed. Infertil. Reprod. Med. Clin. N. Am. **5**(3)**:** 405–411.
7. Noedenskjold, F. & M. Ahlegren. 1984. Interfimbrial adhesion detection and treatment of an easily overlooked cause of infertility. J. Reprod. Med. **29**(8)**:** 595–596.
8. Mahadevan, M.M., D. Wiseman, A. Leader, *et al.* 1985. The effects of ovarian adhesive disease upon follicular development in cycles of controlled stimulation for in vitro fertilization. Fertil. Steril. **44:** 489–492.
9. Molloy, D., M. Martin, A. Speirs, *et al.* 1987. Performance of patients with a frozen pelvis in in vitro fertilization program. Fertil. Steril. **47:** 450–455.
10. The American Fertility Society. 1988. The American Fertility Society classifications of adnexal adhesions, distal tubal occlusion, secondary to tubal ligation, tubal pregnancies. Mullerian anomalies and intrauterine adhesions. Fertil. Steril. **49**(6)**:** 944–955.

11. FAYEZ, J. & P. SCHNEIDER. 1987. Prevention of pelvic adhesion formation by different modalities of treatment. Am. J. Obstet. Gynecol. **157:** 1184–1188.
12. DIAMOND, M.P., J.F. DANIELL, J. FESTE, *et al.* 1987. Adhesion reformation and de novo adhesion formation after reproductive pelvic surgery. Fertil. Steril. **47:** 864–866.
13. NISSOLE, M. & J. DONNEZ. 1990. CO_2 laser laparoscopy in infertile women. Arch. Gynecol. Obstet. **247:** 565–569.
14. SARAVELOS, H.G., T. LI & I.D. COOKE. 1995. An analysis of the outcome of microsurgical and laparoscopic adhesiolysis for infertility. Hum. Reprod. **10:** 2887–2894.
15. REICH, H. 1987. Laparoscopic treatment of extensive pelvic adhesions including hydrosalpinx. J. Reprod. Med. **32:** 736–740.
16. GOMEL, V. 1983. Salpingo-ovariolysis by laparoscopy in infertility. Fertil. Steril. **40:** 607–611.
17. DONNEZ, J., M. NISOLLE & F. CASANAS-ROUX. 1989. CO_2 laser laparoscopy in infertile women with adnexal adhesions and women with tubal occlusion. J. Gynecol. Surg. **5:** 47–53.
18. TULANDI, T. & M. BUGNAH. 1995. Operative laparoscopy: surgical modalities. Fertil. Steril. **63:** 237–245.
19. THORNTON, M. & G.S. DIZAREGA. 1996. Using barriers to prevent adhesions. Contemp. Obstet. Gynecol. **41:** 107–109.
20. SEKIBA, K. 1992. The Obstetrics and Gynecology Adhesion Prevention Committee: Use of Interceed (TC7) to reduce post-operative adhesion reformation infertility and endometriosis surgery. Obstet. Gynecol. **79:** 518–522.
21. MYOMECTOMY ADHESION MULTICENTER STUDY GROUP. 1995. Gore-tex surgical membrane reduces post myomectomy adhesion formation. Fertil. Steril. **63:** 491–493.
22. SINGHAL, V., T.C. LI & I.D. COOKE. 1991. An analysis of factors influencing the outcome of 232 consecutive tubal microsurgery cases. Br. J. Obstet. Gynecol. **98:** 628–636.
23. MINASSIAN, S.S. & C.H. WU. 1992. Chlamydia antibody and severity of tubal factor infertility. Fertil. Steril. **58:** 1245–1247.
24. MURPHY, A.A. 1992. Reconstructive surgery of the oviducts. Female reproductive surgery. J.A. Rock, A.A. Murphy & H.W. Jones, Eds.: 146–169. Williams and Wilkins. Baltimore.
25. MILINGOS, S., G. KALLIPOLITIS, D. LOUTRADIS, *et al.* 2000. Factors affecting post-operative pregnancy rate after endoscopic management of large endometriomata. Int. J. Gynecol. Obstet. In press.
26. BOER-MEISEL, M.E., E.R. TEVELDE, J.D.F. HABBEMA & J.W.P.F. KARDAUM. 1986. Predicting the pregnancy outcome in patients treated for hydrosalpinx. A prospective study. Fertil. Steril. **45:** 23–29.
27. BRUHAT, M.A., G. MAGE, H. MANHES, *et al.* 1983. Laparoscopy procedures to promote fertility ovariolysis and adhesiolysis: results of 93 selected cases. Acta Eur. Fertil. **14:** 113–117.
28. DAMEWOOD, M.D. 1996. Tubal reconstructive surgery. *In* Reproductive Endocrinology, Surgery and Technology. E.Y. Adashi, J.A. Rock, Z. Rosenwaks, Eds. Vol. 2, **110:** 2091–2104. Lippincott-Raven Publishers. Philadelphia, PA.
29. LUNDORFF, P., M. HAHLIN, B. KALLFELT, *et al.* 1991. Adhesion formation after laparoscopic surgery in tubal pregnancy. A randomized trial versus laparotomy. Fertil. Steril. **55:** 911–915.
30. NEZHAT, C., D.A. METZGER, F. NEZHAT, *et al.* 1990. Adhesion formation following reproductive surgery by videolaseroscopy. Fertil. Steril. **53:** 1008–1011.
31. OPERATIVE LAPAROSCOPY STUDY GROUP. 1991. Post-operative adhesion development after operative laparoscopy. Evaluation at early second look procedures. Fertil. Steril. **55:** 700–704.
32. RIMBOS-KEMPER, T.C.M., J.B. TRIMBOS & E.V. VAN HALL. 1985. Adhesion formation after tubal surgery: results of the 8 day laparoscopy in 188 patients. Fertil. Steril. **43:** 395–400.
33. LUCIANO, A.A. & M. MONTAMINO-OLIVA. 1994. Comparison of post-operative adhesion formation. Laparoscopy versus laparotomy. *In* Adhesions. R.E. Leach, Ed. Infertil. Reprod. Med. Clin. N. Am. **5**(3): 437–444.

34. STRANDELL, A., I. BRYMAN, P.O. JANSON & J. THORBURN. 1995. Background factors and scoring systems in relation to pregnancy outcome after fertility surgery. Acta Obstet. Gynecol. Scand. **74:** 281–287.
35. ADAMSON, G.D., L.L. SUBAK, D.J. PASTA, *et al.* 1992. Comparison of CO_2 laser laparoscopy with laparotomy for treatment of endometriomata. Fertil. Steril. **57:** 965–973.
36. FILMAR, S., V. GOMEL & P.F. MCCOMB. 1987. Operative laparoscopy versus open abdominal surgery. A comparative study on post-operative adhesion formation in the rat model. Fertil. Steril. **48:** 486–490.
37. LUCIANO, A.A., D.B. MAIER, E.I. KOCH, *et al.* 1989. A comparative study of post-operative adhesions following laser surgery by laparoscopy versus laparotomy in the rabbit model. Obstet. Gynecol. **74:** 220–224.
38. MAIER, D.B., J.C. NULSEN, A. KLOCK, *et al.* 1992. Laser laparoscopy versus laparotomy in lysis of pelvic adhesions. J. Reprod. Med. **37:** 965–968.

Chlamydia Screening—Yes, but of Whom, When, by Whom, and with What?

PER-ANDERS MÅRDH[a]

Department of Obstetrics and Gynecology, Lund University, Lund, Sweden

ABSTRACT: The importance of screening programs in reducing the prevalence of genital chlamydial infections is stressed by the fact that the majority of infected persons are more or less asymptomatic. The use of oral contraceptives may mask infections affecting the upper genital tract. This imposes selective screening and rescreening of women with a history of pelvic inflammatory disease. The recent knowledge that vaginal introital samples will provide a detection rate equal to or even higher than that of cervical samples collected in the same women opens up the possibility of screening women in health units lacking a gynecological examination chair. It also opens up the possibility of outpatient screening programs, for example, home sampling and mailing samples to laboratories that will perform analyses. The use of nucleic acid–based assays means increased sensitivity and specificity compared with earlier used techniques such as ELISA. These former methods can also be used in low-prevalence populations with acceptable positive predictable value, but may be misleading if used in post-therapy check-ups because the antigen may persist in microbiologically cured cases.

INTRODUCTION

Chlamydia trachomatis is an important pathogen that may affect the genital tract, the eyes, and the joints.[1] In all communities where it has been monitored in a surveillance program, it has been found to be widespread.[2] In some countries, however, a decrease in prevalence has been registered in recent years, including associated complications such as pelvic inflammatory disease (PID).[3] Pathologic conditions like gonorrhoea and genital chlamydial infections are often asymptomatic or at least show such mild symptoms that they will not drive the infected to consult medical help.[4] It is still not established whether in this respect there may be a difference between the genders in their efforts toward seeking medical assistance.

The introduction of commercially available nucleic acid–based test kits for *C. trachomatis*[5–10] and also of analytic robots has made mass screening for genital chlamydial infections possible.

There has been a change in recommended procedure to switch away from the use of enzyme-linked immunoassays (ELISA) (even if used when employing confirmation tests of positive samples),[11] immunofluorescence (IF) tests,[12,13] and cultures and toward the use of polymerase (PCR)[6,8] and ligase chain reaction (LCR) tests[7] or, as recently proposed, to transcription-mediated amplification (TEM).[14] The use of

[a]Address for correspondence: Prof. P.-A. Mårdh, Department of Obstetrics and Gynecology, Lund University Hospital, SE-221 85 Lund, Sweden. Phone: 46 46 17 13 20; fax 46 46 15 78 68.

nucleic acid–based tests has led to a marked increase in sensitivity (in most settings by 10–50%) and specificity, compared to subjective tests like IF direct tests of clinical samples and microscopic manual reading of tissue cultures (in contrast to the general belief that this is an objective test).[2,10] Particularly in low-prevalence populations, LCR and PCR have proved to give an acceptably high positive predictive value in contrast to ELISA, even if confirmatory ELISA tests are used.[4,12]

Not only have the recommended methods for detection of genital chlamydial infections changed recently, but also the optimal type of sample to be tested. Thus there has been a change over time, occurring in the order mentioned, from urethral samples in men and cervical ones in women to cervical plus urethral samples, followed by voided urine and most recently by introital vaginal samples.[15]

A number of matters that concern screening are still under debate, for example, which groups to include in mass screening campaigns and at what stage in life to conduct them; how often screening should be repeated (maybe never because of economic restrictions), and whether the health provider considers her or himself to be at risk for having acquired a sexually transmitted infection, such as those caused by *C. trachomatis*.

WHOM TO SCREEN AND WHEN?

Most published screening studies have involved young persons, that is, in their late teenage years. Girls have been tested more often than boys. When using sensitive techniques (for example, PCR), genital chlamydial infections can be detected with a rather similar prevalence in women up to approximately 35 years of age, at least in women attending European family-planning clinics for contraceptive advice.[16] The use of such sensitive techniques can lead to detection of even chronic chlamydial infections with few elementary bodies of *C. trachomatis* that might not have been diagnosed when using ELISA. It is likely that chronic low-grade infections become more frequent with increasing age.

As a result of economic restrictions and also limited laboratory capacities, screening has usually been performed selectively, that is, the health provider focuses attention on certain groups in which all persons, without exception, are tested. A large number of groups to screen were identified two decades ago by the Swedish Board of Health and Welfare (TABLE 1)[17] and also in the United States[18] and the United Kingdom.[19] Groups listed in TABLES 1 and 2 have been regarded as at high risk of acquiring genital chlamydial infections. Also identified as high-risk groups were infants with conjunctivitis and pneumonia. With the extended testing possibilities for *C. trachomatis*, it might be advisable to test either everybody within a selected age span attending a clinic or a particular subunit of the age span.

From an epidemiological standpoint, a benefit is gained when screening programs for STDs are combined with counselling, at least of persons found positive. A natural connection with screening for other conditions or situations usually facilitates acceptance of chlamydia screening, for example, screening for cervical neoplasia and pregnancy testing.

TABLE 1. Groups of women suggested for selective screening for *Chlamydia trachomatis*

Women,
Who themselves consider to have been at risk to have acquired an STD
Who have had any STD diagnosed
Who report a sexual partner with signs/symptoms of a genital infection
Who are notified because an STD has been diagnosed in a partner
With signs/symptoms suggestive of:
cervicitis
endometritis
salpingitis
periappendicitis
perihepatitis
proctitis
peritonitis in PID cases
unexplained lower abdominal pain
conjunctivitis with unilateral debut
reactive arthritis
uveitis
nonbacterial urinary tract infection

TABLE 2. Groups of men proposed for selective screening for *Chlamydia trachomatis*

Men,
Who consider themselves to have been at risk to have acquired an STD
Who have had any STD diagnosed
Who report a sexual partner with signs/symptoms of a genital infection
Who are notified because an STD has been diagnosed in a partner
With signs/symptoms suggestive of:
urethritis
vaseitis
epididymitis
proctitis
conjunctivitis with unilateral debut
uveitis
reactive arthritis
Reiter's syndrome

WHICH TEST AND WHICH SAMPLE TYPE?

Different kit producers have been engaged in combat over the potential advantage to use of just their nucleic acid–based test kits. Studies exist that conclude one test is better than the other, and other studies make the opposite claim. The differences have usually not been statistically significant, but show only a numerical advantage for one kit under study over another.

The persistence of chlamydial antigen, even for two weeks after finishing therapy, renders antigen detection tests ineffective in post-antibiotic therapy testing. Thus the results of LCR, PCR, ELISA, and IF tests may persist as positive for at least two weeks in microbiologically cured cases. Laboratories that have closed down their culture diagnostic possibilities in favor of antigen detection tests have deprived themselves of being able to perform accurate tests within the indicated post-therapy period.

Laboratory analysis of urine involves dealing with a relatively large-volume sample type that often has an unpleasant odor and requires extra steps in sample preparation. In addition, it is potentially infectious compared to urethral and cervical swabs. Furthermore, the sample is not suitable for culture studies and is often difficult to read in IF tests in which is produces potentially misleading artifacts.

The extent to which chlamydial infections can persist in the upper genital tract despite treatment with conventional antibiotic dose regimens is poorly understood. The existence of chronic tubal chlamydial infections has been demonstrated,[20] for example, on the basis of *in situ* hybridization studies. Endometrial infections also exist. Diagnosis might not be possible by cercvical samples alone, but if might require endometrial or tubal aspiration, or endometrial and tubal biopsies. Chronic upper genital tract infections by *C. trachomatis* seem to be difficult to eradicate by the so-far recommended antibiotic regimens. It is also not known how frequently such chronic infections may flare up and cause symptoms or contribute to abdominal pain. This also raises the question whether, and if so how frequently, women with proven genital chlamydial infection should be rescreened.

Oral contraceptives may mask symptoms of genital chlamydial infection, including PID,[21] which heightens the importance of screening women on the pill.

SELF-SAMPLING AND HOME TESTING

The possibility of using vaginal samples collected by means of a tampon or introital samples collected with a swab,[22] or by flushing the vagina, apart from voided urine, has opened up self-sampling as an alternative to sampling done by health providers. Almost any epidemiological data of chlamydial infections in women collected before the possibility of using urine as the test sample existed were restricted to samplers who had access to a gynecological examination chair. This is likely to have given a skewed view of the true epidemiology of these infections in female populations.

It should be noted that the detection rate of *C. trachomatis* in introital vaginal samples has been numerically higher, although not significantly higher, than in cervical samples. In some studies this has also been true for samples collected by the patient herself after receiving instruction about how to proceed.

Self-sampling has also made it possible to initiate home sampling with subsequent mailing of the specimen to a laboratory for analysis.[22] However, such a procedure means loss of control over sample quality and identification (which may be particularly important when chlamydial infections are included in laws for STDs, e.g., as in Finland and Sweden).

Studies of the acceptance rates among women of different types of sampling methods have shown that self-sampling is acceptable, but there is a small preference for giving away a voided urine sample. Women of some religious and ethnic backgrounds have, however, strong objections to touching their genitalia for any reason.

SURVEILLANCE OF SCREENING RESULTS

In order to be able to correctly interpret monitored data from surveillance studies, it is essential to indicate which method and also which type of sample has been used, that is, interpret the meaning to judge the likely proportion of false negative and false positive samples and to calculate the likely positive and negative predictive values in a series of monitored tests. If "homemade" nucleic acid–based kits have been used, it is also important to know whether closed sample devices have or have not been employed. Furthermore, commercial kits—in contrast to "in-house" kits—may contain inadequate Taq-polymerase anti-inhibitory substances that may decrease the detection rate, for example, because of the presence of hemin and phosphatases.[9] To know the type of samples analyzed may also be essential for correct interpretation of the results of screening studies. For example, if urine has been analyzed by culture the sensitivity is only approximately 30%.

COST-EFFECTIVE AND COST-BENEFICIAL CALCULATIONS

The cost-effectivenes of a screening test depends on which costs and savings are considered for the calculations.[23–25] Such a calculation may simply look into the direct cost for the laboratory tests and the influence on saved case managements of acute infections and their complications. However, the costs saved from the management of the sequalae may outpace the former savings. The costs for the management of these sequalae may include drug and consultation costs for chronic abdominal pain, infertility workup, *in vitro* fertilization, and gynecological operations aiming to increase chances to conceive. Other, even less easily estimated costs (which may be greater than all the former ones) are those that are related to broken marriages with separate living expenses and the resulting increased costs for child care, adoption of children, and so forth. With regard to chlamydial PID, the proportion of silent tubal infections is unknown. Likewise, it is not known what proportion of tubal infertility cases can be attributed to a previous chlamydial infection. These factors make it difficult to estimate the influence of such sequalae on the cost-effectiveness of chlamydial screening programs.

The prevalence of genital chlamydial infections representing the cut-off level for cost-effective screening programs in women has been estimated to be 6% when the computer model does not include any unknown factor.[23] When including an estimated rate of silent PID, the cut-off level may be only 3%.[24]

SCREENING OF MALE PARTNERS

The success of any screening program depends on whether or not the partners of women found to be chlamydia-positive are notified. More than half of the partners will also be positive even when using the less sensitive test methods like ELISA. The possibility of letting the woman bring a voided urine specimen from her sexual partner to the gynecologist when she has been found to be a carrrier of *C. trachomatis* should be considered.

Screening of voided urine for *C. trachomatis* in men, as in women, has been demonstrated to be cost effective,[25] taking into account a calculated reduction of complications of chlamydial infections in the female population in the region where the program in men has been undertaken.

SUMMARY

Initiating screening programs often means motivating the medical society, health authorities, politicians, and the general population, which may explain the slow movement so far toward introducing such preventative programs as chlamydia screening.[26] Screening for chlamydial infections should be performed and should involve a broader age span than has been the rule so far. Vaginal introital samples (vaginal fluid collected by vaginal flushing) can be used in women with the same or even marginally better sensitivity than cervical samples, and they can obtained by self-sampling.

REFERENCES

1. MÅRDH, P.-A., J. PAAVONEN & M. PUOLAKKAINEN. 1989. Chlamydia. Plenum Press. New York.
2. MÅRDH, P.-A. 1998. Epidemiological aspects of *Chlamydia trachomatis* genital infections. Gynecol. Forum **3:** 21–23.
3. WESTRÖM, L. 1988. Decrease in incidence of women treated in hospital for acute salpingitis in Sweden. Genitourin. Med. **64:** 59–63.
4. MÅRDH, P.-A., K. TCHOUDOMIROVA & D. HELLBERG. 1998. Symptoms and signs in single and mixed genital infections in attendees of family planning and youth clinics. Int. J. Gynecol. Obst. **63:** 145–152.
5. JASCHEK, G., C.A. GAYDOS, L.E. WELSH, *et al.* 1993. Direct detection of *Chlamydia trachomatis* in urine specimens from symptomatic men by using a rapid polymerase chain reaction assay. J. Microbiol. **31:** 1209–1212.
6. DOMEIKA, M., M. BASSIRI & P.-A. MÅRDH. 1994. Diagnosis of genital *Chlamydia trachomatis* infections in asymptomatic males by testing urine by PCR. J. Clin. Microbiol. **32:** 2350–2352.
7. LEE, H.H., M.A. CHERNESKY, J. SCHACHTER, *et al.* 1995. Diagnosis of *Chlamydia trachomatis* genitourinary infection in women by ligase chain assay of urine. Lancet **345:** 213–216.
8. BASSIRI, M., P.-A. MÅRDH, M. DOMEIKA, *et al.* 1997. Multiplex Amplicor® screening PCR kit for *Chlamydia trachomatis* and *Neisseria gonorrhoeae* in women attending non-sexually transmitted disease clinics. J. Clin. Microbiol. **35:** 2556–2560.
9. MÅRDH, P.-A. & M. DOMEIKA. 1996. Application of DNA-based technologies in the diagnosis of sexually tract diseases. *In* Sexually Transmitted Infections: Advances in Diagnosis and Treatment. P. Elsner & A. Eichman, Eds.: 174–183. Karger. Zürich.
10. SCHACHTER, J. 1998. Evaluation of diagnostic tests for *Chlamydia trachomatis*. Gynecol. Forum **3:** 26–28.
11. MÅRDH, P.-A., A.N. ELBAGIR & K. STENBERG. 1990. Use of blocking reagent to confirm enzyme immunoassay results in samples from patients with chlamydial conjunctivitis. Eur. J. Clin. Microbiol. Infect. Dis. **9:** 292–293.
12. COUDRON, P.E., D.P. FEDORKO, M.S. DAWSON *et al.* 1986. Detection of *Chlamydia trachomatis* in genital specimens by the MicroTrak Direct Specimen test. Am. J. Clin. Pathol. **85:**89–92.
13. GENC, M., Y. DUTERTRE, M. BJÖRK *et al.* 1992. Detection of *Chlamydia trachomatis* in first void urine to identify asymptomatic male carriers. APMIS **100:** 645–459.

14. PASTERNACK, R., P. VUORINEN & A. MIETTINEN. 1997. Evaluation of the GenProbe *Chlamydia trachomatis* transcription-mediated amplification assay with urine specimens from women. J. Clin. Microbiol. **35:** 836–838.
15. STARY, A., B. NAJIM & H.H. LEE. 1997. Vulval swabs as alternative specimen for ligase chain reaction detection of genital chlamydial infection in women. J. Clin. Microbiol. **35:** 836–838.
16. MÅRDH, P.-A, M. BASSIRI, G. CREATSAS, *et al.* Infectious gynecological health in women attending family planning clinics in Europe. Eur. J. Contracept. Reprod. Health Care, in press.
17. ALLMÄNA RÅD FRÅN SOCIALSTYRELSEN. Förebyggande åtgärder mot chlamydia. SOS, Stockholm (Sweden).
18. HANDSFIELD, H.H., L.L. JASMAN, P.L. ROBERTS, *et al.* 1986. Criteria for selective screening for *Chlamydia trachomatis* infection in women attending family planning clinics. JAMA **255:** 1730–1734.
19. CMO´S EXPERT ADVISORY GROUP. 1998. *Chlamydia trachomatis*. Summary and conclusions. Department of Health, Health Promosion Division. London.
20. WOLNER-HANSSEN, P., N.B. KIVIAT & K.K. HOLMES. 1999. Atypical pelvic inflammatory disease: subacute, chronic, or subclinical upper genital tract infection in women. *In* Sexually Transmitted Diseases. K.K. Holmes, F. Sparling, *et al.*, Eds.: 615–620. McGraw Hill. New York.
21. MÅRDH, P.-A. & B. HOGG. 1998. Are oral contraceptives masking symptoms of chlamydia cervicitis and pelvic inflammatory disease? Eur. J. Contracept. Reprod. Health Care **3:** 41–43.
22. ÖSTERGAARD, L., J.K. MÖLLER, B. ANDERSEN, *et al.*. 1996. Diagnosis of urogenital *Chlamydia* infection in women based on mailed samples obtained at home: multipractice comparative study. Br. Med. J. **313:** 1186–1189.
23. GENC, M. & P.-A. MÅRDH. 1996. A cost effectiveness analysis of screening and treatment for *Chlamydia trachomatis* infection in asymptomatic women. Ann. Intern. Med. **124:** 1–7.
24. PAAVONEN, J., M. PUOLAKKAINEN, M. PAUKKU, *et al.* 1998. Cost-benefit analysis of first-void urine *Chlamydia trachomatis* screening program. Am. J. Obst. Gyn. **92:** 293–298.
25. GENC, M., L. RUUSUVAARA & P.-A. MÅRDH. 1993. An economic evaluation of screening for *Chlamydia trachomatis* in adolescent males. JAMA **17:** 2057–2064.
26. MÅRDH, P.-A. 1997. Is Europe ready for STD screening? Genitourin. Med. **73:** 96–98.

Update on *Chlamydia trachomatis*

S. GUASCHINO AND F. DE SETA[a]

Department of Obstetrics and Gynecology "B. Garofolo," University of Trieste, Trieste, Italy

ABSTRACT: *Chlamydia trachomatis* is one the most important sexually transmitted diseases; it can cause serious sequelae despite the absence of symptoms in some people. It's estimated that about 25% of women who have acute salpingitis become infertile, and chlamydial infection is the commonest cause. The introduction of screening programs for its detection are still a topic of discussion. The literature shows that the total cost of examination and treatment of complications known to be associated with genital chlamydial infection (PID, chronic pelvic pain, tubal factor infertility) is generally higher than the total cost of a large-scale *Chlamydia* screening program. The selection of a diagnostic test for detection of chlamydial genital infection depends on availability, local expertise, and prevalence of *Chlamydia trachomatis* in the test population. Cell culture is too expensive in nonendemic regions, so the use of non-culture techniques is very attractive. PCR (polymerase chain reaction) and LCR (ligase chain reaction) are actually the two most commonly used alternatives to conventional methods for detecting STD agents. In fact, PCR and LCR have proved useful for detection of *Chlamydia trachomatis* in cervical and urethral samples both in symptomatic and asymptomatic women. Recently, testing of first-void urine (FVU) specimens with these techniques has shown that the amplification tests are as sensitive as tests with endocervical swab cultures.

For the past two decades, a virtual revolution has occurred in the field of sexually transmitted diseases (STDs). Not only are we in the midst of an epidemic of STDs, but the recognition of this epidemic has focused increased attention on STDs. As is well known, concern about the traditional venereal diseases, such gonorrhea and syphilis, has evolved into the current emphasis on syndromes associated with *Chlamydia trachomatis*, herpes simplex virus (HSV), human papilloma virus (HPV), and, more recently, the different pathologic conditions caused by human immunodeficiency virus (HIV).

Chlamydia trachomatis, in particular, is the most common sexually transmitted disease in Western countries. In the United States over 4 million new cases of infection are estimated to occur each year, 10 million new infections occur in Europe, and 89 million cases occur worldwide. Worldwide, the next most common is gonorrhea, with 62 million cases, and syphilis, with 12 million (excluding trichomoniasis).[1]

[a]Address for correspondence: F. De Seta, Department of Obstetrics and Gynecology "B. Garofolo," Via dell'Istria 65/1, 34100 Trieste, Italy. Phone: 0039-040-3785351/352; fax: 0039-040-761266.

frdeseta@tin.it

In Italy the prevalence of infection differs from region to region, with a higher prevalence in the south than in the north.. The National Institutes of Health (U.S.) reports a prevalence of 2–6% in the female general population, 2–15% ın pregnant women, and 11–30% in women attending STD centers. The European Collaborative Study[2,3] has found that in Italy there is a lower prevalence in women attending the Centers for Contraceptive Advice (2.3%) than in the East European countries (3–5%) and in the United Kingdom (4.2%).

It is not easy to interpret these data because, unfortunately, many chlamydial infections of the lower genital tract in women are asymptomatic. In fact different authors[4,5] have suggested that the failure in controling chlamydial infections and the consequent increase in incidence of these infections can be attributed to several factors: (a) the nonspecific signs and symptoms of chlamydial infection; (b) the mild or absent signs and symptoms of chlamydial infection; (c) inadequate laboratory facilities for detection of *Chlamydia trachomatis*; (d) the expense and technology associated with testing for *Chlamydia trachomatis*; (e) the lack of familiarity clinicians have with chlamydial infections; (f) the fact that at least seven days of multiple-dose therapy was required (until very recently); and (g) the inadequate resources directed at screening high-risk patients and locating and screening partners.

Chlamydia trachomatis causes important diseases in men, women, and infants. In women, it is responsible for urethritis, cervicitis, pelvic inflammatory disease (PIID), and the sequelae of these conditions, such as infertility, ectopic pregnancy, and chronic pelvic pain. In men, infection by *Chlamydia trachomatis* can cause arthritis and epididymitis, which may result in urethral obstructions and decreased fertility in rare cases. Neonates passing through the birth canal of an infected woman can become infected, leading to chlamydial conjunctivitis and pneumonia.[6]

Chlamydia trachomatis is an obligatory intracellular bacterium that contains DNA and RNA; however, it differs from bacteria but is similar to viruses because it is an intracellular parasite. It may be regarded as a bacterium that has adapted to an intracellular environment. Three major groups of infections are related to different *Chlamydia trachomatis* serotypes. The L serotypes (L1, L2, L3) cause lymphogranuloma venereum (LGV); the A, B, and C serotypes are the agents responsible for endemic blinding trachoma; and the remaining serotypes (D, E, F, G, H, I, J, K) are the oculogenital and sexually transmitted strains that cause inclusion conjunctivitis, newborn pneumonia, urethritis, cervicitis, epididymitis, salpingitis, acute urethral syndrome, and perinatal infections.

A number of studies have shown that the same populations at risk for other STDs are at the highest risk for chlamydial infections.[7] Age, socioeconomic status, number of sexual partners, and use of oral contraceptives are predictors of chlamydial genital infections. The rate of incidence of theses infections is inversely related to age and directly related to the number of sexual partners. Lower socioeconomic status has been associated with an increased risk for infection. Risk factors for chlamydial cervical infection in pregnant women include unmarried status, age below 20 years, and presence of other STDs. Also, women who seek prenatal care late and presence of mucopurulent endocervicitis or abacteriuric pyuria represent high risk factors.

More recently, as well as in the past, many studies investigating the cost-effectiveness of screening and treatment *Chlamydia trachomatis* infections have been done. The literature about screening and treatment in family-planning clinics is associated with a reduced incidence of *Chlamydia* sequelae, but whom to screen and by which test remains unclear.

Universal screening aimed at detection of disease among asymptomatic sexually active women has been proposed as a control measure for chlamydial infection and its sequelae. Although the widespread availability of antigen detection tests has reduced the cost of documenting chlamydial infection, universal screening is not an economically feasible alternative for most public clinics. Selective screening with predefined criteria to identify patients at increased risk is far less expensive but is less effective in identifying all infected women.[8] Ideally, all selected women should be screened for *Chlamydia trachomatis*. However, current resources preclude achieving such a goal. All women suspected of having chlamydial genital tract infection should have specific diagnostic testing. This includes women with symptoms, signs, or history of exposure to *Chlamydia* such as pelvic inflammatory disease (PID), endometritis, or acute urethritis and those whose partners have nongonococcal urethritis (NGU). Also, high-risk groups of asymptomatic women (prenatal clinics, abortion clinics, family-planning clinics) and women who have specific risk factors associated with chlamydial infections (adolescents with a new sexual partner or multiple sexual partners) should be screened for *Chlamydia trachomatis*.

The selection of a diagnostic test for detection of chlamydial genital infection depends on availability, local expertise, and prevalence of *Chlamydia trachomatis* in the test population. For screening to be effective along the causal pathway, not only does the presence of the disease need to be demonstrated but there must also be evidence that treatment will lead to prevention of complications. This prevention outcome has only been shown in the screening of women at high risk for infection and of pregnant women. Mass screening has the potential disadvantages of increased cost or unnecessary treatment of patients with false positive test results. Over the past few decades a number of techniques have been used to detect chlamydial infection. The isolation in McCoy cells, combined with staining the cell culture with fluorescein-labeled monoclonal antibodies, was until recently considered the "gold standard" in diagnosis of chlamydial infection. Later, antigen detection tests, such as the direct immunofluorescence test (DIF) and enzyme immunoassay (EIA), have been applied to their detection.

Phillips *et al.*,[9] using decision analysis to estimate the clinical and economic implications of testing asymptomatic women for cervical chlamydial infection, compared a strategy of no routine testing with one involving routine testing with use of culture or of nonculture tests (DFA test or ELISA). They concluded that screening with the nonculture tests would reduce overall costs if the prevalence of infection was 7% or greater, and that screening with culture would reduce costs if the prevalence rate was 14% or more.

Many have found that nucleic acid detection assays, such as nonamplification and, lately, amplification assay (e.g., PCR and ligase chain reaction [LCR]), posses higher sensitivities than the detection methods used earlier.[10] Thus, PCR and LCR have proved useful for detection of *Chlamydia trachomatis* in cervical and urethral samples both in symptomatic and asymptomatic women. Recently, testing with first-void urine (FVU) specimens by these techniques have shown that the amplification tests are as sensitive as tests with endocervical swab cultures.

The European Collaborative Study,[2] performed on women attending European health care units for contraceptive advice or pregnancy termination, have considered the need of screening for *Chlamydia trachomatis* in conjunction with regular gynecological examinations. A PCR kit was used as a screening tool for the detection of *Chlamydia trachomatis* and *Neisseria gonorrhoeae* in FVU specimens from 3340 asymptomatic women. On the basis of the results it is not possible now to recommend routine screening of asymptomatic women. Evaluations based on cost-effectiveness of establishing universal or target screening programs for asymptomatic women attending different health care unit are warranted.

The US Centers for Disease Control and Prevention in Atlanta have recently suggested screening women with mucopurulent cervicitis, sexually active women less than 20 years of age and women 20 to 24 years of age who are inconsistent in their use of barrier contraceptives or have had a new sexual partner or more than one partner during the last 3 months.[11] Screening may offer an additional strategy for the control of *Chlamydia trachomatis* infection, but selective screening based on single historical or clinical risk factors was found to have a relatively low predictive value.

The contribution of a predictor to the proportion of cases detected in screening programs depends on the magnitude of the association and the prevalence of the predictor in the population. Variables linked to less than 15% of cases or more than 85% of all individuals are of limited value as selection criteria, because they cannot discriminate properly between cases and healthy individuals.

Most women with chlamydial disease remain untreated because their infection is either asymptomatic or not manifest. In general, one-half to two-thirds of chlamydial infections of the cervix are asymptomatic. If not treated the infection can persist for several years and subject those infected to the risks of spread of *Chlamydia trachomatis* to the upper genital tract, with subsequent infertility and ectopic pregnancy.

Over 1 million women acquire PID each year in the USA; 20–50% of these cases are associated with *Chlamydia trachomatis*.[12,13] All the women with previous PID are exposed to a significantly increased risk for infertility and ectopic pregnancy. Although STD organisms are clearly involved in the etiology of STD-related PID, the role of sexual behavior in the development of PID remains poorly defined. Several aspects of sexual behavior have been proposed to be associated with an increased risk of PID. These include (a) multiple sex partners; (b) high frequency of sexual intercourse; (c) rate of acquisition of new sex partners within the previous 30 days, and (d) age at first sexual intercourse.

It is generally held that chlamydial salpingitis, like gonococcal salpingitis, results from the intracanalicular spread of *Chlamydia trachomatis* from the endocervix to the endometrium and thence to the fallopian tube. Chronic, subacute, or latent endometrial and tubal infection is probably present in a large number of women, but a consensus definition of these clinically subtle infections is lacking.

The two major sequelae of acute PID, tubal infertility and ectopic pregnancy, have been associated with prior chlamydial infection. Silent salpingitis probably accounts for the major proportion of tubal infertility.[14] Nearly all investigators have found that more than half of the women with documented tubal occlusion report no history of previous PID despite serologic evidence of past chlamydial infection. Moreover, morphologic and physical analyses of tubal epithelium from women with distal tubal obstruction found extensive ultrastructural damage, even in those without knowledge of previous PID.

The value of serology in detecting upper genital tract infections is still debatable.[15] A high antichlamydial immunoglobulin (Ig) G titer, although often detected in upper genital tract infections, cannot be considered proof of current infection. Antichlamydial IgA has been shown to be significantly associated with acute salpingitis, ectopic pregnancy, and tubal factor infertility. Antichlamydial IgM is considered to be a marker of recent or current infection; however, only a few authors have detected positive antichlamydial IgM in chlamydial intrapelvic gynecologic infections. Because the women with tubal infertility have a high prevalence of circulating antibody to *Chlamydia trachomatis*, Mol *et al.*,[16] after a meta-analysis of studies comparing *Chlamydia* antibody titers and laparoscopy for tubal patency and peritubal adhesions on 2729 patients, concluded that *Chlamydia* antibody testing is more appropriate than hysterosalpingography (HSG) in the selection of patients for laparoscopy. In contrast with laparoscopy and HSG, the mechanism of *Chlamydia* antibody testing is based on the detection of previous infection, thereby providing no information on the severity of tubal disease. For this reason, *Chlamydia* antibody testing is unlikely to be a useful tool in the prognosis of fertility. Nevertheless we have to take into account that 80% of women with documented tubal infertility and antibody to *Chlamydia trachomatis* never had symptoms of an upper tract infection or STDs.

Our understanding of the pathogenic mechanisms of *Chlamydia salpingitis* that leads to the development of tubal scarring and infertility is minimal. Unlike most bacterial infections, in which tissue damage results from the direct effect of bacterial replication, the damage and scarring associated with *Chlamydia trachomatis* is the result of the host immune response to the infection. Patton *et al.*[17] demonstrated in a monkey model that primary chlamydial infection is associated with a mild to moderate inflammation with an influx of polymorphonuclear cells. This is a self-limited infection that peaks by 2 weeks and resolves within 5 weeks. Repeated inoculations with *Chlamydia trachomatis* result in an infection and inflammation characterized by mononuclear cells and formation of lymphoid follicles. In the monkey model, these repeated infections can cause extensive tubal scarring, distal tubal obstruction and peritubal adhesions. These observations about the primates and the model of conjunctival infections caused by *Chlamydia trachomatis* in humans suggest that reinfection and the host's immune response are important. In particular, the immune response to a 57-kDa chlamydial heat-shock protein, hsp60, has been associated with the pathogenesis of *Chlamydia* infection. In 1989, Morrison *et al.*[18] demonstrated that the single antigen Hsp 60 has been shown to induce a delayed hypersensitivity response in guinea pigs that were previously infected with *Chlamydia*. Following this study Dorothy Patton[19] suggested in 1994 that the pathogenesis of tubal infertility following *Chlamydia trachomatis* salpingitis is similar to that of blindness caused by ocular chlamydial infection. Both are the results of tissue damage from immunopathologic reactions from chronic or repeated infection. In fact, to being the pathology of chronic salpingitis in infertile women and *Chlamydia*-infected animals, characterized by mononuclear cell infiltrated similar to those observed in trachoma, chlamydial hsp60 has been hypothesized to play a basic role in the pathogenesis of *Chlamydia*-associated tubal infertility.

Toye *et al.*[20] determined the prevalence of antibody to *Chlamydia trachomatis* hsp60 in women with tubal infertility. The results show a strong association between an antibody response to C-hsp60 and development of *Chlamydia*-associated tubal infertility consistent with an immunopathogenetic mechanism. Prospective studies are needed to determine the clinical utility of a C-hsp60 assay a predictor of tubal disease in women presenting with infertility or as a marker of poor fertility outcome in women with *Chlamydia*-associated PID.

Besides damage-related hsp60 response, the tubal damage can be linked to the cytokines that are important in expression of pathogenic antigens and activation of the systemic immune response. Ault *et al.*[21] have shown that the production of TNF-α in response to chlamydial infection could promote the production of other cytokines (interleukin-1 and interleukin-6) and immune-mediated damage of the fallopian tube.

Witkin and Ledger[22] report that immune system activation and cytokine production in response to chlamydial antigens may interfere with embryo implantation or regulatory mechanisms that protect the fetus from attack by the maternal immune system. Alternatively, a past chlamydial infection may have damaged the endometrium sufficiently that successful embryo implantation becomes less likely. Another possibility involves the induction of an autoimmune response as a result of long-term exposure to *Chlamydia trachomatis* antigens. The hsp60 is also one of the first proteins produced by a developing embryo. Therefore sensitization of T lymphocytes to the C-hsp60 may result in the generation of lymphocytes that can also react with the analogous human hsp that can be expressed by the embryo or maternal cells in the pregnant uterus. The resultant immune system activation might directly destroy the embryo or interfere with the immune regulatory system. Continued testing for high-titer *Chlamydia* IgG antibody could lead to improved identification and characterization of this subgroup of women whose recurrent abortions or infertility is currently unexplained. On the other hand, Rae *et al.*[23] report no association between immunoglobulin G antibodies to *Chlamydia trachomatis* and recurrent spontaneous abortion. They conclude that prior chlamydial infection is irrelevant to fetal loss in recurrent aborters in general, whereas relevance to a minority of patients, although not supported by this study, has not been excluded.

We could briefly summarize the pathogenesis of tubal damage as follows: primary infection by *Chlamydia trachomatis* may induce a generation of sensitized lymphocytes that, in the case of long-standing infection or reinfection of chlamydial antigen, can reactivate and respond to epitopes present in the homologous human hsp and cause tissue damage on on immunological basis. In the same way, the abortion could be due to sensitization of lymphocytes by a primary infection, expression of endometrial hsp, and subsequent attack against the embryo.

What about male infection? Several clinical studies have demonstrated an association between WBC in semen and sperm dysfunction. In fact, there is an inverse relationship between elastasi and spermatozoa. Nevertheless, Witkin *et al.*[24] tested 28 infertile males with PCR who had been negative to culture and DNA probes; they found 11 cases positive for *Chlamydia* and about 50% of these had antisperm antibody. They explain these findings with the hypothesis that *Chlamydia* may be present at a concentration below the threshold of culture and DNA probes. This is probably a result of the increased sensitivity of PCR in detecting *Chlamydia trachomatis*. The increased prevalence of an autoimmune response to sperm in men with this organism in their semen suggests that a subclinical chlamydial infection may activate an immune response to sperm. A similar association between *Chlamydia trachomatis* in semen and circulating antisperm antibodies in female partners indicates the possibility that the women could develop an immune response to sperm.

Perhaps a screening program to detect the microorganism in semen from symptom-free, sexually active young men and the prompt treatment of infected persons and their partner(s) could have a greater rate of success in reducing the incidence of unexplained infertility.

Given the morbidity associated with chlamydial infections, some efforts at control measures are indicated. A first step would be introducing chlamydial diagnostic techniques in the management of genital tract complaints in women. A second step would be to administer appropriate therapy with tetracycline or azithromycin (in pregnancy). The appropriate therapy is basicly to prevent, if possible, the greater risk for developing serious complications of this infection and to restrict vertical and horizontal transmission.

The literature shows that the total cost of examination and treatment of complications known to be associated with genital chlamydial infection (PID, chronic pelvic pain, tubal factor infertility) is generally higher than the total cost of a large-scale *Chlamydia* screening program.

Education (primary prevention) and more, less-selective screening of asymptomatic populations (secondary prevention) are the prerequisites for avoiding the costly complications of *Chlamydia* infections. The data from a cost–benefit analysis of a *Chlamydia* screening program are inconclusive. Cost–benefit analysis should place monetary values on both the input (cost) and outcome (benefits) of health care. Although the data clearly show that *Chlamydia* screening is cost-effective in populations with a high prevalence of chlamydial infection, the performance of the diagnostic laboratory tests used in such screening programs should also be carefully evaluated in low-prevalence populations.

REFERENCES

1. SCIARRA, J.J. 1997. Sexually transmitted diseases: global importance. Int. J. Gynecol. Obstet. **58:** 107–119.
2. BASSIRI, M., P.A. MARDH, M. DOMEIKA & EUROPEAN CHLAMYDIA EPIDEMIOLOGY GROUP. 1997. Multiplex AMPLICOR PCR detection of *Chlamydia trachomatis* and *Neisseria gonorrhoeae* in women attending non-sexually transmitted disease clinics. J. Clin. Microbiol. **35:** 2556–2560.
3. GUASCHINO, S., E. GRIMALDI, F. DE SETA, *et al.* 1997. Detection of *Chlamydia trachomatis* in urine of asymptomatic women. *In* Collected Abstracts of the 3rd Congress of the European Society for Gynecologic and Obstetric Investigation. No. FC20. Madonna di Campiglio. Italy.
4. *Cates,* W. *et al.* 1991. Genital chlamydial infections: epidemiology and reproductive sequelae. Am. J. Obstet. Gynecol. **164:** 1771–1778.
5. STAMM, W.E. *et al.* 1990. *Chlamydia trachomatis* infections of the adult. *In* Sexually Transmitted Diseases. K.K. Holmes *et al.*, Eds.: 184–194. McGraw Hill. New York.
6. GENC, M. & A. MARDH. 1996. A cost-effectiveness analysis of screening and treatment for *Chlamydia trachomatis* infection in asymptomatic women. Ann. Intern. Med. **124**(1)**:** 1–7.
7. SWEET, R.L. & R.S. GIBBS. 1995. Infectious diseases of the female genital tract. Third edit. William & Wilkins. Baltimore.
8. FINELLI, L. *et al.* 1996. Selective screening versus presumptive treatment criteria for identification of women with chlamydial infection in public clinic: New Jersey. Am. J. Obstet. Gynecol. **174:** 1527–1533.
9. PHILLIPS, R. *et al.* 1987. Should tests for *Chlamydia trachomatis* cervical infection be done during routine gynecologic visits? An analysis of the costs of alternative strategies. Ann. Intern. Med. **107:** 188–194.

10. BASSIRI, M., M. DOMEIKA, *et al.* 1994. Detection of *Chlamydia trachomatis* in urine specimens from women by ligase chain reaction. J. Clin. Microbiol. **33:** 898–900.
11. MORBIDITY AND MORTALITY WEEKLY REPORT. 1993. Recommendations for the prevention and management of *Chlamydia trachomatis* infections, 1993. **42**(RR-12)**:** 1–39.
12. ORR, P., E. SHERMAN, *et al.* 1994. Epidemiology of infection due to *Chlamydia trachomatis* in Manitoba, Canada. Clin. Inf. Dis. **19:** 876–883.
13. WASSERHEIT, J.N. *et al.* 1986. Microbial causes of proven pelvic inflammatory disease and efficacy of clindamycin and tobramycin. Ann. Intern. Med. **104:** 187.
14. CATES, W. JR., *et al.* 1984. Sexually transmitted organisms and infertility: the proof of the pudding. Sex. Transm. Dis. **11:** 113–116.
15. HENRY-SUCHET, J. *et al.* 1994. Post-therapeutic evolution of serum chlamydial antibody titers in women with acute salpingitis and tubal infertility. Fertil. Steril. **62:** 296–304.
16. MOL BEN, W.J. *et al.* 1997. The accuracy of serum chlamydial antibodies in the diagnosis of tubal pathology: a meta-analysis. Fertil. Steril. **67:** 1031–1037.
17. PATTON, D.L. *et al.* 1983. Host response to primary *Chlamydia trachomatis* infection of the fallopian tub in pig-tailed monkeys. Fertil. Steril. **40:** 829–840.
18. MORRISON, R.P. 1995. *S*erologic response of infertile women to the 60-kd chlamydial heat shock protein (hsp60). Fertil. Steril. **64:** 730–735.
19. PATTON, D.L. *et al.* 1994. Demonstration of delayed hypersensitivity in *Chlamydia trachomatis* salpingitis in monkeys. A pathogenic mechanism of tubal damage. J. Infect. Dis. **169:** 680–683.
20. TOYE, B. *et al.* 1993. Association between antibody to the *Chlamydia* heat-shock protein and tubal infertility. **168:** 1236–1240.
21. AULT, K.A. *et al.* 1996. Tumor necrosis factor-α response to infection with *Chlamydia trachomatis* in human fallopian tube organ culture. Am. J. Obstet. Gynecol. **175:** 1242–1245.
22. WITKIN, S.S. & W.J. LEDGER. 1992. Antibodies to *Chlamydia trachomatis* in sera of women with recurrent spontaneous abortions. Am. J. Obstet. Gynecol. **167:** 135–139.
23. RAE, R. *et al.* 1994. Chlamydial serologic studies and recurrent spontaneous abortion. Am. J. Obstet. Gynecol. **170:** 782–785.
24. WITKIN, S. *et al.* 1993. Detection of *Chlamydia trachomatis* in semen by the polymerase chain reaction in male members of infertile couples. Am. J. Obstet. Gynecol. **168:** 1457–1462.

PID: Clinical and Laparoscopic Aspects

JEANINE HENRY-SUCHET

Chargée d'enseignement à l'Hôpital Saint Louis Paris, Responsable du département de coelio-chirurgie de l'Hôpital Jean Rostand, 141 Grand-rue, Sèvres, France

ABSTRACT: Clinical signs of pelvic inflammatory disease (PID) are not constant and are often limited to slight pelvic pain. Laparoscopy can lead to a rapid and correct diagnosis of PID. Intrapelvic bacteriologic samples can be obtained so as to administer the proper antibiotic. The exact nature of the lesions can be evaluated, and in severe cases, recent abscesses can be treated with good results for fecundity. Because the results in cases of long-standing abscess are not so good, laparoscopy should be performed at the onset of infection and not be reserved until after some weeks of inefficient medical treatment, especially in young women who have not completed their family. In primary chronic salpingitis, the lack of any clinical signs usually leads to a delay in diagnosis until women consult for fertility problems. The ideal point would be to detect some biologic or clinical change that may lead to diagnosis such as a positive anti-*Chlamydia trachomatis* (CT) serology or, in the future, positive anti-CT Hsp 60 antibody could be the key to detecting and treating silent salpingitis in young women, CT being the main microorganism involved in chronic salpingitis. Screening for *C. trachomatis* low genital tract infection is mandatory in young people in order to control the epidemic.

INTRODUCTION

Pelvic inflammatory disease (PID) includes: (1) acute or subacute salpingitis (AS) and/or endometritis, which may cause various degrees of pelvic pain and clinical or biologic signs of inflammation in women aged 15–25 years; and (2) chronic salpingitis (CS), which may be primary or secondary to AS and is usually silent and only diagnosed years later because of infertility in woman aged 25–35.[1]

CLINICAL SIGNS

The clinical diagnosis of AS is usually based on the presence, in a young sexually active woman, of three or more clinical or biologic signs: recent and acute pelvic pain, fever of 38°C or higher, tender adnexal swelling, and elevated leukocyte count, ESR, and/or CRP.

Unfortunately, all these signs are not always present. The frequency of their occurrence in laparoscopic proven AS was evaluated with similar results in Sweden[2,3] and some years later in France[4–6] (TABLE 1). This explains why the clinical picture in about half the cases is not characteristic and frequently simulates other conditions. Although pelvic pain is almost universal, isolated pain, pain on one side only, and bleeding due to associated endometritis are frequent. Lack of inflammatory signs occurs 50% of the time; ESR and/or CRP may be normal in 25% of cases. Pelvic

TABLE 1. Frequency of the different signs of acute salpingitis (%)

Authors	Jacobsen 1969 Sweden	Henry-Suchet 1977 France	Blum 1979 France	Paillault 1979 France
Total cases	623	117	100	77
Pelvic pain	93.9	98	99	89.6
Pelvic pain on side only	—	23	38	28.5
Vaginal discharge	54.6	—	32	65
Temperature 38°C or more	41.3	47.8	76	31
Bleeding	35.5	44	46	42.8
Urinary signs	18.6	—	16	23
ESR 15 or more	75.9	76.9	—	69
Leukocyte count @ 10,000	—	47.8	—	44.7

sonography usually gives normal results. It may show some peritoneal fluid in the cul-de-sac, a valuable sign in women under estro-progestative treatment.

Even in severe cases, diagnosis may be difficult in occlusive forms, pseudoappendicitis forms, or adnexal mass. A special form is the Fitz-Hugh-Curtis syndrome, with elevated fever and pain in the highest right part of the abdomen due to perihepatitis of chlamydial origin in most cases;[7] the associated salpingitis is usually silent.

If the diagnosis is based on clinical and biologic signs only, the risk of false-positive diagnosis is 35% (TABLE 2) and that of false-negative diagnosis 15%. Even if three or more clinical criteria are present, the risk of false diagnosis is 20–30% according to Jacobson.[3] Hospitalized AS patients who have undergone laparoscopy have decreased in number over the last 10 years according to a multicentric French study.[8] Once a women undergoes laparoscopy, the risk of false-positive diagnosis is about the same (30%). The risk of false-negative diagnosis is greater than it was 20

TABLE 2. Clinically suspected acute salpingitis; laparoscopic diagnosis

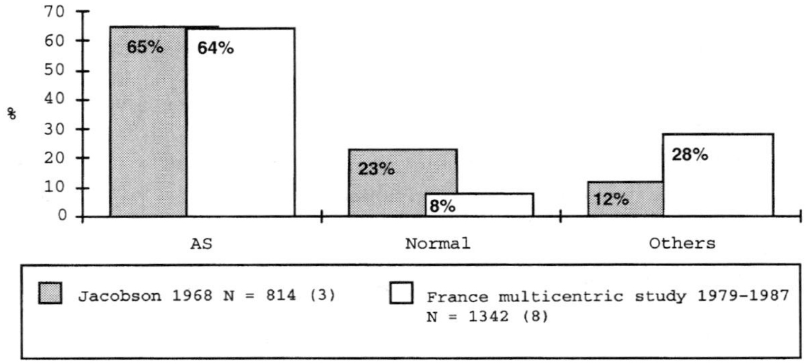

years ago (50%). The other diagnoses are unexplained pelvic pain (30%), adnexal mass (10%), endometriosis (7%), and post-PID adhesions (12%).

LAPAROSCOPIC SIGNS

The indications for laparoscopy in AS are especially strong in young women when early diagnosis is essential to preserve future fertility. Laparoscopy is indicated in mild cases with moderate symptoms in order to confirm the diagnosis and in severe cases for treatment.[9] However, laparoscopy, an invasive technique, necessitates hospitalization and general anesthesia and is expensive. It is therefore not always indicated in women who have completed their family and who have clearcut clinical signs (three or four symptoms of which one is a biologic sign of infection) or a moderate form of the condition (for instance, women with AS wearing an IUD or AS after a legal abortion). In such cases, a diagnosis based on conventionally accepted symptoms is valuable, and outpatient medical treatment can be given initially,[10] with laparoscopy being reserved for those patients who obtain no improvement after 5–7 days.

Laparoscopy is carried out on the first day of hospitalization after bacteriologic samples from the low genital tract and urine have been obtained along with a leukocyte count, ESR, CRP, and serology for *Chlamydia trachomatis* including evaluation of IgG, IgA, and IgM.[11]

Laparoscopy permits[12] immediate and complete diagnosis on the presence of red and swollen adnexae, adhesions and purulent fluid in the pouch of Douglas. Before touching these infected organs, the laparoscope should be rotated towards the liver in search of exudates or adhesions. The Fitz-Hugh-Curtis syndrome with typical violin-string adhesions between liver and diaphragm is found in 5–10% of PID cases, even with no history of hepatic pain. If pain is localized or predominantly on the right side, inspection of the appendix is mandatory, an association between appendicitis and PID being not uncommon. After these maneuvers, the laparoscope is turned down towards the pelvis, and a probe or forceps can be used to manipulate the adnexae to completely evaluate the lesions.

One can differentiate the following:

- recent AS without adhesions, with uterus and tubes only slightly red and swollen, normal fimbriae, normal ovaries, and a turbid exudate in the cul-de-sac;
- severe AS with purulent discharge from the fimbriae and in the cul-de-sac, pyosalpinges, and in some cases adnexal abscesses;
- subacute AS with gelatinous red adhesions, and sometimes the typical aspect of a viscous pelvis: yellow liquid in the cul-de-sac and yellow pseudocysts around tubes and ovaries;[13]
- cases of long-standing duration or recurrent forms with fibrous and dense adhesions and occluded tubes with possible hydrosalpinges or pyosalpinges.

The latter two aspects can be found similarly in women with PID signs or in infertile women without clinical signs or a past history of pelvic pain.

Laparoscopic diagnosis may occasionally be difficult: (1) in severe cases in which the bowels are adherent to the adnexae by adhesions too dense to be lysed with a probe. In such cases, diagnosis must possibly be reconsidered, because other diseases such as ovarian tumors may have the same aspect. Other diagnostic methods, such as vaginal punction under sonographic control, can be used; (2) in mild forms with only very slight inflammation of the tubes which may seem normal: in such cases, biopsy of the fimbriae is mandatory to eliminate or assess the diagnosis of PID.

Laparoscopy allows bacteriologic, histologic, and cytologic samples to be taken from the pouch of Douglas, swabs or, better, microbiopsy from the fimbriae, large biopsies from adhesions. Samples are immediately placed in culture broth for aeroanaerobics, specific transport mediums for mycoplasmas, and chlamydia detection by polymerase chain reaction or in formol for histologic study.

Laparoscopy also allows aspiration of purulent discharge and treatment of abscesses.[9] Recent abscesses are frequently caused by purulent fluid accumulating between the tube (external wall of the abscess), uterus (anterior wall), ovary (lower wall), and bowels (upper wall). The fresh friable adhesions between these organs and the different locations can be broken up with the probe under direct vision; purulent fluid can be aspirated away; the newly freed adnexae on bowels can be washed. Abscesses of the pouch of Douglas can be similarly treated. If the purulent discharge is completely removed, it is not necessary to use a drain. Thus, in most severe cases, the surgeon can use a blunt laparoscopic probe to carry out the same local treatment as he would have done with his fingers at laparotomy, but with far less trauma during this acute phase.

In cases of long-standing abscess with a thick capsule, the adnexae often appear as a dense mass that is difficult to distinguish between a pyosalpinx and an ovary and to determine if an ovarian abscess exists. Puncture of the mass with a needle probe allows aspiration of purulent fluid and insertion of antibiotics directly into the abscess cavity.

The risk of laparoscopic treatment is in the spread of infection either generally or locally. General disseminated infection with septicemia and septic shock from gram-negative bacteria is avoided by starting intensive, broad spectrum intravenous treatment with antibiotics during laparoscopy or, in some cases, beforehand. Localized dissemination with recurrent abdominal infection is a risk if the purulent fluid is not removed entirely. This can be avoided if the limits of laparoscopic treatment are fully understood. If the bowel cannot easily be removed from the pelvic organs by gentle manipulation of the probe or if each location cannot be destroyed, it is preferable to perform a vaginal punction under sonography or a laparotomy.

Surgery, if necessary, should take place after several days or weeks of medical treatment, and therefore it will more likely be conservative.

CLINICAL AND LAPAROSCOPIC FOLLOW-UP AFTER TREATMENT

The patient is usually discharged after clinical signs return to normal (3 days in mild forms, 6–8 days in severe forms). Residual tenderness of the adnexae and a persistent accelerated ESR is common in severe cases. A gynecologic checkup and repeat ESR and CRP are useful on a weekly basis during the first month and then every

TABLE 3. Tubo-ovarian abscesses: laparoscopic treatment — short-term evolution

Authors	Country	*N*	Recovery	Laparoscopy
Henry-Suchet	France	80	72	8
Abeille	France	10	10	0
Mintz	France	50	49	1
Reich	USA	27	26	1
Adducci	USA	7	7	0
Freistadt	USA	4	4	0
Muzsnai	USA	13	12	1
Raiga	France	39	39	0
Total		230	219 (95%)	11 (5%)

TABLE 4. Tubo-ovarian abscesses: laparoscopic treatment — long-term follow-up

Abscess duration before laparoscopy	*N*	Clinical recovery (%)	Chronic pain (%)
< 3 weeks	38	34 (89)	4 (11)*
> 3 weeks	28	22 (78)	6 (22)*
Total	66	56 (85)	10 (15)

* $p < 0.05$.

month for 3 months. Serologic IgG levels for *C. trachomatis* IgG and IgA should be evaluated after 6 weeks and then 3 months. The persistence or recurrence of pelvic pain or abnormal ESR may lead to a reconsideration of the quality of recovery and a change in antibiotic treatment. Clinical evolution after laparoscopic treatment of tubo-ovarian abscess shows a quick and complete recovery in 90% of patients according to our experience[14] and that of others[15–20] (TABLE 3). Of our 80 patients, 66 had long-term follow-up; 56 (85%) of these had made a clinical recovery and 10 (15%) had chronic pain (TABLE 4). This chronic pain was observed in 11% of patients treated for recent abscess versus 22% of those treated for chronic abscess. The difference is significant ($p < 0.05$).

A second-look laparoscopy may be indicated after 3–6 months, especially in severe cases with adhesions or abscesses and particularly if later fertility is desired. The risk of infertility after treatment is 17%: 15% after one, 30% after two, and 60% after three or more.[21] During this second laparoscopy, cytologic and histologic samples should be taken from the peritoneal fluid and fimbriae to detect a residual, chronic evolving infection, particularly after PID due to *C. trachomatis*. Control laparoscopy[22,23] in women clinically cured shows ongoing infection in 20–30%. In the absence of signs of infection, an injection of methylene blue can be made via the uterus to evaluate tubal patency, and reparative surgery may be performed, in most cases via laparoscopy.

After laparoscopic treatment of recent abscesses, the aspect of pelvis is normal in most cases in our experience (TABLE 5); in contrast, after treatment of abscesses

TABLE 5. Tubo-ovarian abscesses: laparoscopic treatment — laparoscopic control

Abscess duration before laparoscopy	*N*	Normal pelvis (%)	Adhesions with tubal obstruction (%)
< 3 weeks	21	18 (85)	3 (15)*
> 3 weeks	16	1 (5)	15 (95)*
Total	37	19 (51)	18 (49)

* $p < 0.0001$.

TABLE 6. Tubo-ovarian abscesses: laparoscopic treatment — fertility after bilateral tubo-ovarian abscess

Abscess duration before laparoscopy	*N*	Pregnancy wanted	Pregnancy obtained
< 3 weeks	18	15	13*
> 3 weeks	12	6	1*
Total	30	21	14

* $p < 0.05$.

of long duration, adhesions usually remain.[17] Thirty-seven patients had second-look laparoscopy 3-6 months later (21 recent abscesses and 16 chronic). Of 21 patients with recent abscess, 18 (85%) had a completely normal pelvis, 1 had unilateral adhesions, and 2 had bilateral adhesions with tubal obstruction. The corresponding figures for 16 patients with chronic abscesses of long duration were 1 (15%), 5, and 10, respectively ($p < 0.0001$). The evolution and sequelae of recent abscesses and those of long duration differed significantly.

Ulterior fertility was evaluated (TABLE 6) in 21 patients who desired to be pregnant and were treated for bilateral abscesses (TABLE 6). Of them, 9 of 15 treated for recent abscesses and 0 of 6 treated for chronic abscess became pregnant without treatment. Four with recent and one with chronic abscess became pregnant after tuboplasty. In total, 13 of 15 with recent and 1 of 6 with chronic abscess became pregnant, with a significant difference ($p < 0.05$). The other patients underwent *in vitro* fertilization. No ectopic pregnancy was observed in this series. Raiga *et al.*[19] also published a series of 39 cases with long-term follow-up and laparoscopic control, and similar results were obtained with anatomic conservation and fertility. Rizk[20] compared medical treatment alone with operative laparoscopy in a randomized series and concluded that laparoscopy significantly improved the long-term outlook for fertility and pregnancy. Other investigators[24–28] recently published data on ultrasound-assisted treatment of tubo-ovarian abscess and obtained short-term similar results, but without second-look laparoscopy or ulterior fertility study. These treatments can be compared successfully with those in other series[29] using antibiotic and then surgical treatment, which results in mutilating surgery in 30–50% of cases.

Chronic salpingitis may develop as a consequence of inadequately treated AS. Primary CS may start without any clinical sign. Among patients operated on for tubal factor infertility, different works[30,31] have shown that although 70% had disease that was histologically of infectious origin, only 30% were treated for AS, 5–10%

had had complicated appendicitis or genital tuberculosis, 10% had undiagnosed subacute salpingitis as shown by a history of nontreated pelvic pain, and 30% had a prior unsuspected infection without any clinical sign; these patients had had "silent salpingitis." Infertility after AS, therefore, is only the "tip of the iceberg" of the infectious causes of tubal factor infertility. The ideal point would be to detect some biologic or clinical change that may lead to diagnosis: a positive anti-*Chlamydia trachomatis* (CT) serology or, in the near future, positive anti-CT Hsp 60 antibody[32] could be the key to the detection and treatment of silent salpingitis in young women, CT being the main microorganism involved with CS. Screening for *C. trachomatis* low genital tract infection is mandatory in young people in order to control the epidemic.[33,34]

REFERENCES

1. Henry-Suchet, J. 1988. Chlamydia trachomatis infection and infertility in women. J. Reprod. Med. **33:** 912–914.
2. Jacobson, L. & L. Westrom. 1969. Objectivized diagnosis of acute pelvic inflammatory disease. Am. J. Obstet. Gynecol. **105:** 1088–1098.
3. Jacobson, L. 1980. Differential diagnosis of acute pelvic inflammatory disease. Am. J. Obstet. Gynecol. **138:** 1006–1011.
4. Henry-Suchet, J. & M. Gayraud. 1977. Annexites non tuberculeuses. Valeur de la coelioscopie dans le diagnostic, le traitement et l'évaluation d'un pronostic tubaire. Infection et Fecondité. :1990–2130. Masson et cie. Paris.
5. Blum, F., D. Pathier, A. Treisser *et al.* 1979. Infections génitales hautes aigues. A propos de 100 cas. Etude clinique et apport de la coelioscopie. J. Gynecol. Obstet. Biol. Reprod. **8:** 711–721.
6. Paillault, C. 1979. Contribution à l'étude des salpingites aigues. Thèse Tours.
7. Wang, S.P., D.A. Eschenbach, K.K. Holmes *et al.* 1980. Chlamydia trachomatis infection in Fitz-Hugh-Curtis syndrome. Am. J. Obstet.Gynecol. **138:** 1034–1038.
8. Henry-Suchet, J., L. Tesquier & J. Berthet. 1992. Coelioscopies pour salpingites aigues et chroniques. Evolution de leur fréquence en France de 1979 a 1987 d'après une étude multicentrique. Contracept. Fertil. Sex. **20:** 357–362.
9. Henry-Suchet, J. 1986. Laparoscopic treatment of tubo-ovarian abscesses. J. Obstet. Gynecol. **6:** S60–S61.
10. Sweet, R.L. 1981. Diagnosis and treatment of pelvic inflammatory disease in the emergency room. Sex. Transm. Dis. **8:** 156–163.
11. Henry-Suchet, J., C. Revol, M. Askienazy-Elbhar *et al.* 1994. Post-therapeutic evolution of serum chlamydial antibody titers in women with acute salpingitis and tubal infertility. Fertil. Steril. **62:** 296–304.
12. Henry-Suchet, J. 1985. Laparoscopic diagnosis and treatment of PID. *In* Infections in Reproductive Health. Common Infections. L.G. Keith, Ed. **1:** 197–208. MTP Press. Boston.
13. Henry-Suchet, J., F. Catalan, V. Loffredo *et al.* 1981. *Chlamydia trachomatis* associated with chronic inflammation in abdominal specimens from women selected for tuboplasty. Fertil. Steril. **36:** 599–605.
14. Henry-Suchet, J., M. Dahan, W. Tannous & M. Askienazy-Elbhar. 1995. Salpingites aiguës non spécifiques. Conduite à tenir. Editions Techniques-Encycl. Méd. Chir. Paris, France **470:** 1–18.
15. Landers, D.V. & R.L. Sweet. 1985. Current trends in the diagnosis and treatment of tuboovarian abscess. Am. J. Obstet. Gynecol. **151:** 1098–1110.
16. Reich, H. & F. McGlynn. 1987. Laparoscopic treatment of tuboovarian and pelvic abscess. J. Reprod. Med. **32:** 747–752.
17. Adducci, J. 1981. Laparoscopy in the diagnosis and treatment of pelvic inflammatory disease with abscess formation. Int. Surg. **66:** 359–360.

18. FREISTADT, H. & T. ROGERS. 1991. Management of pelvic abscess by laparoscopically placed Jackson-Pratt drain. AAGL XX meeting, abstracts. Las Vegas.: 1994.
19. RAIGA, J., S. DENOIX, M. CANIS *et al.* 1995. Laparoscopic treatment of adnexal abscesses. A series of 39 patients. J. Gynecol. Obstet. Biol. Reprod. **24:** 381–385.
20. RIZK, P. 1995. Operative laparoscopy in the management of tubo-ovarian abscess. J. Am. Assoc. Gynecol. Laparos. **2:** 546.
21. WESTROM, L. 1980. Incidence, prevalence and trends of acute pelvic inflammatory disease and its consequences in industrialized countries. Am. J. Obstet. Gynecol. **138:** 880–891.
22. BOUDOURIS, O., F.X. PARIS, A. BEDRAN *et al.* 1987. Controle coelioscopique après traitement de salpingites aigues. A propos de 74 cas. Gynecologie **38:** 173–175.
23. POULY, J.L., G. MAGE, B. DUPRE *et al.* 1985. Coelioscopie de controle précoce après salpingite. J. Gynecol. Obstet. Biol. Reprod. **14:** 989–995.
24. CASOLA, G., E. VAN SONNENBERG, H.B. D'AGOSTINO *et al.* 1992. Percutaneous drainage of tubo-ovarian abscesses. Radiology **182:** 399–402.
25. SHULMAN, A., R. MAYMON, A. SHAPIRO & C. BAHARY. 1992. Percutaneous catheter drainage of tubo-ovarian abscesses. Obstet. Gynecol. **80:** 555–557.
26. HSU, Y.L., J.M. YANG & K.G. WANG. 1995. Transvaginal ultrasound-guided aspiration in the treatment and follow-up of tubo-ovarian abscess: a report of 2 cases. Chung Hua I Hsueh Tsa Chih **56:** 211–214.
27. CASPI, B., Y. ZALEL, Y. OR *et al.* 1996. Sonographically guided aspiration: an alternative therapy for tubo-ovarian abscess. Ultrasound Obstet. Gynaecol. **7:** 439–442.
28. PEREZ-MEDINA, T., M.A. HURTAS & J.M. BAJO. 1996. Early ultrasound-guided transvaginal drainage of tubo-ovarian abscesses: a randomized study. Ultrasound Obstet. Gynecol. **7:** 435–438.
29. GINSBURG, D.S., J.L. STERN, K.A. HAMOD *et al.* 1980. Tubo-ovarian abscess: a retrospective review. Am. J. Obstet. Gynecol. **138:** 1055–1058.
30. HENRY-SUCHET, J., A. RUDELLE, A. COCHINI & A. COLVEZ. 1986. Epidémiologie des causes des stérilités tubaires terminales. Facteurs de prévention. "Recherches récentes sur l'épidemiologie de la fertilité." :191–203. Masson Editeur. Paris.
31. ROSENFELD, D., S. SEIDMAN, R. BRONSON & M. SCHOLL. 1983. Unsuspected chronic pelvic inflammatory disease in the infertile female. Fertil. Steril. **39:** 44–48.
32. STAMM, W.A., R.W. PEELING, D. MONEY *et al.* 1994. Prevalence and correlates of antibody to Chlamydial HSP-60 in *C. trachomatis* infected women. Chlamydial infections. J. Orfila Edit. :614–617. Esculapio. Bologna, Italy.
33. HENRY-SUCHET, J., A. SLUZHINSKA & D. SERFATY. 1996. *Chlamydia trachomatis* screening in Family Planning Centres. A review of cost/benefit evaluations in different countries. Eur. J. Contracept. Reprod. Health Care **1:** 301–309.
34. GENC, M. & P.A. MARDH. 1996. Cost effectiveness analysis of screening and treatment for *C. trachomatis* infection in asymptomatic women. Ann. Intern. Med. **124:** 1–7.

Conservative Management of PID

KOSTIS GEORGILIS[a]

Department of Clinical Therapeutics, University of Athens School of Medicine, "Alexandra" Hospital, 80 Vas. Sofias Avenue, Athens 11528, Greece

ABSTRACT: The goals in the management of pelvic inflammatory disease (PID) are not only treatment of the infection and prevention of immediate complications, but also prevention of its long-term consequences. There are criteria for hospitalization, but patients who do not meet them can be safely treated as outpatients. A variety of sexually transmitted and other microorganisms can cause this infection, but the most important are *Chlamydia trachomatis* and *Neisseria gonorrhoeae*. Regimens with activity against gonococci, chlamydiae, streptococci, gram-negative bacteria, and anaerobes should be administered. Several such antimicrobial regimens have shown very good clinical and microbiologic efficacy. However, their efficacy in preventing long-term complications, such as infertility, has not been established. Close follow-up is an important part of management. Evaluation of male sexual partners is imperative to prevent reinfection. Better diagnostic techniques and treatment modalities for PID must be developed to prevent its long-term consequences.

INTRODUCTION

The most common infection of the female upper genital tract is acute salpingitis with or without concurrent endometritis. This very important condition is also known as pelvic inflammatory disease (PID) and causes both immediate as well as long-term morbidity for many women worldwide. It is imperative to understand that the goals in the management of PID are not only treatment of the infection and prevention of immediate complications. Equally important goals are prevention of the long-term consequences of the infection, such as infertility, recurrence, ectopic pregnancy, and chronic pelvic pain. A large Swedish long-term study has shown that patients with any number of episodes of acute salpingitis have a 21% rate of infertility compared to 3% in the control population.[1] These patients also have a sixfold increase in the incidence of ectopic pregnancy. Moreover, it was demonstrated that the rate of infertility rises in direct association to the number of episodes of salpingitis (TABLE 1). In another large prospective study, the increasing severity of PID was shown to correlate with the decreasing probability of achieving a live birth within 12 years.[2] Subsequent episodes have a greater impact on women with severe disease at the index episode of PID than on those with milder disease (TABLE 2).

[a]Address for correspondence: Dr. Kostis Georgilis, Department of Clinical Therapeutics, University of Athens School of Medicine, "Alexandra" Hospital, 80 Vas. Sofias Avenue, Athens 11528, Greece. Phone: 011-301-7252524, 011-301-7794841; fax: 011-301-7770473, 011-301-7219326.

athena@otenet.gr

TABLE 1. Effect of PID on the rate of infertility[a]

Number of episodes	Rate
Control population	3%
≥1	21%
1	11%
2	34%
≥3	54%

[a]Data from Reference 1.

TABLE 2. Effect of PID severity and of subsequent episodes of PID on the probability of a live birth in 12 years[a]

	Mild	Moderate	Severe
Overall			
	90%	82%	57%
Subsequent episodes			
No	91%	90%	60%
Yes	88%	63%	25%

[a]Data from Reference 2.

Most women with PID are treated as outpatients, but it is widely thought that hospitalization with parenteral treatment with high doses of antimicrobial agents is more beneficial than outpatient management with oral antibiotics. In fact, there have been few studies comparing inpatient and outpatient management in similar groups of patients.[3] According to published guidelines of the Centers for Disease Control and Prevention (CDC) of the United States, hospitalization is recommended (TABLE 3) when the diagnosis is uncertain, surgical emergencies such as appendicitis and ectopic pregnancy cannot be excluded, pelvic abscess is suspected, the patient is pregnant, the patient is an adolescent, severe illness or nausea and vomiting preclude outpatient management, the patient is unable to follow or tolerate an outpatient regimen, the patient has failed to respond to outpatient therapy, clinical follow-up within 72 hours of starting antibiotic treatment cannot be arranged, or the patient is HIV infected.[4]

Today we understand that most serious upper genital tract infections are probably caused by lower genital tract infection. Increasing evidence indicates that the organisms responsible for upper genital tract infections commonly originate in the lower genital tract. Several investigations have demonstrated an association between development of PID and preceding bacterial vaginosis.[5,6] A variety of sexually transmitted and other microorganisms can cause PID (TABLE 4). The most important are *Chlamydia trachomatis* and *Neisseria gonorrhoeae*, because more than half of the cases are caused by one or both of these sexually trasmitted microorganisms.[3] Women with endocervical infection with gonococci or chlamydiae have a significantly increased risk of PID. Other microorganisms have been implicated in PID, such as

TABLE 3. Recommendations for hospitalization in acute PID

1. Diagnosis is uncertain
2. Surgical emergencies are possible
3. Pelvic abscess is suspected
4. Patient is pregnant
5. Patient is an adolescent
6. Severe illness precludes outpatient management
7. Patient unable to follow or tolerate outpatient regimen
8. Patient has not responded to outpatient therapy
9. Clinical follow-up within 72 h cannot be arranged
10. Patient is HIV-infected

TABLE 4. Causative agents of PID

• *Chlamydia trachomatis*
• *Neisseria gonorrhoeae*
• *Escherichia coli*
• Other enteric gram-negative bacteria
• *Bacteroides* species
• *Peptostreptococcus* species
• *Prevotella* species
• Other anaerobic microorganisms
• *Mycoplasma hominis*
• *Ureaplasma urealyticum*

Escherichia coli and other enteric organisms as well as organisms recovered from lower genital tract cultures of women with bacterial vaginosis, such as *Bacteroides* species, anaerobic cocci, *Mycoplasma* species, and *Ureaplasma urealyticum*.[3,5] PID from these organisms apparently follows an alteration of the normal vaginal flora, which consists mostly of lactobacilli. Whether the patient is going to be hospitalized or not, endocervical specimens should be examined for *N. gonorrhoeae* and *C. trachomatis*. However, examination of vaginal or cervical material for anaerobes, mycoplasmata, or other microorganisms that can be recovered from the lower genital tract of normal women is not warranted.[3] Relevant studies in women with acute PID have shown a poor correlation between cultures of endocervical specimens and intraabdominal cultures (of peritoneal fluid or fallopian tube exudate) obtained through transvaginal culdocentesis or laparoscopy.

Because a variety of microorganisms can be involved in PID and a specific microbial diagnosis cannot be made before the initiation of antimicrobial therapy, treatment must be empiric and provide broad-spectrum coverage.[3,4] Monotherapy with penicillins or tetracycline or cephalosporins alone is insufficient, mostly because it fails to eliminate *C. trachomatis* and anaerobes. Therefore, regimens of drugs with activity against gonococci, chlamydiae, streptococci, facultative gram-negative bac-

TABLE 5. Regimens recommended by the CDC for the treatment of hospitalized women with PID

1. Cefoxitin 2 g i.v. q6h
   + doxycycline 100 mg i.v. or p.o. q12h

   or cefotetan 2 g i.v. q12h
   + doxycycline 100 mg i.v. or p.o. q12h

2. Clindamycin 900 mg i.v. q8h
   + gentamicin 2 mg/kg i.v. or i.m. (loading dose)
   and then 1.5 mg/kg i.v. or i.m. q8h

— Give for ≥ 48h after substantial clinical improvement
— Then give doxycycline 100 mg p.o. b.i.d. until day 14
   or clindamycin 450 mg p.o. q.i.d. until day 14

TABLE 6. Comparative efficacy of regimens recommended by the CDC for the treatment of hospitalized women with acute PID[a]

	Cefoxitin/doxycycline (n = 94)	Cefotetan/doxycycline (n = 94)	Clindamycin/gentamicin (n = 104)
Cure	75 (79.8%)	84 (89.4%)	87 (83.6%)
Improvement	14 (14.9%)	4 (4.2%)	11 (10.6%)
Failure	5 (5.3%)	6 (6.4%)	6 (5.8%)

[a]Data from Reference 8.

teria, and anaerobes should be administered.[3,4] Several such antimicrobial regimens have shown very good clinical and microbiologic efficacy, with pooled rates 75–94% and 71–100%, respectively.[7] The most recent recommendations of the U.S. Public Health Service for the treatment of women with acute PID consist of two regimens for hospitalized women and two regimens for outpatients.[4]

The two recommended regimens for hospitalized women with acute PID are shown in TABLE 5. The first regimen consists of doxycycline and either cefoxitin or cefotetan and the second consists of clindamycin and gentamicin. These regimens were compared in a six-center, prospective, open-label trial involving 344 women, of whom 292 were clinically evaluable.[8] There were no differences in the microbial isolates recovered in cultures from endometrial or endocervical specimens taken before therapy. The evaluated antibiotic combinations were found similarly effective, producing almost identical cure rates (TABLE 6). In addition, no clinically significant adverse effects were noted with any of the regimens.[8] A more recent study evaluating two CDC-recommended regimens and the conventional triple-drug combination of ampicillin/gentamicin/clindamycin has come to a similar conclusion.[9]

The two regimens currently recommended by the U.S. Public Health Service for outpatient treatment of women with acute PID[4] are shown in TABLE 7. The first regimen consists of ceftriaxone and doxycycline and the second consists of clindamycin

TABLE 7. Regimens recommended by the CDC for outpatient treatment of PID

1. Cefoxitin 2 g i.m. as a single dose
   + probenecid 1 g p.o. as a single dose
   + doxycycline 100 mg p.o. q12h for 14d

   or ceftriaxone 250 mg i.m. as a single dose
   + doxycycline 100 mg p.o. q12h for 14d

2. Ofloxacin 400 mg p.o. q12h for 14d
   + clindamycin 450 mg p.o. q6h for 14d

   or ofloxacin 400 mg p.o. q12h for 14d
   + metronidazole 500 mg p.o. q12h for 14d

TABLE 8. Comparative efficacy of two regimens recommended by the CDC for outpatient treatment of women with acute PID[a]

	Ceftriaxone/doxycycline ($n = 64$)	Clindamycin/ciprofloxacin ($n = 67$)
Cure	49 (76.6%)	57 (85.1%)
Improvement	12 (18.7%)	8 (11.9%)
Failure	3 (4.7%)	2 (3.0%)

[a]Data from Reference 10.

TABLE 9. Management of pelvic inflammatory disease

- Hospitalization (where needed)
- Treatment with antibiotics
- Close follow-up and reassessment
- Surgical intervention if needed
- Removal of intrauterine devices
- Evaluation and treatment of male sexual partners

and ofloxacin. In a recent multicenter prospective double-blind study the two regimens were compared in outpatients with mild-to-moderate PID diagnosed by laparoscopy.[10] In this study, which involved 138 women, of which 131 were evaluable, a clindamycin dosage of 600 mg t.i.d. was used instead of the recommended 450 mg q.i.d., and ciprofloxacin at 250 mg b.i.d. was used instead of the recommended ofloxacin. The two regimens were equally efficacious with a success rate of 95% for ceftriaxone/doxycycline and 97% for clindamycin/ciprofloxacin (TABLE 8). Also, the two regimens were similarly safe.[10]

Although all regimens just discussed have been associated with elimination of the major pathogens, gonococci and chlamydiae, and with a good clinical response in most cases, their efficacy in preventing long-term complications, such as infertility, has not been established. We need to investigate whether outcome will further improve with more aggressive treatment directed against microorganisms that are not susceptible to the currently recommended antibiotics. In addition, the issue of adjunctive medications, such as corticosteroids and other antiinflammatory agents, in reducing long-term complications is still unsettled.

The key points in the management of PID are outlined in TABLE 9. The statement "treatment with antibiotics" should be interpreted as "prompt initiation of antibiotics." It has been shown that delayed care of PID results in increased risk of infertility and ectopic pregnancy; this association is more prominent in chlamydial infections.[11] Before any type of treatment is initiated, a pregnancy test should be performed routinely to minimize the possibility of overlooking a tubal pregnancy. Close follow-up of patients is an important part of management. Patients should be reassessed 24–48 hours after treatment is begun. Substantial clinical improvement should be apparent within 3–5 days of initiation of therapy. The absence of improvement or the worsening of the condition should alert us to the possibility that the diagnosis of PID may not be correct. Laparoscopy or ultrasonography should also be considered, as well as hospitalization, if the patient was managed as an outpatient.

Conservative management will suffice in most cases. Surgical intervention to drain pelvic abscess is infrequently required. If intrauterine devices are present, they should be removed after initiation of antimicrobial treatment. Such devices should be avoided in women who have had any number of episodes of PID unless no other method of contraception can be applied.[3]

Evaluation of the male sexual partners of women with PID is imperative, because of the risk of reinfection. The men should be examined for all sexually transmitted infections. However, chlamydial and gonococcal infections in men may be asymptomatic, and tests for detection of these organisms are not very sensitive. Therefore, male sexual partners should be treated empirically with drugs against uncomplicated infections with *N. gonorrhoeae* and *C. trachomatis*, even if the etiology of the PID episode in the woman is thought to have been determined.[4]

The current rates of infertility and ectopic pregnancy result in part from an increased prevalence of PID.[12] Therefore, effective public health measures must be taken for the control of sexually transmitted diseases, which are the major cause of this infection. Prevention of infertility relies also on early diagnosis and prompt institution of appropriate antibiotic regimens. Therefore, better diagnostic techniques, including culture procedures, and treatment modalities for PID are needed to prevent its long-term consequences.

REFERENCES

1. WESTROM, L. 1980. Incidence, prevalence and trends of acute pelvic iflammatory disease and its consequences in industrialized countries. Am. J. Obstet. Gynecol. **138:** 880–892.
2. LEPINE, L.A., S.D. HILLIS, P.A. MARCHBANKS *et al.* 1998. Severity of pelvic inflammatory disease as a predictor of the probability of live birth. Am. J. Obstet. Gynecol. **178:** 977–981.
3. MCCORMACK, W.M. 1994. Pelvic inflammatory disease. N. Engl. J. Med. **330:** 115–119.
4. CDC. 1993. Pelvic inflammatory disease. MMWR **42:** 75–81.

5. Sweet, R.L. 1995. Role of bacterial vaginosis in pelvic inflammatory disease. Clin. Infect. Dis. **20**(Suppl. 2)**:** S271–S275.
6. Peipert, J.F., A.B. Montagno, A.S. Cooper & C.J. Sung. 1997. Bacterial vaginosis as a risk factor for upper genital tract infection. Am. J. Obstet. Gynecol. **177:** 1184–1187.
7. Walker, C.K., J.G. Kahn, A.E. Washington *et al.* 1993. Pelvic inflammatory disease: metaanalysis of antimicrobial regimen efficacy. J. Infect. Dis. **168:** 969–978.
8. Hemsell, D.L., B.B. Little, S. Faro *et al.* 1994. Comparison of three regimens recommended by the Centers for Disease Control and Prevention for the treatment of women hospitalized with acute pelvic inflammatory disease. Clin. Infect. Dis. **19:** 720–727.
9. McNeely, S.G., S.L. Hendrix, M.M. Mazzoni *et al.* 1998. Medically sound, cost-effective treatment for pelvic inflammatory disease and tuboovarian abscess. Am. J. Obstet. Gynecol. **178:** 1272–1278.
10. Arredondo, J.L., V. Diaz, H. Gaitan *et al.* 1997. Oral clindamycin and ciprofloxacin versus intramuscular ceftriaxone and oral doxycycline in the treatment of mild-to-moderate pelvic inflammatory disease in outpatients. Clin. Infect. Dis. **24:** 170–178.
11. Hillis, S.D., R. Joesoef, P.A. Marchbanks *et al.* 1993. Delayed care of pelvic inflammatory disease as a risk factor for impaired fertility. Am. J. Obstet. Gynecol. **168:** 1503–1509.
12. Jossens, M.O.R., J. Schachter & R.L. Sweet. 1994. Risk factors associated with pelvic inflammatory disease of differing microbial etiologies. Obstet. Gynecol. **83:** 989–997.

Surface Morphology of the Human Endometrium

Basic and Clinical Aspects

GEORGE NIKAS,[a,e] ANTONIS MAKRIGIANNAKIS,[b,d] OUTI HOVATTA,[a] AND HOWARD W. JONES, JR.[c]

[a]*Division of Obstetrics & Gynaecology, Huddinge Hospital, Karolinska Institute, Stockholm S-18164, Sweden*

[b]*Department of Obstetrics & Gynecology, University of Pennsylvania Medical Center, Philadelphia, Pennsylvania, USA*

[c]*The Howard and Georgeanna Jones Institute for Reproductive Medicine, Norfolk, Virginia 23507-1912, USA*

ABSTRACT: The human endometrium is an extremely sensitive target for steroid hormones. During the menstrual cycle, this tissue undergoes dynamic changes that are reflected on the surface morphology of the epithelium and that can be followed by scanning electron microscopy. The morphologic changes peak at the midsecretory phase, with the formation of the so-called pinopodes. Increasing evidence suggests that these pinopodes are accurate markers for endometrial receptivity, and their detection may be of high clinical utility in the preparation of endometrium before embryo transfer. This article recapitulates published figures of endometrial ultrastructure and presents some unpublished data from ongoing studies.

INTRODUCTION

The onset of human conception occurs when a blastocyte about 1 week old attaches to and begins to penetrate the endometrium. This is followed shortly by the appearance of hCG in serum, and it signals a moment of immense joy for thousands of infertile couples undergoing *in vitro* fertilization (IVF). Regrettably, a much greater number of patients undergoing embryo transfer will fail to experience this feeling.[1] To explain the high incidence of implantation failure, attention has been focused on the quality of the embryo. Nevertheless, the probability of a positive pregnancy test remains inexplicably low, even after the transfer of expanded blastocysts.[2] In addition, implantation can occur in the absence of a viable conceptus, giving rise to an unembryonic pregnancy (blighted ovum).

Clearly, it is not the embryo quality alone that determines the success of implantation. In animals such as mice or rats, with an invasive type of placentation, implan-

[d]Current address: Division of Obstetrics & Gynaecology, ICSM, Hammersmith Hospital, London W12 ONN, UK

[e]Address for correspondence: Division of Obstetrics & Gynaecology, Huddinge Hospital, Karolinska Institute, S-14186, Sweden. Fax: +46858587575.
yorgos.nikas@klinvet.ki.se

tation only starts when the endometrium, after appropriate hormonal preparation, has reached a phase of receptivity for blastocyst implantation. This phase is short and needs to coincide with zygote development to the blastocyst stage. Accordingly, this phase defines a bifactorial, transient period when implantation can commence, called implantation or nidation window.[3] Theoretically, such regulation could ensure that the complex mechanisms that control trophoblast invasion and protect the maternal tissues may already be on guard if receptivity is achieved. Given the highly invasive type of human implantation, the existence of a short and precisely regulated receptive phase is likely. Consequently, insufficiently or untimely developed receptivity could lead to implantation failure in assisted reproduction.

Experimentally tested traits of a receptive endometrium are lacking in the human, and therefore any assumption on this topic remains speculative. However, there are a number of candidate markers whose relevance to implantation is supported by animal studies and by the their pattern of expression in humans. One such marker is the change in morphology of the apical plasma membrane of the endometrial epithelial cells as seen in scanning electron microscopy (SEM). In these cells, the microvilli (mv) transform to large and smooth projections, protruding towards the uterine cavity. In rodents, these projections perform pinocytosis,[4] hence the name "pinopodes." Pinopodes are progesterone-dependent structures detectable only at the time of blastocyst attachment.[5,6] Consistent with this fact, they follow displacement of receptivity by the administration of antiprogestin,[7] whereas high doses of estrogen inhibit both pinopode formation and implantation.[8] Similar projections were found in the midsecretory phase human endometrium.[9,10]

SURFACE MORPHOLOGY OF THE HUMAN ENDOMETRIUM

We have used SEM to study the temporal changes of cell surface morphology in the human endometrium throughout the menstrual cycle. We examined consecutive biopsies taken at 48-hour intervals from normal, controlled ovarian hyperstimulation (COH) and hormone-controlled (HC) cycles.[11–13] The subjects participating in these studies were enrolled in egg donation programs and volunteered to give two to four biopsies. According to our findings, all cycles show a similar pattern in the evolution of surface morphology, as follows: During the proliferative phase, the cells vary greatly in size, and their shapes are either elongated or polygonal. Bulging is minimal, the intercellular clefts are barely marked, and the mv are short and slender. There were no differences between mid- and late proliferative phases. By contrast, during the early and mid-secretory phase the morphologic changes are distinct and may allow dating of the tissue in a 24–48-hour interval. Taking an ideal 28-day cycle as reference, an increase in mv density and length is noticed on days 15 and 16, and the cells begin to bulge, mainly at the central part of their surface. Smooth apical projections, usually smaller than pinopodes, are occasionally seen in small groups in the endometrial folds. On day 17, bulging increases involving the entire cell apex and the microvilli reach their maximum development, being long, thick, and upright. On day 18, the mv start to diminish in size and their tips may appear swollen. On day 19, there is pronounced and generalized cell bulging. The mv decrease further in number and length by fusing together or disappear. Smooth and slender membrane

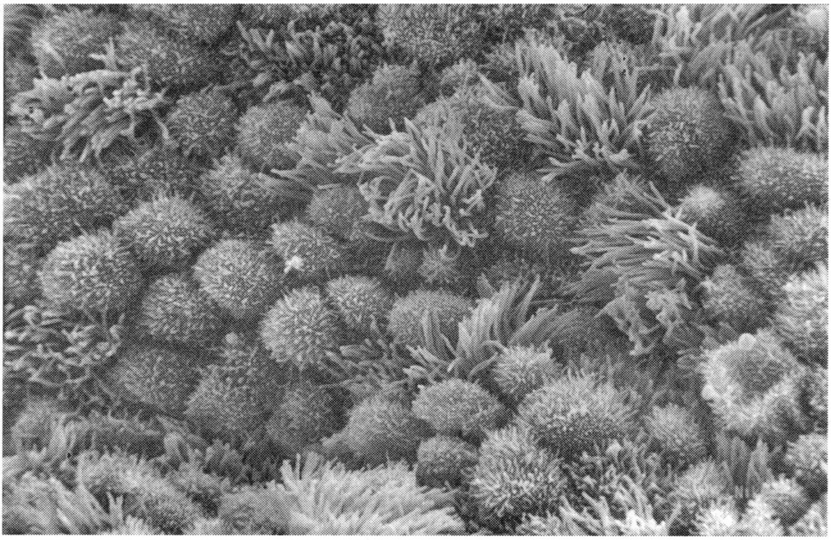

FIGURE 1. SEM micrograph of endometrial epithelium on day LH +5 of a natural cycle. The secretory cells are bulging and covered with short and slender microvilli which in some cells appear fusiform. Ciliated cells are also seen.

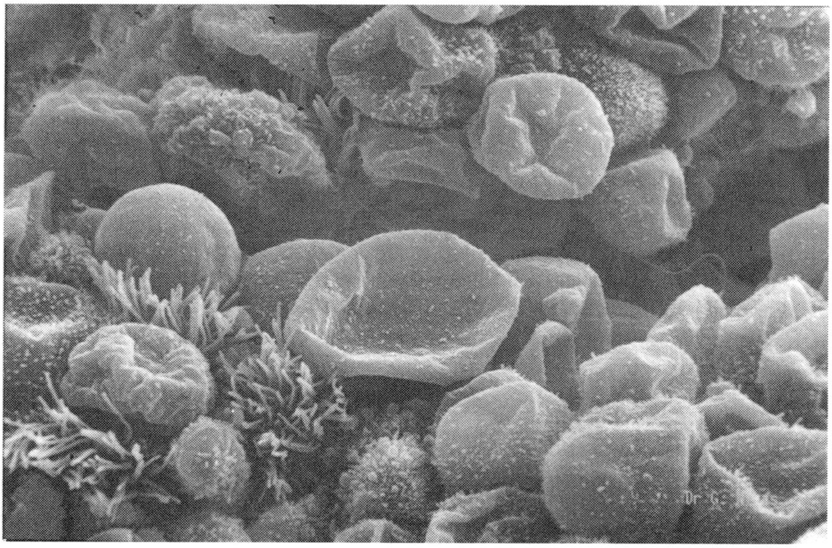

FIGURE 2. SEM micrograph of endometrial epithelium on day LH +7 from the same patient as in FIGURE. 1. Most secretory cells bear fully developed pinopodes, almost covering some of the ciliated cells.

projections begin to form, arising from the entire cell apex (developing pinopodes). By day 20, the mv are virtually absent and now the membranes protrude and fold maximally (fully developed pinopodes). Fully developed pinopodes assume many shapes, resembling mushrooms or flowers. On day 21, bulging decreases and small tips of mv reappear on the membranes, which are now wrinkled, and the cell size starts to increase (regressing pinopodes). By day 22, the pinopodes have virtually disappeared and the mv have became more numerous. Day 23 is characterized by a further increase in the size of cells which by day 24 begin to appear dome-shaped and covered with short, stubby mv (FIGS. 1 and 2).

This sequence of changes consistently appeared in all type of cycles, and fully developed pinopodes were always confined to one biopsy, indicating a short lifespan of less than 48 hours. However, the actual cycle days when pinopodes formed were variable, depending on both the hormonal treatment applied and the patient's individual response.[14] In natural cycles, fully developed pinopodes formed on day 19, 20, or 21, peaking in most patients on day 20 (day of luteinizing hormone surge designates day 13). In HC cycles, they formed on day 20, 21, or 22, peaking in most cases on day 21 (day of progesterone start designates day 15). In COH cycles, more variations and pinopodes formed from day 18 to day 22, peaking in most cases on day 19 (day of oocyte pickup designates day 14). These data are summarized in FIGURE 3. In addition to the interindividual variations in the timing of pinopode formation, the number of pinopodes also varied between patients, some showing plentiful and others only sparse pinopodes. More interestingly, the number of pinopodes correlated strongly with implantation success after embryo transfer in a subsequent cycle.[15,16]

These data argue positively for the relevance of pinopodes in implantation and also for the similarity of menstrual cycles in the same individual. We have some di-

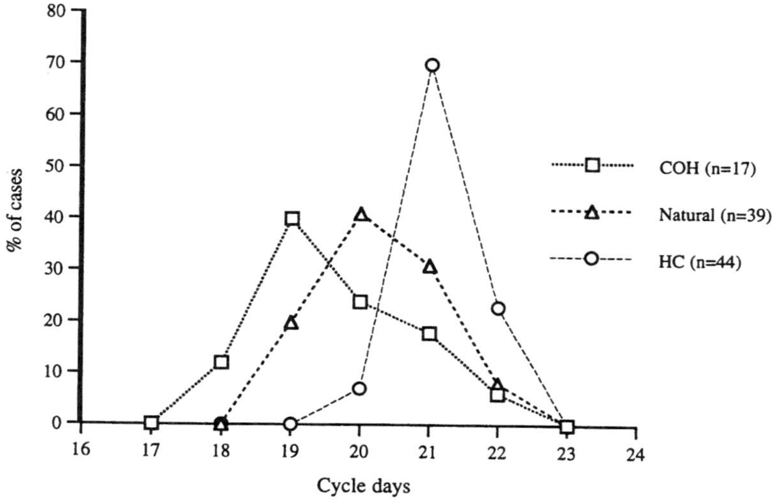

FIGURE 3. Differential expression of pinopodes in COH natural and HC cycles. For details see text.

rect evidence for that as well, deriving from observations on two repeated cycles studied in the same individuals (n = 5) under the same hormone regimen. Not surprisingly, the surface endometrial morphology during the second cycle was similar to the first cycle (Nikas *et al.*, unpublished data). In a larger series of egg donors (n = 14) with a history of repeated implantation failure and low pinopode number, a second HC cycle under an increased estrogen and progesterone dosage was studied. More pinopodes were present in the second cycle, and a delay in the timing of their formation by at least 1 day was noted (Nikas *et al.*, unpublished data). Many of these patients became pregnant after embryo transfer during the high dosage HC cycle. Pinopodes were plentiful in most COH cycles studied,[12] providing additional evidence that high hormone levels do not necessarily inhibit pinopode formation. The reported detrimental effect of high estrogen levels on implantation in IVF[17] may therefore be due to other reasons, such as a likely increase in uterine contractility with subsequent expulsion of embryos from the uterine cavity.[18] Another finding in our studies of IVF cycles was a shift in the timing of pinopode formation.[12] We hypothesize that this may reflect a shift in the window of receptivity, which in turn may affect implantation rates. In natural cycles, we may assume an inherent synchrony between the maturing uterus and the developing embryo, ensuring that both will meet at the right stage. In IVF cycles, embryonic development is probably delayed because of the *in vitro* condition,[19] whereas the uterus may be advanced, resulting in early closure of the nidation window before the zygote eventually reaches a stage capable of initiating implantation.

We attempted to correlate surface ultrastructure with other parameters of endometrial function. In all types of menstrual cycle studied, no correlation was found between pinopode numbers and/or the timing of their formation with serum hormone levels at the time of biopsy. A premature (day 13) increase in serum progesterone in COH cycles above a cut-off value of 6 ng/ml, however, correlated strongly with accelerated pinopode formation. This correlated very significantly with the concomitant disappearance of epithelial progesterone receptors from both the glandular and the surface epithelia.[20] In the same biopsies, conventional histologic study of hematoxylin and eosin stained sections showed that if the endometrial surface is carefully examined, the pinopodes are visible as smooth protrusions of the cell apices.[21] It is not possible to judge pinopode abundance or stage of development; nevertheless, this observation can provide a rough idea of the presence or absence of pinopodes on routine histologic examination.

Another interesting morphologic feature that occurs in the secretory phase endometrium is apoptotic cell death. Extensive apoptosis was observed at the implantation sites of rat and mouse endometrial epithelium.[22] The expression of associated genes, such as the bcl-2 family, are regulated by sex steroids. In the human, antiprogestin administration inhibits the progesterone downregulation of steroid receptors in endometrial glands, resulting in persistent proliferation and bcl-2 secretion, which blocks the apoptotic pathway and promotes cell survival.[23] Coincident with the onset of apoptosis, the bcl-2 homologous antagonist/killer (BAK) protein localizes at the glandular epithelial cells.[24] Apoptosis was studied mainly at the late secretory phase in connection with the onset of menstrual shedding. However, recent evidence suggests that regulated apoptosis may be important during the window of receptivity: On days 19–20, apoptosis is detectable in the glands of the basalis, sub-

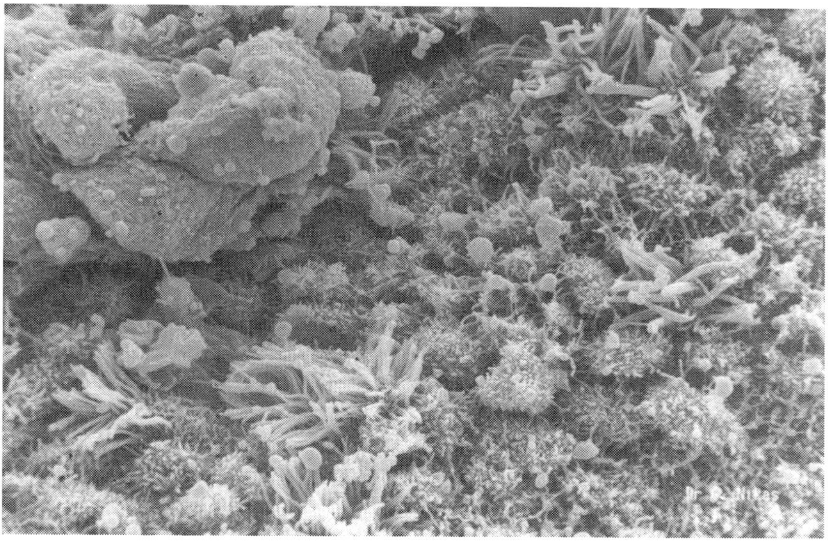

FIGURE 4. SEM micrograph of endometrial epithelium on day 18 of a natural cycle. A cluster of detaching, apoptotic cells is seen (*top left*). Their plasma membranes appear degenerated, bearing no cilia or microvilli, but many blebs.

sequently extending to the functionalis.[25]. According to our SEM observations (unpublished), apoptotic cells, sometimes forming rows, are not uncommon in midsecretory biopsies. These cells are discernible by the loss of apical mv, formation of blebs, and partial cell detachment (FIG. 4). The significance of this finding in relation to the opening of the implantation window is under investigation. SEM is very suitable in the detection and quantification of apoptosis on the endometrial surface.

Our direct aim is to evaluate the clinical utility of the detection of pinopodes in biopsies as a method to assess endometrial receptivity before an embryo transfer. This could help in optimizing the endometrial preparation and the timing of embryo transfer for better embryo-endometrial synchronization. Optimization is possible in embryo recipients awaiting transfer of donor or frozen embryos, for in these cases the endometrium and/or the embryonic age can be manipulated. A multicentric study is currently being carried out as follows[26]: The recipients go through an assessment natural or HC cycle. Two endometrial samples are taken on cycle days 20 and 22 and examined by SEM. A diagnosis is made on the basis of the following parameters: (1) number of pinopode present, scored in three grades: I for abundant, II for moderate, and III for few or absent, depending on the percentage of the endometrial surface occupied by pinopodes (>50%, 20–50%, and <20%, respectively). (2) stage of pinopode development: developing, fully developed, and regressing. The most receptive day of the cycle corresponds to "fully developed" pinopodes or is postulated to be one day before "regressing" or one day after "developing" pinopodes are observed. A transfer cycle follows when synchronization with the donor is arranged, so that the predicted most receptive day coincides with embryonic age day 6. We assume by that

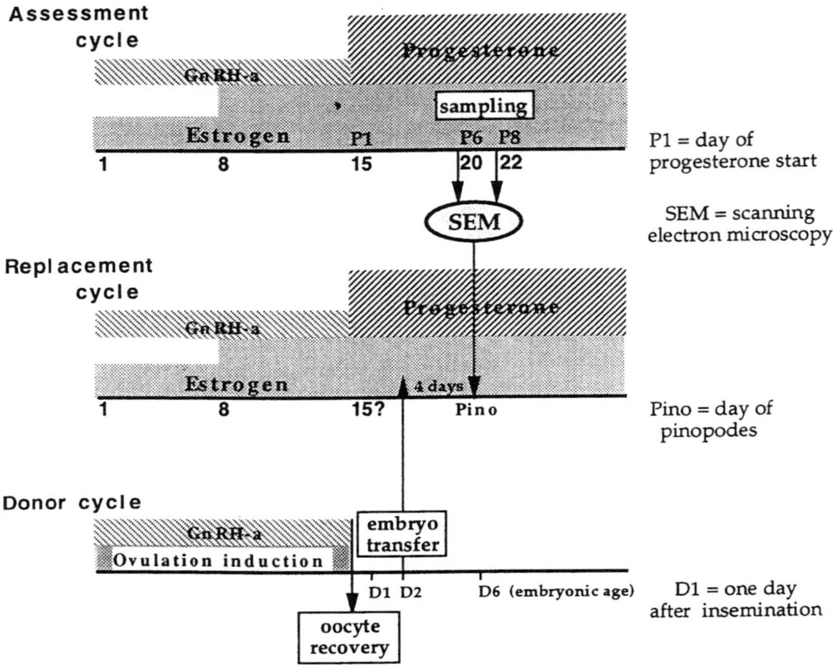

FIGURE 5. Assessment of uterine receptivity and timing of embryo transfer in HRT cycles, using the detection of pinopodes in endometrial samples. For details see text.

time the IVF embryo is ready to implant (FIG. 5). Preliminary results of these studies support the use of SEM in monitoring endometrial maturation and timing embryo transfer on an individual basis.

CONCLUSIONS

Examination of endometrial morphology in SEM can give valuable information on the hormone status and features associated with uterine receptivity. Given the clinical significance of the latter during assisted reproduction, SEM appears to be a precious tool for assessing and optimizing the end tissue response in order to improve the chances of getting pregnant in assisted reproduction.

REFERENCES

1. EDWARDS, R.G. 1985. Causes of early embryonic loss in human pregnancy. Hum. Reprod. **1:** 185–198.
2. TSIRIGOTIS, M. 1998. Blastocyst stage transfers: pitfalls and benefits. Hum. Reprod. **13:** 3285–3295.

3. PSYCHOYOS, A. 1986. Uterine receptivity for nidation. Ann. N.Y. Acad. Sci. **476:** 36–42.
4. ENDERS, A.D. & D.M. NELSON. 1973. Pinocytotic activity of the uterus of the rat. Am. J. Anat. **138:** 277–300.
5. PSYCHOYOS, A. & P. MANDON. 1971. Scanning electron microscopy of the surface of the rat uterine epithelium during delayed implantation. J. Reprod. Fertil. **26:** 137–138.
6. PSYCHOYOS, A. & P. MANDON. 1971. Etude de la surface de l'épithélium utérin au microscope électronique à balayage. Observation chez la ratte au 4ème et 5ème jours de la gestation. C. R. Acad. Sci. Paris **272:** 2723–2729.
7. SARANTIS L., D. ROCHE & A. PSYCHOYOS. 1988. Displacement of receptivity for nidation in the rat by the progesterone antagonist RU 486: a scanning electron microscopy study. Hum. Reprod. **3:** 251–255.
8. MARTEL, D., M.N. MONIER, D. ROCHE & A. PSYCHOYOS. 1991. Hormonal dependence of pinopode formation at the uterine luminal surface. Hum. Reprod. **6:** 597–603.
9. NILSSON, O. 1962. Correlation of structure to function of the luminal cell surface in the uterine epithelium of mouse and man. Z. Zellforsch. Microsk. Anat. **56:** 803–808.
10. MARTEL, D., C. MALET, J.P. GAUTRAY & A. PSYCHOYOS. 1981. Surface changes of the luminal uterine epithelium during the human menstrual cycle: a scanning electron microscopic study. *In* The Endometrium: Hormonal Impacts.: 15-29. Plenum Press. New York.
11. NIKAS, G., P. DRAKAKIS, D. LOUTRADIS *et al.* 1995. Uterine pinopodes as markers of the "nidation window" in cycling women receiving exogenous oestradiol and progesterone. Hum. Reprod. **10:** 1208–1213.
12. NIKAS, G., O.H. DEVELIOGLU, J.P. TONER & H.W. JONES, JR. 1998. Endometrial pinopodes indicate a shift in the window of receptivity in IVF cycles. Hum. Reprod. **14:** 787–792.
13. NIKAS, G. 1999. Cell-surface morphological events relevant to human implantation. Hum. Reprod. **14** (Suppl.)**:** 37–44.
14. NIKAS, G. 1999. Pinopodes as markers of endometrial receptivity in clinical practice. Hum. Reprod. **14** (Suppl.)**:** 99–106.
15. NIKAS, G., N. REDDY & R.M.L. WINSTON. 1996. Implantation correlates highly with the expression of uterine pinopodes in ovum recipients under HRT: a preliminary study. Abstr. (FR21) at the IX World Congress in Human Reproduction. May 29–June 1, 1996. Philadelphia, PA.
16. REDDY, N., T.A. RYDER, M.A. MOBBERLEY *et al.* 1997. Positive correlation of pregnancy with the presence of endometrialpinopodes in oocyte recipients: a preliminary study. (Abstr.) Hum. Reprod. **12**(Suppl.)**:** 0–070.
17. SIMON, C., F. CANO, D. VALBUENA *et al.* 1995. Clinical evidence for a detrimental effect on uterine receptivity of high serum oestradiol concentrations in high and normal responder patients. Hum. Reprod. **10:** 2432–2437.
18. FANCHIN, R., C. RIGHINI, F. OLIVENNES *et al.* 1998. Uterine contractions as visualized by ultrasound alter pregnancy rates in IVF and embryo transfer. Hum. Reprod. **13:** 1968–1974.
19. LOPATA, A. 1996. Implantation of the human embryo. Hum. Reprod. **11**(Suppl. 1)**:** 175–184.
20. DEVELIOGLU, O.H., J.G. HSIU, G. NIKAS *et al.* 1999. Endometrial estrogen and progesterone receptor and pinopodeexpression in stimulated cycles in oocyte donation. Fertil. Steril. **71:** 1040–1047.
21. DEVELIOGLU, O.H., G. NIKAS, J.G. HSIU *et al.* 2000. Assessment of endometrial pinopodes by light microscopy. Fertil. Steril. In press.
22. PARR, E.L., H.N. TUNG & M.B. PARR. 1987. Apoptosis as the more of uterine epithelial cell death during embryo implantation in mice and rats. Biol. Reprod. **36:** 211–225.
23. CHRITCHLEY, H.O., S. TONG, S.T. CAMERON *et al.* 1999. Regulation of bcl-2 gene family members in human endometrium by antiprogestin administration *in vivo*. J. Reprod. Fertil. **115:** 389–395.
24. TAO, X.L., R.A. SAYERGH, J.L. TILLY & K.B. ISAACSON. 1998. Elevated expression of the proapoptotic BCL-2 family member, BAK, in the human endometrium coincident with apoptosis during the secretory phase of the cycle. Fertil. Sreril. **70:** 338–343.

25. VON RANGO, U., I. CLASSEN-LINKE, C.A. KRUSCHE & H.M. BEIER. 1998. The receptive endometrium is characterized by apoptosis in the glands. Hum. Reprod. **13:** 3177–3189.
26. NIKAS, G., J. GARCIA-VELASCO, A. PELLICER & C. SIMON. 1997. Assessment of uterine receptivity and timing of embryo transfer using the detection of pinopodes (Abstr.). Hum. Reprod. **12**(Suppl.)**:** 0–069.

Biological Factors in Culture Media Affecting *in Vitro* Fertilization, Preimplantation Embryo Development, and Implantation

D. LOUTRADIS,[a,b] P. DRAKAKIS,[b] K. KALLIANIDIS,[b] N. SOFIKITIS,[c] G. KALLIPOLITIS,[b] S. MILINGOS,[b] N. MAKRIS,[b] AND S. MICHALAS[b]

[b]*IVF Unit, Alexandra Maternity Hospital, 1st Dept of Obstetrics/Gynecology, Athens University Medical School, Athens, Greece*

[c]*Reproductive Physiology and IVF Center, Department of Urology, Tattori University School of Medicine, Yonago 683, Japan*

ABSTRACT: Optimal culture conditions are of paramount importance for *in vitro* fertilization of gametes, preimplantation embryo development, and implantation for all species. Water is the basis of all culture media, and ultrapure water should be employed. The main energy sources of a medium are lactate, pyruvate, and glucose. The concentrations of the first two vary in different media, whereas the latter is necessary mainly for the later stages (morula to blastocyst) of development. A fixed nitrogen source is essential for implantation embryo development whether this is provided by amino acids, albumin, or serum. Suboptimal culture conditions can block development. Pronuclear zygotes of most species (but not human) arrest at some point between the two-cell and the 16-cell stage. Modifying culture conditions can lead the embryos to develop through this block. Hypoxanthine also causes a two-cell block to mouse pronuclear zygotes, and this again depends largely on culture conditions. Simple culture media are bicarbonate-buffered systems with pyruvate, lactate, and glucose. Complex media, such as Ham's F-10, contain in addition amino acids and other elements found in serum. Human tubal fluid simulates the fallopian tube microenvironment. EDTA, gonadotropins, growth factors, and other substances can be included in the media to stimulate development. Coculture of embryos with oviductal cells has shown promising results.

INTRODUCTION

Optimal culture conditions for human embryos that are universally accepted and employed have not yet been established, as is demonstrated by the variety of media and protein supplementation methods used for human programs around the world. A lot of research has been done on mouse embryo development *in vitro* (as well as in rabbits), and this system has been employed to investigate the effect of a wide variety of *in vitro* culture situations.

The first demonstration of *in vitro* development of fertilized mouse ova took place in Germany in 1941. The embryo was cultured on a blood clot with an extract of oviduct tissue.[1] In 1949, Hammond used a medium composed mainly of serum or egg

[a]Address for correspondence: Prof. D. Loutradis, 62, Sirinon Street, 17561 P. Faliro, Athens, Greece. Phone: +301-9833576; fax: +301-7786537.

white.[2] Subsequent attempts for *in vitro* culturing of mouse embryos showed that eight-cell embryos could develop into blastocysts under a variety of conditions *in vitro*, even in a serum-free medium consisting mainly of Krebs-Ringer bicarbonate[3]; whereas two-cell embryos did not develop beyond the two- or four-cell stage in the defined buffered-salts culture media.[2,4,5] A major breakthrough was the addition of lactate in the serum-free medium, which allowed two-cell embryos to develop to the blastocyst stage.[6] Still, development of zygotes to blastocysts could be achieved only for a few inbred strains of mice, whereas the majority arrested at the two-cell stage.[7–9] Since the first reports on *in vitro* development of mouse zygotes or two-cell embryos, extensive research has been undertaken in order to improve the culture media used by modifying standard components, the energy or nitrogen sources, or by supplementing them with other substances that are believed to improve blastocyst development. The criterion of "percent blastocyst formation" from mouse zygotes or two-cell embryos is used routinely in many laboratories for testing the quality of the media prepared for human IVF programs. Data on the effect of variations of different parameters or components of such media on blastocyst development can provide valuable information on improved rates of development and implantation for human embryos. Moreover, using such a system, one can investigate the mechanisms that control early embryo development and reveal the delicate pathways involved.

WATER AND PHYSICAL PROPERTIES OF CULTURE MEDIA

Water is the major constituent of all culture media. It is an excellent solvent, gathering contaminants from everything it comes in contact with, and it is able to support microbial growth easily. There are five basic groups of contaminants found in water: Dissolved ionized and nonionized solids and gases, particulate matter, microbials, and pyrogens. The use of ultrapure water, free from contaminants, is imperative for the development of good quality embryos of all species. The importance of using appropriate water was shown by Fukuda, who used five different water preparations of BWW culture medium[8] for *in vitro* fertilization and development of mouse ova. Fertilization rate ranged from 4.8% to 68.0%, blastocyst development from 20.9% to 69.4%, and percentage of hatched blastocysts from 4.7% to 51.0%.[10] The earlier the stage at which mouse embryos were started in culture, the more evident was the influence of water quality on development, particularly on the hatching process.

The basic methods for purifying water are distillation, deionization, filtration, reverse osmosis, adsorption, and ultrafiltration. By means of distillation, a broad range of impurities is removed. Deionization removes ions and minerals from water with synthetic resins, which have an affinity for dissolved, ionized salts. Filtration by a screen or membrane filter accomplishes absolute removal of all bacteria with the use of 0.2-μm filters, because the smallest known bacterium is about 0.3 μm. Reverse osmosis removes a high percentage of contaminants and is used as a pretreatment method. By means of adsorption, organic impurities and chlorine are removed. Finally, ultrafiltration is a recently developed post-treatment of purified water, which effectively removes pyrogens by the use of an internal membrane with a pore size of 0.05 μm.[11]

The most reliable physical parameter of water quality for successful oocyte fertilization and development *in vitro* seems to be the electrical conductivity of water, which should be as close to 0.06 μsec/cm as possible[10] or its reciprocal, resistivity, with a value of 18.3 Megohm-cm.

Another important factor for embryo culture is the pH of the medium. During oocyte retrieval, examination, and manipulation under the microscope and embryo transfer, human oocytes and embryos are subjected to broad pH changes of the bicarbonate-buffered systems as a response to changes in CO_2 environments. John and Kiessling have shown that suboptimal high pH levels, caused mainly by exposure to atmospheric air (0.03% CO_2) during observation and manipulation of the embryos, can affect later events in mouse embryo development, such as compaction of the morula and blastocele formation. They found that mouse embryo development was not affected over a pH range of 7.17 (8.4% CO_2) to 7.37 (5.3% CO_2) if serum was not included in the medium, whereas addition of the latter (resulting to embryo stress) caused impaired embryo development at the lower (7.17–7.27) and higher (around 7.50) pH values.[12] A pH range from 7.30 to 7.45 is used for the culturing of human and other embryos in most laboratories. Osmolarity, which has been shown to affect embryo development *in vitro,*[13] is generally arranged to be between 275 and 285 mOsm, which is considered the optimum range.[13,14]

ENERGY SOURCES

The best combination of energy sources for culturing two-cell and, especially, pronuclear stage embryos has been the object of extensive research. As far back as 1965, Brinster had shown that, although glucose, fructose, and other hexoses, as well as acetate, citrate, and most intermediates of the tricarboxylic acid (TCA) cycle could not support development of two-cell mouse ova if employed alone in the culture medium, other compounds, such as pyruvate, lactate, oxaloacetate, or phosphoenolpyruvate did allow development of two-cell ova into blastocysts when used as the sole energy source.[15]

The interaction between various energy sources in a culture medium is complex and, in many cases, not well understood. Lactate and pyruvate are two compounds that are of fundamental importance for the development of preimplantation embryos and the addition of lactate to culture media was a major step.[6] Lactate is reversibly converted to pyruvate by lactate dehydrogenase. The optimum concentration of each compound when they are present together in the medium is different from their optimum concentration when employed alone, and Brinster found optimum concentrations of 0.25 mM pyruvate and 30 mM lactate.[16] Pyruvate's concentration is similar to that found in blood (0.1 mM), whereas that of lactate is ten times more.[17] The provision of both substrates, with lactate being 100 times higher in concentration, most probably produces redox equilibrium favorable to development considering the high lactate dehydrogenase levels in the mouse embryo.[16,18–20]

Pronuclear stage embryos are more sensitive to energy sources of culture conditions. Lactate alone cannot support the first cleavage division,[21] whereas by lowering its concentration the zygotes of some random-bred mice can go through this division, although their later development is impaired.[22] A deleterious effect of high lactate concentration on early embryonic development has been reported.[23] Pyruvate alone or pyruvate with lactate can support preimplantation development of mouse embryos until the morula stage, but they cannot support the transition to blastocysts without the addition of glucose.[20] Glucose, on the other hand, which has traditionally been used as a third energy (carbon) source,[8,24] seems to be necessary to rescue embryos from this "morula stage block"; but it doesn't seem to play any role in supporting embryo development before the four-cell stage, and it may be detrimental if present during the initial stages.[25,26] The inhibitory effect of glucose has been attributed to the generation of the "Crabtree effect,"[27] that is, stimulation of glycolysis, which competes with mitochondrial respiration for phosphate, thus reducing energy generation. It may also be due, though, to repression by glucose of specific metabolic genes transcribed in response to changes in the availability of different carbon sources.[22]

Metabolism of early cleavage states seems to be closely related to that in the oviduct. High concentrations of lactate were found in rabbit oviductal fluid, and this concentration increased during the first three days of ovulation.[28] It has also been found that the mucosa of the human oviduct converts, under aerobic conditions, over 60% of the glucose in the medium into lactic acid.[29]

Other substrates have been shown to be beneficial if employed in the culture medium during the early stages of development; for example, glutamine was shown to be preferred to glucose as an energy substrate for these early stages, rescuing pronuclear stage zygotes of certain mouse strains from developmental block at the two-cell stage.[30]

NITROGEN SOURCES

The protein requirements of preimplantation embryos have been investigated for several years. A fixed nitrogen source has been found to be essential for the development of two-cell embryos into blastocysts since 1965.[15] Bovine serum albumin (BSA) has been the most commonly used protein source in culture media.[15,31] Fetal calf serum has also been employed,[32] but a decrease in the number of normal fetuses obtained after uterine transfer of those embryos was observed.[32,33] Human maternal and fetal cord sera have been used extensively for human IVF programs,[34,35] with the latter giving better results in some studies.[36]

There is great variability in the capacities of different serum samples to support embryo development,[34] and Menezo has shown that there is no advantage in using serum instead of albumin in the culture media for human IVF.[37] Moreover, it seems that serum fractions of different molecular weights have different effects on embryo culture and some fractions (<1000 or >30,000 MW) contain embryo growth inhibitory proteins.[38] Given the additional fact that human sera do not support development of *in vitro*–fertilized mouse embryos successfully,[34,39] it is not certain whether protein or amino acids play an important nutritive role in culture media.[40] Indeed, blastocyst development of two-cell mouse embryos has been achieved in the absence of any amino groups[32] or with the addition of polyvinylpyrrolidone.[41]

Mouse pronuclear stage zygotes can develop to blastocysts *in vitro* in the absence of protein but in the presence of amino acids.[12] Caro and Trounson reported a successful pregnancy after IVF using a culture medium containing no protein.[42] The chelating agent ethylenediaminetetraacetic acid (EDTA)[43] can support zygote to blastocyst development in a relatively simple medium, such as Earle's balanced salts solution (EBSS[44]).[40,45–47] This supports the assumption that the ligand function of proteins may be more important to early embryo development than their nutritional effects.[40,47] Nevertheless, it has been shown that amino acids are needed for outgrowth from the mouse blastocyst, and their presence in the culture medium at fertilization and during the first 48 hours of cleavage is beneficial for postimplantation development of fetuses.[47]

BLOCKS TO PREIMPLANTATION EMBRYO DEVELOPMENT UNDER SUBOPTIMAL CULTURE CONDITIONS

Mouse embryos, with the exception of certain inbred strains[7,48] when cultured from the pronuclear zygote stage, arrest at the two-cell stage, a phenomenon known as the "two-cell block."[23,49,50,51] *In vitro* developmental arrest is not unique to the mouse. Cattle embryos arrest at the 8- to 16-cell stage,[52] porcine and rat embryos at the four-cell stage,[53,54] and hamster embryos at the two-cell stage,[25] although human embryos are an exception.[55] This block is reversed by transfer of cytoplasm from a nonblocking strain,[56,57] suggesting that the latter contain factors absent or at subeffective concentrations in blocking strains. One example might be enzymes or their mRNAs that may be considered responsible for rescuing *in vitro*–arrested two-cell embryos by overcoming glucose repression, as mentioned previously.[22,58] In the absence of any evidence that such a developmental block occurs *in vivo*, the two-cell block seems to be due to *in vitro* stresses resulting from suboptimal culture conditions, since it can be overcome by improving these conditions. Indeed, transfer of arrested embryos to explanted oviducts in organ culture[59]; supplementation of EBSS with lactate, pyruvate, and EDTA[40]; or substitution of glucose with glutamine in a balanced salts medium with BSA and EDTA (CZB medium)[30] rescues pronuclear mouse zygotes from the two-cell block. In addition, the appropriate adjustment of the concentrations of NaCl, KCl, KH_2PO_4, and $NaHCO_3$, besides those of pyruvate and glucose, also results in passage through this block, providing evidence that blocks to development can be caused by inappropriate concentrations of some of the common constituents of media that are currently employed.[60,61]

A similar phenomenon is the hypoxanthine-induced two-cell block to the development of mouse embryos. Micromolar concentrations of hypoxanthine, as well as adenosine and inosine, but not guanosine, block the second or third cleavage of several strains of mouse embryos if cultured *in vitro* from the pronuclear or early two-cell stage.[45,62] This arrest is maternally controlled, and it occurs late in the S phase or during the G2 phase of the cell cycle.[62,63] Embryonic transcription and translation are not blocked by the purines,[63] and the latter seem to inhibit a cAMP-dependent process because compounds that elevate cAMP alleviate the hypoxanthine-induced inhibition.[63,64] The importance of culture conditions for development though the block was also demonstrated by the report that the embryos are extremely sensitive to hypoxanthine if glucose is present in the medium, but the arrest is reversed by glutamine and high levels of lactate.[26] It is noteworthy that hypoxanthine inhibits embryo cleavage regardless of whether albumin, amino acids, or EDTA is present in the culture medium.[63]

The importance of employing appropriate culture media for human IVF by extending the knowledge obtained from mouse embryo cultures was demonstrated in two recent reports, in which culturing of human gametes in the complex medium Ham's F-10 (HF-10) without hypoxanthine yielded higher fertilization and embryo cleavage rates compared to culturing them in HF-10 with hypoxanthine.[65,66]

SIMPLE AND COMPLEX CULTURE MEDIA

Culture media can be divided into simple and complex. Simple media are bicarbonate-buffered systems that contain basic physiologic saline with pyruvate, lactate and D-glucose. The main differences among various types of simple media are variations in their ion concentrations of lactate and pyruvate. M16[18] has been the basis for various modifications for improved embryo development and for rescuing through the two-cell block.[61,67] CZB contains glutamine and EDTA instead of glucose,[30] and it was shown to support mouse embryo development through the two-cell block. The same is true for EBSS with EDTA.[47] Human tubal fluid (HTF) is a medium that simulates the human fallopian tube milieu.[68] All of these media are supplemented with serum or albumin when used for human IVF. Penicillin and streptomycin are also added.

Complex media contain, in addition to the basic components of simple media, amino acids, vitamins, and other substances, mainly in levels at which they are found in serum. Their fundamental difference from simple media is that fixed nitrogen is present as free amino acids. The most widely used complex medium, especially in the United States, is Ham's F-10.[69] It consists of a Kreb's-Ringer bicarbonate buffer system supplemented with pyruvate, lactate, amino acids, vitamins, trace elements, and other substances found in serum, such as thymidine and hypoxanthine. Penicillin and streptomycin are also added to it, as is albumin or serum for the reasons discussed previously. The recent findings about the deleterious effects of hypoxanthine on human IVF outcome[65,66] along with the previous reports about the induced two-cell block on mouse preimplantation embryos[45,62] suggest that hypoxanthine should not be included in its composition for human IVF.

IMPROVEMENT OF CULTURE CONDITIONS

Increasing the *in vitro* developmental potential of early embryos by supplementing the culture medium with various components has been given considerable attention by many workers. The effect of EDTA on mouse embryo development has already been mentioned.[40,43,45,47] The addition of the β–amino acid in HTF results in a significantly higher rate of mouse blastocyst formation.[70] Glutamine has also been shown to have a beneficial effect whether or not glucose is present in the medium.[30,71]

Human menopausal gonadotropin and human chorionic gonadotropin were shown to rescue mouse pronuclear zygotes through the hypoxanthine-induced two-cell block.[64] Gonadotropins have also been shown to increase the developmental potential of mouse embryos from *in vitro*–matured oocytes.[72] Insulin[73,74] and insulin-like growth factor-1,[75] as well as growth hormone,[76] have been shown to exert a positive effect on preimplantation mouse embryos. The role of platelet-activating factor,[77,78] low molecular weight oviductal factors,[79] and epidermal growth factor[77,80,81] are also under investigation.

The effect of incubation volume and embryo density on embryonic development has also been looked at. Decreasing the volume and increasing the number of embryos has been reported to exert a beneficial effect,[82,83] although no statistical differences have been found by others.[84]

A culture medium based on the composition of human fallopian tube fluid (HTF) with high potassium levels has also been employed in order to investigate development of embryos *in vitro* in an environment similar to the milieu of the human oviduct.[68] Results were contradictory because more clinical pregnancies were reported by some workers,[68] whereas others did not observe any statistically significant improvement in the IVF outcome of this fluid over other media.[85,86] A further step was the co-culturing of embryos with oviductal and/or uterine cells. Reports with mouse[87] and human embryos[88] have shown beneficial effects on embryo development and on clinical pregnancy and implantation rates. Differences among species have been observed regarding the preparations of these media. For some species (cattle), a medium preconditioned with oviductal cells has beneficial effects on embryonic development, whereas for others (sheep, pig) direct contact between embryos and cell monolayers is necessary.[89] For human IVF, free-floating cells, pretreated with trypsin, are preferred to an intact monolayer because the sperm bind to the latter reducing the fertilization rate.[88] The discovery that monolayers of Vero cells have a rescuing effect on poor-quality human embryos is also of great interest.[90]

Finally, one should bear in mind that *in vitro* conditions cannot fully support fertilization and early cleavage of preimplantation embryos[39,91,92] and that even the highest quality media have not improved success rates of IVF programs significantly. The existence of a variety of media indicates by itself that none is optimal for embryo culturing. A combination of the various media is often used in order to achieve specific end-points, and the choice of medium is most frequently determined historically.

REFERENCES

1. KUHL, W. 1941. Untersuchungen uber die cytodynamik der furchung und fruhentwicklung des eis der weissen maus. Abb. Senchenb. Naturforsch. Ges. **456:** 1–17.
2. HAMMOND, J. 1949. Recovery and culture of tubal mouse ova. Nature **163:** 28–29.
3. KREBS, H.A. & K. HENSELEIT. 1932. Untersuchungenuber die Harnstoffbildung im Tierkorper. Z. Phys. Chem. **210:** 33–66.
4. WHITTEN, W.K. 1956. Culture of tubal mouse ova. Nature **177:** 96–97.
5. MCLAREN, A. & J.D. BIGGERS. 1958. Successful development and birth of mice cultivated in vitro as early embryos. Nature **182:** 877–878.
6. WHITTEN, W.K. 1957. Culture of tubal ova. Nature **179:** 1081–1082.
7. WHITTEN, W.K. & J.D. BIGGERS. 1968. Complete development in vitro of the preimplantation stages of the mouse in a simple chemically defined medium. J. Reprod. Fertil. **17:** 399–401.
8. BIGGERS, J.D., W.K. WHITTEN & D.G. WHITTINGHAM. 1971. The culture of mouse embryos in vitro. *In* Methods of Mammalian Embryology. J.C. Daniel, Jr., Ed.: 86-116. Freeman. San Francisco.
9. SHIRE, J.G.M. & W.K. WHITTEN. 1980. Genetic variation in the timing of first cleavage in mice: effect of maternal genotype. Biol. Reprod. **23:** 369–376.

10. FUKUDA, A., Y. NODA, S. TSUCUI, *et al.* 1987. Influence of water quality on in vitro fertilization and embryo development for the mouse. J. IVF Embryo Transf. **4:** 40–45.
11. BARNSTEAD. Ed. 1991. The Water Book. Barnstead/Thermolyne Corporation. p.80.
12. JOHN, D.P. & A. KIESSLING. 1988. Improved pronuclear mouse embryo development over an extended pH range in Ham's F-10 medium without protein. Fertil. Steril. **49:** 150–155.
13. BRINSTER, R.L. 1965. Studies on the development of mouse embryos in vitro. I. The effect of osmolarity and hydrogen ion concentration. J. Exp. Zool. **158:** 49–57.
14. NAGLEE, D.L., R.R. MAURER & R.H. FOOTE. 1969. Effect of osmolarity on in vitro development of rabbit embryos in a chemically defined medium. Exp. Cell Res. **58:** 331–333.
15. BRINSTER, R.L. 1965. Studies on the development of mouse embryos in vitro. II. The effect of energy source. J. Exp. Zool. **158:** 59–68.
16. BRINSTER, R.L. 1965. Studies on the development of mouse embryos in vitro. IV. Interaction of energy sources. J. Reprod. Fertil. **10:** 227–240.
17. LONG, C. 1961. Biochemist's Handbook. D. Van Nostrand Company. Princeton, New Jersey.
18. WHITTINGHMAM, D.G. 1971. Culture of mouse ova. J. Reprod. Fert. (Suppl.) **14:** 7–21.
19. KAYE, P.L. 1986. Metabolic aspects of the physiology of the preimplantation embryo. *In* Experimental Approaches to Mammalian Embryonic Development. J. Rossant & R.A. Pedersen, Eds.: 267–292. Cambridge University Press. Cambridge.
20. BROWN, J.J.G. & D.G. WHITTINGHAM. 1991. The roles of pyruvate, lactate and glucose during preimplantation development of embryos from F1 hybrid mice in vitro. Development **112:** 99–105.
21. WHITTINGHAM, D.G. 1969. The failure of lactate and phosphoenolpyruvate to support development of the mouse zygote in vitro. Biol. Reprod. **1:** 381–386.
22. BROWN, J.J.G. & D.G. WHITTINGHAM. 1992. The dynamic provision of different energy substrates improves development of one-cell random-bred mouse embryos in vitro. J. Reprod. Fertil. **95:** 503–511.
23. CROSS, P.C. & R.L. BRINSTER. 1973. The sensitivity of one-cell mouse embryos to pyruvate and lactate. Exp. Cell Res. **77:** 57–62.
24. BRINSTER, R.L. 1971. Uptake and incorporation of amino acids by the preimplantation mouse embryo. J. Reprod. Fertil. **27:** 329–338.
25. SCHINI, S.A. & B.D. BAVISTER. 1988. Two-cell block to development of cultured hamster embryos is caused by phosphate and glucose. Biol. Reprod. **39:** 1183–1192.
26. DOWNS, S.M. & M.P. DOW. 1991. Hypoxanthine-maintained two-cell block in mouse embryos: dependence on glucose and effect of hypoxanthine phosphoribosyltransferase inhibitors. Biol. Reprod. **44:** 1025–1039.
27. CRABTREE, H.G. 1929. Observations on the carbohydrate metabolism of tumors. Biochem. J. **23:** 536–545.
28. MASTROIANNI, L. & R.C. WALLACH. 1961. Effect of ovulation and early gestation on oviduct secretions in the rabbit. Am. J. Physiol. **200:** 815–818.
29. MASTROIANNI, L., W.W. WINTERNITZ & N.P. LOWI. 1958. The in vitro metabolism of the human endosalpinx. Fertil. Steril. **9:** 500–505.
30. CHATOT, C.L., C.A. ZIOMEK, B.D. BAVISTER, *et al.* 1989. An improved culture medium suports development of random-bred 1-cell mouse embryos in vitro. J. Reprod. Fertil. **86:** 679–688.
31. KANE, M.T. & D.R. HEADON. 1980. The role of commercial bovine serum albumin preparation in the culture of one-cell rabbit embryos to blastocyst. J. Reprod. Fertil. **60:** 469–475.
32. CARO, C.M. & A. TROUNSON. 1984. The effect of protein on preimplantation mouse embryo development in vitro. J. IVF Embryo Transf. **1:** 183–187.
33. ARNY, M., L. NACHTIGALL & J. QUAGLIARELLO. 1987. The effect of preimplantation culture conditions on murine embryo implantation and fetal development. Fertil. Steril. **48:** 861–865.
34. SHIRLEY, B., J.W. EDWARD-WARTHAM, JR., J. WITMYER, *et al.* 1985. Effects of human serum and plasma on development of mouse embryos in culture medium. Fertil. Steril. **43:** 129–143.

35. MELDRUM, D.R., R. CHETKOWSKI, K.A. STEINGOLD, *et al.* 1987. Evolution of a highly successful in vitro fertilization–embryo transfer program. Fertil. Steril. **48:** 86–93.
36. LEUNG, P.C.S., M.J. GRONOW, G.N. KELLOW, *et al.* Serum supplement in human in vitro fertilization and embryo development. Fertil. Steril. **41:** 36–41.
37. MENEZO, Y., J. TESTART & D. PERRONE. 1984. Serum is not necessary for human in vitro fertilization, early embryo culture and transfer. Fertil. Steril. **42:** 750–755.
38. OGAWA, T., T. ONO & R.P. MARRS. 1987. The effect of serum fractions on single-cell mouse embryos in vitro. J. IVF Embryo Transf. **4:** 153–159.
39. HAN, H-D. & A.A. KIESSLING. 1988. In vivo development of transferred mouse embryos conceived in vitro in simple and complex media. Fertil. Steril. **50:** 159–163.
40. FISSORE, R., K.V. JACKSON & A.A. KIESSLING. 1989. Mouse zygote development in medium without protein in the presence of ethylenediamintetraacetic acid. Biol. Reprod. **41:** 835–841.
41. CHOLEWA, J.A. & W.K. WHITTEN. 1970. Development of two-cell embryos in the absence of a fixed-nitrogen source. J. Reprod. Fertil. **22:** 553–555.
42. CARO, C.M. & A. TROUNSON. 1986. Successful embryo development and pregnancy in human IVF using a chemically defined culture medium containing no protein. J. IVF Embryo Transf. **3:** 215–217.
43. ABRAMCZUK, J., D. SOLTER & H. KOPROWSKI. 1977. The beneficial effect of EDTA on development of mouse one-cell embryos in chemically defined medium. Dev. Biol. **61:** 378–382.
44. EARLE, W.R. 1943. Production of malignancy in vitro. IV. The mouse fibroblast cultures and changes seen in the living cells. J. Nat. Cancer Inst. **4:** 165–212.
45. LOUTRADIS, D., D. JOHN & A.A. KIESSLING. 1987. Hypoxanthine causes a 2-cell block in random-bred mouse embryos. Biol. Reprod. **37:** 311–316.
46. JACKSON, K.V. & A.A. KIESSLING. 1989. Fertilization and cleavage of mouse oocytes exposed to the conditions of human oocyte retrieval for in vitro fertilization. Fertil. Steril. **51:** 675–681.
47. MEHTA, T.S. & A.A KIESSLING. 1990. Development potential of mouse embryos conceived in vitro and cultured in ethylenediaminetetraacetic acid with or without amino acids or serum. Biol. Reprod. **43:** 600–606.
48. BIGGERS, J.D. 1971. New observations on the nutrition of the mammalian oocyte and the preimplantation embryo. *In* The Biology of the Blastocyst. R.J. Blandau, Ed.: 319–327. University of Chicago Press. Chicago.
49. COLE, R.J. & J. PAUL. 1965. Properties of cultured preimplantation mouse and rabbit embryos, and cell strains derived from them. *In* Preimplantation Stages of Pregnancy. G.E.W. Wolstenholme & M. O'Connor, Eds.: 82–122. Churchill. London.
50. GODDARD, J.M. & H.M.P. PRATT. 1983. Control of events during early cleavage of the mouse embryos: an analysis of the "2-cell block." J. Embryol. Exp. Morphol. **73:** 111–113.
51. BIGGERS, J.D. 1987. Pioneering mammalian embryo culture. *In* The Mammalian Preimplantation Embryo. B.D. Bavister, Ed.: 1–22. Plenum Press. New York.
52. THIBAULT, C. 1966. In vitro culture of cow eggs. Ann. Biol. Anim. Biochim. Biophys. **6:** 159–164.
53. WHITTINGHAM, D.G. 1975. Fertilization, early development and storage of mammalian ova in vitro. *In* The Early Development of Mammals. M. Balls & A.E. Wild, Eds.: 1–24. Cambridge University Press. Cambridge.
54. DAVIS, D.L. & B.N. DAY. 1978. Cleavage and blastocyst formation by pig eggs in vitro. J. Anim. Sci. **46:** 1043–1053.
55. PURDY, J.M. 1982. Methods for fertilization and embryo culture in vitro. *In* Human Conception in Vitro. R.G. Edwards & J.M. Purdy, Eds.: 135–148. Academic Press. London.
56. MUGGLETON-HARRIS, A., D.G. WHITTINGHAM & L. WILSON. 1982. Cytoplasmic control of preimplantation development in vitro in the mouse. Nature (London) **299:** 460–462.
57. PRATT, H.P.M. & A.L. MUGGLETON-HARRIS. 1988. Cycling cytoplasmic factors that promote mitosis in the cultured 2-cell mouse embryo. Development **104:** 112–120.
58. MUGGLETON-HARRIS, A.L. & J.J.C. BROWN. 1988. Cytoplasmic factors influence mitochondrial reorganization and resumption of cleavage during culture of early mouse embryos. Hum. Reprod. **3:** 1020–1028.

59. WHITTINGHAM, D.G. & J.D. BIGGERS. 1967. Fallopian tube and early cleavage in the mouse. Nature **213:** 942.
60. LAWITTS, J.A. & J.D. BIGGERS. 1991. Optimization of mouse embryo culture media using simplex methods. J. Reprod. Fertil. **91:** 543–556.
61. LAWITTS, J.A. & J.D. BIGGERS. 1991. Overcoming the 2-cell block by modifying standard components in a mouse embryo culture medium. Biol. Reprod. **45:** 245–251.
62. NUREDDIN, A., E. EPSARO & A.A. KIESSLING. 1990. Purines inhibit the development of mouse embryos in vitro. J. Reprod. Fertil. **90:** 455–464.
63. FISSORE, R., S. O'KEEFE & A.A. KIESSLING. 1992. Purine-induced block to mouse embryo cleavage is reversed by compounds that elevate cyclic-adenosine monophosphate. Biol. Reprod. **47:** 1105–1112.
64. LOUTRADIS, D., P. DRAKAKIS, S. MICHALAS, *et al.* 1994. The effect of compounds altering the cAMP level on reversing the 2-cell block induced by hypoxanthine in mouse embryos in vitro. Eur. J. Obstet. Gynecol. Reprod. Biol. **57:** 195–199.
65. BASTIAS, M.C., S. MCGEE, S.H. BRYAN & J.M. VASQUEZ. 1992. Deleterious effect of hypoxanthine in culture medium for human in vitro fertilization. Fertil. Steril. Abstracts of the 48th Annual Meeting of the AFS, p. S149.
66. LOUTRADIS, D., A.A. KIESSLING, K. KALLIANIDIS, *et al.* 1993. A preliminary trial of human zygote culture in Ham's F-10 without hypoxanthine. J. Assoc. Reprod. Genet. **10:** 271–275.
67. MENEZO, Y. & C. KHATCHADOURIAN. 1990. Implication de l' activite glucose 6 phosphate isomerase (EC 5.3.1.9) dans l' arret de al segmentation de l' oeuf de souris au stade 2 cellules in vitro. CR Acad. Sci. Paris **310** (serie III): 297–301.
68. QUINN, P., J.F. KERIN & G.M. WARNES. 1985. Improved pregnancy rate in human in vitro fertilization with the use of a medium based on the composition of human tubal fluid. Fertil. Steril. **44:** 493–498.
69. HAM, R.G. 1963. An improved nutrient solution for diploid chinese hamster and human cell lines. Exp. Cell Res. **29:** 515–526.
70. DUMOULIN, J.C.M., J.L.H. EVERS, J.A. BAKKER, *et al.* 1992. Temporal effects of taurine on mouse preimplantation development in vitro. Hum. Reprod. **7:** 403–407.
71. PETTERS, R.M., B.H. JOHNSTON, M.L. REED & A.E. ARCHIBONG. 1990. Glucose, glutamine and inorganic phosphate in early development of the pig embryo in vitro. J. Reprod. Fertil. **89:** 269–275.
72. JINNO, M., B.A. SANDOW & G.D. HODGEN. 1989. Enhancement of the developmental potential of mouse oocytes matured in vitro by gonadotropins and ethylene diaminetetraacetic acid (EDTA). J. IVF Transf. **6:** 36–40.
73. HARVEY, M.B. & P.L. KAYE. 1988. Insulin stimulates protein synthesis in compacted mouse embryos. Endocrinology **122:** 1182–1184.
74. TRAVERS, J.P., L. EXELL, B. HUANG, *et al.* 1992. Insulin and insulin-like growth hormone factors in embryonic development. Effects of a biologically inert insulin (guinea pig) on rat embryonic growth and development in vitro. Diabetes **41:** 318–324.
75. HARVEY, M.B. & P.L. KAYE. 1992. Insulin-like growth factor-1 stimulates growth of mouse preimplantation embryos in vitro. Mol. Reprod. Dev. **31:** 195–199.
76. DRAKAKIS, P., D. LOUTRADIS, S. MICHALAS, *et al.* 1995. A preliminary study of the effect of growth hormone on mouse preimplantation embryo development in vitro. Gynecol. Obstet. Invest. **40:** 222–226.
77. COLVER, R.M., A.M. HOWE, P.G. MCDONOUGH & J. BOLDT. 1991. Influence of growth factors in defined culture medium on in vitro development of mouse embryos. Fertil. Steril. **55:** 194–199.
78. NAKATSUKA, M., N. YOSHIDA & T. KUDO. 1992. Platelet activating factor in culture media as an indicator of human embryonic development after in vitro fertilization. Hum. Reprod. **7:** 1435–1439.
79. MINAMI, N., K. UTSUMI & A. IRITANI. 1992. Effects of low molecular weight oviductal factors on the development of mouse one-cell embryos in vitro. J. Reprod. Fertil. **96:** 735–745.
80. HARPER, K.M. & B.G. BRACKETT. 1993. Bovine blastocyst development after in vitro maturation in a defined medium with epidermal growth factor and low concentrations of gonadotropins. Biol. Reprod. **48:** 409–416.

81. DRAKAKIS, P., D. LOUTRADIS, S. MILINGOS, *et al.* 1996. The in vitro development of mouse embryo beyond the blastocyst stage into the hatching and outgrowth stage using different energy sources. J. Assist. Reprod. Genet. **13:** 786–792.
82. PARIA, B.C. & S.K. DEY. 1990. Preimplantation embryo development in vitro: Cooperative interactions among embryos and role of growth factors. Proc. Natl. Acad. Sci. USA **87:** 4756–4760.
83. LANE, M. & D.K. GARDNER. 1992. Effect of incubation volume and embryo density on the development and viability of mouse embryos in vitro. Hum. Reprod. **7:** 55–562.
84. TASSIOULA, E., K. SERTA, D. LOUTRADIS & A.A KIESSLING. 1992. Mouse embryo development is not improved by group culture or small volumes. Fertil. Steril. Abstracts of the 48th Annual Meeting of the AFS, p. S146.
85. CUMMINS, J.M., T.M. BREEN, S.M. FULLER, *et al.* 1986. Comparison of two media in a human in vitro fertilization program: lack of significant differences in pregnancy rate. J. IVF Embryo Transf. **3:** 326–330.
86. GARDNER, D.K. & H.J. LEESE. 1990. Concentrations of nutrients in mouse oviduct fluid and their effects on embryo development and metabolism in vitro. J. Reprod. Fertil. **88:** 361–368.
87. SAKKAS, D. & A.O. TROUNSON. 1990. Co-culture of mouse embryos with oviduct and uterine cells prepared from mice at different days of pseudopregnancy. J. Reprod. Fertil. **90:** 109–118.
88. BONGSO, A., S-C. NG, C-Y. FONG, *et al.* 1992. Improved pregnancy rate after transfer of embryos grown in human fallopian tubal cell coculture. Fertil. Steril. **58:** 569–574.
89. BONGSO, A., S-C. NG, C-Y. FONG & S. RATNAM. 1991. Cocultures: a new lead in embryo quality improvement for assisted reproduction. Fertil. Steril. **56:** 179–191.
90. MENEZO, Y.J.R., J.F. GUERIN & J.C. CZYBA. 1990. Improvement of human early embryo development in vitro by co-culture on monolayers of Vero cells. Biol. Reprod. **42:** 301–305.
91. BOLTON, V., S.M. HAWES, C.T. TAYLOR & J.H. PARSONS. 1989. Development of spare human preimplantation embryos in vitro: an analysis of the correlations among gross morphology, cleavage rates and development to the blastocyst. J. IVF Embryo Transf. **6:** 30–35.
92. KIESSLING, A.A., H.W. DAVIS, C.S. WILLIAMS, *et al.* 1991. Development and DNA polymerase activities in cultured preimplantation mouse embryos: comparison with embryos developed in vivo. J. Exp. Zool. **258:** 34–47.

Intracytoplasmic Sperm Injection

Survey of World Results

BASIL C. TARLATZIS[a] AND HELEN BILI

1st Department of Obstetrics and Gynecology, Aristotle University of Thessaloniki, Thessaloniki, Greece

ABSTRACT: The widespread application of intracytoplasmic sperm injection (ICSI) has raised concern about the efficacy and safety of this novel technique. The European Society of Human Reproduction and Embryology (ESHRE) has established an ICSI Task Force to collect annually the clinical results, the outcome of pregnancy, and the follow-up of children after ICSI using ejaculated, epididymal, and testicular sperm in order to address these important issues in a relatively short time. Over a 3-year span (1993–1995), the number of centers for ICSI increased from 35 to 101, and the total number of ICSI cycles per year rose from 3,157 to 23,932. The incidence of oocytes damaged by the procedure remained low (<10%), whereas the fertilization rates obtained with ejaculated, epididymal, and testicular spermatozoa for 1995 were 64%, 62%, and 52%, respectively. Thus, 86–90% of the couples had embryo transfer, and the viable pregnancy rate was 21% for ejaculated, 22% for epididymal, and 19% for testicular sperm, while the incidence of multiple gestations was 29%, 30%, and 38%, respectively. It is noteworthy that no difference was found in ICSI results concerning the etiology of azoospermia, for example, obstructive (congenital or acquired) or nonobstructive. Furthermore, 3,149 transfers of frozen-thawed embryos after ICSI with ejaculated, epididymal, or testicular sperm were performed, and in 11%, 9%, and 7% of them, respectively, a viable pregnancy was achieved. The ICSI results were similar during this 3-year period, irrespective of the origin of the sperm. The perinatal outcome of children born after ICSI was not different from that after *in vitro* fertilization or natural conception and was only affected by multiplicity. Moreover, the incidence of major or minor malformations was not increased, but the chromosomal, especially the sex chromosomal, aberration rate was slightly elevated (~2%). Therefore, ICSI has opened new horizons in the treatment of male infertility. The achievement of pregnancy after ICSI using ejaculated, epididymal, or testicular sperm is very satisfactory. The procedure seems to be safe, but further follow-up of the children is necessary to more accurately assess its safety.

INTRODUCTION

Intracytoplasmic sperm injection (ICSI) has revolutionized the treatment of male infertility, because pregnancy can be achieved with severely compromised spermatozoa.[1] From the beginning, it became obvious that the method could be applied in a wide variety of male infertility problems, ranging from oligoteratoasthenozoospermia (OTA) to azoospermia. This, in combination with very good results, led to rapid

[a]Address for correspondence: Prof. Tarlatzis, Geniki Kliniki Gravis 2, Nea Paralia, 54 645 Thessalonki, Greece. Phone: 00-30-31-892127; fax: 00-30-31-89511.

spreading of ICSI worldwide and to its establishment as a routine procedure in most *in vitro* fertilization (IVF) programs.

The advent of ICSI technology and its wide application necessitate that particular attention be paid to the safety of this novel technique, because with ICSI the never proven selection of spermatozoa by the zona pellucida and/or oolemma is bypassed.[2] On the other hand, gathered experience from previous years, albeit limited, seems encouraging.[3] Thus, in the near future collaborative efforts should be directed at clarifying the perinatal outcome, possible genetic risks, or other adverse effects in children born after ICSI. The ICSI Task Force of the European Society of Human Reproduction and Embryology (ESHRE) was first established in 1994, focusing on gathering data from worldwide centers practicing ICSI in order to accumulate sufficient information to address the issues of safety and efficacy of this procedure.

Five forms were used to collect data: (1) those referring to the clinical experience with ICSI, (2) those concerning the follow-up of children born after ICSI, (3) those aimed at evaluating children with congenital malformations, and (4,5) two forms referring to the results of cryopreservation after ICSI using ejaculated, epididymal, and testicular spermatozoa and also to the follow-up of children born after transfer of frozen-thawed ICSI embryos.[3] In this survey the overall results of ICSI for the years 1993-1995 using ejaculated, epididymal, and testicular sperm are presented.[4]

INDICATIONS AND NUMBER OF CYCLES

Although ICSI was originally developed to treat male infertility, it is currently also used for other disorders. Abnormal semen quality was the main indication for ICSI (101 centers), followed by failed IVF (96 centers), obstructive azoospermia (73 centers), nonobstructive azoospermia (63 centers), preimplantation diagnosis (8 centers) as well as globozoosperrnia, antisperm antibodies, idiopathic infertility, etc (23 centers).

The 101 clinics performing ICSI reported a total of 39,675 cycles (36,774 with ejaculated, 1,748 with epididymal, and 1,153 with testicular sperm). Over the last 3 years, an impressive rise in the application of this technique has been observed.[3] Similarly, the number of centers performing higher number of cycles per year also increased in 1995, although variations between centers still existed.

FERTILIZATION AND EMBRYO TRANSFER

Using ejaculated spermatozoa, from the 255,861 metaphase II (MII) oocytes injected, 24,502 (9.6%) were damaged during the ICSI procedure and 157,381 (61.5%) were normally fertilized, resulting in 109,197 (42.6%) good quality embryos that could be transferred or frozen (FIG. 1). These led to 27,502 embryo transfers (87.9%) and 7,327 cycles (23.4%) with embryo freezing.[4]

In the cycles with epididymal sperm, from the 14,784 MII oocytes injected, 1,204 (8.1%) were damaged and 8,511 (57.6%) fertilized, leading to 5,852 (39.6%) embryos that were available for transfer or freezing (FIG. 1). Thus, 1,403 embryo transfers (87.1%) and 359 cycles with freezing (22.3%) were accomplished. Moreover, the ICSI results were similar when classified according to the etiology of obstruction, congenital or acquired (FIG. 2).

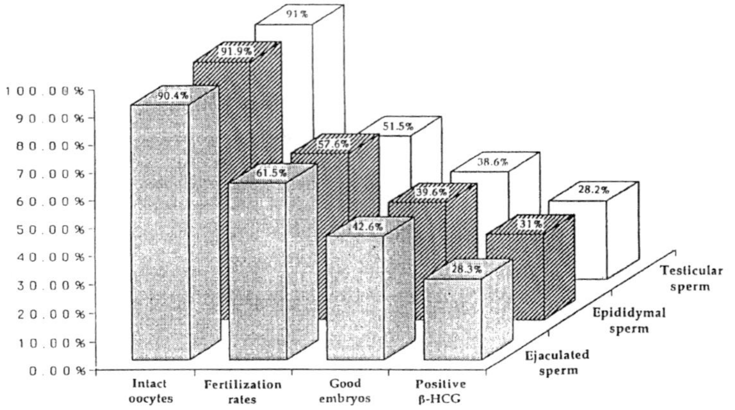

FIGURE 1. ICSI results (1993–1995) according to the origin of the sperm. Reproduced with permission from Tarlatzis and Bili.[4]

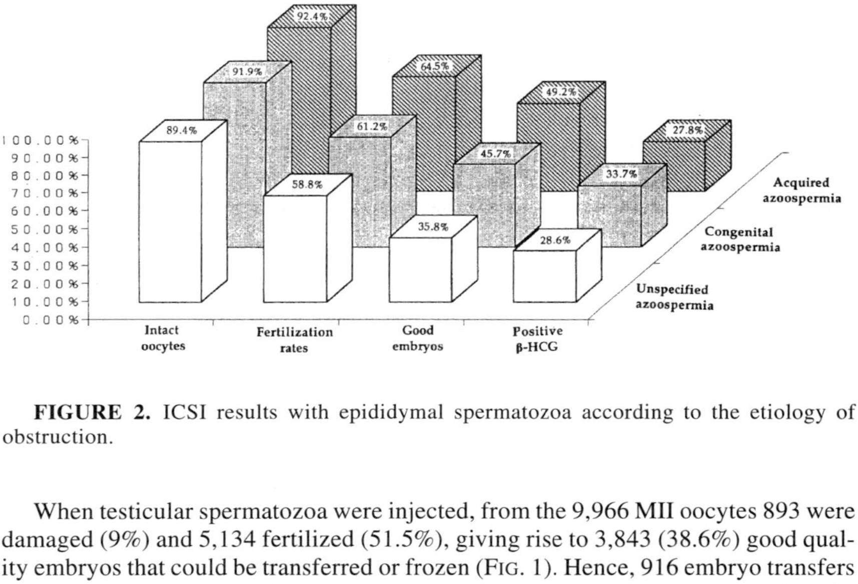

FIGURE 2. ICSI results with epididymal spermatozoa according to the etiology of obstruction.

When testicular spermatozoa were injected, from the 9,966 MII oocytes 893 were damaged (9%) and 5,134 fertilized (51.5%), giving rise to 3,843 (38.6%) good quality embryos that could be transferred or frozen (FIG. 1). Hence, 916 embryo transfers (90.2%) and 274 embryo freezings (30%) were done. On the other hand, when the ICSI data were analyzed according to the etiology of azoospermia, patients with nonobstructive azoospermia had lower fertilization and embryo transfer rates than did obstructive cases (FIG. 3). This was probably due to the smaller chances of finding spermatozoa at all or in sufficient numbers in patients with nonobstructive lesions. According to a recent study, this is possible in approximately 50% of these patients.[5]

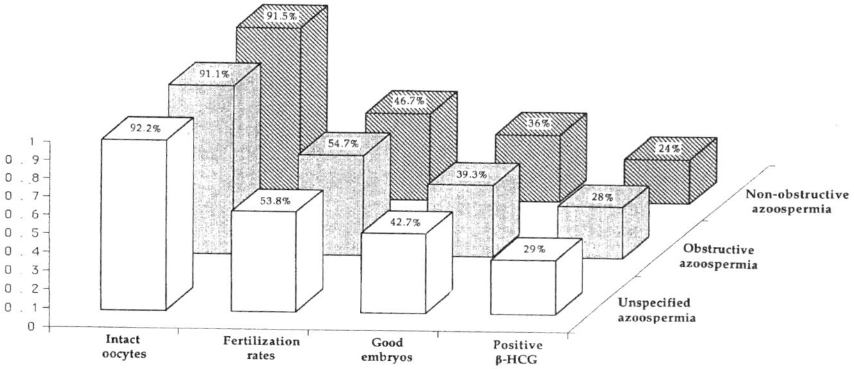

FIGURE 3. ICSI results with testicular spermatozoa according to the etiology of azoospermia.

Therefore, it is evident that in cases of male infertility, fertilization rates after ICSI, even with severely impaired sperm, are significantly higher than those with classical IVF.[6] Moreover, most of the fertilized oocytes (67.9–75.2%) develop into high quality embryos that can be either transferred or frozen. Thus, even in cases of non-obstructive or obstructive azoospermia, 84.7 and 91.1% of the patients, respectively, will have embryo transfer, which is impossible with classical IVF or any other assisted reproduction technique, whereas 22.6 and 26.2% of the aforementioned categories of patients, respectively, are expected to have a frozen/thawed embryo transfer as well.

It is noteworthy that the incidence of oocytes damaged during the procedure in 1995 ranged between 8.3% and 9.3%, and it did not differ from that observed in previous years.[7] Hence, oocyte damage seems to be an inherent drawback of the ICSI procedure per se. Moreover, the incidence of fertilization and good quality embryo development in 1995 was similar to that in 1994, except for cases with epididymal sperm where more oocytes were fertilized (62.5 and 52.5%, respectively) and more good quality embryos (61.7 and 73.1% of fertilized oocytes, respectively) were available in 1995, possibly indicating the accumulated experience.

ACHIEVEMENT OF PREGNANCY

The main factor determining the effectiveness of an assisted reproduction technique, such as ICSI, is obviously the achievement of pregnancy and especially of a viable one.

In total, a fresh embryo transfer was performed in 27,502 ICSI cycles (87.9%) with ejaculated sperm, resulting in 8,811 positive β-HCG tests (28.2% per cycle) and 6,571 viable pregnancies (FIG. 1), from which 3,514 were ongoing and 3,057 were delivered. In cases of ICSI with epididymal spermatozoa, a fresh embryo transfer was performed in 1,403 cycles (87.1%), leading to 499 positive β-HCG tests (31% per cycle) and 361 viable pregnancies (FIG. 1), from which 163 were ongoing and

198 delivered.[4] On the other hand, in cases of ICSI with testicular spermatozoa, 916 fresh embryo transfers (90.2%) were accomplished, resulting in 287 positive β-HCG tests (26.2% per cycle) and 199 viable prengancies (FIG. 1).

The overall results for ejaculated, epididymal, and testicular spermatozoa in 1995 were similar to those recorded in 1993–1994.[3] Nevertheless, the results using testicular sperm showed a slight decline in positive β-HCG and in viable pregnancy rates, possibly due to the larger number of cycles performed and the wider application of this procedure in less favorable cases.

Regarding frozen/thawed embryo transfers after ICSI, a total of 3,363 cycles were recorded during 1995 from 57 centers.[3] Of those, 2,990 embryo transfers were done in 3,146 cycles after ICSI using ejaculated sperm, giving rise to 525 positive β-HCG tests (16.7%) and 341 viable pregnancies (64.9%). With frozen/thawed embryos using epididymal sperm, 91 transfers were performed in 144 cycles, leading to 22 positive β-HCG tests (15.3%), from which 13 were viable pregnancies (59.1%). On the other hand, 68 frozen/thawed embryo transfers after testicular sperm injection were done in 73 cycles, resulting in 8 positive β-HCG tests (11.0%) and 5 viable pregnancies (62.5%).

EARLY LOSS OF PREGNANCY AND ECTOPIC PREGNANCY

The implantation rate after IVF and ICSI, even with good quality embryos, remains relatively low despite progress in ovarian stimulation and culture conditions. Moreover, the implantation as well as the miscarriage rate is significantly affected by the woman's age and therefore primarily oocyte and embryo quality.[8]

In cases in which ejaculated spermatozoa were used, from the 8,811 positive β-HCG tests, 888 (10.1%) were biochemical pregnancies, 1,278 (14.5%) clinical abortions, and 132 (1.5%) ectopic pregnancies (FIG. 4). On the other hand, with epididymal sperm, from the 499 positive β-HCG tests, 67 (13.4%) were biochemical

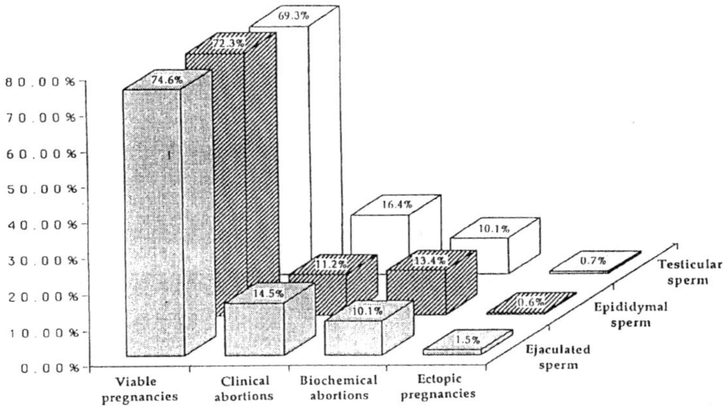

FIGURE 4. ICSI pregnancies (1993–1995) according to the origin of the sperm. Reproduced with permission from Tarlatzis and Bili.[4]

pregnancies and 56 (11.2%) clinical abortions, whereas 3 ectopic pregnancies (0.6%) were observed (FIG. 4). With testicular sperm (FIG. 4), from 287 positive β-HCG results, 29 (10.1%) were biochemical pregnancies, 47 (16.4%) clinical abortions, and 2 (0.7%) ectopic pregnancies.[4] The incidence of early pregnancy loss after ICSI is similar to that after IVF,[8] whereas the incidence of ectopic pregnancy (ranging from 0.6 to 1.5%) is lower than that observed in standard IVF (4.3%), possibly because most women undergoing ICSI have normal tubes in contrast to those undergoing classical IVF.[9]

The outcome of pregnancy after frozen/thawed embryo transfer was similar to that after fresh embryo transfer. Thus, using frozen/thawed embryos from ejaculated sperm, 72 biochemical pregnancies (13.7%), 83 clinical abortions (15.8%), and 10 ectopic pregnancies (1.9%) were observed, whereas with epididymal spermatozoa, 3 biochemical (13.6%), 2 clinical abortions (9.1%), and no ectopic pregnancies were obtained. In addition, using embryos from testicular sperm, 22 biochemical pregnancies (10.1%), 34 clinical abortions (15.6%), and 1 ectopic pregnancy (0.5%) were recorded.[3]

PERINATAL OUTCOME AND ICSI PREGNANCY

The overall incidence of multiple pregnancies after ICSI was approximately the same for ejaculated, epididymal, and testicular sperm (28.6%, 30.2%, and 32.7%, respectively), whereas similar results were also reported after transfer of frozen/thawed ICSI embryos. From them, 21.0–23.8% were twins and 1.6–4.2% were triplets or more (FIG. 5). These findings confirm the good quality of ICSI embryos and further support the need to reduce the number of replaced embryos.[10]

The perinatal outcome of children born after ICSI was not compromised, because the mean gestational age and mean birth weight for single pregnancies were similar to those observed in the general population, whereas they were significantly lower in high order multiple pregnancies.[4] These findings for ICSI babies agree with those observed by Wisanto *et al.*[11,12] but also with those reported for IVF babies from cer-

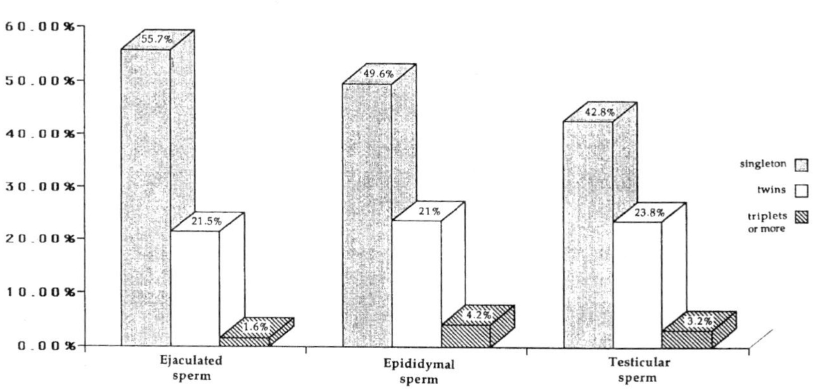

FIGURE 5. Multiple pregnancies after ICSI for 1995 according to the origin of the sperm.

tain registries.[13] It is noteworthy that no significant differences in perinatal outcome were observed between children born after ICSI using ejaculated, epididymal, or testicular sperm and those born using frozen/thawed embryos.[3,4]

GENETIC AND MALFORMATION RISKS

It has been claimed that fertilizing spermatozoa are somehow selected and that only normal spermatozoa achieve fertilization.[14] Yet, with the possible exception of sperm morphology and motility, there is no evidence in humans or in animals to support this selection procedure.[14] Nevertheless, if such a selection mechanism exists, it is important to examine what the implications might be when these selective barriers are bypassed using ICSI. Thus, the follow-up of children born after ICSI is of great significance, but it is a very difficult project, because it requires special arrangements at the centers and substantial funding in order to be done properly.[3,4] Hence, only 17 of the 101 centers that submitted ICSI results up to 1995 were performing a prospective follow-up of the children and only 9 as part of a special project, whereas another 46 centers were trying to collect information by contacting the infertility specialist, pediatrician, or nurses.

Concerning the incidence of congenital malformations, among 2,486 children born after ICSI with ejaculated sperm, 47 major (1.9%) and 185 minor (7.4%) malformations were reported, whereas no major and 3 minor (2.5%) ones were observed in 119 babies born from epididymal sperm and 3 major (4.8%) and 2 minor (3.2%) malformations in 63 babies from testicular sperm. Similar results were also recorded in children born with frozen/thawed ICSI embryos, but the numbers for epididymal and testicular spermatozoa were too small. This incidence of major and minor congenital malformations using sperm of all categories is consistent with the ones reported previously for ICSI[11,15,16] and IVF,[15,16] but it is also within the range observed in the general population.[17,18] However, the definition of major and minor malformations is of critical importance. Thus, according to the definition used by Bonduelle *et al.*[16] and adapted by the ESHRE ICSI Task Force,[19] major malformations are those that generally cause functional impairment or require surgical correction. Recently, Kurinczuk *et al.*,[20] using the definition of the British Paediatric Association's ICD-9 system and the Centers for Disease Control and Prevention in the USA, recalculated the incidence of major malformations reported by Bonduelle *et al.*[21] and found them to be significantly increased (TABLE 1). However, as pointed out by Bonduelle *et al.*[22] in their response, the higher rate is probably due to the different definitions as well as to overestimation of certain transient cardiac defects in ICSI babies due to extensive investigation.

On the other hand, prenatal genetic screening of 539 fetuses born after ICSI with ejaculated, epididymal, and testicular sperm revealed 11 abnormal karyotypes (2%), whereas the postnatal screening of 99 babies showed 2 abnormal karyotypes (2%). Furthermore, in 27 prenatal karyotypes of fetuses from frozen/thawed embryos, one (3.7%) was abnormal, but these numbers are too small to draw any conclusions.[3,4]

In a recent paper, Bonduelle *et al.*[23] studied a total of 1,082 prenatal tests carried out by amniocentesis and chorionic villus sampling. In these 1,082 tests, they observed 18 (1.66%) de novo chromosomal aberrations; 9 of these (0.83%) were sex chromosomal aberrations and another 9 (0.83%) were autosomal aberrations (triso-

TABLE 1. Prevalence of major malformations in children born after intracytoplasmic sperm injection according to different classifications

Classifications	Prevalence	Confidence interval
Belgian classification[21]	3.33%	1.99 to 5.55%
Western Australian classification[20]	7.38%[a]	5.04 to 10.31%
Recalculation by Belgian group[22]	5.23%[b]	—
General Australian population	3.78%[c]	3.67 to 3.90%

NOTE: *a* versus *c*: odds ratio 2.03, $p < 0.0002$; *b* versus *c*: odds ratio 1.406, p = NS.

mies and structural). This rate of sex chromosomal aberrations is significantly increased in ICSI children compared to the general neonatal population.[24] The incidence of autosomal aberrations is also higher in those children, partly because of increased trisomies at higher maternal ages and partly because of an incease in the structural de novo aberrations observed (0.36% compared to 0.07% in the general neonatal population).[24] In addition, Bonduelle *et al.*[23] found a higher incidence of inherited abnormalities mostly derived from the fathers.

This distinction of chromosomal abnormalities cannot be applied to the data collected by the ICSI Task Force, because they were not recorded separately. However, the total incidence of 2% observed in this report, which probably includes both types of abnormalities, is close to the 2.5% reported by Bonduelle *et al.*[23] It seems, therefore, that the rate of chromosomal aberrations in children after ICSI is slightly elevated. This is probably related to the problem of male infertility per se. For this reason, performing karyotypes of the male partners is recommended to detect the preexisting aberrations. Furthermore, because the available data indicates that the rate of de novo chromosomal aberrations of 1.6% is higher than the risk of amniocentesis (0.5%), it seems justified to counsel couples to have prenatal screening until this issue is resolved with higher numbers.

CONCLUSIONS

All gathered data concerning ICSI during the period 1993–1995 show a high success rate of fertilization and achievement of pregnancy irrespective of the origin of sperm. Moreover, the risk of major or minor congenital malformations apparently is not increased, but a slight increase in chromosomal aberrations, especially of the sex chromosomes, is observed. Undoubtedly, this database is not large enough to allow definite conclusions, and this further supports the need to continue the follow-up of children born after ICSI. Centers should be encouraged to join collective efforts such as the ESHRE Task Force on ICSI.

REFERENCES

1. PALERMO, G., H. JORIS, P. DEVROEY & A.C. VAN STEIRTEGHEM. 1992. Pregnancies after intracytoplasmic injection of single spermatozoon into an oocyte. Lancet **340:** 17–18.
2. BUTLER, D. 1995. Spermatid injection fertilizes ethics debate. Nature **377:** 277.
3. TARLATZIS, B.C. & H. BILI. 1998. Survey on intracytoplasmic sperm injection: report from the ESHRE ICSI Task Force. Hum. Reprod. **13:** 165–177.

4. TARLATZIS, B.C. & H. BILI. 1998. Clinical outcome of ICSI: results of the ESHRE Task Force. *In* Treatment of Infertility: The New Frontiers. M. Filicori & C. Flamigni, Eds. :301–308. Communications Media for Education. New Jersey, USA.
5. TOURNAYE, H., G. VERHEYEN, P. NAGY *et al.* 1997. Are there any predictive factors for successful testicular sperm recovery in azoospermic patients? Hum. Reprod. **12:** 80–86.
6. TOUMAYE, H., P. DEVROEY, M. CAMUS *et al.* 1992. Comparison of in-vitro fertilization in male and tubal infertility:a 3 year survey. Hum. Reprod. **7:** 218–222.
7. TARLATZIS, B.C. 1996. Report on the activities of the ESHRE Task Force on Intracytoplasmic Sperm Injection. *In* Genetics and Assisted Human Conception. A. Van Steirteghem, P. Devroey & I. Liebaers, Eds. Oxford University Press. Hum. Reprod. **11** (Suppl. 4)**:** 160–186.
8. LANCASTER, P., E. SHAFIR & J. HUANG. 1995. Assisted conception Australia and New Zealand 1992 and 1993. AIHW National Perinatal Statistics Unit: Assisted Conception Series No. 1, Sydney.
9. MARCUS, S.F. & P.R. BRINSDEN. 1995. Analysis of the incidence and risk factors associated with ectopic prengancy following in vitro fertilization and embryo transfer. Hum. Reprod. **10:** 199–203.
10. STAESSEN, C., Z.P. NAGY, J. LIU *et al.* 1995. One year's experience with elective transfer of two good quality embryos in the human in-vitro fertilization and intracytoplasmic sperm injection programmes. Hum. Reprod. **10:** 3305–3312.
11. WISANTO, A., M. MAGNUS, M. BONDUELLE *et al.* 1995. Obstetric outcome of 424 pregnancies after intracytoplasmic sperm injection. Hum. Reprod. **10:** 2713–2718.
12. WISANTO, A., M. BONDUELLE, M. CAMUS *et al.* 1996. Obstetric outcome of 904 pregnancies after intracytoplasmic sperm injection. *In* Genetics and Assisted Human Conception. A. Van Steirteghem, P. Devroey & I. Liebaers, Eds. Oxford University Press. Hum. Reprod. **11:** 121–130.
13. LANCASTER, P.A.L. 1996. Registers of in-vitro fertilization and assisted conception. *In* Genetics and Assisted Human Conception. A. Van Steirteghem, P. Devroey & I. Liebaers, Eds. Oxford University Press. Hum. Reprod. **11** (Suppl. 4)**:** 89–109.
14. YANAGIMACHI, R. 1995. Is an animal model needed for intracytoplasmic sperm injection (ICSI) and other assisted reproduction technologies? Hum. Reprod. **10:** 2525–2526.
15. BONDUELLE, M., S. DESMYTTERE, A. BUYSSE *et al.* 1994. Prospective follow-up study of 55 children born after subzonal insemination and intracytoplasmic sperm injection. Hum. Reprod. **9:** 1765–1766.
16. BONDUELLE, M., J. LEGEIN, M.-P. DERDE *et al.* 1995. Comparative follow-up study of 130 children born after intracytoplasmic sperm injection and 130 children born after in-vitro fertilization. Hum. Reprod. **10:** 3327–3331.
17. OFFICE OF POPULATION CENSUSES AND SURVEYS. 1988. Congenital malformation statistics: perinatal and infant social and biological factors. Nos 18 and 20, 1985 and 1986. London. HMSO (OPCS series DH3).
18. NEW YORK STATE DEPARTMENT OF HEALTH. 1990. Congenital malformations registry annual report. Statistical summary of children born in 1986 and diagnosed through 1988.
19. KURINCZUK, J.J. & C. BOWER. 1997. Birth defects in infants conceived by intracytoplasmic sperm injection: an alternative interpretation. Br. Med. J. **315:** 1260–1265.
20. BONDUELLE, M., A. BUYSAC, E. VAN AASCHE *et al.* 1996. Prospective follow-up study of 877 children born after intracytoplasmic sperm injection ICSI with ejaculated, epididymal and testicular spermatozoa and after replacement of cryopreserved embryos obtained after ICSI. Hum. Reprod. **11:** 131–155.
21. BONDUELLE M., P. DEVROEY, I. LIEBAERS & A. VAN STEIRTEGHEM. 1997. Commentary: Major defects are overestimated. Br. Med. J. **315:** 1265.
22. BONDUELLE, M. (Editorial) 1998. Incidence of chromosomal aberrations in children born after assisted reproduction through intracytoplasmic sperm injection. Hum. Reprod. **13:** 781–782.
23. JACOBS, P.A., C. BROUNE, N. GREGSON *et al.* 1992. Estimates of the frequency of chromosome anomalies detectable using moderate levels of banding. J. Med. Genet. **29:** 103–110.

Assessing the Outcome of IVF

ALLAN TEMPLETON

Department of Obstetrics & Gynaecology, University of Aberdeen, Aberdeen Maternity Hospital, Cornhill Road, Aberdeen, AB25 2ZD, Scotland

INTRODUCTION

The importance of *in vitro* fertilization (IVF) as a treatment option has become apparent at a time when there is increasing recognition that many previously used treatments are ineffective or less effective. However, IVF is not effective in all situations and circumstances. Treatment still strongly depends on the skill and expertise of the staff involved. Certain groups of women, particularly older women, have consistently poor success rates, and it is now acknowledged that other characteristics having to do with the couple are important in determining outcome. Furthermore, it is common practice to replace several embryos in an attempt to enhance pregnancy rates, but the risk of multiple pregnancy is considerable, and the wisdom of this approach is being questioned. Finally, IVF can only be described as effective if it can be shown to do better than no treatment, and study of background spontaneous pregnancy rates indicates that this might not always be the case. Each of these issues is addressed.

VARIATION IN SUCCESS RATES AMONG CLINICS

The literature is replete with studies purporting to show improvements in success rates, arising out of developments in clinical and scientific techniques. What has never been clear, however, is why similar clinics, apparently employing the same methods, can have such varying results. In the UK, the live birth rates per cycle started vary from 0–28%[1] with an average rate of 15%. The equivalent average figure in the US is nearly 20%,[2] and there is also wide variation in results.[3] Clearly, more could be learned by examining the practices and individual expertise provided in those clinics recording consistently higher than average pregnancy rates.

PATIENT CHARACTERISTICS AFFECTING OUTCOME

Age

Female age is the single most important factor in determining spontaneous fertility, and the effect of age is equally apparent, if not enhanced, when the outcome of all forms of fertility treatment is considered. The effect is particularly strong when the outcome of IVF treatment is considered.[4–6] Using the database established in 1991 by the Human Fertilisation and Embryology Authority (HFEA), Templeton *et al.*[7] examined the relation between age and IVF outcome. Pregnancy rates were highest between the ages of 25 and 35 years. Prior to 25 years, there was a very slight reduction in success rates, which so far remains unexplained. After 35 years, there was a steep decline in success, such that no pregnancies (using the patient's own eggs) were recorded in patients over the age of 45 years.

The effects of age are also apparent in the recently published 1995 Assisted Reproduction Technology Success Rates from the United States and Canada,[8] where 77% of women having assisted reproduction (IVF and GIFT) are between 30 and 40 years of age. Success rates are fairly constant (around 25% live births per cycle) until the age of 34 years, when there is a steep decline. Again no pregnancies were recorded among women over the age of 46 years.

DURATION OF INFERTILITY

It is well established that the duration of infertility is a major factor in determining the likelihood of spontaneous pregnancy in untreated infertile patients,[9,10] and this effect has been quantified to some extent in the study by Collins *et al.*[11] However, in relation to treatment, few studies have been sufficiently large to assess the separate effects on outcome of duration of infertility *and* age. Using the HFEA database, it has been possible to show a highly significant effect of duration of infertility (adjusted for woman's age) on the outcome of IVF treatment. For example, at 1–3 years' duration of infertility, the percentage of live births per cycle was 15.3% (95% CI 14.6–16.1), and at greater than 12 years it was 8.6% (7.4–10.1), that is, nearly halved. Information on duration of infertility is not available from the US Registry.

PREVIOUS PREGNANCY HISTORY

The existence of a previous pregnancy, and particularly a previous live birth, improves the likelihood of a spontaneous pregnancy in subfertile couples.[11] Analysis of the HFEA database indicated that any pregnancy will enhance the likelihood of a live birth following IVF treatment. This effect is considerably enhanced if the prior pregnancy ended in a live birth and is further enhanced if the live birth was the result of prior IVF treatment. A similar effect was noted in the US database, with enhancements of 16–25% in success rates, depending on the age group, associated with a previous live birth.

PREVIOUS CYCLES OF TREATMENT

HFEA data indicate that couples have the highest chance of becoming pregnant in the first IVF cycle and that there is a slight but significant decrease in the live birth rate for each subsequent cycle (age adjusted). This finding is in contrast to that documented in the French Registry[12] where a similar decrease was noted, which was no longer significant after adjusting for age and which was in turn significantly related to the rank of the attempt. Data on the effect of the number of previous unsuccessful attempts are not available in the American Registry.

CAUSE OF INFERTILITY

Before the advent of intracytoplasmic sperm injection (ICSI), male infertility was recognized to significantly comprise the outcome of IVF treatment.[4,5] Recent successful assisted reproductive techniques (SART) database reports on male infertility treated by conventional IVF suggest reductions of around 10% when female age was less than 39 years.

There is, however, continuing uncertainty about the effect of female causes of infertility and also of unexplained infertility on IVF outcome. The HFEA database failed to demonstrate any evident association between an individual cause of infertility and overall outcome when adjusted for age and duration of infertility. When live births per *embryo transfer* were calculated, however, there was a significant difference when comparing tubal disease with unexplained infertility. This finding may be consistent with the suggestion that women with tubal disease, particularly hydrosalpinges, have reduced *implantation rates.* (For a recent review of the literature, see ref. 13). Indeed, it has been claimed that the presence of a hydrosalpinx could halve implantation rates.[14] What is less clear at this stage, although Nackley and Muasher[13] claim the evidence is strong, is whether surgical removal of the hydrosalpinx improves IVF success rates. Such an assertion will require the completion of a randomized, controlled study.

FACTORS AFFECTING THE OUTCOME OF ICSI TREATMENT

The introduction of ICSI treatment has revolutionized treatment of the male by making assisted reproductive techniques available to this group of infertile couples. ICSI has encouraged the introduction of surgical sperm recovery techniques which has further increased the options in this area. Both the HFEA and SART databases indicate that ICSI now seems to be more successful than conventional IVF treatment. To answer this question we analyzed the results from all UK centers doing more than 50 treatment cycles during the period July 1994–April 1996. Live birth rates were then adjusted for factors found to affect outcome in a logistic regression model. A comparison was then made between live birth rates per embryo transfer in the two groups. The Odds Ratio was 0.936 (95% CI, 0.86–1.02), indicating no significant difference in live birth rates when adjusted for these factors.

EFFECT ON OUTCOME OF NUMBER OF EMBRYOS TRANSFERRED

The high rate of multiple births following IVF treatment remains a major concern and is a direct consequence of the number of embryos transferred. Morbidity and costs associated with multiple birth are considerable, to the extent that multiple pregnancy is increasingly felt to be an unacceptable consequence of the pressures experienced by patients and clinicians to maximize pregnancy rates. Centers in many countries have adopted two-embryo transfer policies to minimize multiple pregnancy.[15–19] Others have argued that a more flexible approach is appropriate, particularly

TABLE 1. Predicting outcome (adjusted live birth rate, %)

Age (yr)	Pregnancy	Duration	Spontaneous 1 Year	IVF
28			21	16
28		Short	36	20
28	Yes	Short	66	26
34			14	14
34		Short	24	17
34	Yes	Short	44	22

in older women, and several countries continue to report high order embryo replacements.[2,20–22]

Using the HFEA database of cycles registered during the period 1991–1995, we studied the factors affecting the likelihood of multiple births following embryo replacement.[23] In a logistic regression it became apparent that woman's age, tubal infertility, four or more previous IVF attempts, and long duration of infertility all significantly reduced both the likelihood of a birth and the likelihood of a multiple birth. However, the most interesting finding related to the number of eggs fertilized and hence available for transfer. In almost all circumstances in which four or more embryos were available, replacement of two as opposed to three embryos resulted in an equivalent live birth rate, while at the same time significantly reducing the likelihood of a multiple birth. This appeared to be so at all ages studied. Thus, the number of embryos *available* for transfer seems to be more important than the number of embryos *actually* transferred.

EFFECTIVENESS OF IVF TREATMENT

The efficacy of IVF can only be accepted if treatment can be shown to do better, in defined circumstances, than other comparative treatments or no treatment at all. In relation to the occurrence of spontaneous pregnancy in subfertile couples, it has been known for some time that woman's age, previous pregnancy, and duration of infertility will each affect outcome. The relative weight of these factors has been quantified in the study by Collins *et al.*[11]

Using these data and data extracted from the HFEA database, we compared the anticipated spontaneous pregnancy rates with those that might be expected following IVF treatment in several instances in which infertility was unexplained (TABLE 1). In a woman aged 28, the effects of previous pregnancy and the short duration of infertility were considered. IVF (assuming one cycle of treatment) could not compete with the spontaneous pregnancy rate expected in the absence of treatment, during a 1-year follow-up. In a woman aged 34, only when infertility was primary and the duration of infertility long would it be expected that IVF could produce comparable results to no treatment.

CONCLUSION

In addition to the expertise of individual clinics, certain patient characteristics, chiefly a woman's age, significantly affect the outcome of IVF treatment. Furthermore, it is clear that in many circumstances replacement of only two embryos can be done without any reduction in overall birth rates. More work is needed, using existing databases, on the effectiveness of IVF treatment in defined circumstances.

REFERENCES

1. HFEA. 1997. Human Fertilisation and Embryology Authority Sixth Annual Report.: 1-45.
2. Centers for Disease Control and Prevention. US Dept. of Health and Human Services. 1997. 1995 Assisted Reproductive Technology Success Rates. National Summary and Fertility Clinic Reports. **3:** 1–23.
3. Chapko, K.M., M.R. Weaver, M.K. Chapko, D. Pasta & G.D. Adamson. 1995. Stability of in vitro fertilization-embryo transfer success rates from the 1989, 1990, and 1991 clinic-specific outcome assessments. Fertil. Steril. **64:** 757–763.
4. Hull, M.G., H.A. Eddowes & U. Fahy. 1992. Expectations of assisted conception for infertility. Br. Med. J. **304:** 1465–1469.
5. Tan, S.L., P. Royston & S. Campbell. 1992. Cumulative conception and livebirth rates after in-vitro fertilisation. Lancet **339:** 1390–1394.
6. Roseboom, T.J., J.P.W. Wermeiden, E. Schoute, J.W. Lens & R. Schats. 1995. The probability of pregnancy after embryo transfer is affected by the age of the patients, cause of infertility, number of embryos transferred and the average morphology score, as revealed by multiple logistic regression analysis. *Hum. Reprod.* **10:** 3035–3041.
7. Templeton, A., J.K. Morris & W. Parslow. 1996. Factors that affect outcome of in-vitro fertilisation treatment. Lancet **348:** 1402–1406.
8. Society for Assisted Reproductive Technology and the American Society for Reproductive Medicine. 1998. Assisted reproductive technology in the United States and Canada: 1995 results generated from the American Society for Reproductive Medicine/Society for Assisted Reproductive Technology Registry. Fertil. Steril. **69:** 389–398.
9. Templeton, A.A. & G.C. Penney. 1982. The incidence, characteristics and prognosis of patients whose infertility is unexplained. Fertil. Steril. **37:** 175–182.
10. Hull, M.G.R., C.M.A. Glazener & N.J. Kelly. 1985. Population study of causes, treatment and outcome of infertility. Br. Med. J. **291:** 1693–1697.
11. Collins, J.A., E.A. Burrows & A.R. Willan. 1995. The prognosis for live birth among untreated infertile couples. Fertil. Steril. **64:** 22–28.
12. FIVNAT (French In vitro National). 1993. French national IVF registry: analysis of 1986 to 1990 data. Fertil. Steril. **593***:* 595.
13. Nackley, A.C. & S.J. Muasher. 1998. The significance of hydrosalpinx in in vitro fertilization. Fertil. Steril. **69:** 373–384.
14. Fleming, C. & M.G. Hull. 1996. Impaired implantation after in vitro fertilisation treatment associated with hydrosalpinx. Br. J. Obstet. Gynaec. **103:** 268–272.
15. Staessen, C., Z.P. Nagy, J. Liu *et al.* 1995. One year's experience with elective transfer of two good quality embryos in the human in-vitro fertilization and intracytoplasmic sperm injection programmes. Hum. Reprod. **10:** 3305–3312.
16. Tasdemir, M., I. Tasdemir, H. Kodama, J. Fukuda & T. Tanaka. 1995. Two instead of three embryo transfer in in vitro fertilization. Hum. Reprod. **10:** 2155–2158.
17. Preutthipan, S., N. Amso, P. Curtis & R.W. Shaw. 1996. The influence of number of embryos transferred on pregnancy outcome in women undergoing in vitro fertilization and embryo transfer (IVF-ET). J. Med. Assoc. Thailand **79:** 613–617.
18. Grochowski, D., S. Wolczynski, M. Kulikowski, W. Kuczynski & M. Szamatowicz. 1997. Prevention of high-order multiple gestations in an in vitro fertilization program. Gynecol. Endocrinol. **11:** 327–330.

19. HORNE, G., J.D. CRITCHLOW, M.C. NEWMAN, L. EDOZIEN, P.L. MATSON & B.A. LIEBERMAN. 1997. A prospective evaluation of cryopreservation strategies in a two-embryo transfer programme. Hum. Reprod. **12:** 542–547.
20. AZEM, F., Y. YARON, A. AMIT *et al.* 1995. Transfer of six or more embryos improves success rates in patients with repeated in vitro fertilization failures. Fertil. Steril. **63:** 1043–1046.
21. WU, M.Y., S.U. CHEN, H.F. CHEN *et al.* 1996. How many embryos should be transferred in in vitro fertilization and tubal embryo transfer? J. Formosan Med. Assoc. **95:** 617–622.
22. SVENDSEN, T.O., D. JONES, L. BUTLER & S.J. MUASHER. 1996. The incidence of multiple gestations after in vitro fertilization is dependent on the number of embryos transferred and maternal age. Fertil. Steril. **65:** 561–565.
23. TEMPLETON, A. & J.K. MORRIS. 1998. Reducing the risk of multiple births by transfer of two embryos after in vitro fertilisation. N. Engl. J. Med. **339:** 573–577.

Autoimmune Antiovarian Antibodies and Their Impact on the Success of an IVF/ET Program

JAN HOŘEJŠÍ,[a] JINDRICH MARTÍNEK,[b] DANA NOVÁKOVÁ,[c] JINDRICH MADAR,[d] AND MILADA BRANDEJSKA[a]

[a]*Department of Obstetrics and Gynecology, 2nd Medical Faculty;* [b]*Department of Histology and Embryology, 1st Medical Faculty;* [c]*Department of Clinical Immunology, 3rd Medical Faculty, Charles University, Prague, Czech Republic*

[d]*Institute of Care for Mother and Child, Prague, Czech Republic*

ABSTRACT: In previous papers, we referred to studies of the influence of antiovarian autoantibodies on menstrual cycle disorders in adolescent girls. We examined autoantibodies against ooplasma, zona pellucida, membrana granulosa, theca folliculi interna, and lutein cells. In infertile women in the IVF/ET program, we studied the positivity of antiovarian antibodies and cytokines, namely, TNF-α and IL-1β, in follicular fluid correlated with the following subgroups, characterized by the outcome of *in vitro* fertilization, as follows: G, pregnant; F, fertilized; N, nonfertilized; and O, no oocyte gained. The presence of autoantibodies corresponds to the success or failure of the IVF/ET program. Our results support the hypothesis that antiovarian autoantibodies play an important role in both the endocrine and the reproductive function of the human ovary and that it can influence them negatively.

INTRODUCTION

The incidence of immunologic infertility is reported to vary between 5 and 79%.[1] *In vitro* fertilization and embryo transfer (IVF/ET) are very important in the treatment of couples[2,3] with unexplained infertility of immunologic origin, but the pregnancy rate remains within the 20–30% range. Comparatively limited data dealing with antiovarian antibodies in the serum and follicular fluid have been reported.[4–7]

Vallotton and Forbes[8] in 1966 were the first to refer to evidence of serum antibodies directed to the ooplasm of differentiating ovarian follicles. Since then, many reports dealing with different antiovarian autoantibodies (AOAs) have been published.[9] The different prevalence of these AOAs in primary and secondary amenorrhea[10] as well as primary and secondary sterility support the hypothesis of their significant role in reproductive function. The findings of AOAs in women's serum supplanted the former suggestion that the ovary represents an immunologically privileged organ. Evidence that immune processes take place in ovarian follicles was confirmed by findings of immunocompetent cells (about one third) in the *in vitro* cultured cellular composition of follicular fluid.[11] Simultaneously, different cytokines were detected in follicular fluid.[12] Because of the close association between the incidence of AOAs and reproductive function, we attempted to confirm these findings under simple repeatable model conditions.

This study examines the presence of AOAs in follicular fluid together with an estimation of some cytokines and compares these results with those of the IVF/ET program.

STUDY DESIGN

Samples of follicular fluid collected from 90 consecutive women in the IVF/ET program were cryopreserved for evaluation of autoantibodies. Retrospective analysis of data indicated that the mean age of these women was 31.7 ± 4.3 years. The patients were divided into four subgroups according to oocyte recovery, fertilization, cleavage, and embryo transfer as follows: (1) patients ($n = 27$) with successful pregnancy after embryo transfer; (2) patients ($n = 40$) without successful nidation of cleaving ova; (3) patients ($n = 15$) in whom oocytes were collected but their fertilization was unsuccessful; and (4) patients ($n = 8$) in whom no oocytes were recovered after follicle aspiration.

Antibodies directed to defined ovarian structures, including ooplasm (OO) and zona pellucida (ZP), as germline ovarian components and to cells of membrana granulosa (MG), theca folliculi interna (TI), and corpus luteum (LC) as steroid-producing components were investigated immunohistochemically. Cryostat sections of rat ovary were used to bind serum autoantibodies to target structures in the first step, and they were detected in the second step by incubation with swine antihuman immunoglobulin labeled by fluoroisothiocyanate (SwAHu/FITC, Sevac, Czech Republic) or by horseradish peroxidase (SwAHu/HRP) in the humidified chamber. Both steps were performed for 30 minutes with thorough washing in phosphate-buffered saline solution throughout the entire procedure.

Interferon-γ (IF-γ), interleukin-1β (IL-1β), and tumor necrosis factor-β (TNF-β) were measured by the standard ELISA method using commercial diagnostic kits. Results were statistically evaluated using Student's *t* test and Spearman's nonparametric test.

RESULTS

The first subgroup of 27 women (mean age 30.1 ± 4.0 years) underwent ultrasonographic implantation followed by biochemically confirmed pregnancy. Spontaneous abortion occurred in five cases in the first trimester; in another five patients, twins were successfully developed. Of note in the oocyte recovery and fertilization rate, 8 ± 5.2 oocytes (mean ± SD) were collected and 5.4 ± 3.7 of them were fertilized. Detectable levels of IL-1β were estimated in eight patients (29.6%) and had a mean value of 2.69 ± 1.23 (SD); TNF-β was indicated in seven patients (25.93%) and had a mean value of 10.71 ± 13.57 (SD). In only three women were both cytokines positive in the follicular fluid samples. Antiovarian autoantibodies were estimated as follows: anti-ooplasm antibodies (OO-Ab) were found in 3.7%; anti-zona pellucida (ZP-Ab) antibodies were not detected; increasing values of autoantibodies directed against steroid-producing-cells were as follows: antibodies to MG (MG-Ab) cells, 18.5%; to TI (TI-Ab) cells, 37%; and to LC (LC-Ab) cells, 70.4%.

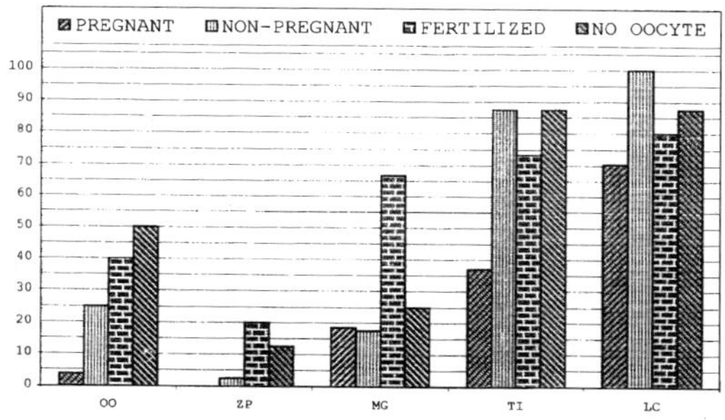

FIGURE 1. Prevalence of antiovarian autoantibodies in follicular fluids of IVF/ET program (in percentage).

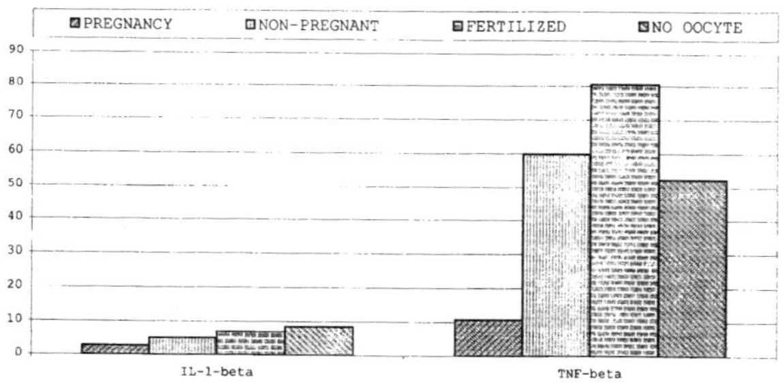

FIGURE 2. Mean level of IL-1-beta and TNF-beta in follicular fluids of IVT-ET program.

The second subgroup was comprised of 40 women whose mean age was 32.7 ± 4.5 years. Oocyte recovery presented a mean number of 5 ova (SD = 2.9) and 3.2 of them were successfully fertilized (SD = 1.9). Pregnancy did not occur after 37 embryo transfers, and in another three cases fertilized oocytes were not successfully transferred. In 77.5% of patients, measurable levels of IL-1β were estimated with a mean value of 4.97 ± 5.9 (SD) and TNF-β was identified in 45% subjects with a mean level of 59.9 ± 45.1 (SD). The prevalence of AOAs was 25% of OO-Ab, 2.5% of ZP-Ab, 17.5% of MG-Ab, and 88% of TI-Ab. LC-Ab were found in all women (100%) in this subgroup (FIG. 1).

The third subgroup contained 15 subjects whose mean age was 31.7 ± 3.3 (SD) years. The average number of aspirated oocytes was 3.1 ± 2.3 (SD) per intervention, but fertilization did not occur. Detectable evidence of IL-1β was ascertained in 60% of patients with a mean level of 7.00 ± 3.46 (SD), and in 66.7% of patients TNF-β was found with an average value of 80.60 ± 73.18 (SD). Antiovarian autoantibodies were present in this subgroup in the following percentages: 40% OO-Ab, 20% ZP-Ab, 66.7% MG-Ab, 73.3% TI-Ab, and 80% LC-Ab. One third of the subjects had four positive ovarian structures, one third had three immunopositive ovarian structures, and only one woman had completely negative follicular fluid (FIG. 2).

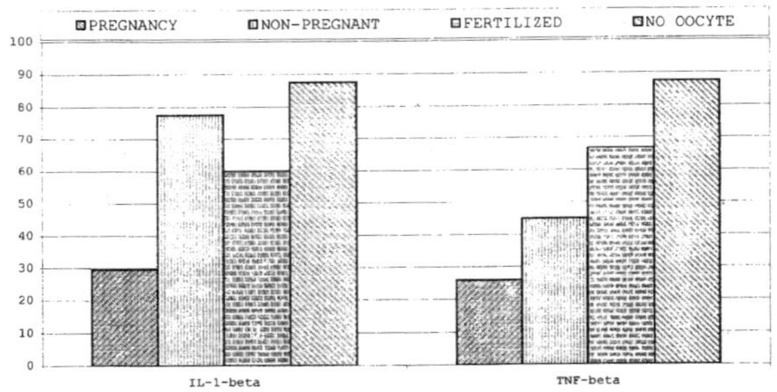

FIGURE 3. Prevalence of IL-1-beta and TNF-beta in follicular fluids of IVF-ET program (in percentage).

The last subgroup consisted of eight patients with a mean age of 32.4 ± 4.6 years. No oocytes were recovered during IVF, and investigation of aspirated follicular fluid indicated an 87.5% incidence of both cytokines (IL-1β, mean value 7.41 ü 5.89; TNF-β, 45.87 ± 35.32). OO-Ab were detected in 50%, ZP-Ab in 13%, MG-Ab in 25%, and TI-Ab and LC-Ab in 87.5% of patients (FIG. 3). Interferon-γ was undetectable in all follicular fluid tested.

DISCUSSION

According to reported data, several factors influence the outcome of IVF/ET, among which are the etiology of infertility, the patient's age, and ovulation induction as well as the quality of embryos and endometrial receptivity. Immunologic disturbances are involved in reproduction failure at all levels of early differentiation (gametogenesis, fertilization, nidation, and embryonic development). The findings of antibodies and their adverse effects on the reproductive process represent one possible mechanism of immunologic sterility.[4,13] Antispermatic[14,15] and antiphospholipid[16,17] antibodies affect the outcome. Antithyroid antibodies also play an important role in reproduction failure.[18,19] Furthermore, cytokines serve as proteinaceous mediators of the immune system. Some data[20,21] also demonstrate an active role of cytokines in the process leading to ovulation as well as in fertilization and early embryonic cleavage. In addition, their production appears to be modulated by gonadal steroids and pituitary hormones.[20,22] Our findings also confirm an increasing prevalence of TNF-β which is significantly linked to the outcome of IFV/ET (FIG. 3). In addition, the greatest prevalence of IL-1β in the subgroup with no retrieved oocytes agreed with the possible alteration of differentiating follicular oocytes due to increased levels of this cytokine in the follicular fluid (FIG. 2).

Results of the incidence of AOAs confirmed the adverse effects of estimated OO-Ab in the follicular fluid on the subsequent pregnancy. The effect seems to be exerted only in the first step of an IVF program, that is, oocyte recovery. ZP-Ab in the follicular fluid had a negative effect on the fertilization rate of harvested oocytes in the IVF program (FIG. 1). TI-Ab and LC-Ab could be associated with a defective luteal phase which is important for implantation of an early embryo. The greatest prevalence of MG-Ab in the subgroup with unsuccessful fertilization lends support to the hypothesis that the binding of that antibody to follicular cells in the cumulus-oocyte complex may be a defective signal in the fertilizing process (FIG. 1).

Evaluation of ovarian autoantibodies can be effective as a prognostic factor in the treatment of infertile patients and for the IVF/ET program. Antibodies against the germline components were significantly linked to oocyte retrieval and fertilization, whereas antibodies directed against steroid-producing-cells indicated a defective luteal phase and altered nidation of the early embryo.

SUMMARY

Collected samples of cryopreserved follicular fluid from 90 consecutive women in an IVF/ET program were studied to evaluate autoantibodies and some cytokines (interferon-γ, interleukin-1β, and tumor necrosis factor-β). Patients (mean age 31.7 ± 4.3 years) were divided into four subgroups according to the effects of oocyte recovery, fertilization, cleavage, and embryo transfer, as follows: (1) successful pregnancy ($n = 27$) after embryo transfer; (2) no successful nidation ($n = 40$) of cleaving ova; (3) unsuccessful fertilization ($n = 15$); and (4) no recovery of oocytes ($n = 8$) after follicle aspiration.

In the first group, anti-ooplasm antibodies (OO-Ab) were found in 3.7%; anti-zona pellucida antibodies (ZP-Ab) were not detected; antibodies to membrana granulosa (MG-Ab) cells were found in 18.5%, to theca folliculi interna cells (TI-Ab) in 37%, and to lutein cells (LC-Ab) in 70.4%; measured levels of IL-1β were estimated in 29.6%; TNF-β was indicated in 25.93%. In the second group the prevalence of AOAs represented 25% of OO-Ab, 2.5% of ZP-Ab, 17.5% of MG-Ab, and 88% of TI-Ab. LC-Ab were found in 100% of patients. Positive findings of IL-1β were exhibited in 77.5% of patients, and TNF-β was identified in 45% of subjects. In the third group, detectable evidence of IL-1β was found in 60% of patients, and in 66.7% TNF-β was found. AOAs were present in following percentages: 40% OO-Ab, 20% ZP-Ab, 66.7% MG-Ab, 73.3% TI-Ab, and 80% LC-Ab. In the fourth group, 87.5% of aspirated follicular fluid was positive for both cytokines (IL-1β and TNF-β) as follows: OO-Ab, 50%; ZP-Ab, 13%; MG-Ab, 25%; and TI-Ab and LC-Ab, 87.5%.

Results of the incidence of AOAs confirmed an adverse effect of OO-Ab in the follicular fluid for the subsequent pregnancy. ZP-Ab acted negatively on the fertilization rate of harvested oocytes in the IVF program. TI-Ab and LC-Ab could be associated with a defective luteal phase, which is important for implantation of an early embryo. The greatest prevalence of MG-Ab in the subgroup with unsuccessful fertilization supports the hypothesis that the binding of that antibody to the follicular cells of the cumulus-oocyte complex may signal a defect in the fertilizing process.

ACKNOWLEDGMENT

This work was supported by Grant NH/56643 from the IGA Ministry of Health, Czech Republic.

REFERENCES

1. Papale, M.L., A. Grillo, E. Leonardi *et al.* 1994. Assessment of the relevance of zona pellucida antibodies in follicular fluid of in-vitro fertilization (IVF) patients. Hum. Reprod. **9:** 1827–1831.
2. Kim, C.H., H.D. Chae, B.M. Kang *et al.* 1997. The immunotherapy during in vitro fertilization and embryo transfer cycles in infertile patients with endometriosis. J. Obstet. Gynaecol. Res. **23:** 463–470.
3. Van Voorhis, B.J. & D.W. Stovall. 1997. Autoantibodies and infertility: a review of the literature. J. Reprod. Immunol. **33:** 239–256.
4. Geva, E, N. Vardinon, J.B. Lessing *et al.* 1996. Organ-specific autoantibodies are possible markers for reproductive failure: a prospective study in an in-vitro fertilization-embryo transfer programme. Hum. Reprod. **11:** 1627–1631.
5. Moustafa, M., M.H. Ozornek, J.S. Krussel *et al.* 1997. The effect of antigamete antibodies on the success of assisted reproduction. Clin. Exp. Obstet. Gynecol. **24:** 67–69.
6. Ulcova-Gallova, Z. & T. Mardesic. 1996. Does in vitro fertilization (IVF) influence the levels of sperm and zona pellucida (ZP) antibodies in infertile women? Am. J. Reprod. Immunol. **36:** 216–219.
7. Crha, I., P. Ventruba, H. Vajciková & Z. Vlašán. 1995. Occurrence of the zona pellucida antibodies in infertile women. Scripta med. (Brno) **68:** 113–119.
8. Vallotton, M.B. & A.P. Forbes. 1966. Antibodies to cytoplasm of ova. Lancet **2:** 264–265.
9. Moncayo, R. & H.E. Moncayo. 1993. Autoimmunity and the ovary. Immunol. Today **13:** 2555–2557.
10. Horejsi, J., D. Nováková & J. Martínek. 1996. Circulating ovarian autoantibodies and FSH levels in adolescent girls with primary menstrual cycle disorders. J. Pediatr. Adolesc. Gynecol. **9:** 74–78.
11. Wang, L.J., M. Brannstrom, V. Pascoe & R.J. Norman. 1995. Cellular composition of primary cultures of human granulosa-lutein cells and the effect of cytokines on cell proliferation. Reprod. Fertil. Dev. **7:** 21–26.
12. Huyser, C., F.L. Fourie, E. Bosmans & P.F. Levay. 1994. Interleukin-1β, interleukin-6, and growth hormone levels in human follicular fluid. J. Assist. Reprod. Genet. **11:** 193–202.
13. Geva, E., A. Amit, L. Letner-Geva & J.B. Lessing. 1997. Autoimmunity and reproduction. Fertil. Steril. **67:** 599–611.
14. Shibahara, H.M., Y. Mitsuo, M. Ikeda *et al.* 1996. Effects of sperm immobilizing antibodies on pregnancy outcome in infertile women treated with IVF-ET. Am. J. Reprod. Immunol. **36:** 96–100.
15. Ford, W.C., K.M. Williams, E.A. McLaughlin *et al.* 1996. The indirect immunobead test for seminal antisperm antibodies and fertilization rates at in-vitro fertilization. Hum. Reprod. **11:** 1418–1422.
16. Balasch, J., M. Creus, F. Fabregues *et al.* 1998. Antiphospholipid antibodies and the outcome of pregnancy after the first in-vitro fertilization and embryo transfer cycle. Hum. Reprod. **13:** 1180–1183.
17. Coulam, C.B., B.D. Kaider, A.S. Kaider *et al.* 1997. Antiphospholipid antibodies associated with implantation failure after IVF/ET. J. Assist. Reprod. Genet. **14:** 603–608.
18. Sher, G., G. Maassarani, C. Zouves *et al.* 1998. The use of combined heparin/aspirin and immunoglobulin G therapy in the treatment of in vitro fertilization patients with antithyroid antibodies. Am. J. Reprod. Immunol. **39:** 223–225.
19. Kim, C.H., H.D. Chae, B.M. Kang & Y.S. Chang. 1998. Influence of antithyroid antibodies in euthyroid women on in vitro fertilization-embryo transfer outcome. Am. J. Reprod. Immunol. **40:** 2–8.
20. Simon, C. & M.L. Polan. 1994. Cytokines and reproduction. West. J. Med. **160:** 429–429.
21. Zolty, M., Z. Ben-Rafael, R. Meiron *et al.* 1991. Cytokine involvement in oocytes and early embryos. Fertil. Steril. **56:** 256–272.
22. Tabibzedeh, S. 1994. Cytokines and the hypothalamic-pituitary-ovarian-endometrial axis. Hum. Reprod. **9:** 947–967.

Ethical Aspects of Reproduction in the Next Century

SOZOS J. FASOULIOTIS AND JOSEPH G. SCHENKER[a]

Department of Obstetrics and Gynecology, Hebrew University, Hadassah Medical Center, Jerusalem 91120, Israel

ABSTRACT: **Doubtless, the technological advancements achieved in the current century in the area of young women's reproductive health care have also led to the evolution of very important ethical issues that will have to be dealt with in the coming century. Abortion, perhaps the most controversial issue of all, continues to raise a number of ethical issues related to the rights of the women versus the rights of the fetus, which, in addition to the risk of sexually transmitted diseases including the human immunodeficiency virus, emphasize the need for adequate family planning and sexual education. Genetic testing for late-onset diseases, disease susceptibilities, and carrier status may offer medical or psychological benefits; however, several complex ethical, legal, and social issues have been revealed with the advent of this new information. New family structures deviating from the traditional heterosexual couple, consisting of either single or lesbian mothers, have appeared, raising serious disputes regarding the welfare of the child. Important demographic changes are expected in the world population in the 21st century, characterized mainly by a significant increase of the older age groups.**

INTRODUCTION

The 21st century offers a bright vision of better health for all. It holds the prospect not merely of longer life, but superior quality of life as well, with less disability and disease. As the new millennium approaches, the global population has never had a healthier outlook. Such an optimistic view must be tempered by recognition of some harsh realities. Nevertheless, unprecedented advances in health during the 20th century have laid the foundations for further dramatic progress in the years ahead. Women's health is given special emphasis. The future of human health in the 21st century depends a great deal on a commitment to investing in the health of women in the world today. Their health largely determines the health of their children, who are the adults of tomorrow.

The recently completed century, and especially the last three decades, are characterized by an amazing and outstanding progress in obstetrics and gynecology, especially in the field of reproduction. *In vitro* fertilization (IVF) and assisted reproductive technology (ART) have become common practice in many countries today, regulated by established legislations, regulations, or by committee-set ethical standards.

[a]Address for correspondence: Joseph G. Schenker, M.D., Professor and Chairman, Department of Obstetrics and Gynecology, Hebrew University, Hadassah Medical Center, P.O. Box 12000, Jerusalem, 91120 Israel.

The rapid evolution and progress achieved in the area of young women's reproductive health care has, however, revealed certain ethical issues that have to be addressed in the coming century.[1] The risk of sexually transmitted diseases, including the human immunodeficiency virus (HIV) and abortion will continue to represent major issues, emphasizing the need for better sex education and contraception planning.[2]

Recent developments in genetic testing enable the physician to screen perspective patients for late-onset diseases, disease susceptibilities, and carrier status. Although this new information may be crucial in the prevention and/or early diagnosis of diseases, it raises serious concerns as it may lead to the social stigmatization of the involved person.[3] New family structures, deviating from the traditional heterosexual couple and including either single or lesbian mothers, have appeared, raising serious disputes regarding the welfare of the child.[4] Demographic changes anticipated in the next century, with the world population reaching about 8 billion by the year 2025 raise serious concerns, especially inasmuch as a significant increase in the older population is expected.[5]

This article presents a discussion about some of the ethical issues involved with the reproduction of young women, as they will appear in the 21st century, providing additional information about the anticipated demographic changes.

REPRODUCTION CONTROL

Recent developments in technology have greatly advanced our ability to control fertility, in terms of both enhancement and regulation. The advance in women's rights has put some of this control in the hands of women. Still, women are often entrenched in difficult situations resulting from the new developments and choices that are before them. Many millions of women in developing countries live in extreme poverty, and their health is negatively affected by the consequences of male domination. A low social status for women, including gender discrimination, exist even in developed countries. There are many ethical issues that derive from the application of reproduction control in young women's health. Young women's health can be enhanced if women are given the opportunity to make their own reproductive choices about sex, contraception, pregnancy, and other important events in their reproductive lives. The goal of improving young women't health will not be met without nondiscriminatory application of human rights principles to the special circumstances of women. These rights are specified in international and national human rights treaties and in national constitutions.

Abortion

Abortion is an intrinsic element of attempts to regulate fertility, expected to continue to have an important role in the 21st century. Induced abortion meets an important human need; it affects women's health and future and has profound demographic implications. No society has achieved low fertility without resource to abortion and, worldwide, close to 50 million abortions have been performed annually since the 1970s.[6] Most abortions are induced because the pregnancy is unintended and unwanted. However, social factors often conceal medical indications, like a pregnancy in adolescence, in women nearing menopause, or in poor women.

It is estimated that over 50% of abortions are obtained by women younger than 25, indicating an unappreciated, but real, problem of unintended pregnancy existing beyond the teenage years. In Western countries abortion rates peak about age 20. Women below 25 years of age obtain 56% of abortions in England and Wales, and 61% of abortions in the United States. Factors contributing to this high abortion rate among young women, include early menarche, early onset of sexual intercourse, sexual activity, single marital status, less frequent use of oral contraceptives, and economic instability, among others.[7]

Many couples cannot achieve a small family with existing contraceptive methods, owing to difficulties such as poor cosntraceptive services, side effects and complications, or misperceptions about risks and benefits. Also, some women may be unable to avoid unwanted pregnancies because of their limited negotiating power within sexual relationships.

The annual worldwide abortion rate is thought to lie between 32 and 46 abortions per 1000 women aged 15–44, varying worldwide from the lowest rate in the Netherlands (5/1000 women in their reproductive years) to the highest rate in the former USSR (186/1000). In the most developed countries, abortion rates vary from about 10 to 30 per 1000 women aged 15–44. This variation is due to differences in contraceptive prevalence, prevailing fertility preferences laws, policies relating to abortion and contraception, and the relation between abortion and contraception. The Netherlands offers a full range of available and cheap contraceptive options, access to sex education and information, and publicly funded abortion services.[8]

The debate on the ethical issues involving abortion carries some extreme views. For those who feel that life begins at conception, abortion will always be equated with murder, in which case there is no middle ground on the key question of abortion itself. Similarly, for those who believe in the absolute autonomy of the woman and her body, there is also no middle ground. Among both extremes are those who agree about the importance of finding ways to decrease the incidence of abortion. Encouraging a delay in the initiation of sexual activity, better sex education in the schools and at home, better information and access to contraceptive services for the sexually active, are but some of these ways.[9]

Even though a pregnancy may not be life threatening, it may be life devastating enough to force women to desperately seek and obtain an abortion by any means possible, even at considerable risk to their own lives. Many women will not accept living with children in poverty, sustaining a pattern of futility of life, living with a deformed or retarded child, or bearing an illegitimate child without paternal support. The difficulty in the ethical debate about abortion results from the lack of compelling analogies for which reasonable solutions have been devised.[10]

Despite the fact that many ethical issues involving abortion remain unresolved, the discussion has been centered on whether abortion should be legal or illegal. There are many countries where abortion is illegal and not regulated, such as several countries in Latin America, often leading to tragic results as some women who, for whatever reason, do not want to be pregnant will seek, often in desperation, the means to terminate the pregnancy.[11]

The most recent estimates from the World Health Organization indicate that 585,000 pregnancy-related deaths occur annually and that over 98% of these deaths occur in developing countries. Of these deaths, about 60,000–120,000 are related to complications of an abortion. As more abortions are undertaken with modern techniques, mortality may fall further, even in countries with restrictive laws. Most deaths from unsafe abortion occur in South Asia, sub-Saharan Africa, and the rural areas of Latin America. Complications of abortion, like hemorrhage, sepsis, and chronic pelvic infections (often associated with infertility) affect hundred of thousands of women each year and drain scarce health-care resources away from other reproductive health services.[12]

Where abortion is legal, available, and carried out under modern aseptic techniques, mortality is exceedingly low. Early termination of pregnancy ranks among the safest and easiest of surgical procedures. Therefore, the debate should be framed in terms of whether abortion should be safe or unsafe. Despite this, the first time abortion appeared on the international agenda was in 1994 at a conference in Cairo, Egypt, where it was recognized that the complications of abortion pose a serious public health threat and recommended that abortion should be provided safely, where it is not against the law.[8]

Teen pregnancy is a serious public health problem in many countries. This may stem in part from the double standard regarding sexuality that dominates society. There is blatant sexuality in advertising, television, and films. On the other hand, sex education in schools and at home is very limited. Countries that have dealt successfully with the problem have advocated increased sex education in the schools and wider access to contraception. Decreasing the incidence of teen pregnancies will undoubtedly decrease the demand for abortions.[13]

Other ethical issues related to abortion will continue to generate attention. They include such difficult issues as abortion for sex selection, a concern at all times but of particular importance in societies in which there is a strong bias towards males, and the concerns of those involved with the rights of the disabled, when abortion is used to terminate a pregnancy in which there is a deformity compatible with life that is in some way undesirable (i.e., Down syndrome).[14]

Access to safe abortion is critical to the health of women worldwide as well as to their social autonomy. The improvement of family-planning services, the availability of contraception, and the expansion of access to safe abortion are important means of achieving a low maternal mortality rate. These are all low-cost interventions, and their provision should be accelerated. Restricting access to abortion results in illegally performed procedures. Good contraceptive practice is a profoundly more efficient method for deterring pregnancy termination. The combination of good family planning and safe abortion will result in fewer embryos being destroyed and lower maternal morbidity and mortality rates.

Contraception

Women all over the world are increasingly taking control of their own fertility. Three major factors account for this evolution. Women are looking beyond a domestic and reproductive role, into playing an economically productive role in their societies. A technological revolution has introduced a range of effective contraceptive methods that are convenient to use. Governments and the international community realized that enabling women to control their fertility and to decrease the number of births is critical for checking rapid population growth and for speeding up the stabilization of the world population, and they are providing and promoting the necessary information and services.[15]

Currently, more than 50% of married women of childbearing age are using a form of contraception. This contraceptive prevalence varies widely between countries, ranging from 1% to 75%.[16] The trend for increasing contraceptive use is, however, universal in developing countries. Between 1960 and 1965 and between 1985 and 1990, the number of contraceptive users in all developing countries has increased from 31 to 381 million, in East Asia from 18 to 217 million, in Latin America from 4 to 44 million, in South Asia from 8 to 94 million, and in Africa from 2 to 18 million, and is anticipated to continue to increase in the next century.[17] Most of these users are women. Worldwide, the number of male users of contraceptive methods is only one third of the number of female users.

The regulation of human fertility will continue to be based on the use of steroids, barriers, sterilization, and abortion well into the 21st century. The oral contraceptive pill has perhaps been subject to more research and more post-marketing surveillance than any other pharmaceutical product. Current low-dose formulations provide positive health care for those under 30 years of age by reducing the risks of ovarian and endometrial cancer. Positive benefits probably continue until the age of 40 years, when balanced against the risks of an unwanted pregnancy. Contraceptive pills of the future (including steroidal formulations delivered as implants or vaginal rings, possibly in combination with nonsteroidal agents) could provide an even more positive approach to health care, with the focus on breast cancer, menstrual dysfunction, and osteoporosis.[18]

Barrier methods are essential for all except those who never change partners, until such time as another means is found to prevent the spread of HIV infection. Recent estimates have indicated that 120 million people, mainly located in Africa, Latin America, India, and Southeast Asia, will be infected by HIV-1 or HIV-2 by the year 2000.[19] Condoms for men and women have the potential to limit exposure to HIV, papilloma virus, and seminal immunosuppressive agents, but their acceptability remains low. Some improvements are now in sight. New designs are needed to enhance sexual pleasure for both men and women, new materials are required to improve shelf life in hot and ozone-polluted environments, and new spermicidal and antiviral agents are required to give added protection.

Voluntary sterilization, already the most widely used method of fertility regulation in the world, will probably continue to increase in importance. Some 140 million women and 65 million men have already undergone tubal occlusion or vasectomy. The medical cost of these procedures, however, continues to be too high for much of the developing world. Immunological and molecular procedures may provide a nonsurgical, low-cost approach.[18] Also, the widespread application of medical procedures based on the use of anti-progestagens could reduce the cost in medical services and patient morbidity.

Controversial ethical issues arise in the area of contraceptive research. Scientific priorities do not always match women's needs. The development of effective reversible contraceptives for women has proceeded faster than the development of similar methods for men. This reflects the prejudice about which sex should bear responsibility for contraception and the reality that many men refuse to use any male contraception. The fact that this trend does not change reflects women's need to gain reproductive control. Contraceptive research has been marred by ethically unacceptable studies, often leading to an unwanted pregnancy.[20] Another problem emanating from contraceptive research was that recommendations were slow to be implemented, thus occasionally exposing women to great risks. Unfortunately, there has been a significant reduction in contraceptive research and development in recent years, mainly as a result of expensive toxicology requirements, poor public image, the fear of litigation, and the lack of insurance. Only major policy changes will solve this paradox.[21]

Because sterilization is associated with the permanent elimination of the possibility for procreation, a number of ethical, legal, and religious issues have arisen often leading to personal misjudgments, legal disputes, and failure in applying family planning. These are heightened in the case of young women seeking sterilization who are motivated by a desire to remain childless. Their wish is often based on adverse emotional experiences in the past that have left them with the belief that they will be unfit mothers or that have engendered a strong desire for independence. The physician is confronted with the ethical dilemma of whether to perform an irreversible procedure, knowing that these young women may change their minds in the future.[22] Involuntary sterilization is currently not practiced, except in cases of severely mentally retarded people, who are unable to appreciate the consequences of their acts or care for their children and who may have a high likelihood of propagating hereditary disease. The issue of informed consent is even more complicated in the mentally retarded who might be candidates for involuntary sterilization. In these cases where voluntary consent cannot be obtained, the law, either by statute or court, should provide the necessary authority for involuntary sterilization. The absence of a specific legislation or court order does not permit the parent or guardian to give the requisite consent. Civil or criminal liability for assault and battery may be imposed on one who sterilizes another without following the procedure required by law.[23]

While the new contraceptive techniques offer better control, they also expose women to the risks and side-effects of long-term use, a hazard that arises from their reproductive roles. In order to achieve effective contraceptive use both in the developed and the developing countries, education campaigns are needed. Education must emphasize that the responsibility for contraceptive use lies not only with the female partner, but also with the male. Dissemination of information about the safety and efficiency of the contraceptive methods is of great importance, as is scientific research into the development of new contraceptive techniques. One group for whom education is especially important is teenagers, so that teenage pregnancies can be prevented, and the rate of abortions reduced.

SEXUALLY TRANSMITTED DISEASES

The dramatic demographic changes that have occurred in recent years have important implications for the sexual behavior of young women. Specifically, age at first marriage has increased, whereas age at sexual maturation and age at first intercourse have decreased. Taken together, these developments signify that a larger proportion of young women are unmarried and sexually active than ever before. This affects the level of sexual activity among young adults (i.e., the average number of partners) and, ultimately, the negative health impact of such activity (i.e., disease transmission, unplanned pregnancy).[24]

Young, sexually active women face an increasing number of sexual risks in their daily lives as evidenced by mushrooming rates of HIV infection and acquired immunodeficiency syndrome (AIDS) among heterosexual women, as well as an epidemic resurgence of sexually transmitted diseases (STDs) such as gonorrhea, herpes simplex virus, human papilloma virus, chlamydia, and syphilis. In addition, sexual transmission has assumed an increasingly important role in the spread of "nontraditional" STDs such as the hepatitis B virus and cytomegalovirus. Sexually transmitted diseases affect people in both developing and industrialized countries with an estimated annual incidence of curable STDs of 333 million new cases per year, an incidence that, unfortunately, is anticipated to increase in the next century.[25]

Sexually transmitted diseases pose significant and serious threats to young women's reproductive health and fertility, to their general well-being, and indeed to their very lives; whereas, in some cases, undiagnosed and untreated STDs may also result in devastating congenital infections in newborns. HIV infection is a transmissible disease with profound social and psychological implications for the woman, her partner, and her family as well as for the healthcare team and society. Vertical transmission from mother to fetus, or to infant via breast milk, may occur. Thus, physicians and healthcare providers have a critical role in preventing and treating sexually transmitted diseases.[26]

The impact of AIDS on society is disastrous. From being virtually absent from the human immunodeficiency virus epidemic in the 1980s, women estimated to be infected by the HIV now number close to 16 million. In 1995 alone, 2.3 million women became infected with HIV—in fact, close to half of all newly infected adults in the world today are women. Each day, 3000 additional women are infected and by the end of the year 2000, over 18 million women will have become infected and 4 million of them will have died.[27]

The primary ethical issues that have been raised revolve around the risk of transmitting the disease and in the case of HIV, the question of HIV testing of young women and, perhaps more complex, the testing of neonates. However, these issues bring sharply into focus the ethical conflict between patient privacy and confidentiality and the need to protect the sexual partners, the healthcare team, and the public.

Preventing the spread of STDs requires that persons at risk of transmitting or acquiring infections change their behaviors. Although we must appreciate the importance of confidentiality and patient privacy, the ethical responsibility of individual patients to prevent harm to others still exists. Every effort should be made through counseling to convince individual patients of their responsibility to others, including the importance of allowing such information to be used to protect sexual partners and healthcare workers.[28]

Because HIV infection has the potential of reaching epidemic proportions, the overriding consideration of infection control for the whole population comes into tension with the limits of individual rights. In addition to aggressive educational programs, other measures that may be considered are mandatory offering of antenatal screening and confidential disclosure of HIV status to sexual partners and to healthcare workers at risk of exposure. Information regarding numbers of seropositive individuals should be made available to public health officials.

The difficulty, and resulting ethical dilemma, is that HIV infection is not like any other infectious disease. Individuals who are informed of positive serostatus suffer severe psychological sequelae including the sense that they have been given a death sentence. Furthermore, discrimination based on seropositivity in regard to housing, jobs, and insurance exists. Physicians have a duty, therefore, to provide not only individual counseling and care for patients but also public advocacy to protect them from unfair and punitive actions.[29]

Informed consent must be obtained before testing for HIV infection and communication of the resultant information. If, in spite of every effort, consent is not obtained and the risk of transmission is high, under certain circumstances, with consultation, it may be justified to override patient confidentiality.

Because assisted reproductive technology requires the elective donation of gametes, embryos, or surrogate carriage of pregnancy and because of the elective nature of this technology, confidential counseling and testing should be included with the procedure. To protect the interests of those at risk of unwanted exposure to HIV, including the potential child, only seronegative individuals should be allowed to participate.[28]

The very high incidence of STDs worldwide (including HIV) is a serious public health issue. The increasing mobility of populations, urbanization, poverty, demographic changes especially in the developing countries, sexual exploitation of women, and changes in sexual behavior are some of the factors that will continue to place an ever-increasing proportion of the population at risk for STD infection in the 21st century. Prevention and control of STDs can be based on the promotion of responsible sexual behavior, general access to condoms at affordable prices, promotion of early resource to health services by people with STDs and by their sexual partners, prompt and appropriate management of STDs, inclusion of STD management in basic health care including maternal and child health, family planning and other reproductive health services, and targeted intervention for people at high risk.

GENETIC TESTING

The recent rapid advances in human genetics, largely fueled by the Human Genome Project, have resulted in an expansion of the number and range of genetic tests. These tests are capable of providing carrier and presymptomatic information, including risk of future disease, disability, and early death. In addition, these tests may reveal genetic information not only about the health of the individual, but also about his or her family members.

Genetic testing, as a means of identifying members of families who encompass a high risk of developing cancer, has been considered to be an area of major medical progress. Uncontrolled access to genetic testing raised a dilemma, however, especially when preliminary reports indicated that there was a strong interest both in the general population and in high-risk families for performing the test.[30] The complexities, and for the time being also uncertainties, of giving or receiving genetic counseling about the results of such tests in addition to complex medical, scientific, and technical matters such as the reliability of genetic screening tests, the interpretability and predictive value of positive test results, and the clinical ability to prevent cancers in presymptomatic individuals who test positive, prompted medical and scientific organizations to set the criteria for appropriate population testing.

Despite the biologic uncertainties, the potential discrimination, and other social and personal problems, biotechnology companies have developed and have already commercialized tests for the detection of gene mutations. The risk of a possible financial and also psychological exploitation of the public on the basis of the results appeared obvious.[31] Test providers explain the commercialization of such tests as being the result of increasing public demand and that argue that the incompleteness of our knowledge and the problems involved in the incorporation of testing into clinical practice do not provide sufficient grounds for withholding information.[32] The well-known principle in cancer diagnosis and treatment which states that "prevention is better than treatment and that early diagnosis is better than late diagnosis" is often used as an argument by these companies, which propose that genetic predisposition testing will aid in both prevention and testing. They conclude that insisting on further research before recommending widespread screening or suggesting that it should not be a decision for the patient alone is seen as unduly cautious or paternalistic.

Although the right of the patient to information is should be seriously considered and respected, several other issues, mainly those related to the ethical, legal, and psychosocial implications of test results, should in no way be ignored. Potentially, misuse of genetic information could have disastrous implications for the patient's psychological well being, family relationships, and future marital status, as well as create difficulty in securing employment and life or health insurance. In a study of the perceptions of 322 members of genetic support groups with one or more of 101 different genetic disorders in the family, it was found that as a result of a genetic disorder 25% of the respondents or affected family members believed they were refused life insurance, 22% believed they were refused health insurance, and 13% believed they were denied or let go from a job. Fear of being socially stigmatized resulted in 9% of respondents or family members refusing to be tested for genetic conditions, 18% not revealing genetic information to insurers, and 17% not revealing information to employers.[33]

As the fear of genetic discrimination exists, consideration of the issues of disclosure of information and confidentiality prove to be essential. Healthcare professionals should actively advocate that genetic testing for BRCA-1 and BRCA-2 and other mutations be used constructively to modify rather than to stigmatize individuals or deprive them of appropriate care.[34]

The American Society of Clinical Oncology, recognizing the danger of the creation of a genetic underclass that might be virtually uninsurable, supported legislation to outlaw discrimination on the basis of genetic characteristics. Various pieces of legislation have been formulated, and at least 24 states in the United States have enacted laws providing some protection against abuse of genetic information, in an insurance or employment setting.[35]

Psychological counseling with regard to carrier status is of great importance and should be included as part of any multidisciplinary team in a genetic test-performing clinic. Several psychological reactions have been observed by persons upon the announcement of the results of a BRCA test, ranging from parental guilt and depression after a positive result, to survivor guilt in the case of a negative result. A prospective study of 279 people with BRCA-1 linked hereditary breast or ovarian cancer showed no increases in depressive symptoms and functional impairment one month after disclosure of test results in BRCA-1 carriers, but those identified as noncarriers showed statistically significant improvement in psychosocial functioning. The need for further studies on the psychological impact of BRCA mutation testing is emphasized.[36]

The inheritance character of the revealed gene mutations also raises the possibility of performing genetic tests on the children of carriers, but currently there is a debate about whether parents have the authority to verify the possible gene status of their child for genetic diseases such as hereditary breast–ovarian cancer or Huntington's disease or any other late-onset genes that do not manifest until adulthood without that child's consent. Because the results of such a study may "stigmatize" an otherwise "normal" child for the rest of his life, the implication is that there should be a limit to parental authority. On the other hand, this scenario makes most desirable the idea of introducing alternative strategies including the early application of preventive measures or even gene correction for the betterment of as many human individuals as possible. Until that possibility appears, the ethical opinion widely accepted now seems to be that parents should not be free to have children screened for late-onset diseases before the children are able to consent.[37]

As the public's awareness for gene mutations enlarges, obstetricians will soon have to deal with requests for prenatal diagnosis of these mutations in possibly affected fetuses.[38] The procedure is relatively straightforward when the exact mutation in a parent is known, and the result is provided within a few days after performing prenatal testing in fetal cells, thus enabling a pregnancy termination if desired. The ethical issues related to abortion are even more complex in such cases, because the justification for aborting a fetus with a mutant gene might seem marginal given that the individual likely will be unaffected by cancer for many decades. The advent of preimplantation genetic diagnosis may provide couples who object to abortion with the opportunity for implanting embryos with normal genes, but again many ethical and religious issues have to be resolved before the application of this procedure in such cases becomes routine.[39]

In this transition period, healthcare professionals from many disciplines will be forced to integrate the rapidly evolving technologies and expanding knowledge base of cancer genetics into their patient care paradigms. Physicians without formal genetics training must begin to prepare for the new era of molecular medicine because they will be forced to advise patients contemplating genetic testing about the need for performing the test and the possibility of testing other members of the family and, most of all, to interpret the receiving results for the benefit of their patients.

REPRODUCTIVE TECHNOLOGIES: FAMILY STRUCTURE AND THE WELFARE OF THE CHILD

In spite of the changes that have taken place in the structure of the family in the latter part of this century, it remains the case that a family headed by two heterosexual, married parents who are genetically related to their children represents the ideal and that deviations from this pattern are commonly assumed to result in negative outcomes for the child. Restriction of IVF to married or cohabitant couples may be explained by the widely accepted public view that children raised in a family framework have an advantage over children living with a single parent.

Further development is anticipated in the next century in the field of *in vitro* fertilization and assisted reproductive technology, which will subsequently lead to a more widespread application of these new technologies. As a result, an increase in the frequency of these new forms of family structure is expected, enhancing further the need for evaluating family functioning and child development in such cases.

Most professional bodies in the various countries recommend that IVF-ART should be restricted to heterosexual couples, legally married or at least living in a stable relationship. In the majority of nations in Europe and in South America, IVF-ART is offered either to married couples or to couples maintaining a stable relationship, often stating that cohabitation of two years fulfills this requirement (e.g. France). In Asia, marriage is usually a requirement, as in many of these countries religion significantly influences social life (e.g., Iran, Saudi Arabia, and Jordan), whereas Hong Kong, India, China, and Israel allow these procedures also for cohabitant couples. Israel is the only country from the Asian region that provides IVF to single mothers. In Europe, this policy is found in Belarus, Italy, Netherlands, Russia, Spain, Ukraine, and the United Kingdom, whereas it is forbidden in South America mainly for religioous reasons. Other nations make no mention of a specific societal relationship for the prospective parents (e.g. Canada). In two nations (Denmark and Argentina) the statute is quite clear, and it specifies that IVF cannot be offered to lesbian or homosexual couples. The welfare of the child, from infancy to adulthood, is gaining worldwide acceptance as a basic factor in evaluating IVF-ART outcome, and thus some countries (e.g., Australia, Belgium, and Denmark) have already established some form of regulation or law regarding this issue.[1, 40]

Families that are the result of assisted reproduction, although continuously increasing in number, may differ from "normal" families, either because one or both parents are not genetically related to the offspring (sperm, egg, embryo donation, surrogacy) or because of structural differences. (It is well known that a growing number of single heterosexual women and lesbian women are opting for assisted reproduction.) In the United States, a woman has the right to decide when and how to conceive.[41] Under the European Convention of Human Rights (1978), a single woman or even a lesbian couple are entitled to have children, even though these children may have no legal father.[42] The creation of these new types of families also raises important questions about the psychological consequences for the children who result, and for this reason many have recommended that follow-up studies of these families should be carried out.[43]

The social recognition and acceptance of these families, their social context, and the processes through which social environments affect family relationships are issues that have received much attention and raised many disputes. It is important to emphasize that negative attitudes may exist toward the reproductive technologies themselves, with procedures such as IVF and donor insemination (DI) sometimes considered immoral or unnatural. As a result, families with a child conceived by assisted reproduction may experience overt prejudice not only from the wider community but also from relatives and friends.[44]

In this respect, sociological studies have shown that several aspects of parenting influence the development of their children; sensitive responding, emotional availability, and a combination of warmth and control are associated with positive outcomes, whereas marital conflict and parental psychiatric disorders have a negative effect.[45] Taking this into account, society is now facing the dilemma of determining the "ideal structure" of families resulting from assisted reproduction, in light of the fact that social groups formerly considered inappropriate for parenting have been reevaluated and their rights have been reconsidered.

A European study (conducted in Italy, the United Kingdom, Spain, and The Netherlands) about family relationships and the social and emotional development of children in families (heterosexual couples) created by IVF and DI compared these families with control groups consisting of families with a naturally conceived child and adoptive families. Mothers of children conceived by assisted reproduction expressed greater warmth towards their children, were more emotionally involved with their children, interacted more with their children, and reported less stress associated with parenting than mothers who conceived their children naturally. Similarly, fathers in assisted reproduction families were found to interact more with their children and to contribute more to parenting than fathers with a naturally conceived child. With respect to the children themselves, no group differences were found for either the presence of psychological disorder or for the children's perceptions of the quality of family relationships.[46]

Previous studies have reported that on average, children in single-parent families do less well than those in two-parent households in terms of both psychological adjustment and academic achievement. They are also less likely to go on to higher education and more likely to leave home and become parents themselves at an early age. In these cases, this rather nonoptimal outcome is explained not only by the fact that the child is raised by a single parent, but also by other factors that seem to play an important role, like economic distress and the psychological influences of being exposed to the conflict and family disruption that are commonly associated with their parents' separation or divorce.[47]

Children born to single mothers following donor insemination differ in important ways from children who find themselves in a one-parent family following divorce, in that they are raised by a single mother from the beginning without experiencing the detrimental effects produced by their parents separation. However, these families still have to face several social adjustment problems as a result of the occasional reluctance of the society to accept single-mother families and because of possible financial scarcity. These children might be forced to be more solitary and isolated as a result of the absence of the father.

Despite the lack of studies on single-mother families resulting from donor insemination, other studies focusing on fatherless or so-called "sole mother families" demonstrate that whether or not these children do less well than those from two-parent homes seems to depend on their financial situation and the extent to which their mother has an active network of family and friends to offer social support. The currently existing information indicates that the best predictor of outcomes for children in these families is the family circumstances rather than single parenthood per se.[48]

Lesbian families, although similar to the ones headed by a single, heterosexual mother in that the children are being raised by women without the presence of a father, do differ in the sexual orientation of the mother. The raising of a child by a lesbian couple encompasses certain disadvantages. First, these children have a higher possibility of developing psychological problems as a result of their family structure and the reactions it raises in society, especially at school. Second, the absence of a father eliminates the traditional father figure of a normal family model, endangering the normal sexual development of these children, that is, boys may be less masculine and girls may be less feminine. This might lead them into homosexuality, an outcome that is often considered undesirable by courts of law, policy-making bodies, and a large part of society.

Earlier studies investigating the outcome of children in lesbian families included women who had become mothers in the context of a heterosexual marriage before adopting a lesbian identity and who were compared with single heterosexual mothers. No differences between these children were identified in emotional well-being, quality of friendships or self-esteem, or in terms of masculinity or femininity. Regarding the parenting ability of the mothers themselves, it has been demonstrated that lesbian mothers were as just as child-oriented, just as warm and responsive to their children and just as nurturing and confident as heterosexual mothers.[49]

Controlled studies of lesbian couples who conceived their child through donor insemination have recently been published. In the UK, 30 lesbian-mother families were compared with 41 two-parent, heterosexual families using standardized interview and questionnaire measures of the quality of parenting and the socio-emotional development of the child.[48] Similarly, Brewaeys *et al.* studied 30 lesbian-mother families in comparison with 68 heterosexual two-parent families in Belgium.[50] These studies proclaim that the children's development, thus far, does not seem to differ from their peers in two-parent heterosexual families in terms of gender development, implying that the presence of the father is not necessary for the development of sex-typed behavior for either boys or girls and that the mother's lesbian identity, in itself, does not have a direct effect on the gender role or behavior of her daughters or sons. In terms of socio-emotional development, the children appeared to be functioning well; there seemed to be no evidence of raised levels of emotional or behavioral problems among the children raised in a lesbian-mother family.

These results show that society, either as expressed through laws or legislation or as influenced by religious or cultural issues, maintains in the majority of cases a more compassionate and supporting role to the normal heterosexual family (marriage or stable relationship) and hesitates to provide full access to other "deviated" groups. On the other hand, findings from recent studies suggest that all these "new" aspects of family structure may matter less for children's psychological adjustment than warm and supportive relationships with parents and a positive family environment.

It is our view that society, as we are progressing into the next century, should not seek to prevent any fertile person, whatever his or her marital status, from reproducing, and neither the n law nor professional bodies should discriminate against any group of the society. Each case should be judged on its merits, leaving aside the question whether or not infertile couples or single persons have an inalienable right to a child whatever the method or cost to society or themselves. A provision, however, should be in place that IVF in unmarried couples not be carried out without the written consent of the man involved. Regulatory bodies in countries dealing with assisted reproduction should set laws or other statutes by means of which the welfare of the offspring can be followed.

DEMOGRAPHIC CHANGES IN THE 21ST CENTURY AND WOMEN'S HEALTH

The world population is expected to face important demographic changes in the 21st century, which doubtlessly will have a significant impact. The global population, which was 2.8 billion in 1955, has reached 6 billion today; and, considering the fact that an increase of nearly 80 million people per year is seen, it is anticipated that by the year 2025, it will reach a total of 8 billion. Every day in 1997, about 365,000 babies were born and about 140,000 people died, giving a natural increase of about 220,000 people a day. Today's population is made of 613 million children under 5, 1.7 billion children and adolescents aged 5–19, 3.1 billion adults aged 20–64, and 390 million over age 65.[51]

Even so, the most important pattern of progress now emerging is an unmistakable trend toward healthier, longer life. Supported by solid scientific evidence of declines in disability among older people in some populations, this has considerable implications for individuals and for societies. The explanation for this trend lies in the social and economic advances that the world has witnessed during the late 20th century—advances that have brought better living standards to many, but not all, people. The world saw a golden age of unparalleled prosperity between 1950 and 1973, followed by an economic slump that lasted 20 years. A global economic recovery has been under way since 1994. The long-term benefits are now becoming apparent. Although they are most evident in the industrialized world, they are slowly but surely materializing in many poorer countries, too.

The average life expectancy at birth in 1955 was just 48 years, in 1995 it was 65 years, and in 2025 it will reach 73 years. It is expected that no country will have a life expectancy of less than 50 years. Today, over 5 billion people in 120 countries have a life expectancy of more than 60 years. Many thousands of people born this year will live through the 21st century and see the advent of the 22nd century. Whereas there were only 200 centenarians in France in 1950, by the year 2050, the number is projected to reach 150,000—a 750-fold increase in 100 years.[51]

This increase in aging has caused a serious change in the proportions among various ages within population groups, however, favoring mainly the older ones, a change that is expected to become aggravated in the 21st century. Specifically, in 1955, there were 12 people aged over 65 for every 100 aged under 20. By 1995, the old-to-young ratio was 16/100, and by 2025 it will be 31/100. The proportion of young people under 20 years will fall from 40% now to 32% of the total population by 2025, despite reaching 2.6 billion—an actual increase of 252 million. On the other hand, the number of people over 65 year of age will rise from 390 million now to 800 million by 2025— reaching 10% of the total population, whereas in many developing countries, especially in Latin America and Asia, increases up to 300% are expected in this specific age group. Globally, the population of children under 5 will grow by just 0.25% annually between 1995 and 2025, while the population over 65 years will grow by 2.6%.[51]

These demographic trends, which have profound implications for human health in all age groups, follow the many positive changes that have occurred in the past 50 years. More people than ever before now have access to at least minimum health care, safe water supplies, and sanitation facilities. Most of the world's children are now immunized against the six major diseases of childhood: measles, poliomyelitis, tuberculosis, diphtheria, pertussis, and neonatal tetanus.

During the same period, there have been steady and sometimes spectacular advances in the control and prevention of other diseases, the development of vaccines and medicines, and countless other medical and scientific innovations. The past decades have seen the final defeat of smallpox, one of the oldest diseases of humanity, and the gradual reduction in several others, including leprosy and poliomyelitis. Globally, adults are now surviving longer, largely because during the past half-century, when they were children, epidemics of infectious diseases such as tuberculosis and respiratory disease were being better controlled. The continuing gains in the survival of infants and young children means that the adult population is increasing.

Population aging raises serious social and ethical concerns. Currently, just over half the population is of working age, 20–64, and by 2025 the proportion will have reached 58%. The health of the adult population of working age will be vitally important if this age group is to support growing numbers of dependants, both young and old.

The proportion of older people requiring support from adults of working age will have increased from 10.5% in 1955 and 12.3% in 1995 to 17.2% in 2025. On the other hand, this highly productive part of the population also seems to be very vulnerable. More than 15 million adults aged 20–64 are dying every year, most of causes that are preventable. Among the most tragic of these deaths are those of 585,000 young women who die each year in pregnancy or childbirth. Also, 2–3 million adults a year are dying of tuberculosis, despite the existence of a strategy that could effectively cure all cases, whereas about 1.8 million adults died of AIDS in 1997. The annual death toll for AIDS is likely to rise. In addition, a decrease in the average number of babies per woman of childbearing age has been observed, from 5.0 in 1955 to 2.9 in 1995 and reaching 2.3 in 2025. Although only three countries were below the population replacement level of 2.1 babies in 1955, there will be 102 such countries by 2025, further aggravating the demographic problem.[51]

Population aging has also immense implications for all countries. In the 21st century, one of the biggest challenges will be how best to prevent and postpone disease and disability and to maintain the health, independence, and mobility of an aging population. Even in wealthy countries, most old and frail people cannot meet more than a small fraction of the costs of the health care they need. In the coming decades, few countries will be able to provide specialized care for their large population of aged persons.

Some European countries already acknowledge that there is insufficient provision to meet with dignity the needs of all those over the age of 75, who currently consume many times more medical and social services than those under 75. Developing countries will face even more serious challenges, given their economic difficulties, the rapidity with which populations age, the lack of social service infrastructures, and the decline of traditional care-giving provided by family members.

Women's health is inextricably linked to their status in society. It benefits from equality and suffers from discrimination. Today, the status and well-being of countless millions of women worldwide remains tragically low. As a result, human well-being in general suffers, and the prospects for future generations are dimmer.

In many parts of the world, discrimination against women begins before they are born and stays with them until they die. Throughout history, female babies have been unwanted in some societies and are at a disadvantage from the moment of birth. Today, girls and women are still denied the same rights and privileges as their brothers at home, at work, in the classroom, or in the clinic. They suffer more from poverty, low social status, and the many hazards associated with their reproductive role. As a result, they bear an unfair burden of disadvantage and suffering, often throughout their lives.

Global population aging is resulting in the evolution toward societies that are, for the most part, female. Yet while women generally live longer than men do, for many of them greater life expectancy carries no real advantage in terms of additional years lived free of disability. The status of women's health in old age is shaped throughout their lives by factors over which they have little, if any, control. If longer lives for women are to be years of quality, policies must be aimed at ensuring the best possible health for women as they age. These policies should be geared toward the problems that begin in infancy or childhood and should cover the whole life span, through adolescence and adulthood into old age.

The health of parents, particularly the mother, before and during pregnancy and the services available to her throughout her pregnancy, especially at delivery, are important determinants of the health status of their children. Infants whose health status is compromised at birth are more vulnerable to various health problems later in life. Girls who are inadequately fed in childhood may have impaired intellectual capacity, delayed puberty, possibly impaired fertility and stunted growth, leading to higher risks of complications during childbirth. Female genital mutilation, of which 2 million girls are at risk every year, and sexual abuse during childhood both increase the risk of poor physical and mental health in later years.

Most reproductive health and family-planning programs have not paid enough attention to the special needs of adolescents. Premature entry into sexual relationships; high-risk sexual behavior; and lack of education, basic health information, and services all compromise the current and future well-being of girls in this age group.

These girls are at increased risk of sexually transmitted diseases, including HIV/AIDS, early pregnancy and motherhood, and unsafe abortion. Adolescent girls are not physically prepared for childbirth, and are much more at risk of maternal death than women in their twenties. Inadequate diet during adolescence can jeopardize girls' health and physical development, with permanent consequences. Iron-deficiency anemia is particularly common among adolescent girls.

The consequences of poor health in childhood and adolescence, including malnutrition, become apparent in adulthood, particularly during the childbearing years. This time is a particularly dangerous phase in the lives of many women in developing countries, where healthcare services, especially reproductive health facilities, are often inadequate and where society puts pressure on couples to have many children. More than 50% of pregnant women in the developing world are anemic.

Where women have many pregnancies, the risk of related death over the course of their lifetime is compounded. The risk of pregnancy-related death in Europe is one in 1400, whereas in Asia it is one in 65, and in Africa, one in 16. Many millions of women are made old before their time by the daily harshness and inequalities of their earlier lives, beginning in childhood. They experience poor nutrition, reproductive ill-health, dangerous working conditions, violence and lifestyle-related diseases, all of which exacerbate the likelihood of breast and cervical cancers, osteoporosis, and other chronic conditions after menopause. In old age poverty, loneliness, and alienation are common.

CONCLUSION

Further development in the area of reproductive health care of young women is anticipated in the next century, and therefore a more thorough review and analysis of the ethical issues is needed. Health professionals involved in the field of public health and reproductive health care of young women must be active and effective participants in these ethical considerations.

REFERENCES

1. SCHENKER, J.G. 1997. Assisted reproduction practice in Europe: legal and ethical aspects. Hum. Reprod. Up. **3:** 173–184.
2. DICZFALUSY, E. 1991. Contraceptive prevalence, reproductive health, and our common future. Contraception **43:** 201–207.
3. MACDONALD, D.J. 1998. Genetic predisposition testing for cancer: effects on families' lives. Holist. Nurs. Pract. **12:** 9–19.
4. COLPIN, H., *et al.* 1995. New reproductive technology and the family: the parent–child relationship following *in vitro* fertilization. J. Child Psychol. Psychiatr. **36:** 1429–1441.
5. WORLD HEALTH ORGANIZATION. 1990. Division of epidemiological surveillance and health situation and trend assessment. Global estimates for health situation assessment and projections. WHO/HST/90.2. World Health Organization. Geneva.
6. TIETZE, C. *et al.* 1986. Induced abortions: a world review, 1986. Alan Guttmacher Institute. New York.
7. DAVID, H.P. 1992. Abortion in Europe, 1920–91: a public health perspective. Stud. Fam. Plann. **23:** 1–22.
8. KULCZYCKI, A. *et al.* 1996. Abortion and fertility regulation. Lancet **347:** 1663–1668.
9. SCHENKER, J.G. & V.H. EISENBERG. 1997. Ethical issues relating to reproduction control and women's health. Int. J. Gynecol. Obstet. **58:** 167–176.
10. RYAN, K.J. 1992. Abortion or motherhood, suicide and madness. Am. J. Obstet. Gynecol. **166:** 1029–1036.
11. ROYSTON, R.W. & J. FERGUSON. 1985. The coverage of maternity care: a critical review of available information. World Health Stat. Q. **38:** 267–288.
12. WHO DIVISION OF REPRODUCTIVE HEALTH, UNSAFE ABORTION. 1998. Global and regional estimates of incidence of and mortality due to unsafe abortion with a listing of available country data. 3rd edit. WHO/RHT/MSM/97.16. World Health Organization. Geneva.
13. HENSHAW, S.K. *et al.* 1989. Teenage pregnancy in the US: The scope of the problem and state responses. Alan Guttmacher Institute Press. New York.
14. REUBINOFF, B.E. & J.G. SCHENKER. 1996. New advances in sex preselection. Fertil. Steril. **66:** 343–350.
15. FATHALLA, M.F. 1993. Contraception and women's health. Br. Med. Bull. **49:** 245–251.
16. UNITED NATIONS POPULATION DIVISION. 1989. Levels and trends of contraceptive use as assessed in 1988. Population study No. 110, ST/ESA/SER.A/110. United Nations. New York.
17. UNITED NATIONS POPULATION FUNDS. 1991. The state of world population. UNFPA. New York.
18. LINCOLN, D.W. 1993. Contraception for the year 2020. Br. Med. Bull. **49:** 222–236.
19. POTTS, M. *et al.* 1991. Slowing the spread of human immunodeficiency virus in developing countries. Lancet **338:** 608–613.
20. NOTMAN, M.T. & C.C. NADELSON. 1980. Women as patients and experimental subjects. International Encyclopedia of Bioethics. pp. 1704–1713.
21. ROSENFIELD, A.G. 1994. Reproductive health: an ethical perspective. J. Reprod. Med. **39:** 337–342.
22. MYERSCOUGH, P.R. 1981. Sterilization. *In* Dictionary of Medical Ethics. 2nd edit. A.S. Duncan, G.R. Dunstan & R.B. Welbourn, Eds.: 417–420. Crossroad. New York.
23. MACKLIN, R. & W. GAYLIN. 1981. Mental Retardation and Sterilization: A Problem of Competency and Paternalism. The Hastings Center. Hastings-on-Hudson, NY.
24. SEIDMAN, S.N. & R.O. RIEDER. 1994. A review of sexual behavior in the United States. Am. J. Psychiatry **151:** 330–341.

25. HUTCHINSON, M.K. 1997. Something to talk about: sexual risk communication between young women and their partners. J. Obstet. Gynecol. Neonat. Nurs. **27:** 127–133.
26. RIZK, B. & S.R. DILL. 1997. Infertility among HIV-positive women. Counseling HIV patients pursuing infertility investigation and treatment. Hum. Reprod. **12:** 415–416.
27. MBOI, N. 1996. Women and AIDS in South and South-East Asia: the challenge and the response. World Health Stat. Q. **49:** 94–103.
28. SCHENKER, J.G. 1997. Prophylactic oophorectomy. FIGO Committee for the study of ethical aspects of human reproduction: Guidelines on the subject of AIDS and human reproduction. Hum. Reprod. **12:** 1619.
29. BAYER, R. 1991. Public health policy and the AIDS epidemic: an end to HIV exceptionalism? N. Engl. J. Med. **324:** 1500.
30. CHALIKI, H. *et al.* 1995. Women's receptivity to testing for a genetic susceptibility to breast cancer. Am. J. Public Health **85:** 1133–1135.
31. HEALY, B. 1997. BRCA genes—Bookmaking, fortunetelling, and medical care. N. Engl. J. Med. **336:** 1448–1449.
32. SKOLNICK, M. 1996. Commentary on the ASCO statement on genetic testing for cancer susceptibility. J. Clin. Oncol. **14:** 1737–1738.
33. LAPHAM, E. *et al.* 1996. Genetic discrimination: perspectives of consumers. Science **274:** 621–624.
34. GARBER, J.E. *et al.* 1996. Testing for inherited cancer susceptibility. JAMA **275:** 1928–1929.
35. MANN, G.B. & P.I. BORGEN. 1998. Breast cancer genes and the surgeon. J. Surg. Oncol. **67:** 267–274.
36. LERMAN, C. *et al.* 1996. BRCA-1 testing in families with hereditary breast–ovarian cancer. A prospective study of patient decision making and outcomes. JAMA **275:** 1885–1892.
37. SCHULMAN, J.D. & R.G. EDWARDS. 1996. Preimplantation diagnosis is disease control, not eugenics. Hum. Reprod. **11:** 463–464.
38. LANCASTER, J.M. *et al.* 1996. An inevitable dilemma: prenatal testing for mutations in the BRCA-1 breast/ovarian cancer susceptibility gene. Obstet. Gynecol. **87:** 306–309.
39. FASOULIOTIS, S.J. & J.G. SCHENKER. 1998. Preimplantation genetic diagnosis: principles and ethics. Hum. Reprod. **13:** 2238–2245.
40. SCHENKER, J.G. & A. SHUSHAN. 1996. Ethical and legal aspects of assisted reproduction practice in Asia. Hum. Reprod. **11:** 908–911.
41. MCGUIRIE, M. & N. ALEXANDER. 1985. Artificial insemination of a single woman. Fertil. Steril. **43:** 182–188.
42. EUROPEAN CONVENTION OF HUMAN RIGHTS. 1978. Art. 12 and 14. Strasbourg.
43. BLYTH, E. & C. CAMERON. 1998. Better the devil you know? An emerging issue in the regulation of assisted conception. Hum. Reprod. **13:** 25–34.
44. GOLOMBOK, S. *et al.* 1995. Families created by the new reproductive technologies: quality of parenting and social and emotional development of the children. Child Dev, **64:** 285–288.
45. RUTTER, M. 1985. Resilience in the face of adversity: protective factors and resistance to psychiatric disorder. Br. J. Psych. **147:** 596–611.
46. GOLOMBOK, S. *et al.* 1996. The European study of assisted reproduction families: family functioning and child development. Hum. Reprod. **10:** 2324–2331.
47. MCLANAHAN, S. & G. SANDEFUR. 1994. Growing up with a single parent: what hurts, what helps. Harvard University Press. Cambridge, MA.
48. GOLOMBOK, S. *et al.* 1997. Children raised in fatherless families from infancy: family relationships and the socioemotional development of children of lesbian and single heterosexual mothers. J. Child Psychol. Psychiatry **38:** 783–791.
49. PATTERSON, C.J. 1992. Children of lesbian and gay parents. Child Dev. **63:** 1025–1042.
50. BREWAEYS, A. *et al.* 1997. Donor insemination: child development and family functioning in lesbian mother families. Hum. Reprod. **12:** 1349–1359.
51. WORLD HEALTH ORGANIZATION. 1998. The World Health Report 1998: Life in the 21st Century—A Vision for All. Geneva.

The Perimenopausal Transition

LEON SPEROFF

Department of Obstetrics and Gynecology, Oregon Health Sciences University, Portland, Oregon 97201, USA

INTRODUCTION

There is only one marker, menstrual irregularity, that is used to define and establish what is called the perimenopausal transition. The *menopause* is that point in time when permanent cessation of menstruation occurs following the loss of ovarian activity. Menopause is derived from the Greek words, *men* (month) and *pausis* (cessation). The years prior to menopause, which encompass the change from normal ovulatory cycles to cessation of menses, are known as the *perimenopausal transitional* years, marked by irregularity of menstrual cycles. *Climacteric* indicates the period of time when a woman passes from the reproductive stage of life through the perimenopausal transition and the menopause to the postmenopausal years. Climacteric is from the Greek word for ladder.

Menstrual cycle length is determined by the rate and quality of follicular growth and development, and it is normal for the cycle to vary in individual women. Our best information comes from two longitudinal studies (with very similar results): the study of Vollman of more than 30,000 cycles recorded by 650 women and the study of Treloar *et al.* of more that 25,000 woman-years in a little over 2,700 women.[1,2] The observations of Vollman and Treloar documented a normal evolution in length and variation in menstrual cycles.

Menarche is followed by approximately 5–7 years of relatively long cycles at first, then by increasing regularity as cycles shorten to reach the usual reproductive age pattern. In the 40s, cycles begin to lengthen again. The highest incidence of anovulatory cycles is under age 20 and over age 40.[3] At age 25, over 40% of cycles are between 25 and 28 days in length; from 25–35, over 60% are between 25 and 28 days. The perfect 28-day cycle is indeed the most common mode, but it totaled only 12.4% of Vollman's cycles. Overall, approximately 15% of reproductive age cycles are 28 days in length. Only 0.5% of women experience a cycle less than 21 days long, and only 0.9% a cycle greater than 35 days.[4] Most women have cycles that last from 24 to 35 days, but at least 20% of women experience irregular cycles.[5]

When women are in their 40s, anovulation becomes more prevalent, and prior to anovulation, menstrual cycle length increases, beginning 2–8 years before menopause.[2] The duration of the follicular phase is the major determinant of cycle length.[6,7] This menstrual cycle change prior to menopause is marked by elevated follicle-stimulating hormone (FSH) levels and decreased levels of inhibin, but normal levels of luteinizing hormone (LH) and slightly elevated levels of estradiol.[8–12]

Contrary to older belief (based on the report by Sherman *et al.*[6]), *estradiol levels do not gradually wane in the years before menopause, but remain in the normal range, although slightly elevated, until 6 months to 1 year before follicular growth and development cease.* The data from Sherman *et al.*[6] were from a small cross-sectional study of one cycle collected from 8 women aged 46–56. More recent longitudinal studies of women as they pass through the perimenopausal transition reveal that estrogen levels do not begin to decline until less than a year before menopause.[12] Indeed, women experiencing the perimenopausal transition actually have higher overall estrogen levels, a response that is logically explained by an increased ovarian follicular response to the increase in FSH secretion during these years.[13]

As noted, most women experience a 2- to 8-year period of time prior to menopause when anovulation becomes prevalent.[2] During this time ovarian follicles undergo an accelerated rate of loss until eventually the supply of follicles is finally depleted.[14,15] In a study of human ovaries, the accelerated loss began when the total number of follicles approximated 25,000, a number reached in normal women at the age of 37–38.[16] This loss correlates with a subtle but real increase in FSH and a decrease in inhibin. The accelerated loss is probably secondary to the increase in FSH stimulation. These changes, including the increase in FSH, reflect the reduced quality and capability of aging follicles and their reduced secretion of inhibin, the granulosa cell product that exerts an important negative feedback influence over FSH secretion by the pituitary gland. Specifically, it is the secretion of inhibin B (composed of the alpha subunit and the $Beta_B$ subunit) that is decreased in older women who have an increase in FSH secretion.[17]

The FSH and inhibin change and inverse relationship indicate that inhibin is a more sensitive marker of ovarian follicular competence and, in turn, that FSH measurement is a clinical assessment of inhibin. Thus, the changes in the later reproductive years (the decline in inhibin allowing a rise in FSH) reflect lesser follicular competence, because the better follicles respond early in life, leaving the lesser follicles for later.[9,10] The decrease in inhibin secretion by the ovarian follicles begins early (around age 35), but accelerates after 40 years of age. This is reflected in the decrease in fecundability that occurs with aging. *Furthermore, the ineffective ability to suppress gonadotropins with postmenopausal hormone therapy is a consequence of the loss of inhibin, and for this reason FSH cannot be used clinically to titer estrogen dosage.*

The perimenopausal years are a time during which postmenopausal levels of FSH (greater than 20 IU/L) can be seen despite continued menstrual bleeding, while LH levels still remain in the normal range. Occasionally corpus luteum formation and function occur, and the perimenopausal woman is not totally safe from the threat of an unplanned and unexpected pregnancy until elevated levels of both FSH (>20 IU/L) and LH (>30 IU/L) can be demonstrated.[11] However, fluctuations can occur, with a period of ovarian failure followed by resumption of ovarian function.[10] *Because variability is the rule, it would be wise to recommend the use of contraception until the postmenopausal state is definitely established.* According to the *Guinness Book of World Records*, a woman from Portland, Oregon, holds the modern record for the oldest spontaneous pregnancy, conceiving when 57 years and 120 days old.

In the longitudinal Massachusetts Women's Health Study, women who reported the onset of menstrual irregularity were considered to be in the perimenopausal period of life.[18] The median age for the onset of this transition was 47.5 years. Only 10% of women ceased menstruating abruptly with no period of prolonged irregularity. The perimenopausal transition from reproductive to postreproductive status was, for most women, approximately 4 years in duration. In the study by Treolar, the average age for entry into the perimenopausal transition was 45.1, and the age range that included 95% of the women was 39–51.[19] The mean duration of the perimenopausal transition was 5.0 years, with a range of 2–8 years.

The most important thing a clinician can offer the perimenopausal woman is the education she wants to make therapeutic choices. This early educational process will help to build a solid relationship with patients, which they will want to continue as they age.

The following recommendations are derived from my own clinical experience:

(1) Provide guidance and education to facilitate a patient's decision-making.

(2) Provide time and an appropriate location for sensitive and uninterrupted discussions.

(3) Use educational materials, especially handouts, but also explain them using your own words.

(4) Involve family members during counseling and educational visits.

(5) Be accessible. Consider designating a member of your staff as the menopause resource person. Encourage phone calls.

(6) Be involved in community and hospital educational programs for the public.

(7) Use an effective, well-trained counselor for patients who need in-depth help in coping with life's trials and tribulations.

Preventive intervention during the perimenopausal years has three major goals. The overall objective is to prolong the period of maximal physical energy and optimal mental and social activity. A specific goal is to detect as early as possible any of the major chronic diseases, including hypertension, heart disease, diabetes mellitus, and cancer, as well as impairments of vision, hearing, and teeth. Finally, the clinician should help perimenopausal women to smoothly traverse the menopausal period of life. Preventive health care and management of the later reproductive years give clinicians an excellent opportunity to function as a woman's primary care provider.

A complete medical history and physical examination should be performed every 5 years, at about age 40, 45, 50, and 55. Annual visits should include a breast and pelvic examination, Pap test, screening for sexually transmitted diseases when appropriate, and hemoccult testing after age 50. At each visit, appropriate testing is scheduled for specific chronic conditions, indicated immunizations are provided, and counseling covers changing nutritional needs, physical activities, injury prevention, occupational, sexual, marital, and parental problems, urinary function, and use of tobacco, alcohol, and drugs.

SMOKING

The relationship of cigarette smoking to coronary heart disease, chronic obstructive pulmonary disease, lung cancer, and other chronic diseases is well established. Smoking has a greater adverse effect on women compared with men,[20] and women who smoke only 1–4 cigarettes per day have a 2.5-fold increased risk of fatal coronary heart disease. Smokers must be repeatedly counseled to quit smoking. Physician persistence pays off! Follow-up visits just for this purpose are worthwhile. The success rate with formal smoking cessation programs increases with repeated usage.

PHYSICAL ACTIVITY

Physical inactivity is well recognized as a coronary artery disease factor in men. There is a significant positive relationship between HDL cholesterol levels and physical activity in postmenopausal women. Furthermore, in women with low HDL cholesterol levels, there is a greater increase in HDL cholesterol with aerobic exercise programs than in women with normal to high levels.

For both cardiovascular reasons and protection against osteoporosis, weight-bearing exercise at least 30 minutes per day 3 times a week should be strongly encouraged. Brisk walking provides sufficient exercise for cardiovascular training, but ordinary walking will not protect bone mass. Weight-lifting is better for the spine than running, but running does help hip bone mass.

IMMUNIZATIONS

All individuals 65 years old and older, all adults (regardless of age) with chronic cardiovascular or pulmonary disorders, and older people who are living in chronic care facilities should be immunized annually with the influenza vaccine. Because the highest number of unprotected people for tetanus are in those over 60, the tetanus-diphtheria toxoids must be administered to older people with the same frequency as recommended for younger adults (every 10 years). It is recommended that the pneumococcal vaccine be offered to all people at age 50 because of its safety, inexpensive cost, and the increased incidence of pneumonia with advancing age. Only a single immunization is necessary for healthy individuals, but high risk individuals should be revaccinated every 6 years. Postexposure prophylaxis should be offered to women exposed to hepatitis A, hepatitis B, tuberculosis, and rabies. Hepatitis B vaccination is recommended for high risk individuals.

HYPOTHYROIDISM

Hypothyroidism increases with aging and is more common in women. The symptoms and signs are very subtle, but the functional impairment can be great. Since the diagnostic tests have very high sensitivity and specificity combined with low cost, older women should be screened for both hypothyroidism and hyperthyroidism with the highly sensitive TSH (thyroid stimulating hormone) assay obtained at age 45 and then every 2 years beginning at age 60 or with the appearance of any symptoms suggesting hypothyroidism.

DIABETES MELLITUS

Periodic fasting plasma glucose measurements are recommended for women who are markedly obese, have a family history of diabetes, and have a history of gestational diabetes.

EXCESS USE OF ALCOHOL

It is estimated that alcoholism affects up to 10% of older women, contributing significantly to functional disability. However, the excess use of alcohol is often overlooked and misdiagnosed. An older woman is at high risk for alcoholism if there is a family history of alcoholism and if there has been personal habitual alcohol use. Heavy drinkers of alcohol have more oral cancer and cancers of the larynx, throat, esophagus, and liver.

The **CAGE** questions are helpful (two positive answers indicate a problem and more than two, probable alcohol dependency).

C - Have you ever felt the need to **C**ut down on your drinking?
A - Have you ever felt **A**nnoyed by criticism over your drinking?
G - Have you ever felt **G**uilty for your drinking?
E - Do you ever have an **E**ye opener?

EXPOSURE TO UNOPPOSED ESTROGEN

Throughout the usual period of life identified with perimenopause (ages 45–55), there is a significant incidence of dysfunctional uterine bleeding. Although the greatest concern provoked by this symptom is endometrial neoplasia, the usual finding is non-neoplastic tissue displaying estrogen effects unopposed by progesterone. This results from anovulation in premenopausal women and from extragonadal endogenous estrogen production or estrogen administration in the postmenopausal woman.

In the absence of organic disease, appropriate management of uterine bleeding is dependent upon the age of the woman and endometrial tissue findings. In the perimenopausal woman with dysfunctional uterine bleeding associated with proliferative or hyperplastic endometrium (uncomplicated by atypia or dysplastic constituents), periodic oral progestin therapy is mandatory, such as medroxyprogesterone acetate 10 mg given daily the first 10 days of each month. If hyperplasia is present, follow-up aspiration curettage after 3–4 months is required, and if progestin is ineffective and histologic regression is not observed, formal curettage is an essential preliminary to alternate therapeutic surgical choices.

If contraception is required, the clinician and the healthy, nonsmoking patient should seriously consider the use of oral contraception. The anovulatory woman cannot be guaranteed that spontaneous ovulation and pregnancy will not occur. The use of a low dose oral contraceptive will at the same time provide contraception and prophylaxis against irregular, heavy anovulatory bleeding and the risk of endometrial hyperplasia and neoplasia.

Clinicians have been made so wary of providing oral contraceptives to older women that a traditional hormone regimen is often utilized to treat a woman with the kind of irregular cycles usually experienced in the perimenopausal years. This addition of exogenous estrogen when a woman is not amenorrheic or experiencing menopausal symptoms is inappropriate and even risky (exposing the endometrium to excessively high levels of estrogen). The appropriate response is to regulate anovulatory cycles with monthly progestational treatment or to utilize low dose oral contraception.

A common clinical dilemma is when to change from oral contraception to postmenopausal hormone therapy. It is important to change because even with the lowest estrogen dose oral contraceptive available, the estrogen dose is four-fold greater than the standard postmenopausal dose, and with increasing age, the dose-related risks with estrogen become significant. One approach to establish the onset of the postmenopausal years is to measure the FSH level, beginning at age 50, on an annual basis, being careful to obtain the blood sample on day 6 or 7 of the pill-free week (when steroid levels have declined sufficiently to allow FSH to rise). Friday afternoon works well for patients who start new packages on Sunday. When FSH is greater than 30 IU/L, it is time to change to a postmenopausal hormone program.

IMPACT OF POSTMENOPAUSAL ESTROGEN DEPRIVATION

Hormone therapy is an option that should be offered to most women as they consider their paths for successful aging. The menopause has been overladen with negative symbolism. Many of the behavioral complaints at the time of the menopause, however, can be explained by psychological and sociocultural influences. That is not to say that important interactions between biology, psychology, and culture do not occur, but it is time to stress the normalcy of this life event. Menopausal women do not suffer from a disease (specifically a hormone deficiency disease). Hormone therapy should be viewed as specific treatment for symptoms in the short-term and preventive pharmacology in the long term.

Part of the reason for our negative stereotypical views of menopause is that the initial characterization of menopause was derived from women presenting with physical and psychological difficulties. In addition, the variability in menopausal reactions makes the cross-sectional study design particularly unsuitable. It is important to educate women and clinicians about the normal events of this time period. Changes in menstrual function are not symbols of some ominous "change." There are good physiologic reasons for changing menstrual function, and understanding the physiology will do much to reinforce a healthy, normal attitude.

During the menopausal years, some women will experience severe multiple symptoms, while most will show no reactions or minimal reactions that can go unnoticed. The differences in menopausal reactions in symptoms across different cultures is poorly documented, and indeed, it is difficult to do so. Individual reporting is so conditioned by sociocultural factors that it is hard to determine what is due to biological vs. cultural variability. Nevertheless, there is reason to believe that the nature and prevalence of menopausal symptoms are common to all women. Data from longitudinal studies uniformly indicate that most women experience menopause without difficulty as a normal physiologic event in their lives.

VASOMOTOR SYMPTOMS

The vasomotor flush is viewed as the hallmark of the female climacteric, experienced to some degree by most postmenopausal women. The term "hot flush" is descriptive of a sudden onset of reddening of the skin over the head, neck, and chest, accompanied by a feeling of intense body heat and concluded by sometimes profuse perspiration. The duration varies from a few seconds to several minutes and rarely for an hour. The frequency may be rare to recurrent every few minutes. Flushes are more frequent and severe at night (when a woman is often awakened from sleep) or during times of stress. In a cool environment, hot flushes are fewer, less intense, and shorter in duration than in a warm environment.[21]

In the longitudinal follow-up of a large number of women, fully 10% of the women experienced hot flushes before menopause, whereas in other studies as many as 15–25% of premenopausal women reported hot flushes.[18,22,23] In the Massachusetts Women's Health Study, the incidence of hot flushes increased from 10% during the premenopausal period to about 50% just after cessation of menses.[18] By approximately 4 years after menopause, the rate of hot flushes declined to 20%. In a community-based Australian survey, 6% of premenopausal women, 26% of perimenopausal women, and 59% of postmenopausal women reported hot flushing.[24]

Although the flush can occur in the premenopause, it is a major feature of postmenopause, lasting in most women for 1–2 years but in some (as many as 25%) for longer than 5 years. In cross-sectional surveys, up to 40% of premenopausal women and 85% of menopausal women report vasomotor complaints.[23] In the US, no difference was noted in the prevalence of vasomotor complaints in surveys of black and white women.[25,26] In a massive review of hot flushing, it was concluded that exact estimates of prevalence are hampered by inconsistencies and differences in methodologies, cultures, and definitions.[27]

The physiology of the hot flush is still not understood, but it apparently originates in the hypothalamus and is brought about by a decline in estrogen. However, not all hot flushes are due to estrogen deficiency. Flushes and sweating can be secondary to diseases, including pheochromocytoma, carcinoid, leukemias, pancreatic tumors, and thyroid abnormalities.[28] Unfortunately, the hot flush is a relatively common psychosomatic symptom, and women often are unnecessarily treated with estrogen. *When the clinical situation is not clear and obvious, estrogen deficiency as the cause of hot flushes should be documented by elevated levels of FSH.*

Premenopausal women experiencing hot flushes should be screened for thyroid disease and other illnesses. A comprehensive review of all possible causes is available.[29] Clinicians should be sensitive to the possibility of an underlying emotional problem. Looking beyond the presenting symptoms into the patient's life will be an important service to the patient and her family that eventually will be appreciated. This is far more difficult than simply prescribing estrogen, but confronting problems is the only way of reaching some resolution. Prescribing estrogen inappropriately (in the presence of normal levels of gonadotropins) only temporarily postpones by a placebo response dealing with the underlying issues.

A striking and consistent finding in most studies dealing with menopause and hormonal therapy is a marked placebo response in a variety of symptoms including flushing. In an English randomized, placebo-controlled study of women being treated with estrogen implants and requesting repeat implants, no difference in outcome was noted in terms of psychologic and physical symptoms comparing women who received an active implant with those who received a placebo.[30]

A significant clinical problem encountered in my referral practice is the following scenario: a woman will occasionally experience an apparent beneficial response to estrogen, only to have the response wear off in several months. This leads to a sequence of periodic visits to the clinician and ever-increasing doses of estrogen.

When a patient reaches a point of requiring large doses of estrogen, careful inquiry must be undertaken to search for a basic psychoneurotic or psychosocial problem. To help persuade a patient that her symptoms are not due to low levels of estrogen, I find it very helpful and convincing to measure the patient's blood level of estradiol and share the result with her.

NEUROPHYSIOLOGIC EFFECTS

The view that menopause has a deleterious effect on mental health is not supported in the psychiatric literature or in surveys of the general population.[22,23,31,32] The concept of a specific psychiatric disorder (involutional melancholia) has been abandoned. Indeed, depression is less common, not more common, among middle-aged women, and menopause cannot be linked to psychologic distress.[33–40] The longitudinal study of premenopausal women indicates that hysterectomy with or without oophorectomy is not associated with a negative psychological impact among middle-aged women.[41] Longitudinal data from the Massachusetts Women's Health Study document that menopause is not associated with an increased risk of depression.[42] Although women are more likely to experience depression than are men, this sex difference begins in early adolescence, not at menopause.[43]

The U.S. National Health Examination Follow-up Study includes both longitudinal and cross-sectional assessments of a nationally representative sample of women. This study found no evidence linking either natural or surgical menopause to psychologic distress.[44] Indeed, the only longitudinal change was a slight decline in the prevalence of depression as women aged through the menopausal transition. Results in this study were the same in estrogen users and in nonusers.

A negative view of mental health at the time of menopause is not justified; many of the problems reported at menopause are due to the vicissitudes of life.[45,46] Therefore, there are problems encountered in early postmenopause that are seen frequently, but their causal relation with estrogen is unlikely. These problems include fatigue, nervousness, headaches, insomnia, depression, irritability, joint and muscle pain, dizziness, and palpitations. Indeed, men and women at this stage of life both express a multitude of complaints that do not reveal a gender difference that could be explained by a hormonal cause.[47]

Attempts to study the effects of estrogen on these problems have been hampered by the subjectivity of the complaints (high placebo responses) and the "domino effect" of what reducing hot flushes does to the frequency of symptoms. Using a double-blind crossover prospective study format, Campbell and Whitehead[48] concluded many years ago that many symptomatic "improvements" ascribed to estrogen therapy result from relief of hot flushes — a "domino" effect.

A study of 2,001 women aged 45–55 focused on the utilization of the health care system by perimenopausal women.[49] Health care utilizers in this age group were frequent previous users of health care, were less healthy, and had more psychosomatic symptoms and vasomotor reactions. These women were more likely to have had a significant previous adverse health history, including a history of premenstrual complaints. This study emphasized that perimenopausal women who seek health care help are different from those who do not seek help, and they often embrace hormone therapy in the hope it will solve their problems. It is this population that is seen most often by clinicians, producing biased opinions regarding menopause among physicians. We must be careful not to generalize to the entire female population the behavior experienced by this relatively small group of women. Most importantly, perimenopausal women who present to clinicians often end up being treated with estrogen inappropriately and unnecessarily. Nevertheless, it is well established that a woman's quality of life is disrupted by vasomotor symptoms, and estrogen therapy provides impressive improvement.[50,51]

Emotional stability during the perimenopausal period can be disrupted by poor sleep patterns. Hot flushing does have an adverse impact on the quality of sleep.[52] Estrogen therapy improves the quality of sleep, decreasing the time to onset of sleep and increasing rapid eye movement (REM) sleep time.[50,53] Perhaps flushing may be insufficient to awaken a woman but sufficient to affect the quality of sleep, thereby diminishing the ability to handle the next day's problems and stresses.

Thus, the overall "quality of life" reported by women can be improved by better sleep and alleviation of hot flushing. However, it is still uncertain if estrogen treatment has an additional direct pharmacologic antidepressent effect or if the mood response is an indirect benefit of relief from physical symptoms and, consequently, improved sleep. Utilizing various assessment tools for measuring depression, improvements with estrogen treatment have been recorded in oophorectomized women.[54,55] In a large prospective cohort study of the Rancho Bernardo retirement community, no benefit could be detected in measures of depression in current users of postmenopausal estrogen than in untreated women.[56] Indeed, treated women had higher depressive symptom scores, presumably reflecting treatment selection bias; symptomatic and depressed women seek hormone therapy. Nevertheless, estrogen therapy is reported to have a more powerful impact on women's well-being beyond the relief of symptoms such as hot flushes.[57] In elderly depressed women, improvements in response to fluoxetine were enhanced by the addition of estrogen therapy.[58]

OSTEOPOROSIS

Osteoporosis is epidemic in the United States, presently affecting 15–20 million individuals. Until about age 40, bone resorption roughly equals formation. Beyond age 40, resorption begins to exceed formation by about 0.5% per year. This adverse relationship accelerates after menopause, and up to 5% of trabecular bone and 1–1.5% of total bone mass loss will occur per year. This accelerated loss will continue for 10–15 years, after which bone loss is considerably diminished. For the first 20 years following cessation of menses, menopause-related bone loss results in a 50% reduction in trabecular bone and a 30% reduction in cortical bone. Indeed 25% of individuals over 70 years of age show radiographic evidence of fractures. Hip fractures begin to occur in the 10–15 years following menopause, and by age 90, 20% of all white women will have developed hip fractures, of which one-sixth will be fatal within 3 months. Hip fractures alone occur in about 240,000 women per year with a mortality of 40,000 annually and an associated cost of billions of dollars.

Should a clinician be concerned about bone loss and consider interventions during the perimenopausal years? Some studies have concluded that calcium supplementation of perimenopausal women retards metacarpal and lumbar bone loss.[59,60] However, the amount of perimenopausal bone loss is small unless estrogen levels are below normal.[61,62] Healthy women (exercisers and nonexercisers) who are anovulatory or have inadequate luteal phase function (and thus are exposed to less progesterone) do not have an increase in bone loss.[63,64] Interventions and treatments to prevent future osteoporosis are not necessary in women who have adequate estrogen levels and who are eating normally.

The primary care clinician should always keep in mind the necessity to monitor thyroid hormone dosage with periodic measurements of thyroid-stimulating hormone (TSH). Postmenopausal women receiving long-term treatment with thyroxine, corticosteroids, anticonvulsants, or heparin should be urged to use estrogen-progestin therapy and calcium supplementation.

CARDIOVASCULAR DISEASE

Diseases of the heart are the leading cause of death for women in the U.S., followed by malignant neoplasms, cerebrovascular disease, and motor vehicle accidents. Of the 550,000 people in the U.S. who die each year of heart disease, 250,000 are women. Nearly one third of heart disease mortality in women occurs before age 65. Most cardiovascular disease results from atherosclerosis in major vessels. The risk factors are the same for men and women: high blood pressure, smoking, diabetes mellitus, and obesity. When controlling for these risk factors, men have a risk of developing coronary heart disease over 3.5 times that of women. Even taking into consideration the changing lifestyle of women (e.g., employment outside the home), women still maintain their advantage in terms of risk for coronary heart disease. However, with increasing age, this advantage is gradually lost, and cardiovascular disease is the leading cause of death in both older women and older men.

There are important differences in lipoprotein risk factors between women and men. LDL cholesterol is more important in men than in women, whereas in women, HDL cholesterol and triglycerides are more important. Diabetes is a more important risk factor in women, perhaps because of effects on the lipoproteins. Lifestyle-induced changes in lipoprotein levels may be more difficult in women. Nevertheless, the major risk factors for coronary disease have predictive value in both men and women, and the overall treatment strategy is the same. Postmenopausal hormone therapy deserves consideration as a legitimate component of preventive health care for older women. One can argue convincingly that protection against cardiovascular disease is the major benefit of postmenopausal estrogen treatment, and the magnitude of this benefit is considerable.

BREAST CANCER

Currently, female American newborns have a lifetime probability of developing breast cancer of 12.5%, about 1 in 8, double the risk in 1940.[65] The incidence increased over the last 4 decades, but it plateaued in 1987 (about 180,000 new cases of invasive breast cancer per year). Mortality rates remained disappointingly constant (44,000 deaths per year) until a decline began in 1990. The 5-year survival rate for localized breast cancer (about 60% of breast cancers) has risen from 72% in the 1940s to 97% in 1997.[65] This is attributed to earlier diagnosis because of the greater utilization of screening mammography and increased use of chemotherapy, and in the late 1990s a continuing decline in mortality should be observed. With regional spread, the 5-year survival rate for breast cancer is 71%; with distant metastases, the rate is 18%. The overall survival rates (all stages combined) are approximately 84% at 5 years after diagnosis, 67% after 10 years, and 56% after 15 years.[65]

The incidence of breast cancer steadily increased until 1990 throughout the world since breast cancer registration began in the 1930s. The increase was almost entirely due to an increasing incidence in women over age 50. This long-term steady increase was present long before the beginning of widespread mammography screening in the 1980s. From 1982 through 1987, a more rapid increase in the incidence of breast cancer occurred due to the detection by screening mammography of early stage, small tumors; the incidence of larger tumors and metastatic tumors actually decreased slightly.[65] For these reasons, the long-term increase (about 1% per year) cannot be explained solely as the result of widespread screening mammography. Because the incidence since 1990 has plateaued, the long-term increase over the last decades is attributed to lifestyle and reproductive changes (diet and exercise; reduced parity, and delayed childbearing). The breast is the leading site of cancer in U.S. women (30% of all cancers) and is now unfortunately (because smoking is obviously the reason) exceeded by lung cancer as the leading cause of death from cancer in women.[65]

About 19% more breast cancers occur in women 40–49 than in women aged 50–59, accounting for approximately 20% of all deaths due to breast cancer.[65] But, it has been questioned whether mammography screening is effective for women under 50.[66,67] The 5-year survival rate for patients under 50 with breast cancers detected by examination was 77% compared to 95% in those patients with breast cancers detected by mammography.[68] In a randomized trial in Gothenburg, Sweden, women aged 39–49 undergoing mammographic screening every 18 months had a 45% reduction in breast cancer mortality.[69] A metaanalysis of 7 randomized clinical trials concluded that in women aged 40–49 offered mammography screening, there was a 24% reduction in breast cancer mortality.[70]

It takes longer for a significant difference in mortality to appear in 40–49-year-old women than in women over age 50. There are two explanations. One is that tumors grow faster in younger women, and the other is the greater difficulty in achieving accurate mammography because of the denser, more glandular breasts in younger women compared to the more fatty breasts in older women. Because the breast density changes gradually, rapid tumor growth must be the more critical factor.

Once detected by mammography, the stage of disease and survival expectations are the same comparing women aged 40–49 with women over age 50.[71] However, cancers that are detected between screenings have lower survival rates (at all ages). Therefore, another reason that it has been difficult to demonstrate an impact of screening in the age group 40–49 is that because of less than annual screening, more of the cancers are detected late (between screenings). This, in turn, reflects the faster tumor growth in younger women.[72] Because the randomized clinical trials have screened younger women at 2-year or longer intervals, it is not surprising that screening has been less effective for these faster growing tumors. It is logical that women aged 40–49 should have annual screening mammography.[73,74]

Younger women without risk factors must understand that approximately 50 of every 1,000 will require further diagnostic procedures, and the yield will be one invasive cancer and one noninvasive tumor.[75] Although false-positive results are more common among younger women, the difference is not so dramatic that the overall effectiveness of screening is impaired.[73]

SCREENING FOR BREAST CANCER

All women should be taught self-examination of the breast by age 20. Because of the changes that occur routinely in response to the hormonal sequence of a normal menstrual cycle, breast examination is most effective during the follicular phase of the cycle and should be performed monthly.

All women over the age of 35 should have an annual breast examination.

Women with a first-degree relative with premenopausal breast cancer should begin annual mammography 5 years before the age of the relative when diagnosed.

Annual mammography should be performed in all women over age 39.

HYPERTENSION

Hypertension is the most common chronic disease in older women and a significant risk factor for stroke, congestive heart disease, and renal disease. Beginning at age 50, hypertension is more common in women than in men, and more common in black patients. Treatment of isolated systolic hypertension (systolic blood pressure of 160 mm Hg or greater) or combined hypertension (systolic blood pressure of 160 mm Hg or greater and diastolic blood pressure of 90 mm Hg or greater) decreases cardiovascular morbidity.

The doses of estrogen and progestin used for postmenopausal hormonal therapy do not cause hypertension (except for the very rare idiosyncratic reaction). Because of the protective impact of appropriate estrogen therapy on the risk of cardiovascular disease, women with controlled hypertension are in need of that specific benefit of estrogen.

SEXUALITY

The decline in sexual activity with aging is influenced more by culture and attitudes than by nature and physiology. Given the availability of a partner, the same general high or low rate of sexual activity can be maintained throughout life. Longitudinal studies indicate that the level of sexual activity is more stable over time than previously suggested. Sexual attitudes and behavior in old age are a continuation of lifelong patterns, and the main reason for declining sexuality in older women is the unavailability of a healthy and willing partner. Sexual desire remains intact. Sexuality is an integral component of everyone's quality of life. Even if the desire or ability to have sexual intercourse is no longer present, the desire to be affectionate and intimate persists.

It will not be uncommon to encounter women who have had surgery that affects sexuality. The list includes hysterectomy, vulvectomy, coronary bypass surgery, and surgery of the breast. Sexual problems however are not limited to surgical procedures and illnesses of the genitalia. Altered self-image can occur with diseases of any site.

Sexual counseling, to be effective, must be provided to couples both before and after surgery. It is not unexpected that the surgeon may not be fully capable of providing this counseling. A major contribution from an older woman's primary physician is to arrange for competent and experienced sexual counseling. Unfortunately most physicians operate on the principle that if no questions are raised, there is no problem. The expert surgeon should be grateful for the help of experts in psychosexual therapy. Seek out the potential for posttreatment sexual morbidity before treatment. Assess the patient's abilities for coping and her sense of body image. Consider the quality of the patient's relationship and be sensitive to the absence of a relationship. This entire effort may take some time. The normal state of presurgical anxiety, fear, and denial hampers good communication.

Antihypertensive agents are frequently responsible for male sexual dysfunction, but little information is available regarding female sexual function. However, remember that vaginal lubrication is the female counterpart to male erection; therefore, vaginal dryness is a likely consequence. Adrenergic blocking agents are especially noted to affect libido and potency in men. Similarly, psychotropic drugs of all categories have been associated with inhibition of sexual function in men. Finally, we should always suspect alcoholism when patients complain of sexual dysfunction.

FAMILY PLANNING

After World War II, the U.S. total fertility rate reached a modern high of 3.8 births per woman. Women born in this period will be reaching their 45th birthday around 2010. For approximately a 20-year period, therefore, there will be an unprecedented number of women in the later child-bearing years. It is estimated that the number of women aged 35–49 will increase 61% between 1982 and 1995.

Worth emphasizing is the series of benefits women can derive from the use of oral contraception including less need for therapeutic abortion and surgical sterilization; less endometrial cancer; less ovarian cancer; less benign breast disease; fewer ectopic pregnancies; more regular menses; less flow; less dysmenorrhea; less anemia; less salpingitis; less rheumatoid arthritis; increased bone density; probably less endometriosis; possibly protection against atherosclerosis; possibly fewer fibroids; possibly fewer ovarian cysts.

Oral contraception is definitely beneficial for: dysfunctional uterine bleeding; dysmenorrhea; mittelschmerz; endometriosis prophylaxis; acne and hirsutism; hormone therapy for hypothalamic anemorrhea; and prevention of menstrual porphyria. It is probaly beneficial for functional ovarian cysts; premenstrual syndrome; and control of bleeding (dyscrasias, anovulation).

It is also worth emphasizing the methods of contraception other than the traditional birth control pill. The progestin-only minipill achieves near total efficacy in women over 40 because of the combination of the minipill's actions and reduced fecundity in older women. Long-acting progestin methods should be considered when estrogen is contraindicated. Most importantly, the copper IUD is an excellent choice for older women.

NUTRITION

Attention to good nutrition is an essential part of preventive health care. At least 20% of American adults (20–30% of women) older than 30 years are more than 20% overweight; the overweight prevalence continues to increase steadily. This degree of excess body weight is sufficient to detrimentally alter biochemical and physiologic function and to shorten life expectancy. Obesity is associated with four major risk factors for atherosclerosis: hypertension, diabetes, hypercholesterolemia, and hypertriglyceridemia.

It is well recognized that women have a greater prevalence of obesity than do men. One reason may be that women have a lower metabolic rate than men, even when adjusted for differences in body composition and level of activity.[76] Another reason that more women might gain weight with age is the postmenopausal loss of the increase in metabolic rate associated with the luteal phase of the menstrual cycle.[76] However, a major impact of menopause on body weight cannot be documented.[77] The major influence on body weight is an individual's lifetime pattern of diet and exercise.

Both men and women tend to gain weight with increasing age. Unfortunately, basal metabolic rate decreases with age. After age 18, the resting metabolic rate declines about 2% per decade. A 30-year-old individual will inevitably gain weight if there is no change in caloric intake or exercise level over the years.

Central body (android) obesity is associated with cardiovascular risk factors including hypertension and adverse cholesterol-lipoprotein profiles. The waist:hip ratio is the variable most strongly and inversely associated with the level of HDL_2, the fraction of HDL cholesterol most consistently linked with protection from cardiovascular disease. Weight loss in women with lower body obesity is mainly cosmetic, whereas loss of central body weight is more important for general health in that improvement in cardiovascular risk is associated with loss of central body fat.

The waist:hip ratio is a means of estimating the degree of upper to lower body obesity; the ratio accurately predicts the amount of intraabdominal fat (which is greater with android obesity). The waist measurement is measured as the smallest circumference (girth) between the rib cage and iliac crests. The hip measurement is the largest circumference between the waist and thighs. Interpretation is as follows: greater than 0.85, android obesity; less than 0.75, gynoid obesity.

Despite various fads and diet books, the best weight-losing diet continues to be a limitation of calories to between 900 and 1200 per day, the actual amount depending on what the individual patient will accept and pursue. When energy intake is less than this, it is very difficult to obtain the recommended levels of vitamins and minerals.

DOMESTIC ABUSE AND VIOLENCE

Domestic violence includes both physical and mental abuse. Recognition of this problem requires a high index of suspicion. Direct questioning is appropriate and recommended. Physicians should be prepared to provide effective counseling for the acute resolution of this problem. This includes legal and social alternatives and resources and the possibility of long-term therapy. It is helpful to incorporate the following questions into an assessment for the presence of abuse:

1. Have you ever been emotionally or physically abused by your partner or someone important to you?
2. Within the last year, have you been hit, slapped, kicked, or otherwise physically hurt by someone?
3. Within the last year, has anyone forced you to have sexual activities?
4. Are you afraid of your partner or anyone?

REFERENCES

1. VOLLMAN, R.F. 1977. The menstrual cycle. *In* Major Problems in Obstetrics and Gynecology. E. Friedman, Ed. W.B. Saunders Co. Philadelphia.
2. TRELOAR, A.E., R.E. BOYNTON, G.B. BORGHILD & B.W. BROWN. 1967. Variation of the human menstrual cycle through reproductive life. Int. J. Fertil. **12:** 77–126.
3. COLLETT, M.E., G.E. WERTENBERGER & V.M. FISKE. 1954. The effect of age upon the pattern of the menstrual cycle. Fertil. Steril. **5:** 437.
4. MUNSTER, K., L. SCHMIDT & P. HELM. 1992. Length and variation in the menstrual cycle — a cross-sectional study from a Danish county. Br. J. Obstet. Gynaecol. **99:** 422.
5. BELSEY, E.M., A.P.Y. PINOL & TASK FORCE ON LONG-ACTING SYSTEMIC AGENTS FOR FERTILITY REGULATION. 1997. Menstrual bleeding patterns in untreated women. Contraception **55:** 57–65.
6. SHERMAN, B.M., J.H. WEST & S.G. KORENMAN. 1976. The menopausal transition: analysis of lh, fsh, estradiol, and progesterone concentrations during menstrual cycles of older women. J. Clin. Endocrinol. Metab. **42:** 629.
7. LENTON, E.A., B. LANDGREN, L. SEXTON & R. HARPER. 1984. Normal variation in the length of the follicular phase of the menstrual cycle: effect of chronological age. Br. J. Obstet. Gynaecol. **91:** 681.
8. BUCKLER, H.M., A. EVANS, H. MAMLORA *et al.* 1991. Gonadotropin, steroid and inhibin levels in women with incipient ovarian failure during anovulatory and ovulatory 'rebound' cycles. J. Clin. Endocrinol. Metab. **72:**116–124.
9. MACNAUGHTON, J., M. BANGAH, P. MCCLOUD *et al.* 1992. Age-related changes in follicle stimulating hormone, luteinizing hormone, oestradiol and immunoreactive inhibin in women of reproductive age. Clin. Endocrinol. **36:** 339.
10. HEE, J., J. MACNAUGHTON, M. BANGAH & H.G. BURGER. 1993. Perimenopausal patterns of gonadotrophins, immunoreactive inhibin, oestradiol and progesterone. Maturitas **18:** 9–20.
11. METCALF, M.G. & J.H. LIVESAY. 1985. Gonadotropin excretion in fertile women: effect of age and the onset of the menopausal transition. J. Endocrinol. **105:** 357.
12. RANNEVIK, G., S. JEPPSSON, O. JOHNELL *et al.* 1995. A longitudinal study of the perimenopausal transition: altered profiles of steroid and pituitary hormones, SHBG and bone mineral density. Maturitas **21:** 103–113.
13. SANTORO, N., J.R. BROWN, T. ADEL & J.H. SKURNICK. 1996. Characterization of reproductive hormonal dynamics in the perimenopause. J. Clin. Endocrinol. Metab. **81:** 1495–1501.
14. RICHARDSON, S.J., V. SENIKAS & J.F. NELSON. 1987. Follicular depletion during the menopausal transition — evidence for accelerated loss and ultimate exhaustion. J. Clin. Endocrinol. Metab. **65:** 1231–1237.
15. GOUGEON, A., R. ECHOCHARD & J.C. THALABARD. 1994. Age-related changes of the population of human ovarian follicles: increase in the disappearance rate of non-growing and early-growing follicles in aging women. Biol. Reprod. **50:** 653–663.
16. FADDY, M.J., R.G. GOSDEN, A. GOUGEON *et al.* 1992. Accelerated disappearance of ovarian follicles in mid-life: implications for forecasting menopause. Hum. Reprod. **7:** 1342–1346.

17. Klein, N.A., P.J. Illingworth, N.P. Groome *et al.* 1996. Decreased inhibin B secretion is associated with the monotropic FSH rise in older, ovulatory women: a study of serum and follicular fluid leavels of dimeric inhibin A and B in spontaneous menstrual cycles. J. Clin. Endocrinol. Metab. **81:** 2742–2745.
18. McKinlay, S.M., D.J. Brambilla & J.G. Posner. 1992. The normal menopause transition. Maturitas **14:** 103–115.
19. Treloar, A.E. 1981. Menstrual cyclicity and the pre-menopause. Maturitas **3:** 249–264.
20. Davis, D.L., G.E. Dinse & D.G. Hoel. 1994. Decreasing cardiovascular disease and increasing cancer among whites in the United States from 1973 through 1987. JAMA **271:** 431.
21. Kronnenberg, F. & R.M. Barnard. 1992. Modulation of menopausal hot flashes by ambient temerature. J. Therm. Biol. **17:** 43–49.
22. Hunter, M. 1992. The South-East England longitudinal study of the climacteric and postmenopause. Maturitas **14:**17–26.
23. Oldenhave, A., L.J.B. Jaszmann, A.A. Haspels & W.T.A.M. Everaerd. 1993. Impact of climacteric on well-being. Am. J. Obstet. Gynecol. **168:** 772–780.
24. Guthrie, J.R., L. Dennerstein, J.L. Hopper & H.G. Burger. 1996. Hot flushes, menstrual status, and hormone levels in a population-based sample of midlife women. Obstet. Gynecol. **88:** 437–442.
25. Schwingl, P.J., B.S. Hulka & S.D. Harlow. 1994. Risk factors for menopausal hot flashes. Obstet. Gynecol. **84:** 29–34.
26. Pham, K.T., J.A. Grisso & E.W. Freeman. 1997. Ovarian aging and hormone replacement therapy. Hormonal levels, symptoms, and attitudes of African-American and white women. J. Gen. Intern. Med. **12:** 230–236.
27. Kronnenberg, F. 1990. Hot flashes: epidemiology and physiology. Ann. N.Y. Acad. Sci. **592:** 52–86.
28. Wilkin, J.R. 1981. Flushing reactions: consequences and mechanisms. Ann. Intern. Med. **95:** 468–476.
29. Mohyi, D., K. Tabassi & J. Simon. 1997. Differential diagnosis of hot flashes. Maturitas **27:** 203–214.
30. Pearce, J., K. Hawton, F. Blake *et al.* 1997. Psychological effects of continuation versus discontinuation of hormone replacement therapy by estrogen implants: a placebo-controlled study. J. Psychosom. Res. **42:** 177–186.
31. Ballinger, C.B. 1990. Psychiatric aspects of the menopause. Br. J. Psychiatr. **156:** 773–787.
32. Schmidt, P.J. & D.R. Rubinow. 1991. Menopause-related affective disorders: a justification for further study. Am. J. Psychiatr. **148:** 844–854.
33. Hällström, T. & S. Samuelsson. 1985. Mental health in the climacteric. The longitudinal study of women in Gothenburg. Acta Obstet. Gynecol. Scand. (Suppl.) **130:** 13–18.
34. Gath, D., M. Osborn & G. Bungay *et al.* 1987. Psychiatric disorder and gynaecological symptoms in middle aged women: a community survey. Br. Med. J. **294:** 213–218.
35. McKinlay, S.M. & J.B. McKinlay. 1989. The impact of menopause and social factors on health. *In* Menopause: Evaluation, Treatment, and Health Concerns. C.B. Hammond, F.P. Haseltine & I. Schiff, Eds. :137–161. Alan R. Liss. New York.
36. Matthews, K.A., R.R. Wing, L.H. Kuller *et al.* 1990. Influences of natural menopause on psychological characteristics and symptoms of middle-aged healthy women. J. Consult. Clin. Psychol. **58:** 345–351.
37. Koster, A. 1991. Change-of-life anticipations, attitudes, and experiences among middle-aged Danish women. Health Care Women Int. **12:** 1–13.
38. Holte, A. 1992. Influences of natural menopause on health complaints: a prospective study of healthy Norwegian women. Maturitas **14:** 127.
39. Kaufert, P.A., P. Gilbert & R. Tate. 1992. The Manitoba Project: a re-examination of the link between menopause and depression. Maturitas **14:** 143.
40. Dennerstein, L., A.M.A. Smith, C. Morse *et al.* 1993. Menopausal symptoms in Australian women. Med. J. Aust. **159:** 232.
41. Everson, S.A., K.A. Matthews, D.S. Guzick *et al.* 1995. Effects of surgical menopause on lipid levels and psychosocial characteristics: the Healthy Women Study. Health Psychol. **14:** 435–443.

42. Avis, N.E., D. Brambilla, S.M. McKinlay & K. Vass. 1994. A longitudinal analysis of the association between menopause and depression. Results from the Massachusetts Women's Health Study. Ann. Epidemiol. **4:** 214–220.
43. Kessler, R.C., K.A. McGonagle, M. Swartz *et al.* 1993. Sex and depression in the National Comorbidity Survey I: lifetime prevalence, chronicity and recurrence. J. Affect. Disord. **29:** 85.
44. Busch, C.M., A.B. Zonderman & P.T. Costa, Jr. 1994. Menopausal transition and psychological distress in a nationally representative sample: is menopause associated with psychological distress? J. Aging Health **6:** 209–228.
45. Dennerstein, L., A.M.A. Smith & C. Morse. 1994. Psychological well-being, midlife and the menopause. Maturitas **20:** 1.
46. Mitchell, E.S. & N.F. Woods. 1996. Symptom experiences of midlife women: observations from the Seattle midlife women's health study. Maturitas **25:** 1–10.
47. Van Hall, E.V., M. Verdel & J. Van Der Velden. 1994. "Perimenopausal" complaints in women and men: a comparative study. J. Women's Health **3:** 45–49.
48. Campbell, S. & M. Whitehead. 1977. Estrogen therapy and the menopausal syndrome. Clin. Obstet. Gynecol. **4:** 31–47.
49. Morse, C.A., A. Smith, L. Dennerstein *et al.* 1994. The treatment-seeking woman at menopause. Maturitas **18:** 161–173.
50. Wiklund, I., J. Karlberg & L.-A. Mattsson. 1993. Quality of life of postmenopausal women on a regimen of transdermal estradiol therapy: a double-blind placebo-controlled study. Am. J. Obstet. Gynecol. **168:** 824–830.
51. Daly, E., A. Gray, D. Barlow *et al.* 1993. Measuring the impact of menopausal symptoms on quality of life. Br. Med. J. **307:** 836.
52. Woodward, S. & R.R. Freedman. 1994. The thermoregulatory effects of menopausal hot flashes on sleep. Sleep **17:** 497–501.
53. Schiff, I., Q. Regestein, D. Tulchinsky & K.J. Ryan. 1979. Effects of estrogens on sleep and psychological state of hypogonadal women. JAMA **242:** 2405–2407.
54. Dennerstein, L., G.D. Burrows, G.J. Hyman & C. Wood. 1979. Hormone therapy and affect. Maturitas **1:** 247–254.
55. Sherwin, B.B. 1988. Affective changes with estrogen and androgen replacement therapy in surgically menopausal women. J. Affect. Disord. **14:** 177–187.
56. Palinkas, L.A. & E. Barrett-Connor. 1992. Estrogen use and depressive symptoms in postmenopausal women. Obstet. Gynecol. **80:** 30–36.
57. Limouzin-Lamothe, M.-A., N. Mairon, C.R.B. Joyce & M. Le Gal. 1994. Quality of life after the menopause: influence of hormonal replacement therapy. Am. J. Obstet. Gynecol. **170:** 618–624.
58. Schneider, L.S., G.W. Small, S.H. Hamilton *et al.* 1997. Estrogen replacement and response to fluoxetine in a multicenter geriatric depression trial. Am. J. Geriatr Psychiatry **5:** 97–106.
59. Baran, D., A. Sorensen, J. Grimes *et al.* 1990. Dietary modification with dairy products for preventing vertebral bone loss in premenopausal women: a three-year prospective study. J. Clin. Endocrinol. Metab. **70:** 264–270.
60. Elders, P.J.M., P. Lips, C. Netelenbos *et al.* 1994. Long-term effect of calcium supplementation on bone loss in perimenopausal women. J. Bone Miner. Res. **9:** 963.
61. Gambacciani, M., A. Spinetti, F. Taponeco *et al.* 1994. Bone loss in perimenopausal women: a longitudinal study. Maturitas **18:** 191–197.
62. Garton, M., J. Martin, S. New *et al.* 1996. Bone mass and metabolism in women aged 45–55. Clin. Endocrinol. **44:** 536–570.
63. Waller, K., J. Reim, L. Fenster *et al.* 1996. Bone mass and subtle abnormalities in ovulatory function in healthy women. J. Clin. Endocrinol. Metab. **81:** 663–668.
64. De Souza, M.J., B.E. Miller, L.C. Sequenzia *et al.* 1997. Bone health is not affected by luteal phase abnormalities and decreased ovarian progesterone production in female runners. J. Clin. Endocrinol. Metab. **82:** 2867–2876.
65. American Cancer Society. 1998. Cancer facts & figures — 1998. http://www.cancer.org/statistics.
66. Eddy, D.M, V. Hasselblad, W. McGivney & W. Hendee. 1988. The value of mammography screening in women under age 50 years. JAMA **259:** 1512.

67. Miller, A.B., C.J. Baines, T. To & C. Wall. 1992. Canadian National Breast Screening Study: 1. Breast cancer detection and death rates among women aged 40 to 49 years. Can. Med. Assoc. J. **147:** 1459.
68. Stacey-Clear, A., K.A. McCarthy, D.A. Hall *et al.* 1992. Breast cancer survival among women under age 50: is mammography detrimental? Lancet **340:** 991.
69. Bjurstam, N., L. Björneld, S.W. Duffy *et al.* 1997. The Gothenburg Breast Screening Trial. First results on mortality, incidence, and mode of detection for women ages 39–49 years at randomization. Cancer **80:** 2091–2099.
70. Smart, C.R., R.E. Hendrick, J.H. Rutledge, III, & R.A. Smith. 1995. Benefit of mammography screening in women ages 40-49 years: current evidence from randomized controlled trials. Cancer **75:** 1619.
71. Curpen, B.N., E.A. Sickles, R.A. Sollito *et al.* 1995. The comparative value of mammographic screening for women 40-49 years old versus women 50-64 years old. Am. J. Roentgenol. **164:** 1099.
72. Kerlikowske, K., D. Grady, J. Barclay *et al.* 1996. Effect of age, breast density, and family history on the sensitivity of first screening mammography. JAMA **276:** 33.
73. Kerlikowske, K., D. Grady, J. Barclay *et al.* 1996. Likelihood ratios for modern screening mammography: risk of breast cancer based on age and mammographic interpretation. JAMA **276:** 39–43.
74. Report of the Organizing Committee and Collaborators, Falun Meeting. 1996. Breast cancer screening with mammography in women aged 40–49 years. Int. J. Cancer **68:** 693–699.
75. Kerlikowske, K., D. Grady, J. Barclay *et al.* 1993. Positive predictive value of screening mammography by age and family history of breast cancer. JAMA **270:** 2444.

Premature Ovarian Failure Is Not Premature Menopause

SOPHIA N. KALANTARIDOU AND LAWRENCE M. NELSON[a]

Section on Women's Health Research, Developmental Endocrinology Branch, National Institute of Child Health and Human Development, National Institutes of Health, Bethesda, Maryland 20892, USA

ABSTRACT: Normal menopause occurs at an average age of 50 and results from ovarian follicle depletion. Normal menopause is an irreversible condition, whereas premature ovarian failure is characterized by intermittent ovarian function in half of these young women. These young women produce estrogen intermittently and sometimes even ovulate despite the presence of high gonadotropin levels. Indeed, pregnancy has occurred after a diagnosis of premature ovarian failure. On pelvic ultrasound examination, follicles were equally likely to be detected in patients more than 6 years after a diagnosis of premature ovarian failure as in patients less than 6 years after the diagnosis. Thus, the probability of detecting a follicle appears to remain stable during the normal reproductive lifespan of these young women. Indeed, pregnancy was reported in a 44-year-old woman 16 years after a diagnosis of premature ovarian failure. No treatment to restore fertility in patients with premature ovarian failure has proved to be safe and effective in prospective controlled studies. Theoretically, these unproved therapies might even prevent one of these spontaneous pregnancies from occurring.

INTRODUCTION

Premature ovarian failure causes amenorrhea, infertility, sex steroid deficiency, and elevated gonadotropins in women younger than 40 years.[1] It affects 1% of women by age 40 and 0.1% by age 30.[2] Premature ovarian failure is not merely early natural menopause. Young women with premature ovarian failure may ovulate intermittently,[3] and, indeed, pregnancies have occurred after a diagnosis of ovarian failure.[4]

Young women with this disorder need thorough assessment, sex steroid replacement, and long-term surveillance to monitor therapy and minimize health risks in later life.[5] In fact, the mortality rate was increased among women with premature ovarian failure compared with women with natural menopause at an average age of 50 (adjusted rate ratios of 1.50, 95% confidence interval 0.97–2.34) in a recent epidemiologic study of more than 3,000 women using data from the National Health and Survey (NHANES) Epidemiologic Follow-up Study.[6] This finding is in agreement with a previous 6-year longitudinal study of more than 5,000 women which

[a]Address for correspondence: National Institutes of Health, Building 10, Room 10N262, 10 Center Drive MSC 1862, Bethesda, Maryland 20892-1862, USA. Phone: + 301-496-4686; fax: + 301-402-0574.

Lawrence.Nelson@nih.gov

showed that premature ovarian failure is associated with a nearly twofold age-specific increase in mortality rate (age-adjusted odds ratio of death 1.95, 95% confidence interval 1.24–3.07).[7]

PATHOPHYSIOLOGY OF PREMATURE OVARIAN FAILURE

Premature ovarian failure is characterized by intermittent ovarian function in half of these young women,[3] whereas normal menopause is an irreversible condition resulting from ovarian follicle depletion at an average age of 50.[8] Young women with premature ovarian failure produce estrogen intermittently and may even ovulate despite the presence of high gonadotropin levels.[3] Indeed, pregnancy has occurred after a diagnosis of premature ovarian failure[4] even in women in whom no follicles were observed on ovarian biopsy.[9] In fact, on pelvic ultrasound examination. we were equally likely to detect follicles in patients more than 6 years after a diagnosis of premature ovarian failure as in patients less than 6 years after the diagnosis.[3] Thus, the probability of detecting a follicle appears to remain stable during the normal reproductive lifespan of these young women.[3] However, the follicles in most cases are not functioning normally.[3] In contrast to normal women, these young women have a poor correlation between follicle diameter and serum estradiol levels.[3] Nevertheless, nearly 20% of these women ovulated during 4 months of observation.[3]

Inappropriate luteinization of graafian follicles appears to be a major pathophysiologic mechanism impairing follicle function in young women with spontaneous premature ovarian failure.[3] In six women with spontaneous premature ovarian failure we performed ovarian biopsies when an antral follicle was detected on ultrasound, and in all six cases, examination revealed follicles with luteinization of the granulosa cells and increased vascularization.[3] A small initial follicle pool or an increased rate of atresia may be responsible for this phenomenon.[10] Normal human ovaries contain approximately 7 million oocytes during gestation month 5.[11] This initial pool of oocytes will last a woman throughout her normal reproductive lifespan. During reproductive years, for every follicle that ovulates, approximately 1,000 undergo atresia. In normal ovaries, factors produced by the entire cohort of follicles, such as inhibin-b,[12] may be necessary for providing sufficient negative feedback to maintain gonadotropins in the normal range. We found few other follicles in the ovaries of our patients. These few "lonely" follicles face inappropriately high luteinizing hormone (LH) levels. Given that inappropriate luteinization takes place,[3] the increased LH appears to impair normal follicle function.

SIGNS AND SYMPTOMS OF PREMATURE OVARIAN FAILURE

Premature ovarian failure may present as either primary or secondary amenorrhea.[5] The majority of the patients develop ovarian failure after having established regular menses.[5] No characteristic menstrual history precedes premature ovarian failure. Approximately 50% of the patients have a history of oligomenorrhea or dysfunctional uterine bleeding (prodromal premature ovarian failure), 25% develop amenorrhea acutely, some postpartum, and some after stopping oral contraceptives.[5]

Primary amenorrhea is not associated with symptoms of estrogen deficiency. Symptoms in cases of secondary amenorrhea may include hot flushes, night sweats, fatigue, and mood changes.[5] Incomplete development of secondary sex characteristics may occur in women with primary amenorrhea, whereas these characteristics are usually normal in women with secondary amenorrhea.[5] These young patients generally have normal fertility before developing premature ovarian failure.[5]

ASSOCIATED AUTOIMMUNE ENDOCRINE DISORDERS

Premature ovarian failure may be associated with other autoimmune endocrine disorders including autoimmune adrenal failure (Addison's disease), hypothyroidism, and diabetes mellitus. Autoimmune hypothyroidism is the most common disorder associated with premature ovarian failure.[13,14] We prospectively evaluated 119 patients with karyotypically normal spontaneous premature ovarian failure at the National Institutes of Health.[14] Of those, 32 had hypothyroidism (27%), 3 had adrenal insufficiency (2.5%), and 3 had diabetes mellitus (2.5%). All the cases of adrenal insufficiency were diagnosed prior to ovarian failure.[14]

ETIOLOGY OF PREMATURE OVARIAN FAILURE

In most cases no etiology of premature ovarian failure can be identified (karyotypically normal spontaneous premature ovarian failure)[5] (TABLE 1). On the basis of serial blood sampling we found that nearly half of these patients have ovarian follicles remaining in the ovary.[3] The follicles function intermittently, and nearly 20% of patients ovulate during 4 months of observation.[3]

Autoimmunity is a well established mechanism of ovarian failure[15–17] and may be a dominant cause of reversible premature ovarian failure (TABLE 1). As a group, patients with premature ovarian failure have increased activation of peripheral T lymphocytes.[18] Autoimmune lymphocytic oophoritis is characterized by inflammatory infiltration of the theca interna of developing follicles and sparing of primordial follicles.[15–17] Lymphocytic infiltration is more prominent in mature follicles.[15–17] Although it has been suggested that the MHC molecule DR3 occurs with greater frequency in patients with spontaneous premature ovarian failure,[19] we were unable to confirm this finding in our patients despite a power of 99%.[20]

Antibodies against membrane-bound receptors are known to cause diseases such as myasthenia gravis[21] and autoimmune hypothyroidism.[22] We used a recombinant system expressing human FSH and LH receptors to look for gonadotropin receptor blocking antibodies.[23] Immunoglobulin G (IgG) from patients with premature ovarian failure did not interfere with either the FSH-receptor or LH-receptor interaction.[23]

In autoimmune polyglandular syndrome (APS) type I, also known as autoimmune polyendocrinopathy-candidiasis-ectodermal dystrophy (APECED), premature ovarian failure develops in up to 60% of the cases.[24] In this syndrome, associated disorders include adrenal failure, hypothyroidism, hypoparathyroidism, and mucocutaneous candidiasis. APS type 1 is an autosomal recessive disease caused by a single gene defect on chromosome 21q22.3.[25,26]

TABLE 1. Etiology of premature ovarian failure

Idiopathic (karyotypically normal spontaneous premature ovarian failure)
Autoimmunity
Autoimmune polyglandular syndrome type I
Gonadotropin and gonadotropin-receptor abnormalities (signal defects)
Enzyme deficiencies (cholesterol desmolase, 17α-hydroxylase, and 17-20 desmolase)
Iatrogenic (chemotherapy, radiation)
X-chromosome abnormalities
Galactosemia
Viral agents

Gonadotropin and gonadotropin-receptor abnormalities (signal defects), usually inherited in an autosomal recessive fashion, may also be a cause of premature ovarian failure. Mutation of the β subunit of FSH has been described in two patients with primary amenorrhea.[27,28] One patient conceived after treatment with FSH.[27] Mutations in the FSH receptor gene may also cause hypergonadotropic primary amenorrhea with variable development of secondary sex characteristics.[29,30] Women heterozygous for the gene have normal fertility.[29,30] Ovarian biopsy specimens from these patients revealed the presence of primordial follicles in all cases.[29,30] Mutations of the LH receptor gene also cause ovarian failure with normal development of secondary sex characteristics.[31–33] Ovarian biopsies in these patients revealed primordial, preantral, and antral follicles, whereas no preovulatory follicles, corpora lutea, or corpora albicans were seen.[31–33]

Enzyme deficiencies impairing estrogen synthesis, such as cholesterol desmolase, 17α-hydroxylase, and 17-20 desmolase, cause amenorrhea and failure to develop secondary sex characteristics despite the presence of developing follicles[34,35] (TABLE 1). Interestingly, fertilizable eggs could be retrieved after ovulation induction for *in vitro* fertilization in patients with either 17α-hydroxylase deficiency or 17-20 desmolase deficiency despite undetectable peripheral estradiol levels.[36]

Premature ovarian failure may also result from chemo- and radiotherapy and the likelihood of developing the disorder depends on age at treatment, drug type, dose, and duration of treatment[37,38] (TABLE 1).

Chromosomal abnormalities are detected in 40–50% of women with primary amenorrhea.[39] Recent studies suggested two genes (*POF1* and *POF2*) important for ovarian function that are localized to Xq21.3-q27 and Xq13.3-q21.1, respectively.[40,41] Also, defects in the human diaphanous gene may be a cause of ovarian failure.[42] In addition, an increase in the familial incidence of ovarian failure was found in women with fragile X premutations, thus indicating that the FMR1 gene (Xq27.3) may influence ovarian function[43,44] (TABLE 1).

Finally, galactosemia may be a rare cause of ovarian failure[45] (TABLE 1). It occurs because of a deficiency in the enzyme galactose-1-phosphate uridyl transferase (GALT). It is an autosomal recessive disorder, causing mental retardation, cataracts, and hepatocellular and renal damage and it becomes clinically apparent due to these disorders.[45]

DIAGNOSIS OF PREMATURE OVARIAN FAILURE

We define premature ovarian failure as the presence of at least 4 months of amenorrhea and two serum FSH values greater than 40 mIU/mL (obtained at least 1 month apart) in women less than 40 years of age.[1] History should be taken regarding prior ovarian surgery, chemotherapy or radiation, and autoimmune disorders. Particular attention should be paid to symptoms of adrenal failure (Addison's disease), such as anorexia, weight loss, abdominal pain, weakness, salt craving, and increased skin pigmentation. Adrenal failure may run a long insidious course before the disease becomes life-threatening.

In patients with primary amenorrhea, particular attention should be paid to breast and pubic hair development according to Tanner stages. In most cases physical examination gives completely normal results. Rarely, pelvic examination may reveal ovarian enlargement in patients with autoimmune premature ovarian failure (lymphocytic oophoritis).[1]

In our view a karyotype should be performed in all patients experiencing premature ovarian failure. Although it has been suggested that chromosomal analysis should only be performed in patients less than 35 years of age, women with X chromosome abnormalities have given birth and developed ovarian failure after this age.[40] Because the risk of gonadal germ cell neoplasia is substantial, patients with ovarian failure and a karyotype containing a Y chromosome should undergo bilateral gonadectomy.[46]

Pelvic ultrasound, ovarian biopsy, and antiovarian antibody testing have no proven clinical benefit in premature ovarian failure.[1] As clinically indicated, work-up should include tests for the diagnosis of other possible concurrent autoimmune disorders, such as hypothyroidism, diabetes mellitus, and Addison's disease. Based on our findings, the most useful evaluation in women with karyotypically normal spontaneous premature ovarian failure includes only serum thyroid-stimulating hormone (TSH), free thyroxine, and fasting glucose.[14] Testing for adrenal insufficiency with the corticotropin stimulation test can be performed as clinically indicated.[14]

MANAGEMENT OF PREMATURE OVARIAN FAILURE

Young women find the diagnosis of premature ovarian failure particularly traumatic, and a carefully planned approach is required when informing patients of this diagnosis. It is important to emphasize that premature ovarian failure can be transient and that in most cases we can never be certain that no follicles remain in the ovary.[5]

Sex Steroid Replacement Therapy

Young women with premature ovarian failure need estrogen/progestin replacement therapy to relieve symptoms of estrogen deficiency, to maintain bone density, and to reduce the risk of cardiovascular disease.[5] We found that two thirds of our patients with karyotypically normal spontaneous premature ovarian failure have a bone mineral density 1 standard deviation (SD) below the mean of similar age women despite taking hormone replacement therapy at least intermittently.[47] Of note, this bone density has been associated with a 2.6-fold increased risk for hip fracture.[48]

All women with premature ovarian failure should fully understand that hormone replacement should be continued at least until the average age of natural menopause (approximately 50 years) and that they should have long-term follow-up by a physician with an interest in this condition. These young women usually require administration of estrogen at a dose equivalent to 1.25 mg of conjugated estrogen, which is greater than the standard dose given to older women experiencing natural menopause. Androgen replacement should also be considered in women experiencing persistent fatigue, poor well being, and low libido despite adequate estrogen replacement.[5] A transdermal testosterone matrix patch, designed to deliver a dose of testosterone equivalent to ovarian testosterone production, is now undergoing evaluation at the National Institutes of Health. Patients with premature ovarian failure should also be informed of the need for adequate calcium intake and physical activity.

Infertility-Related Therapy

Women with premature ovarian failure have intermittent ovarian function,[3] and they have a 5–10% chance of spontaneous pregnancy.[9] There is no treatment to restore fertility in young patients with premature ovarian failure that has been proven safe and effective in prospective controlled studies. Theoretically, these unproved therapies might even prevent one of these spontaneous pregnancies from occurring. Hormone replacement therapy does not prevent conception,[4] and indeed these young women may even conceive while taking the oral contraceptive.[49] Attempts at ovulation induction in these patients using clomiphene citrate,[50] human menopausal gonadotropins,[51] and a combination of gonadotropin-releasing hormone analog with purified urinary FSH[52] resulted in no greater ovulation rates than those seen in untreated patients.[13] Our controlled studies show no benefit to a period of ovarian rest induced by gonadotropin-releasing hormone analog[53] or danazol.[54] For women with premature ovarian failure desiring fertility, oocyte donation is an option,[55] and in fact this treatment is as successful in older women as it is in younger women.[56]

Anecdotal reports have suggested that glucocorticoid treatment may restore ovarian function in women with premature ovarian failure.[57] Nevertheless, we know that nearly 20% of women with karyotypically normal spontaneous premature ovarian failure ovulate intermittently.[3] Therefore, ovulation and pregnancies achieved using ovulation induction and/or immunosuppression may represent spontaneous remissions that could have occurred with mere observation.[1] These methods have no proven benefit; in fact, major complications such as iatrogenic Cushing's syndrome, osteonecrosis, and corticosteroid-induced osteoporosis can occur. A prospective study of alternate-day prednisone therapy for lymphocytic oophoritis is now underway at the Clinical Center of the National Institutes of Health. In this study, because no diagnostic serum marker is available, histologic confirmation of the disease is a prerequisite for prednisone administration. In our view, treatment to restore fertility in young women with premature ovarian failure should be limited to investigational protocols carefully designed to prove safety and efficacy.

FOLLOW-UP OF PATIENTS WITH PREMATURE OVARIAN FAILURE

Young women with premature ovarian failure should be monitored annually regarding their compliance with hormone replacement therapy.[5] Moreover, these patients should be followed up for the presence of signs and symptoms of associated autoimmune endocrine disorders, such as hypothyroidism, adrenal insufficiency, and diabetes mellitus.[14] Additional testing should be performed as clinically indicated.

CONCLUSIONS

Normal menopause occurs at an average age of 50 and results from ovarian follicle depletion.[8] Normal menopause is an irreversible condition, whereas premature ovarian failure is characterized by intermittent ovarian function in half of these young women.[3] These young women produce estrogen intermittently and sometimes even ovulate despite the presence of high gonadotropin levels.[3] Indeed, pregnancy has occurred after a diagnosis of premature ovarian failure.[4] No treatment to restore fertility in young patients with premature ovarian failure has been proven safe and effective in prospective controlled studies. Theoretically, these unproved therapies might even prevent one of these spontaneous pregnancies from occurring.

Early loss of ovarian function has both significant psychosocial sequelae and major health implications.[5] Young women with premature ovarian failure have a nearly twofold age-specific increase in mortality rate.[6,7] They need a thorough assessment, sex steroid replacement, and long-term surveillance to monitor their therapy.[5] Also, these young patients should be followed up annually for the presence of associated autoimmune endocrine disorders such as hypothyroidism, adrenal insufficiency, and diabetes mellitus.[14]

ACKNOWLEDGMENT

Dr. Sophia N. Kalantaridou is the recipient of a scholarship from the "Alexandros S. Onassis" Public Benefit Foundation/Group T-034.

REFERENCES

1. Nelson, L.M., J.N. Anasti & M.R. Flack. 1996. Premature ovarian failure. *In* Reproductive Endocrinology, Surgery, and Technology. E.Y. Adashi, J.A. Rock & Z. Rosenwaks, Eds.:1394–1410. Lippincott-Raven Publishers. Philadelphia, PA.
2. Coulam, C.B., S.C. Adamson & J.F. Annegers. 1986. Incidence of premature ovarian failure. Obstet. Gynecol. **67:** 604–606.
3. Nelson, L.M., J.N. Anasti, L.M. Kimzey *et al.* 1994. Development of luteinized graafian follicles in patients with karyotypically normal spontaneous premature ovarian failure. J. Clin. Endocrinol. Metab. **79:** 1470–1475.
4. Alper, M.M., E.E. Jolly & P.R. Garner. 1986. Pregnancies after premature ovarian failure. Obstet. Gynecol. **67**(Suppl)**:** 59–62.
5. Kalantaridou, S.N., S.R. Davis & L.M. Nelson. 1998. Premature ovarian failure. Endocrinol. Metab. Clin. N. Am. **27.** In press.
6. Cooper, G.S. & D.P. Sandler. 1998. Age at natural menopause and mortality. Ann. Epidemiol. **8:** 229–235.

7. SNOWDON, D.A., R.L. KANE, W.L. BEESON *et al.* 1989. Is early natural menopause a biologic marker of health and aging? Am. J. Public Health **79:** 709–714.
8. RICHARDSON, S.J. & J.F. NELSON. 1990. Follicular depletion during the menopausal transition. Ann. N.Y. Acad. Sci. **592:** 13–20.
9. REBAR, R.W. & H.V. CONNOLLY. 1990. Clinical features of young women with hypergonadotropic amenorrhea. Fertil. Steril. **53:** 804–810.
10. DUNCAN, M., L. CUMMINGS & K. CHADA. 1993. Germ cell deficient (gcd) mouse as a model of premature ovarian failure. Biol. Reprod. **49:** 221–227.
11. BAKER, T.G. & O.W. SUM. 1976. Development of the ovary and oogenesis. Clin. Obstet. Gynecol. **3:** 3–26.
12. BURGER, H.G., N. CAHIR, D.M. ROBERTSON *et al.* 1998. Serum inhibins A and B fall differentially as FSH rises in perimenopausal women. Clin. Endocrinol. **48:** 809–813.
13. REBAR, R.W. & M.I. CEDARS. 1992. Hypergonadotropic forms of amenorrhea in young women. Endocrinol. Metab. Clin. N. Am. **21:** 173–191.
14. KIM, T.J., J.N. ANASTI, M.R. FLACK *et al.* 1997. Routine endocrine screening for patients with karyotypically normal spontaneous premature ovarian failure. Obstet. Gynecol. **89:** 777–779.
15. IRVINE, W.J., M.M.W. CHAN, L. SCARTH *et al.* 1968. Immunological aspects of premature ovarian failure associated with idiopathic Addison's disease. Lancet **2:** 7574–7890.
16. BANNATYNE, P., P. RUSSELL & R.P. SHERMAN. 1990. Autoimmune oophoritis: a clinicopathologic assessment of 12 cases. Int. J. Gynecol. Pathol. **9:** 191–207.
17. SEDMAK, D.D., W.R. HART & R.R. TUBBS. 1987. Autoimmune oophoritis: a histopathologic study of involved ovaries with immunologic characterization of the mononuclear cell infiltrate. Int. J. Gynecol. Pathol. **6:** 73–89.
18. NELSON, L.M., L.M. KIMZEY, G.R. MERRIAM *et al.* 1991. Increased peripheral T lymphocyte activation in patients with karyotypically normal spontaneous premature ovarian failure. Fertil. Steril. **55:** 1082–1087.
19. WALFISH, P.G., I.S. GOTTESMAN, A.B. SHEWCHUK *et al.* 1983. Association of premature ovarian failure with HLA antigens. Tissue Antigens **21:** 168–169.
20. ANASTI, J.N., S. ADAMS, L.M. KIMZEY *et al.* 1994. Karyotypically normal spontaneous premature ovarian failure: evaluation of association with the class II major histocompatibility complex. J. Clin. Endocrinol. Metab. **78:** 722–723.
21. LINDSTROM, J.M., M.E. SEYBOLD, V.A. LENNON *et al.* 1976. Antibody to acetylcholine receptor in myasthenia gravis. Prevalence, clinical correlates, and diagnostic value. Neurology **26:** 1054–1059.
22. DREXHAGE, H.A., G.F. BOTTAZZO, L. BITENSKY *et al.* 1981. Thyroid growth-blocking antibodies in primary myxoedema. Nature **289:** 594–596.
23. ANASTI, J.N., M.R. FLACK, I. FROEHLICH *et al.* 1995. The use of human recombinant gonadotropin receptors to search for immunoglobulin G-mediated premature ovarian failure. J. Clin. Endocrinol. Metab. **80:** 824–828.
24. AHONEN, P., S. MYLLÄRNIEMI, I. SIPILÄ *et al.* 1990. Clinical variation of autoimmune polyendocrinopathy-candidiasis-ectodermal dystrophy (APECED) in a series of 68 patients. N. Engl. J. Med. **322:** 1829–1836.
25. THE FINNISH-GERMAN APECED CONSORTIUM. 1997. An autoimmune disease, APECED, caused by mutations in a novel gene featuring two PHD-type zinc-finger domains. Nature Genet. **17:** 399–403.
26. NAGAMINE, K., P. PETERSON, H.S. SCOTT *et al.* 1997. Positional cloning of the APECED gene. Nature Genet. **17:** 393–398.
27. MATTHEWS, C.H., S. BORGATO, P. BECK-PECCOZ *et al.* 1993. Primary amenorrhoea and infertility due to a mutation in the beta-subunit of follicle-stimulating hormone. Nature Genet. **5:** 83–86.
28. LAYMAN, L.C., E.J. LEE, D.B. PEAK *et al.* 1997. Delayed puberty and hypogonadism caused by mutations in the follicle-stimulating hormone beta-subunit gene. N. Engl. J. Med. **337:** 607–611.
29. AITTOMÄKI, K., J.L.D. LUCENA, P. PAKARINEN *et al.* 1995. Mutation in the follicle-stimulating hormone receptor gene causes hereditary hypergonadotrophic ovarian failure. Cell **82:** 959–968.

30. AITTOMÄKI, K., R. HERVA, U.H. STENMAN *et al.* Clinical features of primary ovarian failure caused by a point mutation in the follicle-stimulating hormone receptor gene. J. Clin. Endocrinol. Metab. **81:** 3722–3726.
31. LATRONICO, A.C., J.N. ANASTI, I.J.P. ARNHOLD *et al.* 1996. Brief report: testicular and ovarian resistance to luteinizing hormone caused by inactivating mutations of the luteinizing hormone-receptor gene. N. Engl. J. Med. **334:** 507–512.
32. ARNOLD, I.J.P., A.C. LATRONICO, M.C. BATISTA *et al.* 1997. Ovarian resistance to luteinizing hormone: a novel cause of amenorrhea and infertility. Fertil. Steril. **67:** 394–397.
33. TOLEDO, S.P.A., H.G. BRUNNER, R. KRAAIJ *et al.* 1996. An inactivating mutation of the luteinizing hormone receptor causes amenorrhea in a 46,XX female. J. Clin. Endocrinol. Metab. **81:** 3850–3854.
34. KATER, C.E. & E.G. BIGLIERI. 1994. Disorders of steroid 17 alpha-hydroxylaxion deficiency. Endocrinol. Metab. Clin. N. Am. **23:** 341–357.
35. ZACHMANN, M. 1995. Defects in steroidogenic enzymes: discrepancies between clinical steroid research and molecular biology results. J. Steroid Biochem. Mol. Biol. **53:** 159–164.
36. PELLICER, A., F. MIRO, M. SAMPAIO *et al.* 1991. In vitro fertilization as a diagnostic and therapeutic tool in a patient with partial 17,20 desmolase deficiency. Fertil. Steril. **55:** 970–975.
37. KOYAMA, H., T. WADA, Y. NISHIZAWA *et al.* 1977. Cyclophosphamide-induced ovarian failure and its therapeutic significance in patients with breast cancer. Cancer **39:** 1403–1409.
38. STILLMAN, R.J., J.S. SCHINFELD, I. SCHIFF *et al.* 1981. Ovarian failure in long-term survivors of childhood malignancy. Am. J. Obstet. Gynecol. **139:** 62–66.
39. SARTO, G.E. 1974. Cytogenetics of fifty patients with primary amenorrhea. Am. J. Obstet. Gynecol. **119:** 14–23.
40. KRAUSS, C.M., R.N. TURKSOY, L. ATKINS *et al.* 1987. Familial premature ovarian failure due to an interstitial deletion of the long arm of the X chromosome. N. Engl. J. Med. **317:** 125–131.
41. POWELL, C.M., R.T. TAGGART, T.C. DRUMHELLER *et al.* 1994. Molecular and cytogenetic studies of an X;autosome translocation in a patient with premature ovarian failure and review of the literature. Am. J. Med. Genet. **52:**19–26.
42. BIONE, S., C. SALA, C. MANZINI *et al.* 1998. A human homologue of the Drosophila diaphanous gene is disrupted in a patient with premature ovarian failure: evidence for conserved function in oogenesis and implications for human sterility. Am. J. Med. Genet. **62:** 533–541.
43. SCHWARTZ, C.E., J. DEAN, P.N. HOWARD-PEEBLES *et al.* 1994. Obstetrical and gynecological complications in fragile X carriers: a multicenter study. Am. J. Med. Genet. **51:** 400–402.
44. CONWAY, G.S., N.N. PAYNE, J. WEBB *et al.* 1998. Fragile X premutation screening in women with premature ovarian failure. Hum. Reprod. **13:** 1184–1187.
45. WAGGONER, D.D., N.R.M. BUIST & G.N. DONNELL. 1990. Long-term prognosis in galactosemia: results of a survey of 350 cases. J. Inherit. Metab. Dis. **13:** 802–818.
46. DAVIS, S.R. 1996. Premature ovarian failure. Maturitas **28:** 1–8.
47. ANASTI, J.N., S.N. KALANTARIDOU, L.M. KIMZEY *et al.* 1998. Bone loss in young women with karyotypically normal spontaneous premature ovarian failure. Obstet. Gynecol. **91:**12–15.
48. CUMMINGS, S.R., D.M. BLACK, M.C. NEVITT *et al.* 1993. Bone density at various sites for prediction of hip fractures. Lancet **341:** 72–75.
49. WRIGHT, C.S.W. & H.S. JACOBS. 1979. Spontaneous pregnancy in a patient with hypergonadotropic ovarian failure. Br. J. Obstet. Gynaecol. **86:** 389–392.
50. SHAPIRO, A.G. & A. RUBIN. 1977. Spontaneous pregnancy in association with hypergonadotropic ovarian failure. Fertil. Steril. **28:** 500–501.
51. JOHNSON, T.R. & E.P. PETERSON. 1979. Gonadotropin induced pregnancy following "premature ovarian failure." Fertil. Steril. **31:** 351–352.
52. VAN KASTEREN, Y.M., A. HOEK & J. SCHOEMAKER. 1995. Ovulation induction in premature ovarian failure: a placebo-controlled randomized trial combining pituitary suppression with gonadotropin stimulation. Fertil. Steril. **64:** 273–278.

53. NELSON, L.M., L.M. KIMZEY, B.J. WHITE *et al.* 1992. Gonadotropin suppression for the treatment of karyotypically normal spontaneous premature ovarian failure: a controlled study. Fertil. Steril. **57:** 50–55.
54. ANASTI, J.N., L.M. KIMZEY, R.A. DEFENSOR *et al.* 1994. A controlled study of danazol for the treatment of karyotypically normal spontaneous premature ovarian failure. Fertil. Steril. **62:** 726–730.
55. LYDIC, M.L., J.H. LIU & R.W. REBAR. 1996. Success of donor oocyte in *in vitro* fertilization-embryo transfer in recipients with and without premature ovarian failure. Fertil. Steril. **65:** 98–102.
56. NAVOT, D., M.R. DREWS, P.A. BERGH *et al.* 1994. Age-related decline in female fertility is not due to diminished capacity of the uterus to sustain embryo implantantion. Fertil. Steril. **61:** 97–101.
57. LUBORSKY, J.L., I. VISINTIN, S. BOYERS *et al.* 1990. Ovarian antibodies detected by immobilized antigen immunoassay in patients with premature ovarian failure. J. Clin. Endocrinol. Metab. **70:** 69–75.

Osteopenic Syndromes in the Adolescent Female

G. P. LYRITIS,[a] E. SCHOENAU,[b] AND G. SKARANTAVOS[a]

[a]*Laboratory for the Research of Musculoskeletal System, University of Athens, KAT Hospital, Kifissia 145 61, Athens, Greece*

[b]*Children's Hospital, University of Cologne, Cologne, Germany*

ABSTRACT: Low bone density in growing girls and mature young women is usually a finding that needs an explanation and further clinical investigation. Population-based epidemiologic studies on osteoporosis in young persons do not exist. As a disease, osteoporosis among children and adolescents is rare, and since 1965 only 100 cases of idiopathic juvenile osteoprososis have been reported. When osteoporosis occurs in children, it is usually secondary to an underlying medical disorder (e.g., anorexia nervosa, leukemia) or to medications, but occasionally no identifiable primary cause can be detected. It may also be the result of a genetic disorder such as osteogenesis imperfecta. On the other hand, osteopenia in growing and young persons seems much commoner and needs further investigation. Adolescence is a period of increased calcium requirement, and girls with an underlying bone disease are at higher risk for bone demineralization. An additional point of interest is the changes in the geometry of bones through their continuous adaptation to simultaneous skeletal and muscular growth. Bones, through the mechanostat mechanism, adapt to mechanical loading by differentiating their geometry. A recent finding in this direction is that before and during the teenage years there is an environmental effect of physical activity and nutrition on hip geometry. Another important finding is an age-dependent increase in bone cross-sectional area and bone strength index in the absence of an increase in volumetric spongiosa bone density and cortical bone density. Girls, in comparison to boys, deposit more calcium in their bones during puberty, thus probably preparing their skeleton for the forthcoming events of pregnancy and lactation.

INTRODUCTION

Osteopenia can develop early in life, especially during the period of rapid bone acquisition when peak bone mass and size are gained.[1,2] In the female skeleton, at least half of peak bone mass is achieved during the second decade of life. Several factors can contribute in attaining and augmenting peak bone mass, including genetic, nutritional, and exercise. Current data suggest that adolescent females have calcium deficiency, and therefore increasing calcium intake may be of value in increasing peak bone mass and size.[3] However, assurance of compliance in increasing calcium intake in the teenage female population is difficult. Several diseases in the adolescent may cause severe osteopenia and consequent disability. Osteoporosis is a known result of anorexia nervosa[4] mainly due to malnutrition, very low body weight, secondary amenorrhea, and cortisol excess. Other disorders, medications, and behaviors that may affect bone mass and produce low bone mass are[5]: *primary disorders* such as juvenile arthritis, osteogenesis imperfecta, malnutrition and malabsorption syndromes, and kidney disease; *reproductive disorders* such as exercise-induced amenorrhea, delayed puberty, and Turner syndrome; *systemic disease* such as cystic fibrosis and acute lymphoblastic leukemia; *endocrine disorders* such as growth hormone deficiency, diabetes mellitus, hyperthyroidism, glucocorticoid excess, and hyperprolactinemia; *medications* such as anticonvulsants (e.g., for epilepsy), glucocorticoids (e.g., for juvenile arthritis and cancer), immunosuppressive agents (e.g., for cancer); and *behaviors* such as prolonged inactivity or immobility, inadequate nutrition (especially calcium and vitamin D), excessive exercise leading to amenorrhea, smoking, and alcohol abuse.

IDIOPATHIC JUVENILE OSTEOPOROSIS

Idiopathic juvenile osteoporosis is a rare form of bone demineralization that occurs during childhood. The mechanism of bone loss is unclear.[6] Although osteoblasts usually are normal, some bone histomorphometric studies have shown osteoblast dysfunction and decreased bone formation in affected patients, whereas others report increased bone resorption. Idiopathic juvenile osteoporosis is very rare, and until now fewer than 100 cases have been reported. The disease is diagnosed after excluding the other causes mentioned. The first sign of idiopathic juvenile osteoporosis is pain in the lower back, hips, and feet, often accompanied by difficulty in walking.[7] Physical deformity such as kyphosis, loss of height, and limp may be present. The disease is usually reversible after 2–4 years. Growth may sometimes be impaired during the acute phase, and in some cases permanent disability such as kyphoscoliosis may remain. Some medications used to treat osteoporosis in adults have been used, such as calcitonin[8] and bisphosphonates.[9] Preventive measures for spinal deformities are essential.

OSTEOGENESIS IMPERFECTA

Osteogenesis imperfecta is a genetic disorder characterised by bones that break easily, often from little or no apparent cause. The disease is caused by imperfect bone collagen development, the result of a genetic defect. There are at least four distinct forms of the disorder, representing extreme variation in severity from one person to another.[10] Approximately 60% of recognized cases of osteogenesis imperfecta are classified as type I, 15% as type II, 20% as type III, and 5% as type IV. The most common features of osteogenesis imperfecta include unexpected fractures of both the axial and peripheral skeleton, small stature, blue sclera, possible hearing loss and in some cases dental problems. The prevalence of the disease is not known, but it is estimated that about 20,000 people in the United States are affected by this disorder.

BODY COMPOSITION AND BONE MASS IN YOUNG FEMALES

Increasing body weight is associated with higher bone mass. The effect of body weight on the development of a higher peak bone mass is mediated by both lean body mass and fat body mass. Lean body mass reflects the condition of the muscular system, as will be discussed. A prerequisite for the onset and maintenance of a normal menstrual cycle is fat that is more than 17% of body composition.[11] This condition is an important factor in the development of a high peak bone mass.[12]

BONE MASS CONTENT AND BONE GEOMETRY IN GROWING FEMALES

Recognition of osteopenia in the first two decades of life is particularly challenging. Interpretation of bone densitometry results in children must take into consideration age, sex, body mass, and pubertal stage. All these factors affect both bone size and geometry, a critical parameter in the interpretation of bone density measurements. DEXA measurements are influenced by bone size in the direction of underestimation of "density" of small bones and exaggeration of "density" of larger bones.[13] Estimations of volumetric bone density have been proposed[14] on the basis of projected (DEXA) measurements without effectiveness to solve the problem. An interesting site for the estimation of bone strength is the hip, where it was found that girls attain a higher proportion of adult hip geometry during their early teenage years.[15,16] Actually, adult hip geometry is achieved by age 15. In twin studies it is suggested that 20% of adult hip axis length is associated with environmental factors, mainly physical activity and nutrition. All these environmental variables influence attainment of femoral axis length and femoral width before midadolescence.

DEVELOPMENT OF THE SKELETAL SYSTEM AND THE INFLUENCE OF MUSCLES

Bone growth during childhood and puberty adapts to fundamental lows of bone physiology. Skeletal acquisition is achieved through the mechanism of bone modeling and only partially through the mechanism of bone remodeling. Both mechanisms exert their action using both osteoblasts and osteoclasts. These bone cells are working co-operatively under the coordination of the mechanostat.[17] The mechanostat interprets mechanical loading, expressed as strain. The zone between 50 (lower setpoint) and 2500 (higher setpoint) microstrains represents everyday physical activity, leading to bone maintenance without loss or gain. Mechanical usage lower than 50 microstrains is interperted by the bone units as disuse and is followed by bone loss. On the other hand, overloading over 2500 microstrains stimulates excessive osteoblastic activity and thus bone formation. Muscles are responsible for the greater part of skeletal loading and body weight only for a much smaller part.[19] Under the influence of muscle force long bones increase the thickness of cortical bone with a continuous subperiosteal accretion.[20] Using modern methods as peripheral quantitative computer tomography (pQCT) it was found that the volumetric density of trabecular and cortical bone is steady during life.

In a study of 14 healthy children aged 6–13 years using pQCT at the distal radius, volumetric spongiosa bone density (SBD), cortical bone density (CBD), bone cross-sectional area (BCSA), cortical area (CA), and bone strength index (BSI) were measured. BSI values were calculated on the basis of the moment of resistance and cortical density using system integrated software. These parameters were correlated with grip strength measurements using a grip dynamometer. Age-dependent increases in BCSA ($r = 0.68$), CA ($r = 0.78$), BSI ($r = 0.79$). SBD, and CBD were found. Grip strength correlated strongly with the parameters of bone geometry BCSA ($r = 0.8$), CA ($r = 0.86$), and BSI ($r = 0.9$) at $p < 0.1$. SBD and CBD showed no significant correlation to grip strength. The results of this study suggested that an increase in cortical thickness and cross-sectional area represents the most important adaptation mechanisms of the growing bones in response to biomechanical usage. These parameters represent the most important factors of bone strength. Volumetric bone density (material characteristic) of spongiosa and cortical bone is an age-independent parameter that does not change significantly with increasing muscular strength in

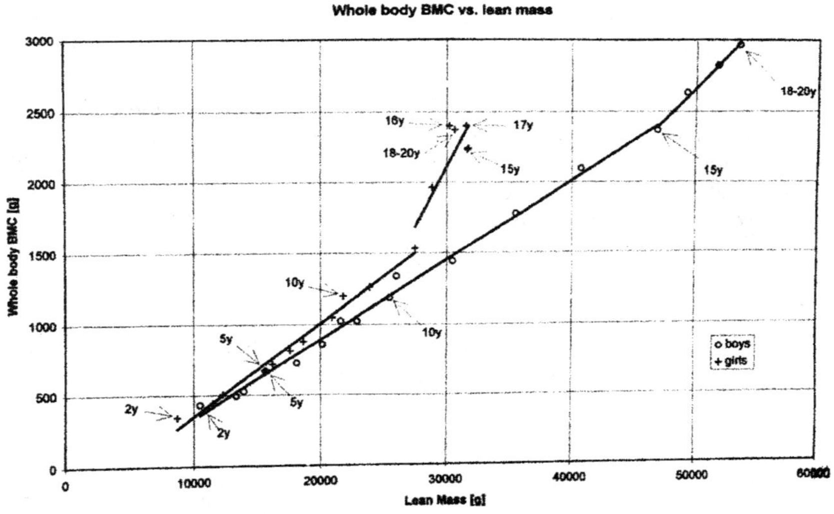

FIGURE 1. This figure plots the grams of bone mineral content (TBMC) on the vertical axis that correspond to the grams of lean body mass (LBM) on the horizontal axis. *Crosses*: girls; *open circles*: boys. It is assumed that the TBMC provides an approximate but useful index of bone strength and the LBM provides an approximate but useful index of muscle strength. *From left to right*, each data point on each curve stands for an age 1 year older than the data point to its left and it shows the mean bone and muscle indices for all subjects in that 1-year age group. The two curves plot the findings in 345 boys and 443 girls. For similar lean body masses (muscle index), around 11–12 years of age bone mass begins to increase faster in girls than in boys. By 14–15 years of age, bone and lean body mass both plateaued in girls, as shown by the closely grouped data points for their 15–20-year age groups on the far right side of their curve. Yet, both indices were still increasing in the 20-year-old males. The 18–20-year age groups for girls were combined in a single data point as well as the data for boys. The data points for girls aged 14 and 15 years overlap. (From Schiessl *et al.*[23] with permission.)

healthy subjects. These relationships must be considered when selecting parameters to be used as success criteria in studies on the influence of physical exercise on bone status.

In an other study using DEXA measurements in 778 healthy caucasian children aged 2–20 years, lean whole body mass was correlated to whole body BMC.[22] Another important finding was that bone mass compared to lean muscle mass began increasing faster in girls after the age of 11–12 and faster in comparison to that of age-matched boys. By 14–15 years of age, muscle index plateaued in girls (FIG. 1). Their bone mass index also plateaued then, at a higher level than that for boys with the same muscle mass index. This finding reveals the estrogen-associated gain in bone mass at puberty, its association with growing lean mass, the difference in this respect between girls and boys with similar lean body masses, and the later plateaus in bone and muscle mass in girls, all of which were predicted earlier.[23] This extra deposit of calcium in girls during puberty (which has no apparent biomechanical purpose) may be a preparation for future biologic needs, such as pregnancy and lactation (H.M. Frost, 1995, personal communication.

REFERENCES

1. BONJOUR, J.P. *et al.* 1991. Critical years and stages of puberty for spinal and femoral bone mass accumulation during adolescence. J. Clin. Endocrinol. Metab. **17:** 555–563.
2. KATZMAN, D.K. *et al.* 1991. Clinical and anthropometric correlates of bone mineral acquisition in healthy adolescent girls. J. Clin. Endocrinol. Metab. **73:** 1332–1339.
3. CHESTNUT, C., III. 1989. Is osteoporosis a paediatric disease? Peak bone mass attainment in the adolescent female. Public Health Rep. **104:** 50–54.
4. BILLER, B.M. *et al.* 1989. Mechanisms of osteoporosis in adult and adolescent women with anorexia nervosa. J. Clin. Endocrinol. Metab. **68:** 548–554.
5. SMITH, R. 1996. Osteoporosis in young people. Osteoporosis Review. J. Natl. Osteoporosis Soc. **4:** 2.
6. BERTELLONI, S. *et al.* 1992. Idiopathic juvenile osteoporosis: evidence of normal osteoblast function by 1,25-dihydroxyvitamin D_3 stimulation test. Calcif. Tiss. Int. **51:** 20–23.
7. VILLAVERDE, V. 1998. Difficulty walking. A presentation of idiopathic juvenile osteoporosis. J. Rheumatol. **25:** 173–176.
8. JACKSON, E.C. *et al.* 1988. Effect of calcitonin replacement therapy in idiopathic juvenile osteoporosis. Am. J. Dis. Child. **142:** 1237–1239.
9. HOEKMAN, K. *et al.* 1985. Characteristics and bisphosphonate treatment of a patient with juvenile osteoporosis. J. Clin. Endocrinol. Metab. **61:** 952–956.
10. BEIGHTON, P. *et al.* 1986 Clinical overview of osteogenesis imperfecta. Am. J. Med. Genet. **29:** 581–594.
11. FRISCH, R.E. *et al.* 1974. Fatness as a determinant of minimum weight for height necessary for their maintenance or onset. Science **185:** 949–951.
12. GEORGIOU, E. *et al.* 1989. Bone mineral loss related to menstrual history. Acta Orthop. Scand. **60:** 192–194.
13. BACHRACH, L.K. 1993. Bone mineralization in childhood and adolescence. Curr. Opin. Pediatr. **5:** 467–473.
14. KROGER, H. *et al.* 1992. Bone densitometry of the spine and femur in children by dual-energy x-ray absorptiometry. Bone Miner. **17:** 75–85.
15. FLICKER, L. *et al.* 1996. Determinants of hip axis length in women aged 10-89 years: a twin study. Bone **18:** 41–45.
16. GOULDING, A. *et al.* 1996. Changing femoral geometry in growing girls: a cross-sectional DEXA study. Bone **19:** 645–649.
17. FROST, H.M. 1990. Structural adaptations to mechanical usage (SATMU): redefining Wolff's Law. The bone modelling problem. Anat. Rec. **226:** 403–413.

18. FROST, H.M. 1990. Structural adaptations to mechanical usage (SATMU): redefining Wolff's Law. The bone remodelling problem. Anat. Rec. **226:** 414–422.
19. WOO, S.L.Y. *et al.* 1981. The effect of prolonged physical training on the properties of long bone: a study of Wolff's law. J. Bone Joint Surg. **63A:** 780–787.
20. GARN, S.M. 1972. The course of bone gain and the phases of bone loss. Paediatr. Clin. N. Am. **3:** 503–520.
21. SCHOENAU, E. *et al.* 1993. Is there an increase of bone density in children? Lancet **342:** 689–690.
22. ZANCHETA, J.R. 1995. Bone mass in children: normative values for the 2–20-year-old population. Bone **16:** 393–399.
23. SCHIESSL, H. *et al.* 1998. Estrogen and bone-muscle strength and mass relationships. Bone **22:** 1–6.

Idiopathic Juvenile Osteoporosis

G.E. KRASSAS[a]

Department of Endocrinology and Metabolism, Panagia General Hospital, Thessaloniki, Greece

ABSTRACT: Osteoporosis in childhood is uncommon, and it may be secondary to a spectrum of diverse conditions. When such causes have been excluded, some patients remain who have a congenital disease (osteoporosis imperfecta) or a disease in which the etiology is obscure, called idiopathic juvenile osteoporosis (IJO). The cause of IJO is unknown, and the diagnosis is based both on the exclusion of other diseases and on its own positive fractures. The basic strategy of treatment is to protect the spine until remission occurs. Sex steroids are contraindicated. Bisphosphonates, calcitriol, fluoride, and calcitonin have been administered therapeuticlly, but the results were equivocal. Usually the disease remits by itself.

Osteoporosis in childhood is uncommon, and it may be secondary to a spectrum of diverse conditions (TABLE 1). When such causes have been excluded, some patients remain who may have an inherited condition called osteoporosis imperfecta (OI) or a disease in which the etiology is obscure. The most severe form of this disorder has been best described by Dent and his colleagues[1–4] under the name of idiopathic juvenile osteoporosis (IJO), although previous descriptions did exist.[5] The disease is rare and mainly affects children between 8 and 14 years old. To date, about 70 cases have been reported in the literature.[6–15] The disease runs an acute course, usually over a period of 2 to 4 years, during which time there is growth arrest and multiple fractures, and then the disease remits. Both the axial and the appendicular skeleton are affected. There is a wide spectrum of severity. The severe cases may have fractures of the vertebrae and the long bones, particularly the metaphyses, that lead to back pain, deformity, and difficulty in walking.[16] They may also present formation of new but osteoporotic bone, characteristically at the metaphyses, but also at other sites of new bone formation, called "neoosseous porosis."[4]

The most remarkable feature of the disease is the almost invariable spontaneous remission. The diagnosis is based both on the exclusion of other diseases and on its own positive features. Any child with fractures and vertebral collapse apparently due to osteoporosis requires investigation for two main reasons: first, to confirm the presence of osteoporosis and if possible to establish its cause; second, and most importantly, to exclude bone infiltration, particularly leukemia. Clinically, it is not difficult to exclude the known causes of osteoporosis, with the important exception of mild OI. Dent and Fiedman[1] stressed that the diagnosis of IJO was best made from its

[a]Address for correspondence: Professor G. E. Krassas, M.D., Endocrine Department, Panagia Hospital, Tsimiski 92, Thessaloniki, Greece 546 22. Phone: 031-447-444; fax: 031-282-476. krassas@the.forthnet.gr

TABLE 1. Secondary forms of juvenile osteoporosis

Endocrine disorders	Gastroinstestinal disorders	Inborn errors of metabolism	Miscellaneous
			Anorexia nervosa
Cushing syndrome	Biliary atresia		Acute lymphoblastic leukemia
Diabetes mellitus	Glycogen storage disease Type 1	Homocystinuria	Anticonvulsant therapy
Thyrotoxicosis	Hepatitis	Lysinuric protein intolerance	Cyanotic congenital heart disease
Glucocorticoid therapy	Malabsorption		Immobilization
Gonadal dysgenesis			

roentgenographic features, which include multiple vertebral compression fractures and fractures of the long bones, especially around the weight-bearing joints. Osteoporotic new bone could be seen in this region and wherever that bone formation was occurring. Patients with mild OI may be distinguished from those with IJO because they usually have blue sclerae and sometimes have dentinogenesis imperfecta and a dominant family history of this disorder. However, none of these features need to be present. TABLE 2 shows the features distinguishing IJO from OI. In practice, it should be very difficult to distinguish OI and IJO by x-ray techniques alone. Repeated fractures with immobilization and surgery can produce remarkable effects on the growing skeleton, and nearly all those changes seen in OI can also develop in IJO. Where it occurs, however, neoosseous osteoporosis seems to be unique to IJO.[16] In the latter, bone formation does not cease and osteoporosis must result from an imbalance between formation and resorption. Jowsey and Johnson[6] and Hoekman *et al.*[7] presented histologic evidence of increased bone resorption, whereas Smith[8] and Reed *et al.*[17] found decreased bone formation to be the major pathophysiologic event in IJO. However, more information from a variety of methods is needed.

Early reports of calcium balance have suggested IJO changes, with initially negative or inappropriately neutral balances[1,3] progressing to positive balance during the healing phase[3] and in response to vitamin D administration. Mader *et al.*[9] and Saggese *et al.*[10] suggested a role for 1,25-dihydroxyvitamin D deficiency in the pathogenesis of IJO. Several reports have also suggested a role for calcitonin deficiency in some patients.[12]

The close relationship of the disease to puberty led Dent[4] to suggest those hormonal factors and especially cortisol might play a role in the pathogenesis of this entity. However, no direct evidence was found for this. The bone loss noted in astronauts undergoing prolonged periods of weightlessness in space might be analogous to IJO, with rapid resorption of weight-bearing bones and suppressed bone formation. Both the bone loss caused by weightlessness and IJO appear to be reversible.[8]

Some have speculated that IJO, like weightlessness, consists of some fundamental disturbance in the mechanical forces that stimulate new bone formation in the growing and young adult skeleton.[18] Because we have no idea why this condition starts or stops, we have no idea how to treat it. The basic strategy of treatment is to protect the spine until remission occurs. Supportive care is instituted promptly (non-

TABLE 2. Differential diagnosis between idiopathic juvenile osteporosis (IJO) and osteogenesis imperfecta (OI)

	IJO	OI
Family history	Negative	May be positive
Onset	Prepubertal	Birth or soon after
Duration	1–5 years	Lifelong
Clinical findings	Metaphyseal fractures	Blue sclerae
		Dentinogenesis imperfecta
		Joint hyperlaxity
		Long bone fractures
Growth rate	Normal	Normal or decreased
Calcium balance	May be negative in acute phase	Positive
Radiological findings	Wedge compressions in spine "Neo-osseous"	Narrow cortex Wormian bones in skull Thin ribs
Connective tissue	Not documented	Mostly, quantitative defect in collagen synthesis

weight-bearing, crutch walking, and physical therapy) in anticipation of spontaneous recovery with the onset of puberty. Sex steroids are contraindicated because of the possibility of early closure of the growth plates. Hoekman *et al.*[7] obtained dramatic results using the bisphosphonate APD. They were able to convert a pretreatment negative calcium balance of –280 mg/day to a positive balance of +356 mg/day after 2 months of treatment in a 13-year-old boy. In addition, Saggese *et al.*[10] demonstrated improvements in bone density and reduced fracture rates in three children treated with calcitriol. Glorieux *et al.*[11] noted an increase in trabecular bone volume and bone formation rate in the patients treated with long-term sodium fluoride therapy. Finally, it has to be mentioned, that Jackson *et al.*[12] found that exogenous calcitonin did not have any therapeutic effect in one patient with calcitonin deficiency and excessive bone resorption.Because the disease remits spontaneously, however, further studies are clearly required before the efficacy of a particular therapeutic regimen can be considered established.

Future investigation should be concentrated on two main topics: First, it is important to identify, as precisely as possible, those patients who have mild OI, not only because of the better prognosis in comparison with patients with severe IJO, but also for genetic counseling. Second, we need more histological studies because it is therapeutically very important to distinguish which bone phase is primarily affected in this disorder, that is, bone formation or resorption. There could be many more etiological factors involved in IJO, which we will only be able to discover when we learn much more about different processes that influence bone formation and resorption.

REFERENCES

1. Dent, C.E. & M. Friedman. 1965. Idiopathic juvenile osteoporosis. Q. J. Med. **34:** 177–210.

2. DENT, C.E. 1969. Idiopathic juvenile osteoporosis (IJO). Birth Defects **5:** 134–139.
3. BRENTON, D.P. & C.E. DENT. 1976. Idiopathic juvenile osteoporosis. *In* Inborn Errors of Calcium and Bone Metabolism. G.H. Bickel & J. Stern, Eds.: 223–238. MTP Press. London.
4. DENT, C.E. 1977. Osteoporosis in childhood. Postgrad. Med. J. **53:** 450–456.
5. CATEL, W. 1954. Pubertatsfischwirbelkrankheit. Kinderaerztl. Prax. **22:** 21–26.
6. JOWSEY, J. & K.A. JOHNSON. 1972. Juvenile osteoporosis: Bone findings in seven patients. J. Pediatr. **81:** 511–517.
7. HOEKMAN, K., S.A. PAPAPOULOS, A.C.B. PETERS & O.L. BIJVOET. 1985. Characteristics and bisphosphonate treatment of a patient with juvenile osteoporosis. J. Clin. Endocrinol. Metab. **61:** 952–956.
8. SMITH, R. 1980. Idiopathic osteoporosis in the young. J. Bone Joint Surg. **62B:** 417–427.
9. MARDER, H.K., R.C. TSANG, G. HUG & A.C. CRAWFORD. 1982. Calcitriol deficiency in idiopathic juvenile osteoporosis. Am. J. Dis. Child. **136:** 914–917.
10. SAGGESE, G., S. BERTELLONI, G.I. BARONCELLI, *et al.* 1991. Mineral metabolism and calcitriol therapy in idiopathic juvenile osteoporosis. Am. J. Dis. Child. **145:** 475–461.
11. GLORIEUX, F.H., N.E. NORMAN, R. TRAVERS & A. TAYLOR. 1993. Idiopathic juvenile osteoporosis. Proceedings of the Fourth International Symposium on osteoporosis and consensus development conference. March 27–April 2. Hong Kong. pp. 200–202.
12. JACKSON, E.C., C.F. STRIFE, R.C. TSANG & H.K. MARDER. 1988. Effect of calcitonin replacement therapy in idiopathic juvenile osteoporosts. Am. J. Dis. Child. **142:** 1237–1239.
13. LAPATSANIS, P., A. KAVADIAS & K. VRETOS. 1971. Juvenile osteoporosis. Arch. Dis. Child. **46:** 66–71.
14. TEOTIA, M., S.P.S. TEOTIA & R.K. SINGH. 1979. Idiopathic juvenile osteoporosis. Am. J. Dis. Child. **133:** 894–900.
15. EVANS, R.A., C.R. DUNSTAN & E. HILLS. 1983. Bone metabolism in idiopathic juvenile osteoporosis. A case report. Calcif. Tiss. Int. **35:** 5–8.
16. SMITH, R. 1979. Idiopathic juvenile osteoporosis. Am. J. Dis. Child. **133:** 889–891.
17. REED, B.Y., J.E. ZESWEKH, K. SAKHAEE, *et al.* 1995. Serum IGF-I is low and correlated with osteoblastic surface in idiopathic osteoporosis. J. Bone Miner. Res. **10:** 1218–1224.
18. NORMAN, M.E. 1996. Juvenile osteoporosis. *In* Official Publication of the American society for Bone and Mineral Research: Primer on the Metabolic Bone Diseases and Disorders of Mineral Metabolism. Third edit. Lippincott-Raven. New York. pp. 275–286.

Alternatives to Estrogen Replacement Therapy

GEORGE B. MAROULIS[a]

Department of Obstetrics and Gynecology, University of South Florida Tampa, Florida 33620, USA

INTRODUCTION

Estrogens exert their influence throughout the body. Estrogens exert many beneficial effects, but there are a few undesirable consequences such as estrogen-related neoplasia and estrogen-induced abnormalities in the uterus, breast, and clotting system.

SELECTIVE ESTROGEN RECEPTOR MODULATORS

We have now realized the creation of estrogens that act on certain organs and not on others. This has been accomplished by designing a group of compounds, called selective estrogen receptor modulators (SERM), that influence in different ways the tissues of interest, that is, bone, heart, blood vessels, breast, uterus, vagina, and brain.[1] These compounds take advantage of the peculiarities of the estrogen receptor and of the effect their binding has on the estrogen receptor.

There are two kinds of estrogen receptors, α (ERα) and β (ERβ). The concentrations of these receptors differ in different parts of the body, and the effectiveness of SERMs depends on (a) how much they are taken up by the various parts of the body and (b) how they bind to the receptors.[2]

The receptors have an -NH_2 (N-terminus), a COOH terminus, a DNA binding domain, and a ligand binding domain. For example, whereas one compound may prevent DNA-receptor interaction, another may prevent or stimulate the ligand binding domain. Once the compounds (ligands) bind on the receptor, they are categorized as type I–IV antiestrogens[3]: type I prevents receptor-DNA interaction (none known); type II inactivates the receptor (i.e., ICI 164); type III causes a partial agonistic effect (i.e., raloxifene); type IV allows conformation of the receptor so that it can bring transcription on a certain number of estrogen-responsive genes (i.e., tamoxifen). Transcription is activated by transcription-activating factors TAF1 and TAF2. TAF1 is on the NH_2 end and TAF2 on the COOH end, which may help create agonistic or antagonistic effects.

Raloxifene (a SERM) can stabilize certain receptor interactions exerting positive effects on the R receptor and is considered a type III antiestrogen. On the other hand, a compound such as tamoxifene stabilizes the estrogen receptor and can allow transcription of a certain number of estrogen receptors.[4] Raloxifene is a benzothiophene and a very interesting compound, because it exerts agonistic and antagonistic activities. Transcription is activated by two different activating factors, TAF1 and TAF2.

[a]Address for correspondence: 5 Neofitou Douka Street, Athens 10674, Greece. Fax: 30-1-7239759.

TABLE 1. Effects of estrogens and SERM on different systems

Compounds	Brain	Uterus	Vagina	Breast	Bone	CV
Estradiol	++	++	++	++	++	++
Raloxifene	–	–	–	–	++	+
Conjugated estrogens	++	++	++	+	++	++
Isoflavones	+	–	+	–	+	+

Therefore, TAF1 interaction may create agonistic activity, whereas TAF2 creates antagonistic activity. Tamoxifen interacts with TAF1 and TAF2 (in the breast). Raloxifene induces different receptor conformations, which explain their variable activity.

Raloxifene was recently marketed for use in postmenopausal women in need of estrogen replacement therapy. The dose of 60 mg is approximately 60% of the equine estrogen dose of 0.625 mg.[5] Raloxifene prevents bone loss (but not as well as do the conjugated estrogens), lowers LDL and cholesterol and triglycerides, but does not increase HDL. Because of its antiestrogenic effects, Raloxifene induces hot flushes and vaginal atrophy and increases the risk of venous thrombosis. Its effect on the cardiovascular system is not yet well established.

TABLE 1 identifies the effects of estrogens and SERM on different systems.[6] Raloxifene's primary use should be in women at risk for breast cancer, who should not use estrogens. Whether the avoidance of risk is worth denying the benefits that estrogens offer, time will tell. Therefore, there is currently no ideal SERM that can act estrogenically and as an agonist on the estrogen receptors of the brain, bone, cardiovascular system, and vagina while having antiestrogenic activity in the breast and uterus.

It should be understood that the effects of SERMs depend on how the SERM interacts with the estrogen receptors which, being of two kinds, differ on location; that is, coronary vessels have ERα and ERβ that may interact differently with the ligands depending on with which of the two they interact. In frontal cortex, ERβ is more abundant than ERα. In the cerebellum, ERβ is expressed.

PHYTOESTROGENS

In addition to man-made SERM, certain naturally existing dietary products act like SERMs. Such are the phytoestrogens, which have been reported to have positive effects on the brain, bone, and cardiovascular system, while not affecting the uterus and breast, and have greater affinity for ERβ.

Phytoestrogens come from plants; they are nonsteroidal substances that have properties similar to those of estrogens.[7] There are two types of phytoestrogens, lignans and isoflavones. Lignans are found in the fibrous husk of whole grains, whereas isoflavones are found in soya and other green plants. The estrogenic effects of the phytoestrogens protect against osteoporosis and heart disease without affecting the uterus and breast.

SYNTHETIC COMPOUND (TIBOLONE)

Finally, there is another compound used as an alternative to estrogen replacement therapy that is not a SERM. The compound is tibolone, a synthetic compound with estrogenic, progestogenic, and androgenic properties. This compound has been shown to alleviate hot flushes, improve mood and insomnia, and improve vaginal dryness, dyspareunia, and libido. The endometrium remains atrophic.[8] However, up to 20% of the women interviewed report breakthrough bleeding. With regard to bone, tibolone is protective and may even lead to an increase in bone mass at the 2.5-mg daily dose. It appears that it suppresses bone remodeling and inhibits bone resportion, as do estrogens.[9]

Its effects on the cardiovascular system are not clearly established. It has been reported to decrease triglyceride, total cholesterol, and HDL levels, while not influencing LDL levels. Its effects on the breast are not yet determined by long-term studies.

In conclusion, these alternatives to estrogen replacement therapy increase our ability to treat women with such needs quite effectively. More improvements are expected in the near future.

REFERENCES

1. Kuiper, G.G., B. Carlsson, K. Grandien *et al.* 1998. Comparison of the ligand binding specificity and transcript tissue distribution of estrogen receptors alpha and beta. Endocrinology **138:** 863–870.
2. Shughrue, P.F., M.V. Lane & I. Merchenthaler. 1997. Comparative distribution of estrogen receptor-alpha and –beta mRNA in the rat central nervous system. J. Comp. Neurol. **388:** 507–525.
3. McDonnell, D.P., D.L. Clemm, T. Hermann *et al.* 1995. Analysis of estrogen receptor function in vitro reveals three distinct classes of antiestrogens. Molec. Endocrinol. **9:** 659–669.
4. McDonnell, D.P. & B.L. Wagner. 1998. The mechanism of action of estrogen and progesterone. In Estrogens and Progesterogens in Clinical Practice. I. Fraser, R. Jansen, R.A. Lobo & M. Whitehead, Eds. Churchill-Livingstone. London.
5. Raloxifene (package insert). International Multicenter Study. 1998. Eli Lilly & Co. Indianapolis.
6. Lobo, R.A. 1998. Designer estrogens: clinical aspects. In Fertility and Reproductive Medicine. R.D. Kempers, J. Cohen, A.F. Haney & J.B. Younger, Eds.: 555–562. Elsevier. New York.
7. Anthony, M.S., T.B. Clarkson, C.L. Hughes, Jr. *et al.* 1996. Soybean isoflavones improve cardiovascular risk factors without affecting the reproductive system of peripubertal rhesus monkey. J. Nutr. **126:** 43–50.
8. Rymer, J.M. 1998. The effects of tibolone. Gynecol. Endocrinol. **12:** 213–220.
9. Rymer, J., M.G. Chapman & I. Fogelman. 1994. Effect of tibolone on postmenopausal bone loss. Osteoporosis Int. **4:** 314–317.

Estrogen Replacement Therapy in the Management of Osteopenia Related to Eating Disorders

VINCENZINA BRUNI, METELLA DEI, ILARIA VICINI, LAURA BENINATO, AND LEONARDO MAGNANI

Department of Obstetrics and Gynecology, University of Florence Medical School, Florence, Italy

ABSTRACT: **The effect of hormone replacement therapy on the bone mineral content of hypoestrogenic subjects depends on the pathogenesis of the disease as well as on the dosage and route of administration. This is particularly true in hypoestrogenism related to eating disorders. We present a longitudinal study of 26 young women with diet-induced amenorrhea compared with a group of subjects with POF. The study protocol included the quantification of weight loss, the endocrine profile (follicle-stimulating hormone, luteinizing hormone, prolactin, E_2, FT3, FT4, thyroid-stimulating hormone, and cortisol), the evaluation of markers of bone turnover (GLA, OSTK-PR, ALP, OHP, and DPYR), and spinal bone density by DEXA at observation and after weight recovery. No hormone replacement therapy was administered. Mean BMD and Z scores before and after recovery do not differ significantly; OHP and DPYR appear significantly higher during basal evaluation, whereas GLA and ALP do not. Data on the impact of oral contraceptive use on bone mineral density are controversial. We particularly discuss the question of long-term treatment with 20 μg ethinyl estradiol pills on peak bone mass acquisition during adolescence.**

INTRODUCTION

The incidence of restrictive eating disorders (diet-induced amenorrhea, anorexia nervosa) in adolescents and young adult women ranges from 1–15% according to different surveys. A serious complication of this abnormal behavior is profound osteopenia of both the trabecular and cortical bone compartments. Longitudinal studies of women with a history of anorexia suggest that after physical recovery, bone density, especially at the appendicular level, may remain below the normal range for their age; the length of amenorrhea, years of physiologic estrogen exposure after weight gain, and body weight as a percentage of ideal body weight independently affect bone recovery.[1,2]

This paper reviews our present knowledge of the pathogenesis of bone loss in anorexia nervosa and highlights the benefits and limitations of hormone replacement therapy as a treatment option for osteopenia.

BONE LOSS IN ANOREXIA NERVOSA

It is now well established that bone loss in eating disorders occurs very early after the onset of amenorrhea, is negatively related to age, weight, and body mass index (BMI), and is positively related to duration of illness. Early onset of amenorrhea, before peak bone mass is reached, is another significant factor. Calcium intake, activity levels, and binge-purging behavior do not greatly contribute to reduced bone density.[3–5] Research on body composition in adolescents with anorexia nervosa demonstrated a strong correlation between bone loss and reduced lean mass and proteins, whereas correlation with the fat component was weaker.[6]

The pathogenesis of reduced bone density is multifactorial and is related to both metabolic and endocrine factors induced by undernutrition. A direct effect of reduced caloric intake on the bone formation rate was demonstated in short-term fasting volunteers[7]; on the other hand, metabolic acidosis, a consequence of nutritional impairment, directly stimulates calcium release from bone tissue and, if prolonged, inhibits osteoblastic activity and enhances osteoclastic activity.[8] Low intake of proteins, calcium, and vitamin D may also contribute to bone loss. Hypoestrogenism has a great impact on bone mineral content especially in girls who have not yet attained their peak bone mass, as it is well known that at bone level, estrogens inhibit the resorptive activity of parathyroid hormone, modulate the action of local growth factors, and, furthermore, facilitate intestinal calcium absorption and reduce renal calcium excretion.[9] In subjects with anorexia nervosa, estrogen deficiency is generally marked, because it is the result of impaired ovarian production, altered metabolism, and reduced peripheral conversion. Elevated cortisol levels decrease bone formation, especially at the trabecular site, inhibiting collagen production and osteoblast precursor differentiation.[4] Low insulin production may reduce calcium absorption.[10] A critical role in bone loss in patients with eating disorders is played by the decreased hepatic synthesis of IGF-1. It has been demonstrated that in bone cells this hormone acts as a modulator of hormonal input and local growth factors and is particularly involved in osteoblastic activity and bone formation rate.[11] The effects of IGF-1 are regulated by at least six different binding proteins, with different sensitivities to metabolic status, and their proteases; the complexity of this system could explain why no direct relation between IGF-1 circulating levels and bone mass was demonstrated in subjects with eating disorders. Interleukin 6 and transforming growth factor-beta (TGF-β) are also both known to stimulate mitosis and differentiation of osteoblasts, and their systemic levels increase in anorectic subjects, but their role in bone loss secondary to starvation is not known. It must be stressed that the extent to which circulating concentrations of growth factors, such as IGF-1 and TGF-β, reflect their bone level remains to be clarified, even if some experimental data on IGF-1 have shown a good correlation of systemic levels with cortical bone formation.[12]

Evaluation of the biochemical markers of bone turnover has contributed more information on the pathogenesis of osteopenia related to eating disorders. Several blood- and urine-specific markers of bone formation and resorption are available; the results of main research studies on bone metabolism in subjects with anorexia nervosa are summarized in TABLE 1. Data derived from measurements of urinary hy-

TABLE 1. Markers of bone turnover in anorexia nervosa

Data	Measurement	Result
Bone formation	Alkaline phosphatase (ALP)	Unchanged [13–17] Elevated [18]
	Osteocalcin (bone GLA protein)	Reduced [7,15,19,20] Elevated [21]
	Procollagen type 1 Carboxylterminal-propeptide (PICP)	Reduced [7]
Bone resorption	Hydroxyproline (HOP)	Unchanged [15,17]
	Deoxypyridinoline (DPYRX)	Elevated [7, 22]
	N telopeptide (NTX)	Elevated [7, 22]
	Cross-laps	Elevated [18]

droxyproline, serum osteocalcin (GLA protein), and alkaline phosphatase[7,13–21] have shown impaired bone formation together with a normal resorption rate, whereas data derived from urinary cross-laps and deoxypiridinoline and serum N telopeptide[7,18,22] have characterized bone metabolism in anorexia nervosa as decreased bone formation associated with increased bone resorption. In any case, the uncoupling of osteoblastic and osteoclastic functions, which in physiologic conditions is strictly related, has been demonstrated as a consequence of undernutrition. One study[20] showed that serum osteocalcin declined, whereas urinary cross-laps increased in proportion to a decrease in BMI in patients whose BMI was below 16.4 kg/m^2. This is the critical value of the index for a positive increase in bone density during recovery.

HORMONE REPLACEMENT THERAPY IN THE TREATMENT OF OSTEOPENIA

Weight rehabilitation is the main factor in normalizing bone metabolism and increasing bone mineral density. Our study on weight recovery has demonstrated that metabolically active hormones (such as cortisol, insulin, IGF-1, and FT_3) return to normal levels with moderate weight gain before reactivation of luteinizing hormone secretion and ovarian follicular estrogen production.[23] Serum levels of IGF-1 seem the best predictors of the restitution of bone mineral content.[24] We recently performed a prospective study of 28 young women with diet-induced amenorrhea (mean weight loss, 13.3 kg) without hormone teatment. Lumbar spine bone mineral density was tested at the first consultation and after resumption of menses or a positive response to the medroxy progesterone acetate test. Weight gain was significant (mean basal BMI, 15.8 kg/m^2; mean BMI after weight recovery, 18.7 kg/m^2), levels of luteinizing hormone, FT_3, and cortisol returned to the normal range, but restoration of bone mass was not significant (mean basal bone mineral density [BMD], 0.90 g/cm^2; mean BMD after weight recovery, 0.93 g/cm^2).[25]

Moreover, we well know that making a real change in eating behavior in these patients is very complex, and persistence of chronic restrictive behavior and, consequently, of a lower than normal bone mass is frequent. Therapeutic strategies used in the treatment of bone loss in postmenopausal women have been suggested for use in women with anorexia nervosa. First, calcium intake should be checked, and, if not sufficient, supplementation is recommended; vitamin D deficiency should be corrected and moderate physical exercise should be encouraged. These recommendations, however, are not sufficient.

Estrogens are potent antiresorptive agents in estrogen-deficient states, but data on their use in subjects with eating disorders are controversial. Preliminary findings on estroprogestin use[26] found a protective effect on lumbar spine BMD, but not at the proximal femur level; this therapeutic effect was later confirmed,[27] but the types of pill used were unreported. Considering estrogen-progestogen replacement therapy, a controlled prospective study on 48 amenorrheic women with anorexia nervosa[28] demonstrated that treatment with conjugated estrogens 0.625 mg + medroxy progesterone 5 mg in sequential regimen does not prevent progressive reduction in trabecular bone density. Another significant result of this study is that estrogen effects differ from one subject to another depending on the percent ideal body weight; patients with the lowest percent ideal body weight had improvement during estrogen administration.

It is possible that young women, just attaining their peak bone mass, require a daily dosage higher than that scheduled for postmenopausal replacement therapy. Moreover, a preliminary study suggested that a transdermal route of estrogen delivery could be more promising than oral administration in the management of osteopenia in adolescents with anorexia nervosa, because it increases IGF-1 levels and partially stimulates osteoblastic function.[29]

Considering our actual knowledge of bone metabolism in anorexia nervosa, an interesting therapeutic perspective could be the association of estrogens, as antiresorptive agents, with drugs able to increase osteoblast function. A possibility is the association with fluoride treatment; this therapy has been tested in a few patients with anorexia nervosa both alone (at a dosage of 11.5 mg/day) and with estroprogestin treatment (at a dosage of 23 mg/day). The results are encouraging; a gain in bone mineral density of 4.5% has been demonstrated after a 6-month period with the first treatment and a 6.3% increase with the combined treatment.[30] Another field of investigation is the therapeutic potential of cytokine regulators. Preliminary study of the effects on bone turnover of recombinant human insulin-like growth factor I[23] demonstrated a dose-dependent effect on markers of bone formation in subjects with anorexia nervosa. Long-term use is actually limited by the need for parenteral administration and the well-known effect of this peptide on many organ systems outside bone; the use of the complex of rhIGF-1 with its natural binding protein-3 has been proposed to target bone tissue.[31] Considering recombinant human TGF-β, its ability to stimulate osteogenic parameters after systemic administration was demonstrated in rats,[32] but data in humans are not yet available.

In conclusion, it is undeniable that the best treatment for eating disorders is an intervention that addresses the underlying psychologic problems and promotes weight rehabilitation. In subjects with long-lasting amenorhea, however, hormonal therapy effective in arresting bone loss and preventing an increased rate of fractures is of great importance. Further controlled studies on estrogen-progestagen treatment are needed, and benefits and limitations of new anabolic agents to increase bone formation should be better understood.

SUMMARY

The high risk of long-lasting osteopenia as a consequence of eating disorders is now well established. Our understanding of this phenomenon has stressed that bone density in subjects with anorexia nervosa is significantly related to sensitive nutritional indices. Nutritional status plays a direct and hormone-mediated profound effect on bone metabolism, inducing decreased bone formation often associated with increased bone resorption. If weight rehabilitation is difficult to achieve, alternative therapeutic options are necessary; hormone replacement therapy at the dosage scheduled for postmenopausal women seems of limited value. Additional studies using different hormone replacement therapy regimens are needed. The effectiveness and safety in long-term experiences of drugs aimed at increasing bone formation (fluoride, rIGF-1, and rTGF-β) are still under discussion.

REFERENCES

1. Herzog, W., H. Minne, C. Deter *et al.* 1993. Outcome of bone mineral density in anorexia nervosa patients 11.7 years after first admission. J. Bone Miner. Res. **8:** 597–605.
2. Brooks, E.R., B. Ogden & D. Cavalier. 1998. Compromised bone density 11.4 years after diagnosis of anorexia nervosa. J. Women's Health **7:** 567–574.
3. Bachrach, L., D. Guido, D. Katzman *et al.* 1990. Decreased bone density in adolescent girls with anorexia nervosa. Pediatrics **86:** 440–447.
4. Biller, B., V. Saxe, D. Herzog *et al.* 1989. Mechanisms of osteoporosis in adult and adolescent women with anorexia nervosa. J. Clin. Endocrinol. Metab. **68:** 548–554.
5. Kiriike, N., T. Iketani, S. Nakanishi *et al.* 1992. Reduced bone density and major hormones regulating calcium metabolism in anorexia nervosa. Acta Psychiatr. Scand. **86:** 358–363.
6. Kooh, S., E. Noriega, K. Leslie *et al.* 1996. Bone mass and soft tissue composition in adolescents with anorexia nervosa. Bone **19:**181–188.
7. Grinspoon, S., H. Baum, V. Kim *et al.* 1995. Decreased bone formation and increased mineral dissolution during acute fasting in young women. J. Clin. Endocrinol. Metab. **80:** 3628–3633.
8. Krieger, N., N. Sessler & D. Bushinsky. 1992. Acidosis inhibits osteoblastic and stimulates osteoclastic activity *in vitro*. Am. J. Physiol. **262:** F442–F448.
9. Prince, R. 1994. Counterpoint: estrogen effects on calcitropic hormones and calcium homeostasis. Endocr. Rev. **15:** 301–312.
10. Rumenapf, G., J. Schmidtler & P. Schwille. 1990. Intestinal calcium absorption during hyperinsulinemic euglycemic glucose clamp in healthy humans. Calcif. Tissue Int. **46:** 73–77.
11. Reed, B., J. Zerwekh, K. Sakhaee *et al.* 1995. Serum IGF1 is low and correlated with osteoblastic surface in idiopathic osteoporosis. J. Bone Miner. Res. **10:** 1218–1224.
12. Danielsen, C. & A. Flyvbjerg. 1996. Insulin-like growth factor I as a predictor of cortical bone mass in a long-term study of ovariectomized and estrogen-treated rats. Bone **19:** 493–498.
13. Crosby, L., F. Kaplan, M. Pertschuk & J. Mullen. 1985. The effect of anorexia nervosa on bone morphometry in young women. Clin. Orthop. Rel. Res. **201:** 271–277.
14. Treasure, J., I. Fogelman & G.F. Russell. 1986. Osteopenia of the lumbar spine and femoral neck in anorexia nervosa. Scott. Med. J. **31:** 206–207.
15. Saggese, G., S. Bertelloni, G.I. Baroncelli *et al.* 1989. Ormoni calciotropi nell'osteoporosi dell'anoressia nervosa. Minerva Pediatr. **41:** 61–65.
16. Matkovic, V., D. Fontana, C. Tominac *et al.* 1990. Factors that influence peak bone formation: a study of calcium balance and the inheritance of bone mass in adolescent females. Am. J. Clin. Nutr. **52:** 878–888.

17. CARMICHAEL, K. & D. CARMICHAEL. 1995. Bone metabolism and osteopenia in eating disorders. Medicine **74:** 254–267.
18. MIRA, M., P. STEWART, J. VIZZARD & S. ABRAHAM. 1987. Biochemical abnormalities in anorexia nervosa and bulimia. Ann. Clin. Biochem. **24:** 29–35.
19. FONSECA, V., V. D'SOUZA, S. HOULDER *et al.* 1988. Vitamin D deficiency and low osteocalcin concentrations in anorexia nervosa. J. Clin. Pathol. **41:** 195–197.
20. HOTTA, M., S. TAMOTSU, K. SATO & H. DEMURA. 1998. The importance of body weight history in the occurrence and recovery of osteoporosis in patients with anorexia nervosa: evaluation by dual X-ray absorptiometry and bone metabolic markers. Eur. J. Endocrinol. **39:** 276–283.
21. MAUGARS, Y. & A. PROST. 1989. Ostèoporose trabèculaire compliquant une anorexie mentale mèconnue. Rev. Rheum. Mal. Osteoartic. **56:** 15–61.
22. GRINSPOON, S., H. BAUM, K. LEE *et al.* 1996. Effects of short-term recombinant human insulin-like growth factor I administration on bone turnover in osteopenic women with anorexia nervosa. J. Clin. Endocrinol. Metab. **81:** 3864–3870.
23. BRUNI, V., M. DEI, A. DIGREGORIO & A. VERNI. 1993. Diet-induced amenorrhea: the effect of moderate recovery of lost weight on endocrine parameters. *In* Recent Developments on Pediatric-Adolescent Gynecology and Endocrinology. G. Creatsas, Ed.: 41–44. Athens.
24. COUNTS, D., H. GWIRTSMAN, L. CARLSON *et al.* 1992. The effect of anorexia nervosa and refeeding on growth hormone-binding protein, the insulin-like growth factors (IGFs), and the IGF-binding proteins. J. Clin. Endocrinol. Metab. **75:** 762–767.
25. BRUNI, V., L. BENINATO, I. VICINI & M. DEI. 1999. Effect of weight recovery on osteopenia related to eating disorders: results of a prospective study. In press.
26. Seeman, E., G. Szmuckler, C. Formica *et al.* 1992. Osteoporosis in anorexia nervosa: the influence of peak bone density, bone loss, oral contraceptive use, and exercise. J. Bone Min. Res. **7:** 1467–1474.
27. MAUGARS, Y., J. BERTHELOT, R. FORESTIER *et al.* 1996. Follow-up of bone mineral density in 27 cases of anorexia nervosa. Eur. J. Endocrinol. **153:** 591–597.
28. KLIBANSKI, A., B. BILLER, D. SCHOENFELD *et al.* 1995. The effects of estrogen administration on trabecular bone loss in young women with anorexia nervosa. J. Clin. Endocrinol. Metab. **80:** 898–904.
29. HAREL, Z. & S. RIGGS. 1997. Transdermal versus oral administration of estrogen in the management of lumbar spine osteopenia in an adolescent with anorexia nervosa. J. Adol. Health **21:**179–182.
30. BAGI, C., E. DELEON, R. BROMMAGE *et al.* 1995. Treatment of ovariectomized rats with the complex of rhIGF-1/IGFBP-3 increases cortical and cancellous bone mass and improves structure in the femoral neck. Calcif. Tissue Int. **57:** 40–46.
31. ROSEN, D., S. MILLER, E. DELEON & A. SOMMER. 1994. Systemic administration of recombinant transforming growth factor beta stimulates parameters of cancellous bone formation in juvenile and adult rats. Bone **15:** 355–358.

Hormone Replacement Therapy and Breast Cancer Risk

GEORGE N. KOUKOULIS[a]

Endocrine Section, 251 Hellenic Air-Force and VA General Hospital, 115 25 Athens, Greece

ABSTRACT: The female breast is subject to a lifetime of hormonal control. After menopause, breast tissue becomes quiescent when estrogens drop to low levels. Menopause-associated hormonal decreases produce short- and long-term consequences that can be treated successfully by hormone replacement therapy (HRT). Despite the beneficial effects of HRT, the potential risk of breast cancer is a concern of both women and physicians. The available data indicate that HRT administered for longer than 5 years moderately increases the risk of breast cancer, but overall the benefits outweigh the potential risk.

INTRODUCTION

Menopause is characterized by drastic changes in the hormonal milieu with a characteristic steady decrease in circulating levels of estrone and estradiol. Menopause-related hormonal alterations produce short- and long-term consequences that can be treated successfully by hormone replacement therapy (HRT). Hot flashes, dyspareunia, atrophic vaginitis, sleep disturbances, and mood changes are among the short-term menopausal symptoms, whereas osteoporosis and cardiovascular disease are the long-term consequences. Life expectancy data indicate that mean age increases worldwide, and considering that natural menopause occurs at approximately 52 years of age, it is clear that women spend the last third of their lives in a postmenopausal state. The quality of life and degenerative diseases in postmenopausal women are two issues of increasing personal, medical, and social importance.

HORMONE REPLACEMENT THERAPY AND WOMEN'S ATTITUDES

It is apparent today that HRT not only relieves climacteric symptoms but also has long-term benefits, including preventing bone loss,[1] reducing the risk of cardiovascular disease,[2] protecting from colorectal cancer,[3,4] and possibly preventing the development of Alzheimer's disease.[5] Although these important benefits have a dramatic effect on morbidity and mortality, HRT is still relatively underused. Despite much published information, it is still sometimes said that HRT is new and that more information is required.

[a]Address for correspondence: Endocrine Section, 251 Helenic Air-Force and VA General Hospital, P. kanelopulu 3 (Katechaki), 115 25 Athens, Greece. Phone: (01) 7799137; fax: (01) 7796568.

The most serious concern about the use of HRT after menopause is the potential oncogenic risk, because endometrial and breast cancer are etiologically linked to the action of steroid hormones. In the UK, only 12% of postmenopausal women actually receive HRT.[6] This low level of use may be explained, to some extent, by adverse events such as fluid retention, weight gain, and breast pain, which are common reasons given for discontinuation, but there are also fears about the risk of endometrial or breast cancer. Fear of the latter is a major reason for the relatively low percentage of persons receiving HRT, and therefore it is important to clarify its overall risks and benefits.

Breast cancer is the most frequent malignant neoplasm in females, accounting for 32% of all female cancers.[7] Breast cancer represents the most feared cancer in women. According to US data, a 50-year-old white woman has a 10% life-time probability of developing and a 3% probability of dying from breast cancer. The median age at which breast cancer is detected is 69 years.[8] However, the frequency of breast cancer increases continuously during a woman's lifespan.[9] After age 50, the incidence of breast cancer increases about 2.1% per year.[10] Breast cancer varies widely in its incidence and associated mortality throughout the world.[11] European sources (from the UK) show a slightly lower life-time probability (6%) of developing breast cancer. Breast cancer makes up 20% of all new female cancers and is responsible for 20% of all female deaths from cancer.

HORMONE REPLACEMENT THERAPY AND BREAST CANCER

Endogenous gonadal hormones have an important role in causing breast cancer, as can be deduced from epidemiologic observations.[12] No abnormality in estrogen excretion was detected in women with breast cancer when it became possible to measure estrogen in urine[13] or later in serum.[14,15] The risk of breast cancer increases in women with early age at menarche and late menopause,[16] with no pregnancy or pregnancy at an older age. Obesity, which is characterized by higher estrogen levels, was also associated positively with moderate elevation in both the incidence of breast cancer and mortality from the disease.[17] However, the influence of lifestyle, genetic factors, physical activity, alcohol consumption, and metabolic or endocrine dysfunction (not related to gonadal steroids) on the relative risk of breast cancer development should not be neglected. Most investigators support the concept that the origin of carcinoma of the breast precedes menopause many years before HRT is proposed to a patient. If that is the case, HRT might influence not only the incidence of breast cancer, but also its clinical evolution.

Studies in premenopausal women indicate that breast mitotic activity peaks when the endogenous progesterone level is highest, which suggests that progesterone may act synergistically with estrogens to accelerate epithelial cell proliferation in breast tissue. Studies from the US suggest that progestogens do not increase the risk of breast cancer, whereas studies from Northern Europe suggest that they may. Epidemiologic information is limited and is based on a small number of patients and different progestogens. The addition of progestin did not reduce the risk of breast cancer associated with estrogen use in postmenopausal women.[18,19] On the other hand, the results of the postmenopausal estrogen/progestin interventions trial (PEPI

TABLE 1. Relative risk of breast cancer in women using hormone replacement therapy from six meta-analyses[a]

Study	No. of studies	Ever used	Long-term use
Armstrong[23]	23	1.01 (0.95–1.08)	—
Steinberg *et al.*[24]	16	1.01 (0.99–1.02)	1.30 (1.20–1.60)
Dupont and Page[30]	31	1.07 (1.01–1.10)	1.09 (0.89–1.50)
Silero-Arenas *et al.*[26]	27	1.06 (1.00–1.12)	1.23 (1.07–1.42)
Grady *et al.* [25]	35	1.01 (0.97–1.05)	1.25 (1.04–1.51)
Colditz *et al.*[27]	34	1.02 (0.93–1.12)	1.23 (1.08–1.40)

[a]The 95% confidence limits are given in parentheses.

study)[20] clearly showed that the risk of adenomatous or atypical endometrial hyperplasia was significantly higher (34%) among women treated with unopposed estrogens, indicating an increased probability of developing endometrial cancer.[21] Thus, although progestins may attenuate the beneficial effects of estrogen on lipoprotein metabolism,[22] the use of estrogen plus progestin is absolutely necessary in postmenopausal women with an intact uterus who choose HRT.

Since 1975, more than 40 studies and 6 meta-analyses[18,23–27] (TABLE 1) on oral contraceptives and HRT and breast cancer risk have been published. Each study has its strengths and limitations that reflect the different study design, number of women studied, and methods for collecting the information. Studies of breast cancer risk are subject to methodologic problems such as noncomparability of groups using or not using the hormonal preparations, a particular problem with HRT. Users tend to be better educated, thinner, and generally healthier than nonusers.[28] Although there are numerous reviews and meta-analyses on both topics, the summary risk estimates and conclusions are inconsistent as to whether oral contraceptives and HRT increase the risk of breast cancer. Studies from Europe show higher risks than do studies from the US,[29] but this could be a function of the particular hormones used and the characteristics of women receiving them. In Europe, estradiol and synthetic estrogens are more commonly used, whereas in the US more than 70% of the estrogen product used is premarin, which is composed of a mixture of estrogens found in mare's urine. In addition, progestin has been used with estrogens in Europe, whereas in the US this combination has only been used in the last decade. Differences in the particular hormones used and the indications for prescribing them may have affected the study results.

Dupont and Page,[30] analyzing 31 studies, concluded that the overall relative risk of breast cancer in menopausal women was not different between estrogen users and nonusers. Another important observation in this study was that unopposed estrogens did not increase the risk of breast cancer in women with benign breast disease. Also, the relative risk of breast cancer associated with conjugated estrogen therapy by dosage (0.625 and 1.25 mg/d) was not significantly different from each other and from controls.

The Nurses' Health Study, a cohort study established in 1976 that follows 120,000 women, has a prospective design and the largest number, two strong points that should eliminate most biases and therefore deserve the greatest attention. Overall, the data are reassuring. Investigators are in substantial agreement that short-term HRT (less than 5 years) is not associated with an increased risk of breast cancer. Meta-analyses found a slight increase in risk only after long-term treatment. In the first analysis of the Nurses' Health Study, a significant increase in breast cancer was observed only in postmenopausal women consuming significant amounts of alcohol.[31] A subsequent analysis[18] published in 1995 raised alarm among physicians and users. In this analysis, the risk of breast cancer was higher in women who were currently using estrogen alone (relative risk [RR] 1.32), estrogen plus progestin (RR 1.41), or progestin alone (RR 2.24) for more than 5 years than in postmenopausal women who had never used hormones. The increased risk of breast cancer was greater among older women. As compared with postmenopausal women who had never taken hormones and after controlling for age at menopause, type of menopause, and family history, the relative risk of postmenopausal women who used hormones was 1.54 for those 55–59 years of age and 1.71 for those 60–64 years of age. Women who stopped taking hormones after 5 or more years were at increased risk of breast cancer for a short period after stopping.

The prognosis of women who developed breast cancer while taking estrogen is reportedly better than that of women not taking it.[32,33] However, this increased survival may reflect better quality of care or earlier diagnosis. This was not the case in the Nurses' Health Study[18] in which the incidence of breast cancer and the risk of dying from it were found to increase at the same rate. Regarding overall mortality among postmenopausal women who use HRT, the results of the third analysis of the Nurses' Health Study[34] showed that mortality, after adjusting for confounding variables, was on average 40% lower in current hormone users (RR 0.63). However, this apparent benefit decreased with long-term use because of a 43% increase in mortality from breast cancer among long-term hormone users (10 years or more). It is important to stress that the largest benefit was derived by users with coronary risk factors (RR 0.151), a fact that should be taken into account when deciding on HRT. The protective effect of hormones was lost 5 years after discontinuing their use.

If the adverse effects of long-term hormone use on the incidence of breast cancer[18,35] and mortality[34] are confirmed by additional research, however, this will argue against the notion that HRT predisposes women to low risk breast tumors, as suggested by studies showing better survival[32] and diagnosis of less advanced disease in hormone users.[36] Substantial reductions in overall mortality among users of the combined regimen as well as users of estrogen alone are indirect evidence against the belief that progestins may diminish the apparent cardioprotective effect of estrogens.[34]

HORMONE REPLACEMENT THERAPY IN WOMEN WITH RISK FACTORS FOR BREAST CANCER

Controversy surrounds the use of HRT in patients who have concomitant risk factors for breast cancer. Kenemans and Scheele,[37] using data from six meta-analyses, failed to demonstrate a consistent synergistic increase in breast cancer risk when HRT was used in women with benign breast disease, nulliparity, a late first pregnancy, natural menopause, and a family history of breast cancer. The increased risk of breast cancer with prolonged HRT is well known, but indirect evidence for the safety of estrogens comes from patients whose pregnancy coincided with or following breast cancer or occurred after taking HRT or oral contraceptives at the time of diagnosis. Neither pregnancy nor oral contraceptive[38] or HRT[39] use has been shown to have an adverse effect on the outcome of breast cancer. This fact is supported by observations in patients with breast cancer who were treated with HRT[32] without any adverse effects. Although these studies describe a limited number of breast cancer patients, the results do not suggest an increase in breast cancer recurrences due to the HRT regimens used. The conventional recommendation is to avoid giving estrogens to women previously treated for breast cancer. However, several investigators now suggest prescribing HRT in previous breast cancer patients who show no present evidence of neoplastic disease but who have significant troublesome menopausal symptoms.

WHY PRESCRIBE HORMONE REPLACEMENT THERAPY?

Given that a white woman's cumulative absolute risk of death from the age of 50–90 years is estimated to be 31% from coronary heart disease, 2.8% from breast cancer, and 2.8% from hip fracture,[40] the benefits of estrogen appear to far outweigh its risks. Long-term hormone users had a 20% reduction in mortality.[41] However, in some women at low risk for breast cancer, the benefits of hormone therapy may not outweigh the risks.[42] Some of the unresolved issues must await the results of ongoing intervention trials of menopausal hormones.

The incidence of osteoporosis is high, with 17.5% of white women over 50 years of age having had a hip fracture.[43] Of women aged 80 years or more, 70% had osteoporosis of the hip, spine, or distal forearm.[44] Coronary heart disease poses an even greater threat to life than does osteoporosis, and a woman is 10 times more likely to die from coronary heart disease than from fracture. Although HRT slightly increases the risk of breast cancer, this event should be considered from the viewpoint that a woman's lifetime risk of death from coronary heart disease is 10 times greater than the risk of dying of breast cancer.

CONCLUSIONS

Despite more than 50 epidemiologic studies of the impact of HRT on the incidence of breast cancer, no consensus has yet been reached. HRT can be given without doubt for 5 years to minimize the risk of breast cancer. Whether this restriction is necessary remains to be proven. It should be stressed that HRT in women whose ovaries are nonfunctional before the age of 50 years does not confer an additional risk. Overall, HRT apparently can be considered safe with respect to breast cancer, with the exception that there is a moderate increase in risk (30–50%) after long-term use. There are currently no convincing data to suggest that combined therapy can prevent this increased risk. Long-term use of HRT must be approached on an individual basis, balancing the benefits against the possible risks, especially in women over 55 years of age. The available data allow the conclusion that the benefits of HRT outweigh the potential risks.

REFERENCES

1. QUIGLEY, M.E.T. *et al.* 1987. Estrogen therapy arrests bone loss in elderly women. Am. J. Obstet. Gynecol. **156:** 1516–1523.
2. GRODSTEIN, F. & M.J. STAMPFER. 1995. The epidemiology of coronary heart disease and estrogen replacement in postmenopausal women. Prog. Cardiovasc. Dis. **38:** 199–210.
3. GRODSTEIN, F. *et al.* 1998. Postmenopausal hormone use and risk for colorectal cancer and adenoma. Ann. Intern. Med. **128:** 705–712.
4. GALLE, E.E. *et al.* 1995. Estrogen replacement therapy and risk of fatal colon cancer in a prospective cohort of postmenopausal women. J. Natl. Cancer. Inst. **87:** 517–523.
5. Consensus on Menopause of the European Menopause Society. 1996. Human Reprod. **11:** 976–979.
6. MCKAY HART, D. 1997. Current attitudes to hormone replacement therapy. Gynecol. Endocrinol. **11**(Suppl 1)**:** 9–12.
7. WINGO, P.A. *et al.* 1995. Cancer statistics. CA. Cancer. J. Clin. **45:** 8–30.
8. Consensus on Menopause of the European Menopause Society. 1996. Human Reprod. **11:** 976–979.
9. Annual Cancer Statistics Review. 1987. Bethesda, MD, National Institutes of Health, III–**36:** NIH publication 88–2789.
10. CUTLER, S.Y. & J.L. YOUNG. 1975. Third National Cancer survey: incidence data. Washington, DC: National Cancer Institute monograph, vol 41.
11. KUBISTA, E. 1997. Current standards of breast cancer treatment in Europe. Gynecol. Endocrinol. **11**(Suppl 1)**:** 23–28.
12. BERNSTEIN, L. & R.K. ROSS. 1993. Endogenous hormones and breast cancer risk. Epidemiol. Rev. **15:** 48–65.
13. JAMMES, V.H.T. & M.J. REED. 1980. Steroid hormones and human cancer. Prog. Cancer Res. Ther. **14:** 471–487.
14. WYSOWSKI, D.K. *et al.* 1987. Sex hormone levels in serum in relation to the development of breast cancer. Am. J. Epidemiol. **125:** 791–799.
15. GARLAND, C.F. *et al.* 1992. Sex hormones and postmenopausal breast cancer: a prospective study in an adult community. Am. J. Epidemiol. **135:** 1220–1230.
16. FEINLEIB, M. 1968. Breast cancer and artificial menopause: a cohort study. J. Natl. Cancer Inst. **41:** 315–329.
17. TRETLI, S. 1989. Height and weight in relation to breast cancer morbidity and mortality: a prospective study of 570,000 women in Norway. Int. J. Cancer **44:** 23–30.
18. COLDITZ, G.A. *et al.* 1995. The use of estrogens and progestins and the risk of breast cancer in postmenopausal women. N. Engl. J. Med. **332:** 1589–1593.
19. EWERTZ, M. 1988. Influence of non-contraceptive exogenous and endogenous sex hormones on breast cancer risk in Denmark. Int. J. Cancer **42:** 832–838.
20. The writing group for the PEPI trial. 1995. Effects of estrogen or estrogen/progestin regimens on heart disease risk factors in postmenopausal women. JAMA **273:** 199–208.
21. ANTURES, C.M.F. *et al.* 1979. Endometrial cancer and estrogen use: report of a large case-control study. N. Engl. J. Med. **300:** 9–13.
22. LOBO, R.A. 1992. The role of progestins in hormone replacement therapy. Am. J. Obstet. Gynecol. **166:** 1997–2004.
23. ARMSTRONG, B.K. 1988. Oestrogen therapy after the menopause—boon or bane? Med. J. Aust. **148:** 213–214.
24. STEINBERG, K.K. *et al.* 1991. A meta-analysis of the effect of estrogen replacement therapy on the risk of breast cancer. J. Am. Med. Assoc. **265:** 1985–1990.
25. GRADY, O. *et al.* Hormone replacement therapy to prevent disease and prolong life in pestmenopausal women. Ann. Intern. Med. **117:** 1016–1041.
26. SILLERO-ARENAS, M. *et al.* 1992. Menopausal hormone replacement therapy and breast cancer: a meta-analysis. Obstet. Gynecol. **79:** 286–294.
27. COLDITZ, G.A. *et al.* *1*993 Hormone replacement therapy and risk of breast cancer: results from epidemiological studies. Am. J. Obstet. Gynecol. **168:** 1473–1480.
28. MATHEWS, K.A. *et al.* 1989. Behavioral antecendents and consequences of the menopause. *In* The Menopause: Biological and Clinical Consequences of Ovarian Failure:

Evolution and Management. S.G. Korenman, Ed. :1–10. Nada, CA. Serono Symposia.
29. HULKA, B.S. 1990. Hormone replacement therapy and the risk of breast cancer. CA. Cancer J. Clin. **40:** 289–296.
30. DUPONT, W.D. & D.L. PAGE. 1991. Menopausal estrogen replacement therapy and breast cancer. Arch. Intern. Med. **151:** 67–72.
31. COLDITZ, GA. 1990. A prospective assessment of moderate alcohol intake and major chronic diseases. Ann. Epidemiol. **1:** 167–177.
32. BERGKVIST, L. *et al.* 1989. Prognosis after breast cancer diagnosis in women exposed to estrogen and estrogen-progestin replacement therapy. Am. J. Epidemiol. **130:** 221–228.
33. HENDERSON, B.E. *et al.* 1991. Decreased mortality in users of estrogen replacement Arch. Intern. Med. **151:** 75–78.
34. GRODSTEIN, F. 1997. Postmenopausal hormone therapy and mortality. N. Engl. J. Med. **336:** 1769–1775.
35. BEGKVIST, L. *et al.* 1989. The risk of breast cancer after estrogen and estrogen-progestin replacement. N. Engl. J. Med. **321:** 293–297.
36. BRINTON, L.A. *et al.* 1986. Menopausal estrogen and breast cancer risk: an expanded case-control study. Br. J. Cancer **54:** 825–832.
37. KENEMANS, P. & F. SCHEELE. 1997. Hormone replacement therapy in patients at high risk of developing breast cancer: the use of a combined risk model. Gynecol. Endocrinol. **11**(Suppl 1)**:** 17–22.
38. ROSNER, D & W. LANE. 1986. Oral contraceptive use has no adverse effect on the prognosis of breast cancer. Cancer **57:** 591–596.
39. DISAIA, P.J. *et al.* 1996. Hormone replacement therapy in breast cancer survivors: a cohort study. Am. J. Obstet. Gynecol. **174:** 1494–1498.
40. CUMMINGS, S.R. *et al.* 1989. Lifetime risks of hip, Colls' or vertebral fracture and coronary heart disease among white postmenopausal women. Arch. Intern. Med. **149:** 2445–2448.
41. BRINTON, L.A. & C.S. SCHAIRER. 1997. Postmenopausal hormone-replacement therapy: time for a reappraisal? (editorial) N. Engl. J. Med. **336:** 1821–1823.
42. COL, N.F. *et al.* 1997. Patient-specific decisions about hormone replacement therapy in postmenopausal women. J. Am. Med. Assoc. **277:** 1140–1147.
43. COOPER, C. & E. BARRETT-CONNOR. 1996. The incidence of osteoporosis epidemiology. *In* Proceedings of the 1996 World Congress on Osteoporosis, Amsterdam, May 18–23. S. Papapoulos *et al.*, Eds. :75–77. Elsevier. Amsterdam.
44. MELTON, L.J. 1996. Global aspects of osteoporosis: epidemiology. *In* Proceedings of the 1996 World Congress on Osteoporosis, Amsterdam, May 18–23. S. Papapoulos *et al.,* Eds. :79–86. Elsevier. Amsterdam.

Gonadotropin-Releasing Hormone Analogues in the Management of Precocious Puberty

BESSIE E. SPILIOTIS[a]

Pediatric Endocrine Unit, Department of Pediatrics, University of Patras Medical School, Patras, 26500 Greece

Gonadotropin-releasing hormone (GnRH) analogues have successfully been used to treat central precocious puberty (CPP) for 20 years.[1–6] By inducing long-term suppression of the pituitary–gonadal axis, these potent agonist analogues of GnRH (GnRHan) have been able to play a major role in allowing the child to return to a prepubertal state "physiologically" and psychologically. Although the success of GnRHan treatment is physically apparent, there have always been concerns regarding two issues: (1) After the cessation of therapy, can the central nervous system mechanisms and the gonads pick up where they left off with reactivation of the process of pubertal maturation? and (2) Can final adult height be improved with the use of GnRHan? These two questions took several years to be answered, but good evidence now available can positively confirm a successful outcome on both counts.

First, preliminary studies in the past showed that the effects of GnRH analogues on sexual maturation in girls are fully reversible,[6] as confirmed by subsequent studies.[7–9] Recently it was shown that menarche occurs 1.2 ± 0.8 years after the cessation of GnRHan therapy with a range of 0.1–4.3 years and that menstrual cycle lengths become increasingly regular, with cycles of 25–35 days' duration reported by 4% of the girls in the first year postmenarche and 65% of the girls studied 3 years postmenarche[7] (FIG. 1). Ovulation was demonstrated in 50% of the girls within 1 year of menarche and 90% of the girls studied 2 years or more postmenarche[7] (FIG. 2). The timing of menarche in girls treated with GnRHan is determined primarily by the decision of when to stop therapy. This decision is usually based on assessment of the young girl for psychologic "readiness" for menarche based on her psycholgic development and the projected height posttherapy based on bone age. Psychologic readiness for menarche is purely subjective and is derived from the parents and the physician's assessment of the child and the child's ability to relate with her peers.

The natural history of CPP includes normal expectations of adult reproductive function,[10] and this was also confirmed in GnRHan-treated patients by the normal pregnancies observed after therapy.[7]

As for the final adult height achieved by the children post-GnRHan therapy, the results of multiple studies show the positive outcome of improved adult height of GnRHan-treated children with CPP.[11–19] To understand the mechanism involved in

[a]Phone: 0030-61-993 948; fax: 0030-061-994 533.
MOC-BERA@med.upatras.gr

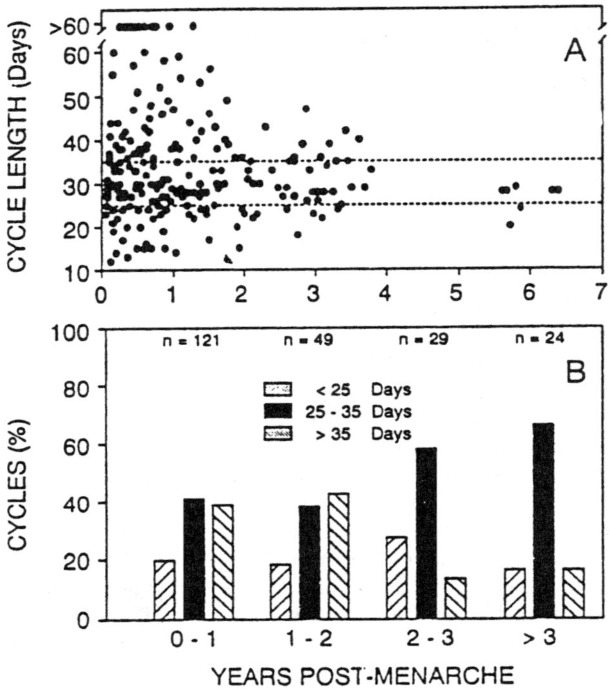

FIGURE 1. Menstrual cycle lengths in 34 girls with central precocious puberty (CPP) after GnRHa therapy plotted relative to time postmenarche. (From Jay *et al.*,[7] reprinted with permission.)

this success, we must remember that growth spurt and bone age advancement in CCP as well as in normal puberty are mediated by an increase in pulsatile GH secretion, which is associated with an increase in testosterone and estradiol[20, 21] and by the direct effects of these sex steroids on the growth plate.[22]

Before the development of the GnRHan, children with CPP had a significantly compromised final height prognosis because of rapid epiphyseal maturation and fusion. Various medications to suppress the secretion of the sex steroids in CPP such as medroxyprogesterone and cyproterone acetate were tried over the years, but they did not alter the height prognosis of children with CPP.[23–25] Although the physical signs of CPP are suppressed with these medications, no difference in growth and bone age advancement was noted between children treated with medroxyprogesterone and cypoterone acetate and those left untreated.

Treatment with the GnRHan started a new era in the therapy of CPP. Until their use, the child with CPP was destined to be short unless she had only slight bone age advancement at the onset of CPP, a slow rate of progression of the physical signs of puberty, and tall parents.[26,27]

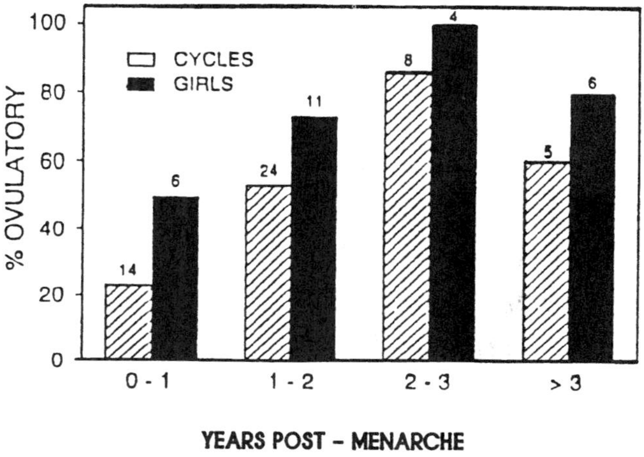

FIGURE 2. Rates of ovulation in girls with central precocious puberty (CPP) after GnRHa therapy plotted relative to time postmenarche. (From Jay *et al.*,[7] reprinted with permission.)

Before initiating GnRHan therapy, the physician must carefully explain to the parents the course of events. The onset of treatment with GnRHan produces an initial stimulation of the gonadotropins before pituitary desensitization, causing an initial rapid increase in growth.[28] The child and parent will notice that during the first 3 months of GnRHan treatment, the physical sings of CPP will progress. When pituitary desensitization to GnRH begins, there is slowing of the growth rate and the bone age and regression of the physical signs of puberty.

Initially it was thought that no long-term difference probably existed in the height achieved by children treated with GnRHan and those left untreated.[29,30] More recent studies have shown a definite improvement in predicted height during treatment with GnRHan, which can range from 2 cm over 2 years to 16 cm over 5 years[30] (TABLE

TABLE 1. Predicted height (PH) in children with central precocious puberty (CPP) treated with GnRHan[30]

Sex	PH (cm) At onset	PH (cm) Follow-up	Drug
Female	156	162	Decapeptyl
Male	174	184	Decapeptyl
Female	162	164	Decapeptyl
Male/female	158	162	Busarelin
Male/female	156	158	Busarelin
Female	145	161	Deslorelin
Female	148	152	Deslorelin or histerelin

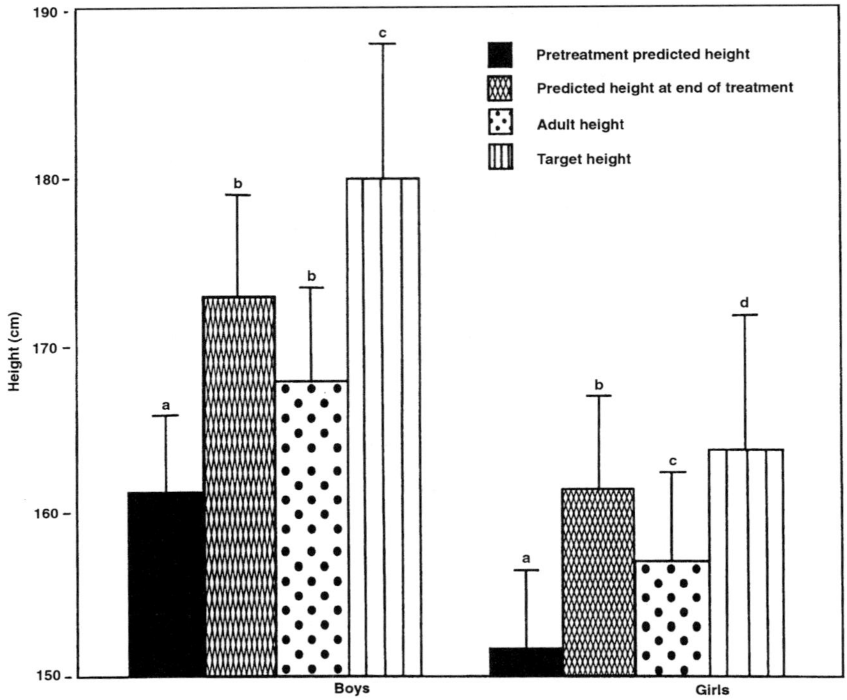

FIGURE 3. Pretreatment predicted height, predicted height at the end of treatment, proximate adult height, and target height in 44 children who received long-term deslorelin treatment for precocious puberty. (From Oerter & Cutler,[30] reprinted with permission.)

1). This occurs because the GnRHan indirectly suppresses sex steroid secretion to the point that bone age advancement is significantly slowed. Of interest is a recent study that showed that the body mass index of children on GnRHan therapy increases during treatment and may remain high on cessation of therapy.[17] Careful dietary instructions must therefore be given to the child, because the child's appetite on initiation of therapy, and without careful and correct eating habits she risks becoming obese.

The good outcome of treatment with the GnRHan as it applies to normal progression of puberty posttherapy with the initiation of menarche, ovulation, and the option for future pregnancies preserved together with a good outlook for final adult height has made therapy with GnRHan the treatment of choice for CPP. The decision to start GnRHan therapy, however, must be made after weighing all the different factors carefully and discussing these at length with the parents. There is good evidence that children who develop CPP at age 7 or 8 often may not need treatment to preserve their height potential,[30] especially if the parental height is good. Some of these children may need their puberty to be suppressed if they are not psychologically mature enough to handle the fact that their physical appearance will differ significantly from that of their peers. Also, parents must take part in the decision-making not only because of their knowledge of the psychologic factors that are important for their child, but also because it must not be forgotten that the GnRH analogues have only been in use less than 20 years. All studies so far have shown no significant side effects, but the decision for treatment must include a risk:benefit ratio so that the physician may make the correct decision for each child.

REFERENCES

1. Crowley, W.F., Jr., F. Comite, W. Vale *et al.* 1981. Therapeutic use of pituitary desensitization with long-acting LHRH agonist: a potential new treatment for idiopathic precocious puberty. J. Clin. Endocrinol. Metab. **52:** 370–372.
2. Styne, D.N., D.A. Harris, C.A. Egli *et al.* 1985. Treatment of true precocious puberty with a potent luteinizing hormone-releasing factor agonist; effect on growth, sexual maturation, pelvic aonography and the hypothalamic-pituitary-gonadal axis. J. Clin. Endocrinol. Metab. **61:** 142–151.
3. Boepple, P.A., M.J. Mansfield, M.E. Wierman *et al.* 1986. Use of potent, long-acting agonist of gonadortropin-releasing hormone in the treatment of precocious puberty. Endocrinol. Rev. **7:** 24–33.
4. Manasco, P.K., O.H. Pescovitz, C. Surimol *et al.* 1989. Six-year results of luteinizing hormone releasing hormone (LHRH) agonist treatment in children with LHRH-dependent pecocious puberty. J. Pediatr. **115:** 105–108.
5. Kaplan, S.L. & M.M. Grumbach. 1990. Pathophysiology and treatment of sexual precocity. J. Clin. Endocrinol. Metab. **71:** 785–789.
6. Ward, P.S., A.W. McNinch *et al.* 1986. Reversible inhibition of central precocious puberty with a long-acting GnRH analogue. Arch. Dis. Child. **60:** 872–874.
7. Jay, N., M.J. Mansfield, R.M. Blizzard *et al.* 1992. Ovulation and menstrual function of adolescent girls with central precocious puberty after therapy with gonadotropin-releasing hormone agonists. J. Clin. Endocrinol. Metab. **75:** 890–894.
8. Manasco, P.K., O.H. Pescovitz, P.P. Feulillan *et al.* 1988. Resumption of puberty after long-term luteinizing hormone-releasing hormone agonist treatment of central precocious puberty. J. Clin. Endocrinol. Metab. **67:** 368–372.
9. Kauli, R., L. Kornreich & Z. Laron. 1990. Pubertal development growth and final height in girls with sexual precocity after therapy with the GnRH analogue D-TRP-6-LHRH. Horm. Res. **33:** 11–17.
10. Murram, D., J. Dewhurst & D.B. Grant. 1984. Precocious puberty: a follow up study. Arch. Dis. Child. **59:** 77–78.
11. Comite, F., F. Cassorla, K.M. Barnes *et al.* 1986. Luteinizing hormone releasing hormone analogue therapy for central precocious puberty: long term effect on somatic growth, bone maturation and height prediction. JAMA **255:** 2613–2616.
12. Drop, S.L.S., R.J.H. Odink, C. Rouwe *et al.* 1987. The effect of treatment with an LHRH agonist (busarelin) on gonadal activity, growth and bone maturation in children with central precocious puberty. Eur. J. Pediatr. **146:** 272–278.
13. Galluzzi, F., R. Satti, A. Albanese *et al.* 1989. Treatment of central precocious puberty with LHRHa (busarelin): long term effect on growth, bone maturation and predicted height. J . Endocrinol. Invest. **12** (suppl 3): 149–150.
14. Manasco, P.K., O.H. Pescovitz, S.C. Hill *et al.* 1989. Six-year results of LHRH agonist treatment in children with LHRH-dependent precocious puberty. J. Pediatr. **115:** 105–108.
15. Boepple, P.P., M.J. Mansfield, J.D. Crawford *et al.* 1991. Final heights in girls with central precocious puberty following GnRH agonist-induced pituitary-gonadal suppression. Pediatr. Res. **29:** 74A.
16. Sippel, W.G., C.J. Partsch, R. Hummelink & F. Lorenzen. 1991. Langzeittherapie mit dem Retard-LHRH-Agonisten Decapeptyl-Depot bei Madchen mit Pubertas praecox vera. Gynakologe **24:** 108–113

17. OERTER, K.E., P. MANASCO, K. BARNES *et al.* 1991. Adult hieght in precocious puberty after long-term treatment with deslorelin. J. Clin. Endocrinol. Metab. **73:** 1235–1240.
18. PAUL, D., F.A. CONTE, M.M. GRUMBACH *et al.* 1995. Long-term effect of gonadotropin-releasing hormone agonist therapy on final and near-final height in 26 children with true precocious puberty treated at a median age of less than 5 years. J. Clin. Endocrinol. Metab. **80(2):** 546–551.
19. OOSTDIJK, W., B. RIKKEN, S. SCHREUDER *et al.* 1996. Final height in central precocious puberty after long term treatment with a slow release GnRH agonist. Arch. Dis. Child. **75(4):** 292–297.
20. HO, K.Y., W.S. EVANS, R.M. BLIZZARD *et al.* 1987. Effects of sex and age on 24-hour profile of growth hormone secretion in man: importance of endogenous estradiol concentration. J.Clin. Endocrinol. Metab. **64:** 51–58.
21. MAURUS, N., R.M. BLIZZARD, K. LINK *et al.* 1987. Augmentation of growth hormone secretion during puberty: evidence for a pulse amplitude-modulated phenomenon. J. Clin. Endocrinol. Metab. **64:** 596–601.
22. ATTIE, K.M., N.R. RAMIREZ, F.A. CONTE *et al.* 1990. The pubertal growth spurt in eight patients with true precocious puberty and growth hormone deficiency: evidence of a direct role of sex steroids. J. Clin. Endocrinol. Metab. **71(4):** 975–983.
23. WERDER, E.A., G. MURSET, M. ZACHMANN *et al.* 1974. Treatment of precocious puberty with cyproterone acetate. Pediatr. Res. **8:** 248–256.
24. STANHOPE, R., K.F. HUEN, F. BUZI *et al.* 1987. The effect of cyporterone acetate on the growth of children with central precocious puberty. Eur. J. Pediatr. **146:** 500–503.
25. KUPPERMAN, H.S. & J.A. EBSTEIN. 1962. Medroxyprogesterone acetate in the treatment of constitutional secual precocity. J. Clin. Endocrinol. Metab. **22:** 456–458.
26. FONTOURA, M., R. BRAUNER, C. PREVOT *et al.* 1989. Precocious puberty in girls: early diagnosis of a slowly progressing variant. Arch. Dis. Child. **64:** 1170–1176.
27. KREITER, M., S. BURSTEIN, R.L. ROSENFIELD *et al.* 1990. Preserving adult height potential in girls with idiopathic true precocious puberty. J. Pediatr. **117:** 364–370.
28. STANHOPE, R., P.J. PRINGLE, C.D.G. BROOK *et al.* 1988. Growth, growth hormone and sex steroid secretion in central precicious puberty with GnRH analogues. Acta Paediatr. Scand. **77:** 525–530.
29. WERDER, E.A., R. ILLIG, M. ZACHMANN *et al.* 1986. Treatment of precocious puberty in girls with intranasal LHRH agonist (Busarelin). Pediatr. Res. **20:** 1185.
30. OERTER, K.E. & G.B. CUTLER, JR. 1993. The decision to treat precocious puberty: height preservation and other considerations. Highlights **1(2):** 5–7.

Current and Potential Application of GnRH Agonists in Gynecologic Practice

JOHN M. TZAFETTAS[a]

3rd University Department of Obstetrics and Gynecology, Hippokrateio Hospital, Thessaloniki, Greece

ABSTRACT: The development of GnRH-a (analogues or agonists) is a major leap forward in the treatment of various hormone-dependent diseases in medicine. Their introduction in reproductive endocrinology, in *in vitro* fertilization/embryo transfer (IVF/ET) and other assisted reproduction techniques had a revolutionary impact. They have been effective in other gynecologic conditions including fibroids, endometriosis, anovulatory disorders, precocious puberty, dysfunctional uterine bleeding, and operative hysteroscopy. Medical castration induced by GnRH-a has become first-line therapy in metastatic breast cancer. Their long-term use, though, has been associated with a variety of adverse effects such as bone loss and decreased cardioprotection. "Steroid add-back" therapy in these cases apparently is an effective alternative. It may allow their safe long-term application beyond 6 months, averting unpleasant side-effects and maintaining bone mass and cardioprotection.

INTRODUCTION

The development of GnRH-a (analogues or agonists) is not only a breakthrough in the field of obstetrics and gynecology, but also a major leap forward in the treatment of various hormone-dependent diseases in general medicine. The importance of their development has been compared to the discovery of oral contraceptives in the 1950s.[1]

Their mechanism of action and influence on the ovarian cycle depend on the mode of application. Single or short-term application may enhance ovulation by inducing a transient rise in supraphysiologic gonadotropin liberation and an increase in GnRH receptor formation (upregulation, flare-up effect). Continued treatment leads to pituitary desensitization and downregulation (decrease in receptor binding site formation), creating a hypoestrogenic condition by suppressing the secretion and production of follicle stimulating hormone (5-fold) and luteinizing hormone (10-fold). This is the result of their strong binding to GnRH receptors (100–200 times higher affinity than the physiologic GnRH). The increased peptidase activity in the degradation of the analogue/receptor complex is not compensated by the physiologic receptor turnover, resulting in suppression of the synthesis and liberation of Gn (desensitization).[2] It has been shown that GnRH-a suppresses growth hormone (GH) release and serum prolactin levels either through a direct effect on pituitary ac-

[a]Address for correspondence: J.M. Tzafettas, MD, FRCOG, 19 Smyrnis Road, Panorama, 55236 Thessaloniki, Greece. Phone: (031) 201300; fax: (031) 218478.
IVFthes@compulink.gr

TABLE 1. Application of GnRH agonists in gynecologic disorders

Treatment	Disorder
Short-term	1. Uterine leiomyomas
	2. Endometriosis
	3. Dysfunctional uterine bleeding
	4. Hyperandrogenism (polycystic ovaries)
	5. Infertility (ovulation induction, *in vitro* fertilization)
Long-term (>6 months)	1. Cancer
	2. Precocious puberty

tivity or as a result of reduced estrogen activity. No further effects on other pituitary hormones have been shown.[3,4]

CLINICAL USE OF GnRH-A IN GYNECOLOGIC CLINICAL PRACTICE

A variety of applications of GnRH-a have recently been used in the treatment of various gynecologic conditions (TABLE 1).

Leiomyomas

Uterine leiomyomas are monoclonal tumors derivied from a single myometrial cell. Although the etiologic mechanism remains unresolved, estrogens have traditionally been considered responsible for promoting their growth.

Prolonged administration of GnRH-a (3–6 months) results in a 40–60% reduction in fibroid volume, often enabling the surgeon to convert an acute condition to a chronic one. Reduction of the size and the blood flow diminishes the need for blood transfusion and facilitates surgical removal, which can often be accomplished transvaginally rather than abdominally, thus shortening hospital stay and improving cost effectiveness.[5]

Doppler ultrasound studies have demonstrated a decrease in arterial blood flow in both the uterus and the fibroids following GnRH-a administration.[6,7] The decreased vascularization caused by the associated estrogonopenia most probably contributes to shrinkage of the myomas and reduction of blood loss during surgery. The decreased blood flow may also induce hyaline degeneration and reduce the cellularity of the fibroid. Furthermore, hypoestrogenism may lead to suppression of intracellular protein synthesis and involution of muscle fibers in the fibroid. In addition, it may be responsible for decreased myometrial and fibroid secretion of IGF-I and IGF-II.[8,9]

GnRH-a may have a place in treating patients not eligible for surgery either because of an other severe medical condition or because of noncompliance.

Endometriosis

Endometriosis has been described as the most debilitating benign gynecologic disease, with an invasive capacity resembling that of malignant tumors. Immunologic factors possibly contribute to the development of the disease, but the disease itself activates the immunologic system, giving rise to both acute and chronic inflammatory reactions, resulting in the formation of adhesions and fibrous tissue. As part of the inflammatory process, the cytokine cascade is initiated and various substances are released such as cytokines, growth factors, and prostaglandins, some of them giving rise to pain, a dominant symptom.

The incidence of endometriosis appears to be increasing and affects more than 30% of women with dysmenorrhea and chronic pelvic pain and more than 50% of patients with unexplained infertility.[10] It has long been known that estrogens and progestagens stimulate endometriosis and that ovariectomy causes regression. On the other hand, it is well understood by now that GnRH-a induce pituitary desensitization and suppress ovarian steroidogenesis, resulting in estrogen deprivation and therefore regression of endometriosis. In suppression of ovarian steroidogenesis, other mechanisms may be involved, such as the absence of LH pulsatility and the direct action on ovarian tissue by reducing the gonadotropin receptors in the ovary.[11]

GnRH-a may reduce adhesion formation by decreasing the plasminogen activator inhibitor which, in turn, decreases fibrin generation and adhesion formation,[12] or by reducing vascularity.

Endometriosis is estrogen dependent for its growth but not for its implantation.[13] It is a progressive disease, and delaying treatment is not justified, particularly in symptomatic cases. Until a few years ago treatment consisted of gestagens and danazol, a rather cumbersome treatment often associated with unpleasant side effects and a high discontinuation rate. Remission rather than cure of the disease can be achieved.[14,15] Recently GnRH-a have become very valuable in the treatment of endometriosis, a typical estrogen-dependent condition. Although there are differences in hormonal activity between danazol and GnRH-a, in terms of disease improvement their effects overlap. However, the androgenic effects of the former (acne, oily skin, and elevated liver enzymes) make GnRH-a a more attractive therapeutic option. Patients on GnRH-a show better compliance, with longer recurrence-free periods from the clinical symptoms.[16,17] Another concern with danazol is its adverse effects on the lipoprotein profile. The reduction of HDL-cholesterol and the increment of LDL-cholesterol worsen the atherogenic profile, with unsure final implications.[18]

According to extensive evaluations of preoperative medical therapies by Donnez *et al.*, a GnRH-a in depot formulation is superior to progestins, danazol, and gestrinome and to the same GnRH-a given as a nasal spray, in terms of reducing inflammation, vascularization, American Fertility Society score, mean endometrioma diameter, and mitotic index.[19]

Before considering such treatment, careful selection of the patients is of paramount importance, best achieved using the revised classification of the American Fertility Society score.[20,21] Contrary to what happens with fibroids, presurgical treatment with GnRH-a is not always preferred in cases of endometriosis, because the lesions may be suppressed and overlooked at surgery or second-look laparoscopy.[22] However, only limited data are available to evaluate the effects of preoperative medical treatment on endometriosis from both the surgical aspect and long-term outcome.[15]

Dysfunctional Uterine Bleeding/Hysteroscopic Surgery

Many studies have shown the efficacy of GnRH-a in treating patients with persistent menorrhagia.[23] Moreover, GnRH-a best prepare the endometrium before ablation, especially compared with danazol. They uniformly reduce edema and thickness and avoid pseudodecidual reaction better than does any other hormonal preoperative treatment. By rendering the endometrium atrophic, there is better visibility, less likelihood of bleeding with less fluid consumption, and more chances of uniform and complete resection, particularly in anemic patients. Even a single depot injection 4–6 weeks before intervention is efficacious for this purpose, a result than can be achieved only with a high dose of danazol (800 mg/day) for 4–10 weeks.[24]

The same advantages are offered in the whole spectrum of hysteroscopic surgery (polyps, submucous fibroids, adenomyomas, intrauterine septa) regardless of the technique used: Nd-YAG laser, resectoscope, loop resection or roller ball, and more recently hot and cold radiofrequency probes.

Assisted Reproduction

There is no doubt that the introduction of gonadotropin-releasing hormone agonists has all but revolutionized the practice of reproductive medicine, particularly IVF/ET. They eliminate the adverse effects caused by premature LH surges and follicular luteinization, resulting in greater recovery of mature oocytes, better quality embryos, and higher pregnancy rates. For the same reasons the cancellation rate is reduced.[25]

The etiologic mechanism that impairs fertility in women with endometriosis is not fully clarified. Among others, it was hypothesized that stable follicular phase and periovulatory hormonal defects caused by subnormal endogenous gonadotropin activity might be responsible, and these can be corrected with GnRH-a in a variety of available protocols. The final results of IVF, as shown in many studies, improve considerably especially in the confirmed presence of premature LH activity.[26] It was shown that GnRH-a combined with an oral contraceptive results in better normalization of the LH/FSH ratio and ovarian volume reduction than does the contraceptive pill alone which is incapable of completely suppressing ovarian steroidogenesis.

A variety of treatment protocols are used in clinical practice including the "short" and "ultra-short" protocols in which the flare-up effect is used and the "long" protocol which leads to complete desensitization and downregulation of the pituitary. The long protocol starts from day 1 (for 10–20 days) or from day 21 of the previous cycle to the day of β-hCG administration. The ultra-long protocol (3–6 months) has proven to be more effective in patients with endometriosis and polycystic ovaries. In the latter, suppression of androgen production and normalization of the LH/FSH ratio induce a significant reduction in hirsutism and hair growth rates. With the addition of exogenous gonadotropins, normal follicular development and synchronization can be established. Furthermore, in anovulatory patients prolonged GnRH-a treatment may restore ovulation spontaneously, at least temporarily.

Recurrent Miscarriage

In a proportion of women recurrent termination of pregnancy remains unexplained, and the use of empiric therapy is unnecessary and should be resisted. No clear evidence exists to support the concept of partner-specific miscarriage or the hypothesis that some women miscarry because they are unable to mount an appropriate protective immune response to prevent rejection of their dissimilar fetus. Hence, in view of the potential complications of immunotherapy, routine tests for HLA type, antipaternal cytotoxic antibody, and the use of immunotherapy are no longer recommended.[27–29]

In our experience and in that of others, more than 40% of patients attending the recurrent miscarriage clinic have polycystic ovaries. Normalization of the hormonal profile of these patients using GnRH-a may prove beneficial in preventing repeat spontaneous abortions.

GnRH-a and Gynecologic Cancer

For many decades, ovarian ablation by either surgery or radiotherapy has been the standard policy in breast cancer, resulting in remission in only one of three cases. This rate was greatly improved with the introduction of methods to measure estrogen and progesterone receptors, allowing selection of patients responsive to treatment and preventing the rest from unnecessary treatment morbidity. This prediction though was proved not quite accurate. About 20–50% of these selected patients may still be ovariectomized unnecessarily, whereas some of the estrogen/progesterone receptor-negative tumors (10%) may respond to hormonal ablation therapy.[30]

Thus, 'medical castration' by 'selective medical hypophysectomy' using GnRH-a has become first-line therapy for hormone-dependent metastatic breast cancer mostly in premenopausal women. In postmenopausal women, only marginal activity occurs, and the mechanism of action of GnRH-a remains unclear. In patients with breast, ovarian, or endometrial cancer refractory to chemotherapy and in view of the absence of deleterious effects with GnRH-a, the latter may have a vital indication despite the fact that only modest remission rates and disease stabilization can be expected, results certainly comparable to those expected with further chemotherapy. In premenopausal women the mechanism of action of GnRH-a can easily be explained through the suppression of estrogens. In postmenopausal women the results may be due to direct inhibition of tumor cell proliferation. In recent years, increasing evidence indicates that in both breast and ovarian cancer there is an autocrine regulatory system based on expression of the GnRH and its receptors that can be a direct target of action for GnRH-a therapy.[31,32] Another explanation for the marginal activity of GnRH-a in postmenopausal patients might be the reduced levels of circulating androgens produced by the postmenopausal ovary through suppression of FSH and LH levels. The androgens, through their peripheral aromatization to estrogens, may exert an indirect endocrine effect, which could explain the efficacy of GnRH-a in postmenopausal patients.

In ovarian cancer, the aforementioned autocrine regulatory system can likely explain the mechanism of action of GnRH-a apart from a previously proposed theory that this cancer is gonadotropin dependent, a theory that is extremely controversial, as many data exist that negate the role of gonadotropins in the pathophysiology of ovarian cancer.[33]

It does appear that GnRH-a are effective in inhibiting the proliferation of human ovarian cell lines that express GnRH receptors, whereas in those who have no such receptors the results are inconsistent and the antiproliferative effects become evident only at extremely increased concentrations.

In patients with endometrial cancer in whom surgery or radiotherapy in contraindicated as well as in young women with adenomatous hyperplasia who have not yet completed their families, the use of GnRH-a could be an interesting approach. However, only very limited or anecdotal data are available on this topic.[34]

It has also been demonstrated that GnRH-a, when combined with chemotherapy and probably radiotherapy, exert a significantly protective effect against irreversible ovarian damage. By modulating some intraovarian factors (inhibin, activin, IGFs, TGFs, etc.), they allow the resting ovarian cells to repair DNA damage induced by cytotoxic agents or radiotherapy.[35]

Add-back Therapy to GnRH-a Treatment

Although there have been reports of prolonged use of GnRH-a for up to 24 months, standard duration does not exceed 6 months, mostly because of the risk of osteoporosis.

There is not much doubt about the mechanism of action of GnRH-a, but what is not well clarified yet is to what extent estrogen needs to be suppressed before therapeutic efficacy is achieved. GnRH-a have a rare characteristic feature: a patient cannot be overdosed and there are no complications from their direct action. However, they cause unpleasant subjective symptoms related to profound estrogen deprivation (hot flashes, mood changes, insomnia, frequency, loss of libido, etc.), but the most worrisome is the less immediately obvious problem of bone loss (decrement in trabecular bone 5.9–8.1%, reported after 6 months of treatment), not totally reversible, and the adverse effects on the cardiovascular system. This is the reason GnRH-a treatment alone was restricted to 6 months until 1990, when Barbieri and Friedman proposed the "estrogen threshold theory." According to this theory, complete down-regulation of the ovaries is not necessary for the treatment of endometriosis and uterine fibroids. The addition of low dose estrogens, to fit into the therapeutic window, can prevent osteoporosis, maintain menstruation, and alleviate the climacteric symptoms.[36,37] Due to variable tissue sensitivity to estrogens, bone, heart, and urogenital tissues can be protected without activation of the relatively insensitive endometriotic or fibroid targets. The concept of the steroid "add-back" therapy is to combat the long-term consequences of the hypoestrogenic state induced by GnRH-a.[38] The big issue is to diminish the adverse effects associated with GnRH-a without compromising therapeutic efficacy.

Following the aforementioned applications of GnRH-a, the potential applications of the steroid (or nonsteroid) add-back therapy are self-evident (TABLES 2 and 3).

Initial studies of the long-term application of GnRH-a in endometriosis used progestins as the add-back steroid of choice, specifically norethisterone (norethidrone, NET) and metroxyprogesterone acetate (MPA). The preference for the progestin-only choice was based on the reluctance of many to give estrogens that might aggravate the disease combined with their ability to exert a direct therapeutic effect. Furthermore, the synthetic progestins have been demonstrated to combat some of the side effects induced by GnRH-a therapy including vasomotor symptoms and bone loss. Comparison between NET and MPA (by pain score and second-look laparoscopy for endometriosis and ultrasonography for fibroids) yielded fundamental differences. Contrary to the combination of GnRH-a/NET, which achieved considerable reduction of endometriotic lesions and uterine volume, MPA appears to inexplicably antagonize the beneficial effects of GnRH-a,[39] a disadvantage not described in later studies.[40]

TABLE 2. Applications of "add-back" therapy

i.	To decrease the side-effects related to GnRH-a therapy
ii.	To provide a medical treatment option to patients at high surgical risk (uterine fibroids, endometriosis, ovarian cysts)
iii.	To delay surgical intervention indefinitely when indicated
iv.	In premenstrual syndrome
v.	In precocious puberty
vi.	In ovarian hyperandrogenism
vii.	In dysfunctional uterine bleeding
viii.	In premenopausal breast cancer

TABLE 3. Regimens of GnRH-a add-back treatment

Agents	Regimen
Steroidal	Progesterone only add-back treatment *(sequential/continuous)*
	Estrogen/Progesterone Add-Back treatment *(sequential/continuous)*
Nonsteroidal	Blockade of bone resorption
	Calcitonin
	Biphosphonates
	Blockade of androgen aromatization
	Supportive measures for bone formation

For conditions other than recurrent endometriosis (persistent bleeding from leiomyomas unsuitable for surgery, hirsutism, premenstrual syndrome, etc.) estrogen/progesterone add-back therapy might be required for a long period of 2 years or more. For instance, GnRH-a (i.m. injection of 3.75 mg) can be combined with orally conjugated estrogen 0.625 mg and MPA 2.5–5 mg daily from day 5 through day 25. The number of days between the last dose of GnRH-a and first menstruation is of importance for the long-term effect of treatment. In postmenopausal women drugs normally used for hormone replacement therapy can be combined with GnRH-a as add-back therapy.[41]

Whatever the case, the ideal circulating E_2 that can achieve treatment of hormone-dependent tissue and at the same time prevent bone mineral loss has yet to be identified.[42]

REFERENCES

1. NIESERT, S. 1996. Leuproelin, an exciting development in the treatment of gynaecological disorders. Hormone Ther. Obstet. Gynecol. **1:** 4–9.
2. REISSMAN, T., R. FELDERBAUM, K. DIEDRICH *et al.* 1995. Development and applications of LHRH antagonists in the treatment of infertility: an overview. Hum Reprod. **10:** 1974–1979.
3. WORD, R.A., M.J. ODOM, W. BYRD & B.R. CARR. 1990. The effect of GnRH-a on growth hormone secretion in adult premenopausal women. Fertil. Steril. **54:** 73–78.

4. WILSON, E.E., B.B. LITTLE, W. BYRD *et al.* 1993. The effect of GnRH-a on adrenocorticotropin and cortisol secretion in adult premenopausal women. J. Endocrinol. Metab. **76:** 162–164.
5. VARCELLINI, P., P.G. CROSIGNANI, C. MANGIONI *et al.* 1998. Treatment with a gonadotrophin releasing hormone agonist before hysterectomy for leiomyomas: results of a multicentre, randomised controlled trial. Br. J. Obstet. Gynaecol. **105:** 1148–1154.
6. MATTA, W.H.M., I. STABILE, R.W. SHAW & S. CAMBELL. 1988. Doppler assessment of uterine blood flow changes in patients with fibroids receiving the GnRH-a buserelin. Fertil. Steril. **49:**1083–1085.
7. ALEEM, F.A. & M. PREDANIC. 1955. The hemodynamic effect of GnRH-a therapy on uterine leiomyoma vascularity:a prospective study using transvaginal color doppler sonography. Gynecol. Endocrinol. **9:** 253.
8. COHEN, D., M.T. MAZUR, M.A. JOZEFCZYK & S.Z.A. BADAWY. 1994. Hyalinization and cellular changes in uterine leiomyomata after GnRH-a therapy. J. Reprod. Med. **39:** 377–380.
9. REIN, M.S., A.J. FRIEDMAN, M.R. PANDIAN & L.J. HEFFNER. 1990. The secretion of IGF-I and II by explant cultures of fibroids and myometrium from women treated with GnRH agonist. Obstet. Gynecol. **76:** 388–394.
10. HOUSTON, D.E. 1984. Evidence for the risk for pelvic endometriosis by age, race and socioeconomic status. Epidemiol. Rev. **6:** 167–191.
11. GUERRERO, H.E., P. STEIN, R.H. ASCH *et al.* 1993. Effect of a GnRH-a on LH receptors and steroidogenesis in ovarian cells. Fertil. Steril. **59:** 803–809.
12. WRIGHT, J.A. & K.L. SHARPE-TIMMS. 1995. GnRH-a therapy reduces postoperative adhesion formation and reformation after adhesiolysis in rat models for adhesion formation and endometriosis. Fertil. Steril. **63:** 1094–1100.
13. BERGQVIST, I.A. 1995. Hormonal endometriosis and the rationales and effects of GnRH-a treatment: a review. Hum Reprod. **10:** 446–452.
14. SAKATA, M., S. OHTSUKA, H. KURATSI *et al.* 1994. The hypothalamic-pituitary-ovarian axis in patients with endometriosis, is suppressed by leuprolide acetate but not by danazol. Fertil. Steril. **61:** 431–437.
15. VARCELLINI, P., A. PISACRETA, O. DE GIORGI *et al.* 1998. Management of advanced endometriosis. *In* Fertility and Reproductive Medicine. R.D. Kempers, J. Cohen, A.F. Haney & J.B. Younger, Eds. :369–386. Excerpta Medica.
16. WHEELER, J.M., J.D. KNITTLE & J.D. MILLER. 1993. Depot leuprolite acetate versus danazol in the treatment of women with symptomatic endometriosis, a multicenter double-blind randomized clinical trial. II. Assessment of safety. Am. J. Obstet. Gynecol. **169:** 26–33.
17. WHEELER, J.M., J.D. KNITTLE & J.D. MILLER. 1992. Depot leuprolide versus danazolin treatment of women with symptomatic endometriosis. I. Efficacy results. Am. J. Obstet. Gynecol. **167:** 1367–1371.
18. FILICORI, M. 1997. Leuprorelin: increasing its role in the management of endometriosis. Obstet. Gynecol. **2:** 4–10.
19. DONNEZ, J., M. NISOLLE, F. CLERCKX *et al.* 1994. Advanced endoscopic techniques used in dysfunctional bleeding, fibroids and endometriosis and the role of GnRH agonist treatment. Br. J. Obstet. Gynaecol. **101:** 2–12.
20. AMERICAN FERTILITY SOCIETY. 1995. Revised American Fertility Society classification of endometriosis: 1995. Fertil. Steril. **43:** 351–352.
21. AHMED, M.S. & R.L. BARBIERI. 1977. Reoperation rates for recurrent ovarian endometriomas after surgical excision. Gynecol. Obstet. Invest. **43:** 53–54.
22. EVERS, J.L.H. 1987. The 2nd look laparoscopy for evaluation of the result of medical treatment of endometriosis should not be performed during ovarian suppression. Fertil. Steril. **47:** 502–504.
23. CANDIANI, G.B., P. VARSELLINI, L. FEDELE *et al.* 1990. Use of goserelin depot, a GnRH agonist, for the treatment of menorrhagia and severe anemia in women with leiomata uteri. Acta Obstet. Gynecol. Scand. **69:** 413–415.
24. KE, R.W. & P.J. TAYLOR. 1991. Endometrial ablation in the treatment of excessive uterine bleeding. Hum. Reprod. **6:** 574–576.

25. LOUMAYE, E. 1990. The control of endogenous gonadotropin secretion with GnRH-a during ovarian hyperstimulation for IVF-ET. Hum. Reprod. **5:** 357–361.
26. TAN, S.L., N. MACONOCHIE, P. DOYLE *et al.* 1994. Cumulative conception live birth rate after IVF-ET with and without the use of short, long or ultrashort regimen of the GnRH-a buserelin. Am. J. Obstet. Gynecol. **171:** 513–516.
27. DAYA, S. & J. GANBY. 1994. The effectiveness of allogeneic immunization in unexplained primary recurrent spontaneous abortion. Recurrent Miscarriage Immunotherapy Trialists Group. Am. J. Reprod. Immunol. **32:** 294–302.
28. THE GERMAN RECURRENT SPONTNEOUS ABORTION/INTRAVENOUS IMMUNOGLOBULIN GROUP. 1994. Intravenous immunoglobulin in the prevention of recurrent miscarriage. Br. J. Obstet. Gynaecol. **101:** 1072–1077.
29. ROYAL COLLEGE OF OBSTETRICIANS AND GYNAECOLOGISTS. 1998. The management of recurrent miscarriage. Guideline No 17. London, UK.
30. EMONS, G. & A.V. SCHALLY. 1994. The use of GnRH agonists and antagonists in gynecological cancers. Hum. Reprod. **9:** 1364–1379.
31. EMONS, G., O. ORTMANN & K.D. SCHULZ. 1996. GnRH-a in ovarian, breast and endometrial cancer. *In* GnRH Analogues, The State of the Art 1996. B. Lunenfeld & V. Insler, Eds. :95–120. Parthenon Publishing. Carnforth. UK.
32. DOWSETT, M., S. JACOBS, J. ATHERNE & J.E. SMITH. 1992. Clinical and endocrine effects of leuprorelin acetate in pre and post-menopausal patients with advanced breast cancer. Clin. Ther. **14:** 97–103.
33. EMONS, G., O. ORTMANN, G. IRMER *et al.* 1996. Treatment of ovarian cancer with LH-RH antagonists. *In* Treatment with GnRH-a: Controversies and Perspectives. M. Filicori & C. Flamigni, Eds.: 165-172. Parthenon. Carnforth. UK.
34. CULLANDER, S. 1992. Treatment of endometrial cancer with GnRH analogs. Recent results. Cancer Res. **124:** 69–73.
35. ATAYA, K., L.V. RAO, E. LAWRENCE & R. KIMMEL. 1995. LHRH agonist inhibit cyclophosphamide-induced ovarian follicular depletion in Rhesus monkeys. Biol. Reprod. **52:** 365–372.
36. FRIEDMAN, A.J., S.M. LOBEL, M.S. REIN & R.L. BARBIERI. 1990. Efficacy and safety considerations in women with uterine leiomyomas treated with GnRH-a: the estrogen threshold hypothesis. Am. J. Obstet. Gynecol. **163:** 1114–1119.
37. BARBIERI, R.L. 1992. Hormone treatment of endometriosis: the estrogen threshold hypothesis. Am. J. Obstet. Gynecol. **166:** 740–745.
38. REGIDOR, P.A., M. REGIDOR, K. KATO *et al.* 1997. Long-term follow-up on the treatment of endometriosis with the GnRH-a buserelin acetate. Eur. J. Obstet. Gynecol. Reprod. Biol. **73:** 153–160.
39. FRIEDMAN, A.J., R.L. BARBIERI, P.M. DOUBLET *et al.* 1988. A randomized double-blind trial of a GnRH-a (leuproralide) with or without metroxyprogesterone acetate in the treatment of leiomyomata uteri. Fertil. Steril. **49:** 404–409.
40. FRIEDMAN, A. & M.D. HORSTEIN. 1993. GnRH-a plus estrogen/progestin "add-back" therapy for endometriosis-related pelvic pain. Fertil. Steril. **60:** 236–243.
41. TAKAYAMA, K., K. ZEITOUN, R.T. GUNBY *et al.* 1998. Treatment of severe postmenopausal endometriosis with an aromatase inhibitor. Fertil. Steril. **69:** 709–713.
42. PICKERSGILL, A. 1998. GnRH-a and add-back therapy: is there a perfect combination? Br. J. Obstet. Gynaecol. **105:** 475–485.

Index of Contributors